Nausea and Vomiting

Overview, Challenges, Practical Treatments and New Perspectives

Nausea and Vomiting

Overview, Challenges, Practical Treatments and New Perspectives

For Primary Care Professionals, Multidisciplinary Students, and all Persons Thoughtful and Curious

Richard H. Blum, PhD
Department of Gynecology and Obstetrics
Stanford University Medical Center, and the Centre for Family Research, University of Cambridge

W. LeRoy Heinrichs, MD, PhD
Department of Gynecology and Obstetrics
Stanford University Medical Center

With consulting editor
Andrew Herxheimer, MB, FRCP
Cochrane Centre, Oxford
(formerly Department of Clinical Pharmacology, Charing Cross and Westminster Medical School, University of London)

W
WHURR PUBLISHERS
LONDON AND PHILADELPHIA

First published 2000 by
Whurr Publishers Ltd
19b Compton Terrace, London N1 2UN, England and
325 Chestnut Street, Philadelphia PA 19106, USA

British Library Cataloguing in Publication Data
A catalogue record for this book is available from the British Library.

ISBN 1 86156 079 6

Printed and bound in the UK by Athenaeum Press Ltd, Gateshead, Tyne & Wear

Contents

Dedication/Preface/ Acknowledgments

To Richard L. Landau, MD

Editor, *Perspectives in Biology and Medicine*

Perspectives in Biology and Medicine, which Dr Landau of the University of Chicago edits, represents the foremost journal for a generative, reflective intellect at work in the biological sciences. (Soon we believe these will be the consolidated 'biopsychological' sciences.) The Journal's approach is one that we ask our students to emulate. In our own way, *Perspectives* is the Form, consonant with Plato's philosophy, upon which this book draws.

Dr Landau, through his editorship, encourages thoughts that are cross-disciplinary, synthesizing, and insightful; they are profoundly enriched by, and also enrich, the humanities and the psychosocial sciences. Through his personal efforts, and with his Board of Editors, replete with Nobel Laureates and other 'thought leaders' as he calls them, critical, erudite perspectives are fostered – some of which are radical or wittily iconoclastic; yet the authors' style is reliably civil and modest. Issues, discoveries in the making, and the correction of unexamined premises, often over decades, are presented in the context of and pertinent to new developments in science and the evidence-based healing arts. His Journal's and his own approach is broadly educated, literate, good-humored, dedicated.

Dr Landau's influence is directly responsible for this book. We had submitted a paper to *Perspectives* about pregnancy nausea and vomiting, with a subtitle indicating a theory that would incorporate psychosomatics. By implication it would be other than reductionism. He wrote back, saying nice enough things about our thoroughness and our approach, but asking pointedly where the integrating theory was. He was right; we had information, categories, and an idea, but nothing synthesizing, let alone elegant. After a year of pondering, he took the trouble to write again, asking where was our resubmission? That was it! Honored by his interest, we went back to work. We began working on nausea and vomiting (NV) as one research topic in the Gyn/Ob 399 Research class that we have co-taught over the past decade.

Now, about 10 years and many gray hairs later, we have done the best that we can. It is not good enough, and yet the best that we can provide about nausea and vomiting, its importance, facts, uncertainty, issues, theory, and therefore perspective.

We would like to acknowledge the help and participation of the following people in the writing of this book.

Gyn/Ob 399 Advanced Research Course student participants: Nisha Acharya, Sarina Behara, Jeannie Chang, Lillian Goldstein, MD; Kate Harding, Joe Hsu, Dana Karlsburg, Chad Hollingsworth, Jane Kim, Charmian Lewis, Melanie Lynch, MD; Deborah Merrill, PaNhia Moua, Sarah Nixon, Ajna Pisani, Bella Shen, Ann Scheck McAlearney, PhD; Craig Thomas, Marcus Torrey.

Statistical Associate: Michael Carley; Student Editor: Chad Hollingsworth; Research Associate: Manjur Patwardhan, MD; Computer Assistance: Robert Pierce.

Advising and/or co-authoring Stanford University Medical Center Faculty or Gyn/Ob Health Promotion Unit professional staff: Joseph Alvarez, MD; John Brock-Utney, MD; Carlos Camargo, MD; Susan Downs, MD; Sarah Donaldson, MD; Gary Fanton, MD; Richard Goode, MD; Gary Gray, MD; Gary Heit, MD; Robert Herner, MD; Halsted Holman, MD; Daniel Kapp, MD; John Kerner, MD; Paul Meyer, MD; Peter O'Hanley, MD; Stanley Schrier, MD; Alfred Spivack, MD; Anne Thrailkill, MSN, FNP, CS; Nelson Teng, MD; Thomas Tayeri, MD; Stephen Peroutka, MD (formerly SUMC, now of Spectra Biochemical); and University of California, San Francisco Medical Center Faculty: William Hilty, MD; Gary Tapin, MD.

We are indebted to Mrs Beverly Roach, a mother whose daughter experienced intractable NV during pregnancy. Through assiduous reading, she rightly concluded how little medicine and psychology understood NV. Reminding us about the high costs of human suffering and the costly burden of this ignorance, she wrote to us, ever so gently, suggesting that investigators in reproductive sciences have a professional duty to become interested in this topic, and she offered a financial gift to sponsor research. Her gift, and another from Mrs Katharine Kent, an avid supporter of women's health, have provided our only funds for conducting the research over the years. For all of its importance to sufferers, which we now see as unique and challenging phenomena, nausea and vomiting are too prosaic to attract funding, except for NASA's motion-sick astronauts and pharmaceutical company-sponsored development of intended antiemetics, which is not successful enough. (Some of these, you will see, turn out, paradoxically, to be emetics as well!)

But it has been our students, as fine a bunch of young folk as ever came down the academic pike, who have sustained us with their bright-eyed interest and labor, and our colleagues, always volunteering and being supportive, who have been there over the few million hours, or so it feels, that this work has taken us. We thank Professor Nelson Teng, MD who directs gynecological oncology in our department at Stanford, C.R.B. Joyce, formerly of CIBA-Geigy and the Department of Pharmacology of London Hospital Medical College, and now Professor of Psychology, Royal College of Surgeons, Dublin, and Professor Martin Richards, formerly Director of Medical Psychology and now of Family Research, and Chair of Political and Social Sciences at the University of Cambridge, for their professional wisdom, friendship, and support for this book.

For the monumental task of typing, and coordination of the many drafts from many authors, we thank Katie Farquharson. James Liu, MLS reference librarian, Stanford Lane Medical Library, has served as an invaluable resource. Chad Hollingsworth served as dedicated student editor, generous with his time and intelligence. To psychologist, Ruth Evans, who did the final editing, we are particularly grateful. Her discerning eye, knowledge of the several disciplines herein, patience, and generosity allowed the book to emerge whole. Michael Carley was our dedicated statistician and Manjur Patwardhan has served as research assistant.

Caveat: So great is the uncertainty about NV and so much in transition is thinking about complex psychobiological events as linear/mechanistic/reductionist vs dynamic/contextual/holistic approaches that, as co-authors, we have sometimes by no means been in agreement. Often the term 'we' is found in this book, but it is an authorial, stylistic 'we.' 'We' did not write it together; one of us may disagree entirely, but, each respecting the other for his apportioned work, we did resolve not to be disputatious, because in this arena certainties are denied.

We beg the reader, particularly our colleagues of one strong set of mind or another, when finding some particularly shocking, or stupid, point of view, to assume it was not your friend, whether Richard or LeRoy, who was responsible for this, but rather that it was written by the one you do not know, and about whom you have no expectations of soundness. Whatever is proposed that is palpably ridiculous, know that the *other* one of us was responsible for it!

Envoi!

Richard R. Blum and W. LeRoy Heinrichs
1999

PART I

INTRODUCING NAUSEA AND VOMITING

CHAPTER 1

What are we about and for whom are we writing?

This book is for health caregivers, teachers, and students attentive to that human discomfort or suffering that is the experience of nausea and/or vomiting. It provides an overview and practical treatment guidance, and it discusses challenges faced in treatment and research. The challenges arise not only from uncertainties found among clinical trial and clinical prevalence study results, but also from the challenges recognized from commonsense observation, animal and drug studies, and from scientific and speculative thought generated in disciplines heretofore far afield from work on nausea and vomiting. These include not only psychology, neuroscience, and evolutionary biology, but also the humanities, because this book occasionally offers piers in the bridge that C.P. Snow sought to build between the humanities and the sciences.

Just as the multidisciplinary student takes joy in intellectual challenge of the sort that stimulates us to offer new questions and new perspectives, many of which are controversial, the practical clinician wants to know what to look for, and what to do when it comes to direct patient care for nausea and/or vomiting. As the importance of providing a remedy for that suffering is great, we offer hands-on practical guidance about optimal treatments. These can be nursing, other supportive, complementary/alternative methods, psychological as well as medical pharmacotherapies, and even music, because studies show its positive effects on nausea and vomiting. We describe illnesses and other conditions in which nausea and/or vomiting may occur, including those that may have significance for differential diagnosis. As nausea and vomiting (henceforth referred to as NV in the plural) are such common side effects from medical treatments and drugs, we provide information about dangers and complications arising from NV themselves. Information about illnesses or other morbidity, in which NV may occur and have significance for differential diagnosis, is also presented. We must employ considerable scientific terminology but, as our concern is with and for primary caregivers, students, and people suffering from NV, we elect the ordinary terminology, the vulgate. We shall try to avoid being pompous, as in our tongue-in-(Latin)-cheek use of 'vulgate.' We shall be as informal as a text on a serious subject allows.

Caregivers and patients, as consumers, will be able to use NV information better if they are aware of deficiencies in existing data and treatments, limitations in advertisements for treatments, and serious problems with current premises about NV. To provide better care, and perhaps become better observers and so contribute to knowledge, the caregiver and student deserve to be able to be thoughtful consumers, as critical analysts of current knowledge, including the limited material (typically a few lines or pages at most) in traditional textbooks.

We join most primary caregivers in our order of primacy concerning caregiving. Our emphasis in NV care is to attribute quality to care when that care makes the patient's quality of life the first priority. A patient-oriented approach, however ordinary, needs to pay particular attention to the patient as the judge of treatment success. It can also mean greater patient control in self-medication, and requires the caregiver to attend to all available treatments in terms of the outcomes that patients care most about, and in conscience will propel the caretaker to an interest in NV because they are endemic, painful, disabling, and sometimes fatal. Furthermore, the field requires the attention of many more to NV's causes, meanings, and processes; this means attention to theory, treatments, and commonsense observation and conclusions.

Our approach seeks to be simple, and to provide survey, overview and guidance that are adequate to the needs of the primary care practitioner. We also favor an informal style, because this book intends to be a conversation with the reader about the materials covered, what they might imply, and the direction of our own thinking on these matters. In addition to data, tables, and guidance, we also allow criticism, commentary, essay, and advocacy. We fall from the grace of simplicity when the material itself is complex, or when inferences drawn from that material are unavoidably complex.

Our aim is to stimulate the practitioner or the student (of either natural or psychosocial sciences), or even a student of philosophy who might wish to reflect upon that profound 'disharmony' (Plato believed the business of the philosopher was to assist harmony) that NV-initiating perturbations can represent. This book may be of particular service as a provocative introduction to problems and to new research directions for advanced scholars/practitioners. We hope it will be useful to academics in oncology, cognitive neuropsychology, obstetrics, olfactory biology, to those who focus on women's health and to holistic medicine practitioners. For the student looking for an Honors thesis, Masters or PhD topic, read on! There are dozens of projects proposed. And for anyone who has read Horgan's *The End of Science* we trust that this book will show it is not so. Indeed, for NV we are at the beginnings.

For the reader who wants to know about the medical details of the somatic processes of perturbation, as derived from neuroanatomical, neuropharmacological, gastroenterological, and related basic bioscience work (i.e., the traditional medical approach), we provide just that – for its own self and as part of the critique and theory. We confess that the wish for simplicity is rarely met, no more so than the wish for certainty. NV are phenomena so complex and probabilistic (although previously sometimes considered simple and only linearly mechanical) that to simplify a subject in which complexity, paradox, and uncertainty are intrinsic would do disservice to the reader, to upcoming students, to sufferers from NV, and to workers in the field.

As NV are best approached as a complex multi-level set of processes, these need to be identified in the best way possible. Their contexts, elements, spheres of action, and implications range from neuromessengers in the brain structures, to enteric systems, to cognitive, mental components; their functions are also in communicative behavior and responses to that behavior – as, for example, pheromones or symbols. Such a review may lead the student reader or professional, who is not in touch with pertinent current issues in neuroscience, psychosomatics, evolutionary biology, or psychological debate about 'mind' or indeed aspects of philosophy bearing on biopsychological theory, to enjoy some updating and introduction to fascinating material with applications far beyond NV. It can be seen that a lot of this is controversial, not simply at the many disciplinary levels addressing how humans function, but sometimes also at broader levels concerning what we, as humans, are about. NV are found, surprisingly, to provide a fine avenue for an approach that yields exciting questions and propositions about humans and their environment.

NV are important enough, insufficiently understood, and indeed insufficiently cared about, to deserve not simply an overview in primary care clinical practice guidance, but also critical thought and the challenge of novel, sometimes revisionist, and quite often unconventional views and speculation. Primarily cross-disciplinary concepts point to theory and encourage new kinds of work. One goal is to suggest perspectives on NV that invite research from other disciplines. We are not at the 'end of science' for NV, as long as we allow for creative fact-based thinking – a kind of hard-headed holism that compels multidisciplinary, multi-level work in open conceptual frameworks, which entertain multiple 'causes,' processes, possible functions (and nonfunctions), and treatments. Our presentation will be a success if it interests caregivers, students, scholars, and practitioners in other disciplines that are becoming relevant, including psychological and social sciences and clinical practices.

Our premises are as follows:

1. NV are insufficiently understood and, in most general texts, are grossly oversimplified and inadequately presented, if not ignored.
2. Treatments are unduly limited and all too often clinical trials are poorly designed or narrowly conceived.
3. Large numbers of practitioners are poorly informed not only as a result of clinical trial deficiencies, but also because there is insufficient attention to teaching about NV as such, including its possible diagnostic–etiologic significance. Furthermore these practitioners, as consumers along with their patients, do not ordinarily receive information setting forth the weaknesses of clinical trial information, and do not consider material that sets forth the cost-effectiveness; different kinds of interventions are also not compared.
4. Pharmaceutical manufacturers are not objective educators but, in marketing, are profit-oriented advertisers. Consumer protection, as a way of thinking about and knowing how to judge the truth of what is published, is required if optimal benefits and least costs are to be enjoyed.
5. Treatment plans/objectives that are patient sensitive will require different success measures and priorities from those commonly now in place. Less attention should be paid to retching episodes than to how the patient feels over time, how much disability is occurring, how the patient herself can participate in self-care, and what complementary comforting strategies may be employed: quality of life is the measure. (More women than men suffer from NV.)
6. Reductionist emphases must be complemented by attention to

multiple levels of NV processes and functions. There is a rationale for person–environment interactive levels of thinking and research. These approaches imply an equal scientific rigor, not a reduced clinical or environmental observational integrity. 'Linear' schemas that are traditional in and appropriate for much of the medical thinking and research in many cases of NV require supplemental or often alternative schematic accounting. Some aspects of NV may be explained using complex, dynamic concepts which accept intrinsic uncertainty, but which also allow the obvious: that for humans consciousness, feelings, and meanings are as essential as the cause, process, and consequence of NV. By extension, nausea, as a higher-level brain experience, whether or not of currently measurable enteric events, requires foremost attention, thus requiring approaches that include the psychosocial and ecological.

7. Attention to NV, because it is an exceedingly common nonadaptive response to diffuse initiating events that involve multiple brain regions, messengers, and levels of activity, may yield insights into other human functions across a range of disciplines, including biological, psychological, and environmental. Maybe evolutionary biology could enjoy some revision.

A great many of the data upon which this work is based rest on traditional work in NV and biomedical science. Yet in seeking to focus on the broad rather than the narrow, and to raise questions rather than to presume certainties, we make radical challenges to conventional assumptions. Take, as example, pregnancy nausea and vomiting (PNV). This natural and discomforting phenomenon (more correctly 'phenomena') remains entirely inexplicable in spite of some years of endocrinological study, too-casual psychogenic accountings and clinical indifference simply because NV are part of normal pregnancy and seem to be (as Greek folk medicine healers would call it) an 'obligatory' condition. Indeed, the attitudes of many caregivers to any NV, including their widespread ignorance of possible treatments, can be attributed to such indifference. Yet, however simple, normal, inevitable, or 'reflexive' NV may seem, it emerges as a most puzzling as well as a clinically underrated phenomenon in terms of patient distress. This situation compels new theories. Our greatest reach of speculation and theory occurs as we consider PNV and its implications for sex differences, evolutionary biology, and the biology of esthetics.

As a result of their much greater vulnerability to NV, we have a special interest in the position of women. Children also require special attention because of their vulnerability, as well as those who are iatrogenically (medically precipitated) and terminally ill. People at greater risk, and contributing to a high prevalence of the phenomena, are also those under stress, in pain, fatigued or suffering from a vast range of sicknesses, from 'flu or migraine to hepatitis or heart attack to cancer. By attending to these disproportionate vulnerabilities, not only is more reliable remedial care likely but future work can explicate these unusual connections and interacting perturbations.

Our audience for this book includes the following groups.

The first group includes primary care providers, whether physicians, physician assistants, nurse practitioners, health psychologists, or ancillary professionals. As the introduction of this audience to NV when in training is through traditional texts, and as examination of these texts shows that information about NV is grossly incomplete, it is essential to supplement information to assure competence.

The second group are those who are responsible for the dissemination of knowledge and thus for improved patient care and research teaching. These are 'opinion leaders,' defined here as men and women who read journals, go to meetings, use on-line computer sources for up-to-date information, and who are active in their local medical, clinical psychological communities and beyond. All teachers of providers are, of course, included. Warren and Mosteller (1993), in their splendid book, *Doing More Good than Harm: the Evaluation of Health Care Interventions*, provide, in a discussion of improving quality of care by effective education (Lomas, 1993), powerful data-based arguments on the diffusion of information as a process of good 'contagion' within closely knit communities of health care providers. Leaders are fewer than one would like; the speed and critical acuity of change based on new information seem to be mostly in their hands. Opinion leaders are initially more likely to read this book, and we hope that this special information leadership audience will become interested in NV care.

The third group are graduate students, whether in medicine or related fields, or in psychological or biological sciences, in which NV will be of greater import with recognition of their consequences and complexity. It is from the student group that we hope to draw tomorrow's committed clinicians and research workers.

The fourth group of undergraduate students is a major audience, although necessarily recruited by those professors who find this a useful text on thinking anew about 'unimportant' and 'we know it all,' painful and disabling human conditions. Our own undergraduate students, not yet ruined by fixed positions, were remarkably innovative, finding the cross-disciplinary approach a way to appreciate and apply a number of disciplinary approaches to the same topic. Many stayed with us and NV for 2 or 3 years.

What is most heartening for students is that discoveries await them, not necessarily through tedious burrowing and benchwork, but through looking for the obvious. Later we recount some findings that have the excitement of discovery, and these may be replicated: a migraine leading to hyperemesis gravidarum (HG) risk; the possibility that severe PNV (not HG) carries a previously unknown obstetric, and therefore population-selective risk; the knowledge that NV risk is a general factor that varies in magnitude among women; or the simple consequence for women of fatigue and stress or for pregnant women of odor, as a precipitant of nausea – the last leads to our intense interest in olfaction and the 'reptilian' brain; only after inquiry, do we discover how painful NV can be for most women, and how much more pervasive N is than V. There are many more discoveries to be found by those who look.

The student asked to consider NV as a field of interest is likely to have a personally repugnant, aversive response – regardless of his objectivity. This unease – we encounter it in discussions with colleagues – seems to be based on our deep experiential recollection of NV: 'revulsion' pure and (not so) simple. That recognition could itself initiate one's own personal speculation and lead to compelling curiosity. What is it, after all, that is so repellent? Could there be a special biologically, as well as evolutionarily, communicated psychological importance for such a common experience, one felt so overwhelmingly and intensely?

The fifth, and final, group is the educated lay person, including the NV sufferers, particularly as that suffering is so widespread, often untreatable, or, when treated, done so in ignorance of best methods. As NV are in such opposition to well-being, as well as being financially expensive, and often iatrogenic as a result of other treatments, patient/families who want to achieve greater relief need to learn enough, and be inquiring and sufficiently assertive to take joint responsibility in their own treatment as knowledgeable partners. Much of a healer's education comes from interacting with patients. Some of the best researchers in clinical trials have characterized the ordinary treatments of doctors that they have observed as uniform, limited, patient inattentive, too expensive, and ignorant of consensus guidelines. We wish to remedy this.

We emphasize that NV interventions must be measured by several outcome criteria. The most important is how the patient herself feels, what her quality of life is, and how urgently she makes others aware of her suffering. There must be shared attention by caregiver and patient to possible side effects from pharmacological treatments of NV. Complementary lifestyle therapies – nutritional and psychosocial, comforting, diverting (the things that nurses and good mothers can do) – and some alternative folk remedies should become part of treatments being tried and tested and their benefit measured by patient preferences.

Costs of NV must be considered and the relative benefits of one compared with another; better still, a group of coherent treatments should be weighed against each other. All too often the practical costs of NV have been ignored, whereas, for antiemetic (AE) medicaments, the tendency has been to overprescribe more expensive drugs rather than rely on the best clinical trials for guidance. With respect to costs, NV impose a surprisingly large burden on the economy as well as the sufferers. For example, postoperative nausea and vomiting (PONV) may increase patient costs by 100–500% above those incurred by room and nursing care (Hirsch, 1994). Total costs may approach 8% of those for cancer.

In consideration of NV a first principle is to accept complexity and ambiguity; in spite of some elegant research, understanding is less and less adequate as one moves away from highly controlled animal surgical experimentation and into the study of human experience, pathology, and behavior. As this study of NV has been medically–psychologically prompted and intends to be practical (although occasionally philosophically indebted), it is human NV with which we are most concerned.

Its management in terms of prevention, control, and relief is empirically more advanced than the underlying scientific knowledge, because treatments owe much to folk medicine, provision of general comfort, and trial and error empirical pharmacotherapies. There are many treatments that work more or less, even though we have no idea at all how they work. In place of acknowledging the incomplete nature of their knowledge, some practitioners and researchers prefer simplicity, like accepting neuropharmacological advocacy for single neurotransmitter messenger systems or a one-brain 'center' as the 'mechanism,' 'place,' or 'cause.' This approach, whether out of reliance on typical textbooks, indifference, or a hope for the simple, ignores inconsistencies in experimental and drug treatment outcomes, or much grosser inadequacies of common assumptions which we shall be considering.

We review a range of clinical trial findings to show that empirical treatment is painfully unreliable, much subject to unknown influences. As Martin (1992) says, there can be over-optimism about compounds that are current or being developed. There is, he says, a 'mythology' – part of which arises because of widespread poor clinical trial research designs that often lead to overestimates – rarely the contrary – of efficacy. The caregiver who is not aware of this bias becomes a manipulated consumer; so does his or her patient and third-party payers. All should know what constitutes good research and about adequately comprehensive trials that go beyond two-drug comparisons and are not randomized controlled trials of large populations.

In Part V there is also information on treatments, but that is of the preceptorial, 'wise old hand,' directly practical sort. There is one chapter for each specialty, or a combined one for related specialties, likely to encounter NV of clinical significance. There is also guidance on important differential diagnosis when NV present themselves as critical signs of conditions that must be correctly identified and treated independently of the NV.

Few, if any, workers to date have thought about NV in a cross-disciplinary, dynamic, nonmechanistic way. This thought has not been necessary as long as workers could expect that traditional neuroanatomical, neuropharmacological research would be explanatory and would lead to efficacious treatments. The success of those research ventures has varied considerably, and a lot of them are overly optimistic when methodologically examined. Nor are new perspectives easily come by until work in other fields has allowed that creative cross-fertilization. Most research work on NV to date has been in neuropharmacology, anatomy, gastroenterology, anesthesiology – oddly enough not oncology, except for drug trials, and, ashamedly for us, almost none in obstetrics – where traditional workers are hardly expected to become familiar with what will be necessary: genetics, ecology, olfactory sensory perception, and cognitive psychology/neuroscience, chemical semiotics, evolutionary biology, even esthetics and natural philosophy.

Here we invite you to look across those fences, open up to ideas and findings. It is difficult enough to be competent in one's own field, let alone escape amateur status as observers in another. Our efforts at perspective and derived theory are inevitably flawed. This should be forgiven only if there is stimulation and sense in what emerges, the 'aha' insight that across the fence there may be solutions to problems that have denied answers for traditionally viewed NV. The reader will decide. Surely there is the risk, as we stray from that current reductionism, itself so productive in animal experimentation, moving out to encompass new approaches and ideas without a substantial body of research behind us, that we may well go wrong. On the other hand, insofar as one rests only upon extant work, it will provide a conventionally acceptable but conceptually terribly insufficient basis for thinking about NV. Convention will deny better new treatments for NV. It is fruitful to maintain a respectful reliance derived from the large body of traditional animal, pharmacological, and clinical research plus perspectives derived from other disciplines, some of which are far removed but lend themselves to placing NV in the context in which these seem to occur.

To this point then, the immediate goals of this text are:

1. To enable the caregiver to be better informed about useful treatments, given some base of knowledge and a conceptually organized view.
2. To stimulate the student and others curious to participate in NV work, including the now largely uninvolved community of psychologists/behavioral scientists acting as researchers or clinicians.
3. To show, especially to undergraduates, that, in NV, science is not, as Horgan claims, dead.
4. To invite, even to prod, the patient with NV to learn more than her caregiver so that she may inform her own treatment.
5. To suggest new approaches to research, and to thinking about NV, particularly to enjoin workers to a theoretical base, perhaps even paradigm shifts (a popular way today of speaking of taking new perspectives).

Pavlov, parallels and *le plus ça change, le plus la même chose*

Lest NV be considered a unique instance of puzzlements, of healing constrained by narrow focus 'models,' consider Pavlov's lesson. That great Nobelist researcher on gastric function understood the need to appreciate the interplay of psychological and physiological factors, thus involving himself in fields that are now psychophysiology, psychosomatics, gastroenterology, cognitive psychology, and animal research methods. Pavlov avoided Descartes' dualism.

Science historian Todes (1997), quotes Tigerstedt who nominated Pavlov for the Nobel Prize in 1904: 'We have here…an example of how organs that are definitely not under the influence of our will can also…be closely dependent on our mental state…' Pavlov also understood that individual differences in animals were important to experimental outcomes, just as we shall see occurs in NV experimentation. Pavlov referred to the 'character' of animals as a variable affecting study outcomes.

Hollis (1997) considers Pavlov's work to have introduced biological function as part of behavioral ecology – what is today the 'ecological perspective.' That perspective is still often missing, most certainly so in NV studies.

Pavlov suffered personal intellectual as well as interpersonal conflicts over moving away from then dominant mechanistic (reductionist, simple causal) ways of thinking, a problem still facing NV workers. Pavlov asked, '…is it possible to include all this apparent chaos of relations within certain bounds…to discover their rules…?' Later we shall ask if dynamic theories, non-linear, not mechanistic but probablistic, interactive, multi-level, thus multi-disciplinary are not a better way to envision NV phenomena. In the meantime, one recognizes in Pavlov a pioneer in work and broader experimental conceptions that yet will guide future NV work.

We add then to (5) opposite, as a goal of this book to lend to those interested in NV work, and its healing, the courage of historical appreciation that broader approaches are not initially popular, although we see they can lead to Nobel prizes.

It is time for a change in how we think about the remarkable phenomena of NV. Until now assumptions about NV have placed them as mere epiphenomena, side effects only. Or if forced to find a Darwinian adaptive role to explain primary NV, then the thoughtless answer is that NV are still functioning in humans and are evolutionarily conserved for 'toxin expulsion.' As for the demand for 'mechanism,' the answer all too ready is 'single neurotransmitter-mediated reflex.' We propose, except for a few primitive exceptions, otherwise.

CHAPTER 2

Caring about nausea and vomiting: an overview of irremediable suffering

The pain and extent

Anyone who has experienced nausea knows that it is an exceedingly uncomfortable, disruptive, and preoccupying experience. Some people speak of it as one of their most painful experiences ever. To the extent that it is uncontrollable through either change of the precipitating condition or some drug, the knowledge of this is likely to make it worse. There have been reports but no studies are cited here about nausea and vomiting (NV) being second only to the common cold as the reason given for employee absenteeism. This assertion of prevalence, beyond an absent primary source, is complicated by the fact that other stress/pain/fatigue may precipitate gastrointestinal (GI) symptoms. Thus reporting of absenteeism may be biased by a specific symptom preference. Even so, we need to allow for a 'humongous' number of painful and disabling NV incidents each year.

For an unknown percentage of patients undergoing chemotherapy or radiotherapy for cancer, N is an indirect cause of fatality. Patients sometimes feel so ill that they give up their treatment rather than experience it. It is typical of the field of study of NV that the various studies show different percentages of such patients dropping out. Bilgrami and Fallon's (1993) study review suggests that up to 10% of cancer patients withdraw from treatment because of NV. We have found no study (although we do have an acquaintance sample) of persons who have elected not to undergo cancer treatments in which the outcomes are uncertain because of NV risk. If they are to die, they say, it is best to do so with acceptance, dignity, and with the least mess (to which goals early onset iatrogenic NV are antithetical).

We cannot transform data on refusals and probably unreliable data on withdrawals into numbers of premature deaths attributable to the nausea-compelled decision. This is because we have not found a study that shows that persons with similar cancers and personal characteristics, who have continued with their treatments, live longer, or have actuarially normal lifespans. The best that we can say is that, if highly efficacious treatments for the several patterns of NV were available, we would surely expect a higher rate of entry and maintenance in therapies.

NV prevalence and some related features

Consider some statistics on prevalence of NV, but first be aware that most research on NV prevalence suffers from unreliability that arises out of population, or situational, differences in risks; there is inconsistency as to which aspect of NV is being measured, by whom and how, and over how long a period. There has been no epidemiological study of NV, except for in one large mental health study (Robins and Regies, 1991; Lydiard et al., 1994) which yields a grossly flawed estimate of lifetime prevalence for V, at 4.2%, with women being more vulnerable. Epidemiology of NV for normal populations is, except for one attempt to identify patterns and correlates, a recollection of lifetime prevalence in some small sample of opportunity conducted by our students, Nixon and Karlsberg.

Most accounts of incidence or prevalence arise from clinical observations; typically they are studies of both prevalence after medical intervention and the efficacy of antiemetic (AE) drugs. These counts suffer considerably when, as most do, post-intervention observations are of short duration and focus on V rather than N. Attention to V is typical because it is easy for the nurse to measure an observable event, and it is not necessary to take the time to talk to a patient or fuss with rating scales. Nevertheless, it is N that matters; it is more disabling, hurts more, matters more to the sufferer and the health economist, and, as we shall propose theoretically for any adaptive dynamic view (the brain as pattern-forming, self-organizing, close to critically unstable flow of environmentally coupled states), the ordinary subjective experience is that it is V that relieves N. It is best then that N has priority in our clinical, scientific, and even philosophical attention.

The difficulty in treating N provides a reason for measurement of N 'control' by drug companies, substituting the restricted and nonoptimal incidence of V in advertising efficacy achievements.

Commonality of NV, including self-induced

Nasser (1993) offers a historical view. Egyptian papyri spoke of the virtues of emesis. Herodotus described frequent self-purging. Hippocrates recommended it monthly and the Arab physician Avicenna proposed that one might use roses as emetics, or feathers, but did warn against it as a habit. Nasser cites a woman's magazine survey which implied that about four-fifths of respondents self-stimulated V. Pollsters were not active in Roman times so we have no figures on vomitoria. Readers of Petronius's *Satyricon* are allowed the inference that feasting at an orgy was followed by feathers and V as a kind of digestif (a vomitorium, however, was a theater exit, not a place to throw up).

Once again, there was N more than V and the N was more important.

To illustrate the dominance of N over V refer to Pater (1994) who questioned a sample of people undergoing cancer treatment about their quality of life. They found a severe disruption as a result of N in 80%, whereas only about 30% reported equivalent distress from V. This is not a reliable ratio, because prevalence varies by sample and condition, and is governed by a host of variables and propensities. In Lindley's (1989) study, using patient diary measures, half of all chemotherapy patients reported N, and about a quarter V. Herrstedt (1994) emphasizes that, when patients are questioned afterwards, they insist that NV are definitely a severe adverse effect in cancer treatments.

Relevant work has been done by Bonneterre et al. (1991); in comparing two AEs, they found that patients preferred one because it reduced N. Their physicians preferred the other because their focus was on the more obvious, physically messy, and more easily 'counted' V. These preferences were independent of the 'hard' criteria of the study which found both drugs to be equivalent. It is evident that the subjective business of patient preference (including the adverse iatrogenic outcomes of procedures as well as the efficacy of AEs), so often ignored by clinicians and so difficult for researchers to deal with, should be paramount in measurement.

Children in chemotherapy: NV and the doctor as problems

AE use in children undergoing treatment, when NV responses are judged to be severe, is 97% (Oster, 1991). However, when examined against a known standard, the clinician's choice of AEs is not up to date. We conclude that the pediatric oncological standard of care for NV is inadequate. We may consider this to be a failure in continuing education, or interest therein. Van Hoff et al. (1991), who followed up on the finding that AE use is a function of judged NV severity, and considered 31 different chemotherapy agents, found that from 17% to 98% of children being treated receive AEs – most frequently cocktails of AEs for severe cases. This shows that milder cases are usually not treated, because of either therapeutic caution or apparent dismissal of patient discomfort when less than extreme. These clinical investigators conclude that most oncologists are unread with respect to NV and the recent AE literature.

Adults in chemotherapy: uncontrolled NV

In a review, Bovbjerg et al. (1990) found that NV incidence in chemotherapy varied from 25% to 75% according to the study. Regarding control by AEs, Bleiberg (1992) found that 33% of cisplatin patients vomited regardless of the AEs given, and for delayed emesis (ordinarily defined as 3 days or more after treatment) there is no control at all. Graves (1992) reported that 30% of all cancer patients have NV that cannot be controlled, regardless of the AEs used. Tonato (1994) found that 30–40% of cisplatin patients have NV regardless of AE treatments. Bleiberg, focusing on 'delayed' NV, asked whether all AEs act only as short-term placebo effects, suppressing later emerging emesis. Clark and Gralla (1993), who found that 90% of chemotherapy patients receiving high cisplatin dosage incurred NV, also observed that it is delayed NV that are refractory to treatment. However, their observations suggest that this reduction in efficacy can begin as early as 16 hours after chemotherapy.

This concern implies that the clinician and researcher must be attentive to delayed NV (the AE trial data suggest that these are pharmacologically untreatable). The literature is in fair agreement that immediate NV after chemotherapy are more common (although NV before the next scheduled chemotherapy may be seen as a continuation). As follow-ups tend to be short, there have been suggestions that delayed NV are more common than realized, particularly as the patient will be at home.

Lindley (1992) reported a 56% NV rate in their sample. The researchers measured quality of life described by the patient and, attentive to delayed NV, they found that, 3 days after outpatient chemotherapy, almost a quarter were unable to go to work and 12% said that they were so sick that they could not care for themselves. This is consistent with the findings of Kaiser (1992), who reported that 78% of a chemotherapy sample incurred NV on the first day in spite of the use of AE compounds (then the more effective serotonin antagonists were not available). By day 5, the quality of life had not recovered, and NV-related hospital admissions and subsequent hospital care costs had increased. Hickok and Morrow (1993) report that, for about 2500 patients, an average of 67% had uncontrolled NV regardless of AEs used. When mild agents were employed, Alba et al. (1989) reported that about a quarter of patients experience NV.

Del Favero (1992) found NV resulting from a cytotoxin (cytarabine) dose, and also a schedule-dependent risk; in their sample there was an invariable first day onset. In some trial groups, NV were uncontrollable by AEs in as many as 86% of patients. Wood (1994) also showed that NV tend to be cytotoxin dose-dependent in cancer. Their important patient follow-up demonstrates that higher doses are optimal to extend survival. If this guideline were to become a consensus to be followed, oncologists would be giving higher-dose regimens. The consequences of this, for cancer populations, will be to increase NV greatly. We would forecast not just greater distress among patients, but more withdrawals and decisions not to enter treatments with an increasingly severe NV risk.

There is already widespread patient/family dissatisfaction with terminal care, where preferences not to engage in heroic and pointless maintenance are ignored by physicians bent on proving what they can do rather than what people want. The study by Wood (1994) may herald this conflict's expansion for nonterminal cancer care. In surgery and radiotherapy, as well as in chemotherapy, NV are the marker – the criteria for 'go/no go' on which patients base their decision. It is a moving marker, a gradient based on intensities of intervention, the efficacy of palliative efforts, and, no doubt, the dominant patient characteristics of a philosophical as well as a psychological kind. Caregivers are advised increasingly to attend to the prevalence and impact of NV, as with the cost–benefits measured in terms of monies, wellness, and time. For cancer patients, particularly women because of their vulnerability, NV are at the heart of quality of life and quality of care issues.

Stratification of NV misery

Chapter 3 lists those aggregates that serve as predictors, risk factors, or predispositions to NV in cancer treatment. As a result of our interest in women as the demographically dominant high-risk group, we emphasize that female NV risks are reported from 'somewhat' to up to four times more than in men (Kucharczyk et al., 1991). The literature for postoperative NV observes a three to four times greater prevalence in women than in men, excluding pregnancy NV. Women's overall NV risk varies with menstrual cycle, pregnancy, age, stress, etc. But women's overall much greater NV vulnerability is not understood at all.

Research workers have attempted to identify some of the variables that (might) account for the greater female propensity for NV.

Terminal patients

Among terminal cancer patients, in two studies, either 77% (Fainsinger et al., 1991) or 62% (Lindley, 1992) found that, next to pain, N is the greatest symptom of acute distress in dying. Gran et al. (1990), also studying patients dying from cancer, found that 44% required efforts at NV control, with no regard to their chemotherapy status. Of these, only 2% reported complete relief. We must ask to what extent the actuality of dying, and of cancer, may color the patients' views on what constitutes 'complete relief.'

Antiemetic treatments may reduce life expectancy among patients being treated for cancer, including possible immune suppression. Bovbjerg et al. (1990) point to a potentially very serious problem.

Anticipatory NV

Anticipatory NV (ANV) occurs when patients who have experienced NV after treatment become nauseous or vomit as they think about, approach, or are prepared for further chemo- or radiotherapy. Pavlovian conditioning is an experimentally supported reason. ANV is a matter of individual autonomic nervous system reactivity (Lerman, 1990; Kvale et al., 1991; Kvale and Hugdahl, 1994). We are told by individuals that they can vomit simply upon hearing the word, imagining the smell, or 'willing' it. Here, perhaps, is an example of spontaneous autonomic learning, i.e., the vegetative becomes conscious (to paraphrase Freud). For MacLean, the smell (i.e., triune or old) brain is where the Unconscious happens.

Individual differences are routinely observed in NV, and also in experimental animals. Some of these differences can be traced to highly specific features. Indeed, great specificity is characteristic of observed experimental variables, such as in animals who have had the brain region or enteric nerve ablated, or in those pre-treated with blocking compounds; in these situations the specifics of the emetic, AE, or molecular structure determine the interactions and outcomes. This is traditional pharmacology at work, yet in NV studies it is frustrated by neural plasticity, regional substitutability, and whether or not the animal was anesthetized. Even different dosages or timing sequences for interventions produce different, if not antithetical, results, as, for example, in Knox's (1993) ferrets. For example, Milano (1991) discovered that cats that were given cisplatin and differed in NV response were found in part to do so as a function of ileal tissue accumulation of serotonin $5HT_3$. (On the other hand, there is work that shows the possibility that neither $5HT_3$ nor the ileum is involved in chemotherapy NV.) If NV are unpredictable at the laboratory level, the clinician who fails to forecast the cause of NV and their solution must understand that the failure is not simply in his or her judgment.

With respect to ANV, Andrykowski et al. (1987) reported that 57% of a sample of women had ANV, whereas Stefanek et al. (1988) found that only 33% reported it, claiming it to be only a mild problem. Lindley's (1992) work, by contrast, found less than 10% with ANV, whereas Redd et al. (1989) found that 70% of his female chemotherapy patients had NV, and 57% had ANV after the sixth chemotherapy round.

Radiation-induced NV

Radiotherapy for cancer commonly induces NV, although less attention has been paid to NV and their treatments in association with this modality. Delay, an implication for slow processes and circulating precipitating compounds, is a hallmark. NV can occur up to 3 weeks after radiotherapy. It is experienced in about 50% of all patients with radiation to abdominal site cancers, in 90% receiving total body radiation, in 80% of those with large field upper abdominal radiation, and in an average of 30% of those receiving lower abdominal site radiation. NV responses to abdominal radiation tend to be rapid. It is not in doubt that all radiation is damaging and causes severe NV. (The studies of Japanese nuclear bombing survivors demonstrate this.) What is challenging is that, with so many years, so many subjects, and so much intelligence having been applied, uncertainty remains as to the 'mechanisms' and processes.

Theories not yet produced

In considering radiation, this is a good place to call attention to the primitive nature of 'theory' as it applies to NV, or indeed to much of biology. It seems that, with such dramatic, and sometimes deadly, effects, and many years of research and practice, there would be a body of thinking that serves to integrate all currently known relationships, and to develop hypotheses critical to the test of an extended theory. Regrettably, we are hardly there.

There are three rough theories as to how the outcome of radiation-initiated NV is processed and precipitated. One invokes ionization, proposing that free radicals do more than protective scavenging; they directly perturb regions such as the chemoreceptor trigger zone (CTZ). However, Cubeddu (1992) found no support for any circulating agents active in provoking chemotherapy NV. As no specific hormonal, neurotransmitter, neuropeptide, or other modulators are proposed as intermediate agents, the general language of irritation may be employed. Another notion (see review by Scarantino, 1992) proposes that the tissue degradation, i.e., destruction inflicted by radiation, yields circulating detritus as the necrotic product of radiation damage which induces NV. We do not rule out unstudied baroreceptor sensitivity to unfamiliar molecules, e.g., a kind of antigen detected that leads to the diffuse NV response.

Scarantino's trial and error application of a serotonin $5HT_3$ antagonist, the popular and expensive AE ondansetron, yielded considerable NV control on radiotherapy days and, apparently 77–90% control thereafter. The ordinary chemotherapy logic of $5HT_3$ antagonist pharmacotherapy assumes that the antagonist blocks receptors present in gastric tissue. These receptors would have otherwise responded to a proposed exaggerated secretion of serotonin that was thought, in turn, to invoke particular vagal or splanchnic afferents to V-inducing brain-stem regions. Out of this theory have come some quite useful AE agents in the form of serotonin blockers, but these do not work consistently and so we infer that other processes are also occurring. It is also the case that $5HT_3$ antagonists will act across the CNS, because serotonin is widely distributed. As is the case with almost all AEs (including placebos), we are not sure how much suppression of NV occurs at local levels (in the GI tract or vagus, or splanchnic nerves) or how much via other depressing or inhibiting actions elsewhere in the brain. As for the serotonin $5HT_3$ gastric action data, there are a few studies whose work shows no difference in post-chemotherapy serotonin levels in gastric tissue.

The reported efficacy of serotonin antagonists when NV are initiated by radiation calls into question the argument of serotonin's specific action on stomach lining receptors (see Cubeddu, 1992). It allows speculation that serotonin antagonists may inhibit CNS processes that are responding to radiation by-products, whether these are free radicals, oxidized or exfoliated tissue, metabolic curiosities, or other factors.

A third notion (Blum, 1988) is based on the finding that radiation energies, even at the lowest levels, are detected by mammalian olfactory apparatus and can lead to learning without awareness – an unconscious 'synesthesia.' Thus, radiation may have an undemonstrated capability to arouse that is equivalent to that of odor molecules (the typical negative hedonistic tone of the reptilian reactive–interpretative olfactory brain). It is this response to odors in pregnancy NV (PNV) that so typically precipitates NV. It is possible, therefore, that radiation NV are mediated via the olfactory apparatus in the reptilian (Hess's 'triune') brain. Even if this were the case, we are no further along in our knowledge of how perturbations initiate these unstable, transforming patterns of activity, or which intermediate (or alternatively region-wide) regions and messengers culminate in NV.

The three theories, none of which is well supported, are not mutually exclusive. We can, with no reductionist elegance at all, simply observe that homeostatic disruptions impose turbulence within the CNS (sensory incongruence, excessive free radicals, circulating tissue detritus, or radiation impacting the olfactory bulb may all be posited as capable of destabilization). These initial stimuli or conditions flow over varying and somewhat unpredictable routes, and via a number of electrochemical messengers. This can yield to N itself, a subjectively disorganizing state or, in just some cases, stimulation of midbrain regions and nuclei – all as action networks generating the motor activity that is V. Insofar as we are tempted to attach a meaning to this dramatic process, or to assume that the biology of it intends function, 'riddance' and 'revulsion' would seem to be good terms. Or, as the classicist Jane Harrison said of the Greeks in the ritual warding off of dangers from the gods, 'apotropaic' at the level of biopsychological function.

Even minimally adaptive accommodation to alien events requires some sensory or synesthetic competence (to sense so as to organize so as to perceive) to initiate response according to some pattern or evolving flow of patterns. When function is implied, plans are then formulated as inherent design capabilities, which are modified by learning. For NV to occur, there must be some recognition and response capability in the organism at a level of organization that is capable of direction toward action. One analogue (and it is only that for it is speculative) is the perception of invasive biologically active materials as 'foreign' or 'unknown' compared with 'self' or 'altered self' which initiates and fails to respect the immune response via specific antigen recognition. Without recognition or protective response capability, an alien invasive particle can disrupt and destroy. The sensory perceptual system is analogous to the adaptive response to environmental patterns. These, once organized as perceptions, allow CNS protective responses to occur when they are deemed necessary. It is obvious, then, that basic and parallel to human interactions with the environment are patterns, information dependent on recognition from the organized response: the old stimulus–response simplification. We may consider it as the basic definition either of life or, granting greater complexity, of intelligence involving information processing, pattern recognition, internal dynamic pattern formations, and such coping responses that enjoy feedback for learning and refinement.

From either view, NV would seem to be a primitive, inefficient, and unrefined capability in humans. For many NV-initiating conditions, including radiotherapy, neither immune nor sensory–perceptual capabilities 'work.' (One need not imply biological competence as a *sine qua non*; people die of immune recognized bacteria or in theaters where 'fire' has been identified.) But the curious thing about NV perturbations is that those associated with pathology and intrusive procedures (radiation, chemotherapy, medications) are not recognized at the level of the CNS where the NV response itself occurs. Brain action levels are not exchanging information that is needed to allow the harmonized anti-NV responses.

The NV system appears to stand, primitively and by itself, in that niche of propelling discomfort. It is perhaps closest to pain or, we think wrongly, seen as equivalent to a withdrawal reflex upon nociception. But because it is ordinarily a more complex process, we must contrast it with other levels of the nonreflexive, differentiated, and interconnected human response schemas. In these one sees that 'plans,' as organized energy-information patterns, are ordered as highly differentiated cells and cell systems present in: the immune response; the automatic homeostatic–vegetative or arousal–survival functions of the ANS; preconscious but learning-favored cerebral problem-solving; and the conscious process in which awareness allows data and task cogitation as solution testing. These show the different levels of intelligence at work, where at least selected actions, choices, and constructive instabilities will occur. Except for N, which is known primarily as an inundating sickness of the self, this 'wisdom of the body' is not readily demonstrated.

But, even for NV, more adaptive patterning can be learned. What is learned is adaptation to perturbations so that they no longer precipitate NV, e.g., as seen in the sailor or during general maturation (of adult compared with child), yielding lower NV risk. (The infant seems curiously immune; one presumes that his NV response apparatus, which we deem to be quite a different response system that is separate from reflux and regurgitation reflux, has not yet matured neurologically.) A different kind of learning about NV occurred among feasting Romans and in bulimic individuals; this was not one of avoidance but of exploitation of a response capability for longer-term purposes: avoiding weight gain, room for more food, and a vision of a socially preferred thin self. Children who vomit to manipulate situations are also quick studies of the voluntary psychosomatic.

Postoperative NV

Claybon (1994) advised that, of about 11 million annual outpatients who receive a general anesthetic, about one-third will experience NV. However, prevalence of postoperative NV (PONV) varies across studies, from 8% to 92% (Camu et al., 1992). For a mid-range example, a study by Ho (1990) reported that 44% of women undergoing laparoscopy experienced NV. As with all iatrogenic NV, their medical control is 'iffy': Claybon's large N study (1000), comparing ondansetron with placebo, found that, even though ondansetron was consistently more effective in controlling retching (albeit with no difference in adverse outcomes or vital signs), 41% of patients had no retching relief. In Kaufmann's (1994) work, 54% of his PONV patients suffered PNV. It is this study that shows a postoperative advantage for women to be able to control the administration of their own analgesics.

As a provocative aside for medical traditionalists, Ho reports that electrical acupuncture was as effective as the AE prochlorperazine in controlling NV. Any theory of NV and its treatments will have to be able to account for (see Chapters 3, 4, and 7) a consistent finding of success with acupuncture – see the work of Dundee and his colleagues, e.g., Dundee et al. (1990a, b) – in NV control. Likewise, apparently contradictory effects for postoperative treatments are reported. For example, Wilkinson (1989) found transdermal hyoscine (scopolamine) to be useful in controlling NV, whereas Tigerstedt (1988) found pharmacologically related scopolamine to be useless. As to the great range of NV incidence found postoperatively, naturally we attribute the variation in part to the immense number of variables that contribute to NV as an outcome, as well as to wide differences in methodology and study quality. There will also be an inherent prediction failure, given that NV are a complex, multilevel, interacting state that is subject to spontaneous phase transitions and unstable boundary conditions. Note that very few studies have made the effort to see how accurate most predictions can be if even a retrospective, i.e., multidiscriminant, analysis is employed. In anesthesiology, we expect that a larger proportion of variance will be explained by known variables. Our as yet undemonstrated prediction is that, case by case, PONV will be more predictable than chemotherapy NV in outpatients. This proposition rests on the assertion that the latter, like pregnancy NV (PNV) or migraine, is situationally much more complex and enduring. We are not then surprised by the findings of Rhodes (1990a) who, conducting a predictive study for patient distress and occurrence of NV, found that only 17% of the variance was accounted for by aggregate risk variables such as type and duration of cytotoxin, patient sex, age, prior NV history, etc. This is a powerful finding which demonstrates just how little is known about dispositions and circumstances leading to NV under one of its most important iatrogenic conditions, cancer therapy.

A parallel work, the largest sample we have encountered in any NV research, was that of Cohen (1994). Recall that efficacy as a function of institution and anesthesia showed here, for 'control' of NV induced by cancer therapy, a broad range for all AEs employed, depending on the institution in which treatment was given. 'Institution' is of course an embracing category with a host of differences, and this simultaneously demonstrates the uncertainty, and as yet rather unimpressive constraints on underlying randomness, that are expressed in the research literature. NV are probabilistic phenomena well beyond the sequential causal logic, comfortably 'nested' in a situation of stable boundary conditions. At the outset, it is essential to realize that one aspect of interpretation of each study, or each therapeutic procedure, is to identify, over a range of persons and conditions, not only what events can be shown to have causal roles, but how much randomness – accident or ignorance – remains. Whatever the level of focus, but particularly when seeking an integrated system involving cells through messengers through brain regions through senses through ecological interactions and personal meanings, we do not expect complex phenomena such as NV to employ anything but probabilistic forecasts for processes or treatments. And it may well be that, among approaches currently available for the consideration of NV psychosomatics, such as ecopsychobiology, it will be the dynamics of chaos theory that will be the most helpful.

Lest this be too worrisome to the clinician – who must nevertheless understand that, although the more comfortable, mechanistic models are inadequate, there are effective things to do – Chapters 3 and 4 deal with risks, side effects, and therapies, and Chapters 15 to 32 provide guidance by clinical specialty. In a kind of anticipatory general summary, it should be known that what one can do with regard to prediction is to aggregate the known risk factors, to anticipate most probable NV outcomes, and to place the patient on a 'risk track,' as is done in obstetrics: for high-risk patients, by procedure, or by personal characteristics relating to pre-treatments. It is also necessary to maximize complementary treatments and to engage in the clinical empirical 'art' that is ready to change AEs, and employ 'cocktail' mixtures, in order to rely on patient preference balanced by professional knowledge of dangers of side effects. Attention should be paid to monetary cost–benefits, and you should not lose sight of old-fashioned bedside empathetic care.

But it is helpful for the clinician engaging in the foregoing not to hold mechanical expectations of a treatment 'ideal.' Martin (1991) spoke of the myths, noting that clinical trial reports overstate good outcomes, which lead to healers expecting more than is likely. Insofar as this discourages the caregiver, it may make NV become a field, like alcoholism, in which the healer prefers either to avoid patients or to handle them at a distance. We also posit a normal aversion to interest because NV continue to present to our minds as a learned revulsion. We do not discount the feelings of the clinician any more than we do those of the patient.

Chapter 3 (p. 53) lists many conditions in which NV are either part of an illness or precipitated. Here, by way of illustration, we mention the self-induced V of bulimia, which again is not a 'simple' psychopathological preference (Nasser, 1993). Broberg's (1990) work on vasopressin levels allows our inference – biased by our own emphasis on the role of olfaction so well characterized by MacLean and also by Hess – that some aspects of bulimia may involve learned, or innate, responses to food tastes and odors. On a more epidemiological note, the work of Drewnowski et al. (1994) suggests that 10% of a sample of college women on a stringent diet could be at risk. For women, the most common adverse effect from estrogen replacement therapy is NV.

Pregnancy NV

NV in pregnancy are 'normal' and common. It should be simple enough at least to carry out prevalence and incidence counts, as opposed to understanding how it comes about, yet there is a definitional problem in the literature. 'Ordinary' pregnancy NV, which we refer to here as 'PNV,' is usually defined as disabling, particularly that occurring in the first trimester, yet it is not a problem that engenders a morbidity risk. Hyperemesis gravidarum (HG), on the other hand, whether defined as NV going on for the second and third trimesters, or that arising in the third trimester, can occur with such severity that the nutritional status of the mother and the safety of both mother and fetus are put at risk. Any life-threatening nutritional condition can be treated by hospitalization with intravenous feeding, but, even when parenteral feeding occurs, outcomes are undesirable; Zibell-Frisk (1990), for instance, reported that 20% of HG-maintained women had pre-term babies, 30% of whom were of low birthweight at full term. As these birth outcomes forecast a higher risk of lifelong health problems, as well as increasing immediate perinatal mortality risk and high hospital costs, we have here further indication of the importance of NV. Intractable V in HG can cause maternal, and thus fetal, death. Treatment by abortion is sometimes done, but does not recommend the 'state of the clinical arts' for HG control. The field of clinical research in NV, we trust we make clear, is in trouble.

As for 'ordinary' PNV, it ranges, for example, from about 66% in adolescents (Behrman, 1990), to about 75% in adults overall (Vellacott, 1988), and, in O'Brien's (1993) sample, to a prevalence of 70%. Weigel and Weigel (1988), in an important epidemiological study, reported that 71% of their group experienced PNV. Jenkins and Shelton (1989) found, in their sample of women with PNV, that about half said that they were 'sick most of the time' for 6 weeks or less, about one-third for 7–10 weeks, and about one-fifth for 11 or more weeks. Almost one-third attested that 'morning sickness' is not a misnomer. In this group, self-care efforts helped; rest, small meals, and avoiding bad smells seemed paramount. Importantly for a theory of PNV, attention from their husbands or partners figured in their comfort. DiLorio and van den Lier (see Funk, 1989), using a diary method with a small and therefore unreliable sample, reported that PNV ordinarily begins in weeks 4–6, with ratings of mild distress for 23 hours per week, moderate distress for about 18 hours per week, and severe for 5 hours per week. Individual patterns differed widely, but fatigue, odors, thoughts of food, hunger, and eating were all precipitants. As for remedies, rest and small meals were used, with drugs not being very useful. One can find studies with a lower or higher prevalence, but this is of little consequence. Paradoxically, the greatest relief was claimed to be when eating.

We conclude that PNV is common, but normal does not mean that the professional caregiver should be indifferent to it; 'common' can also be very unpleasant. Over a quarter of women in O'Brien's sample reported that NV made inroads into their quality of living. But, happily, all of the sample, using self-care via rest and diet, were able to control their PNV. In looking at such patient-centered work, one can use the study by Lindley (1992) as an example of how patients feel when NV adversely altered specific measures: cancer chemotherapy patients' ability to do household chores, enjoyment of meals, being with others, engaging in recreation, and maintaining daily functions. In the Lindley study, it was NV together, i.e., with the V component, that was rated more debilitating than N.

PNV in men

'*Couvade*' (from the French, 'hatching') was described by the anthropologist Tyler in 1865 to be a practice in West China and the Pyrenees where a woman in labor went off in hiding while her husband noisily enacted labor. Reported in other groups as well as by Frazer in 1910 and by Levi Strauss in 1964, the rationale for this behavior was that the demons would be diverted to him, and away from the vulnerable woman and her baby. What we read, however, is conflicting; the practice may be only the repetition of a false tale told by the ancient geographer Strabo (born 60 BC). What does occur is that modern men can get symptoms in pregnancy. These can include at least N if not V. Trethowan and Colon (1965) found NV in English men, along with other GI disorders, depression, and third-trimester hyperpseudogravidarum (our term). Deriving a difficult-to-calculate statistic from Liebenberg (1969), 15% in one sample of husbands appear to have had GI NV symptoms. Liebenberg (1969), citing Borgen, also found a higher frequency of symptoms in the third than in the first trimester for men. And Masoni et al. (1994) found, reassuringly for women and obstetricians' statistics, that women reported more NV and GI symptoms than did their mates. On the other hand, women's GI distress declined after the first trimester, whereas their partner's risk increased. Clinical experience tells us that the period of pregnancy is one of partner closeness, yet not without the characteristics of anxiety, diminished ego boundaries, depression, concerns about support, possible olfactory contagion from vomitus, vulnerable GI systems, and, for some women (our research in progress), profound and novel olfactory aversions to their partners. This is a burgeoning research field.

Head injuries and migraine

Gula et al. (in DiIorio and van der Lint [see Funk, 1989]) found that about one sixth of all head-injured persons suffer from V, and that this is unrelated to clinical assessment of injury severity. For brain tumors, about 40% develop V. For the 25 million migraine sufferers, the predisposition to which Peroutka expects to find genetic links, most experience N and some V.

The foregoing instances of NV by no means exhaust a list of medically recognized conditions in which they are present. It does, however, present data on prevalence that one uses to argue the importance of the phenomena. Chapter 3 (p. 53) offers a larger list of NV-associated conditions and precipitants. Given human plasticity and the idiosyncrasies of learning and individual morphology, and based on the dynamics of neuro- and psychobiology, it appears that NV may be a response to any perception, experience, or condition. We concentrate, however, on its most common, discomforting, and not easily 'unlearnable' and dangerous presentations.

CHAPTER 3

Nausea and vomiting matter: an overview

We see, from patient reports of disability, pain, and work loss, and from the few studies of drop-out rates in cancer treatment, that nausea and vomiting (NV) exact costs defined in terms of quality of life, unprevented cancer morbidity and mortality, and, among women with hyperemesis gravidarum (HG), the risk – and, if untreated, the reality – of fetal loss. Morbidity and mortality costs arise from cancer deaths attributable to dropping out of treatment because of nausea and vomiting. There are also serious costs from overprescription of more expensive – and not necessarily effective – antiemetic (AE) compounds for treatment. Later we offer cost estimates in dollars. NV pose other medical risks, as seen, for example, postoperatively, in tissue damage, or (we have no numbers) the bulimia that becomes anorexia, which itself creates health and sometimes fatal risks; people can also break bones while vomiting or can die as a result of suffocation from aspirated vomitus.

On the other hand, NV are not always unwelcome: bulimics intentionally vomit, children employ it manipulatively, and our small study of NV in pregnancy (PNV) finds that it works to recruit partner/other social support. Later we also ask whether PNV may have other important pheronomic communicative functions, which are, in turn, linked to immunologically consequential olfactory functions.

There are no large-scale epidemiological studies of NV that offer data about specific prevalence and incidence in normal populations. There is no thorough work on etiological risks, or any of changing NV rates as environmental and population characteristics change. Two research endeavors do provide important data: one is the National Health Survey and the other was conducted by our students Sarah Nixon and Dana Karlsberg.

The National Health Survey

The National Health Interview Survey (the last available to us was done in 1993) provides inadequate data, but is set forth here because, if certain assumptions are met, it suggests important demographically linked risk factors. The Survey interview inquired about 'indigestion, nausea and vomiting.' As a result of the nature of the question, the tables summarizing the replies do not discriminate when the householder was talking about NV or perhaps only about 'indigestion' with no NV. Nor were questions asked about NV associated with anything other than acute indigestion. Here we make the convenient assumption that the NV that occurred in most of the incidents reported by respondents included 'indigestion, nausea, and vomiting.'

Householders' reports (a householder is typically a responsible adult at home when an interviewer arrived) yield an annual figure of 5.3% overall. As symptoms that have already been diagnosed or labeled as encompassing conditions tend not to be reported independently (for a review, see Blum, 1960) and the question 'pulls' toward episodes of acute indigestion, it is very likely that other NV incidents (such as that experienced in cancer treatment or, postoperatively, in its terminal stages, or in PNV, motion sickness, toxic smoke inhalation, exercise or other fatigue, high-altitude sickness, brain tumor, drunkenness, migraine headaches, etc.) will not appear in the 'acute indigestion' category. If so, then an approximately 5% annual incidence number of about 8.5 million Americans is a low estimate, probably a *very* low estimate.

A breakdown by age and family shows that indigestion NV are reported most frequently in the ages 18–44 with low (under $10 000) incomes at 7.8 per 100. The lowest rate is among those with incomes higher than $10 000 and over 45 years at 2.1. In the mid-range of 4–5 incidents per 100 are the high- and low-income persons under 18 years, and the high-income persons aged 18–44. These rather dramatic differences introduce the pervasive factor of NV risk variation as a function of personal status variables, in this case demographic. Clinical studies generally report low risk among older persons. Ignoring differences in reporting tendencies about any kind of event that occurs by age, this statistic introduces us to the likely difference in NV rates between spontaneous gastrointestinal (GI) disorders and iatrogenic conditions, and to the ever-present discrepancies depending on how, for what purpose, and from whom NV data are gathered.

The fact that a significant NV risk (keep in mind the definitional problem) arises from poverty and yet is not reported in clinical studies immediately warns us of the lack of psychosocial focus in clinical studies. The survey finding is entirely consistent with epidemiological socioeconomic conclusions made over the years, which show that poverty is a general illness risk. Typically adverse conditions of nutrition, contagion, trauma, sanitation, environmental exposure, hygienic knowledge, psychological distress, work stress, dangers, etc., contribute. Yet the reversal among the poor shown here, where younger adults are more at risk of nonspecific GI NV than children, at a rate that is almost three times that of poor older adults (2.8 vs 7.8), also demands a question. We ask, speculatively, are there special risks for acute GI dis-orders or events that induce NV among exceedingly low-paid workers or those in homeless environments (the study excludes institutionalized persons)? Think of the food gleaned from garbage cans, and the factory toxins exposing the unprotected worker, whose income of maybe $5 an hour buys neither health education, nor medicines, nor even food re-frigeration, and the answer could be, 'How can they not?'

It may well be that NV are sensitive indicators of the interaction of socioeconomic status with the environment in the Survey (if it is a good measure), yielding quite unusual differences in risk. Keep this apparent interaction in mind, because it becomes central to a 'theory' of NV. Future investigators may be able to use NV as an environmental risk marker, once the characteristics of a group or of a person's illness and exposure situation are defined. Clinicians in any event should be sensitive to a patient's socioeconomic conditions because these pose disease, dietary, psychosocial, and other related risks. As is the case in social or public health medicine, a palliative treatment may yield only short-term results and return visits, whereas preventive interventions based on a comprehensive understanding are the ideal for health maintenance. In this instance the Survey data suggest that NV and other GI disorders may be serious health–environmental problems for underpaid young workers. Were we to think of the occurrence of NV in a group as a 'sentinel event,' we would move NV from clinical medicine to public health, thence to ecology, and thence to economics.

Regarding disability linked to age, the Survey shows an average rate of 7.8 restricted activity days as a result of indigestion – including NV across all ages. The greatest activity loss, not being able to 'do stuff' – that 'Ziggy' theorem applied by Kaplan (1994) to the characterization of health-related quality of life – occurs among those aged 5–17 (9.7 days lost) and 45–64 (9.6). The least loss is reported among the very young. Days lost depend on the persons experiencing them – or here the adult reporting on other household members' experiential importance – and on what important functions are lost, or consequential activity restricted. The distribution here can be rationalized, but its significance is not really known. One may propose that the very young have little of consequence to be lost to them from acute GI NV, whereas those in school, or those at work, would be viewed as suffering a consequential NV-induced disability, affecting life's duties and work.

The much higher risk for women over men of restricted days from indigestion NV is much more important: the rate is almost 3 to 1 (in rounded numbers: 5700 actual restricted days for men, 14 200 for women). Indigestion makes a minor contribution to days lost compared with those lost as a result of respiratory conditions (in rounded numbers: 385 300 or second ranked, injuries at 206 900). The fact that the 3:1 ratio, women:men, reported here for disability, mirrors the 3:1 or 4:1 figures for NV risk by sex indicates a consistent relationship of incidence to activity loss.

The household survey reports selected chronic conditions, because these diagnoses are known to and reported by householders. Respiratory conditions are ranked first with respect to prevalence, second to cardiovascular conditions, and a distant third to a mix of organ system disorders. Among the last, however, migraine is the most common, a condition in which NV are often present. Again, in the Survey, as in other studies, women suffer from migraine more than men, at a rate of more than 3 to 1. In both groups migraine, and therefore NV, are most prevalent in the youngest, where the 'young category' embraces all those aged under 45 years, although in women the proportionate difference between this age group and those aged 45–64 is less (men: about 4:1; women: about 2:1). Thus, not only do more women than men suffer from migraine and its associated NV but they suffer these for a longer time over their lives (five times more women than men reporting it in the 45–65 age group). We shall see later that the relationship between migraine and NV may be a powerful one for etiological theory, because migraine may be reduced after the menopause – the age category may fail to show a premenopausal peak. The research question still remains.

Study of women's lifetime NV prevalence and patterns

We sought data on the lifetime prevalence of NV, the experiences giving rise to it, the treatments used for it, and the associations between experiencing one or another kind of N or V measured by precipitating experiences. Our students, Sarah Nixon and Dana Karlsburg, completed work begun by others. Planned as a large-scale study, it was frustrated during recruitment of subjects. The design called for comparison of women attending four clinics at Stanford University Medical Center (SUMC) – medicine, pediatrics (also mothers), general surgery, and obstetrics – with one another and with women graduate students, as well as hospital staff. As we could recruit only a small sample ($n = 163$), its findings are at best provocative. An ideal next-round study would sample at least 1200 women randomly or a census quota would be selected. In this initial work, as with all interview/questionnaire studies, errors arise from failures of memory, definition, verbal skills, or interests. Outcome statistics are biased by unanswered questions. The general rule is that, unless there are trends consistent with one another or with theory, or quite large differences given a small sample, it is necessary to take the results as suggestive and to refrain from reliance on particular percentages as accurately generalizable.

Life situation and N precipitation

We expected differences in NV experience to be extensive depending on the life situation. This has already been shown rather dramatically in the Survey data discussed above. In the limited, but more NV-focused, study discussed here, we could test only for differences arising from patient status in the clinic groups – for example, in pediatrics, being a mother of a patient – as well as for nonpatient status, for example, graduate student or hospital staff status. We were surprised to find that few differences achieved significance when these groups were contrasted; the differences were in fact so few that, given the number of association tests made, we admit the likelihood that any significant differences were by chance (with 100 tests of association, five are expected to be significant by chance). The demographic differences found, which are significant among the youngest women in the surgical group and the oldest patients in the general medicine group, make sense given the age and different illnesses (for medicine) and the accident or elective surgery for younger women. Dramatic but unsurprising are the differences for education ($p = 0.0001$). The nonstudent sample consisted primarily of women who were graduates; in contrast, a number of the women in the patient groups had not completed high school.

We now describe the significant differences among groups with respect to what we consider to be our most important inquiry variable: the self-reported causes of N.

Consider that, at $p \leq 0.01$ (of occurring by chance), 'anxiety/nervousness' is much more commonly reported as a cause of N for the nonpatient group than in any/all of the patient group. This is not independent of education, which covaries; so it is also the case that more educated women are more likely to report anxiety/nervousness leading to N. It may be that this finding is explicable in terms of the greater health self-awareness, and thus possibly more insight/awareness of anxiety among educated women, even though their illness risk is lower because of their higher socioeconomic class. (See Blum and Heinrichs, 1988, for a review and discussion of this literature.) Age associates with, and thus predicts, the likelihood of reporting stress as a precipitant, whereas patient versus nonpatient status shows only a trend in the same direction as anxiety, for reporting by students/staff (Pearson: $p = 0.09$; but Mantel Hanszel: only $p = 0.29$). Although not tested for association, but being a part of the general interview inquiry, 25% say that their work situation gives rise to NV. One would expect risk, as a subjective verbalized insight, to correlate with higher education and socioeconomic class. (Penebaker's paradox: the poor are more ill, more educated women more self-health sensitive.)

Women in our sample report work-related NV causes as: stress: 13% (we have included 'competition' here); foul odors: 4%; poor eating habits: 3%; being 'too high up': 1%. One person in each category reported: overheating and 'spinning around.' (What job did this woman have? Was she speaking figuratively?) In any event, for a quarter of women to find their work a source of N – for that is more common than V – is a commentary on today's workplace for women, and a troubling commentary on the nature of work in the USA.

A strong association links reported over-exertion to N in the nonpatient group; this is consistent with its much greater appearance in the most educated (nonpatient) group. As exercise can precipitate N, and one may posit an education = exercise self-care via exercise lifestyle in students and hospital staff, this makes some sense. Again, careful discrimination in those responding appears to discriminate exertion from stress, although in physiological rather than psychological terms this would, if exercise is the variable here, be a faulty one. We do not know if exertion at work that is not self-defined as 'stress' also operates. The fault lies in our question. Yet nonpatients do, to some extent, discriminate between 'stress' versus 'anxiety' as a cause of N.

There is a powerful association (all tests at $p = 0.00005$) for second trimester PNV and education, with the educated group being at much greater risk. This is not an explicable finding and must be regarded with caution and serious curiosity. Our own theories of PNV, to be presented later, do not account for it, unless again one is dealing only with the self-health sensitivity shown in more educated women. A provocative finding is that mothers of young patients have last trimester (thus 'normal') PNV, rather than hyperemesis gravidarum (HG), more often than other clinic groups, including women in obstetric clinics. This is odd, because one would expect women in obstetric clinics to report more PNV simply because they are more conscious of current pregnancy events. This is not the case. This prompts us to ask whether mothers of children being brought to a pediatrician are more sensitive to adverse risk. In an earlier study (Blum et al., 1972) we found that mothers of children identified as having drug problems recalled these children (compared with their nonproblematic peers) as having had more associated pregnancy/infancy/childhood disorders. As no work to date suggests higher illness risk for children of women with PNV, we suspect that there is a sensitivity in the sense of 'worried recollection' or 'sick child, thus PNV baby' and this leads to a carryover factor. There are no data to suggest that PNV babies are more ill as children, that PNV mothers are more hypochondriacal on behalf of their PNV babies, or that PNV more frequently predisposes mothers to seek pediatric advice. One must be very doubtful, in the absence of prior evidence of PNV, of a delayed teratogenic risk (except an unreplicated claim for male cancer).

Nausea precipitated by headache has a demographic component for the middle years of 21–50, as does fasting/dieting. More education predicts more reports of N precipitated by menstrual periods. Whether this is artifact or perhaps some education-linked self-sensitivity we do not know. Alcohol-induced N occurs more often in the nonpatient group, and is consistently found more frequently in the 21–50 age group and in more educated women (with a strong trend). Given a body of literature on alcohol which shows that there is more drinking in the younger years, this appears to be an exposure variable.

NV general inquiries/general health in our sample

When asked about their general lifetime health, 93% (percentages are rounded to the nearest integer) of all the women said that they were healthy and 90% said that their appetites were generally good. Surprisingly, then, being a clinic patient did not mean that they viewed themselves as ill. We asked whether their health varied with life periods: childhood, adolescence (12–20), early and middle adulthood, older middle age, and when elderly. Only about one-third (36%) saw their health as varying with these periods. When asked about migraine or other severe headache, 36% nevertheless said that they suffered from these. Obviously their presence in an SUMC clinic as patients with severe headache does not mean that these women think of themselves as generally ill; furthermore, most characterize their health as stable and, if appetite is a measure of GI function, as not suffering any chronic GI disorder. We do not characterize these women as a particularly illness-sensitive, symptom-prone or hypochondriacal group, and we conclude that their replies about their NV are not exaggerated.

Lifetime NV experience

Ninety-eight per cent of the population indicate that they have experienced N; 97% say that they have had V (Figure 3.1). (There are some inconsistencies in questionnaire replies, a few saying 'no' to the initial question and then responding 'yes' with respect to specific precipitants for N in their lives; thus these figures represent our summary of NV positive replies.) Altogether only 2% of the population say that they have not had N or V. Within the last 6 months, 43% have been nauseous on more than three occasions, and 21% have vomited on more than three occasions. N is, then, almost universal for women and frequent N is common. For what we might call a large NV-sensitive group – approaching half of our population – it occurs twice as often as V. A minor paradox is the slightly higher life experience with V over N.

NV: emergence of different pattern

In terms of the patterns of particular instances over a lifetime, 27% have vomited without first experiencing N. On inquiry as to whether it was usual for them to vomit upon becoming nauseous, or not to vomit 'most of the time' (we limited our analysis to the 84% who could answer definitively; we assume that the remainder have mixed patterns), we found that 34% habitually have a combined N then V pattern, whereas 66% most commonly do not vomit even though nauseous. The researcher will, of course, want to know how these women differ, and what the components are, at every level from ecological to G-cell protein messengers, in the patterns emerging. Importantly, this report of a normal population tells us that N and V

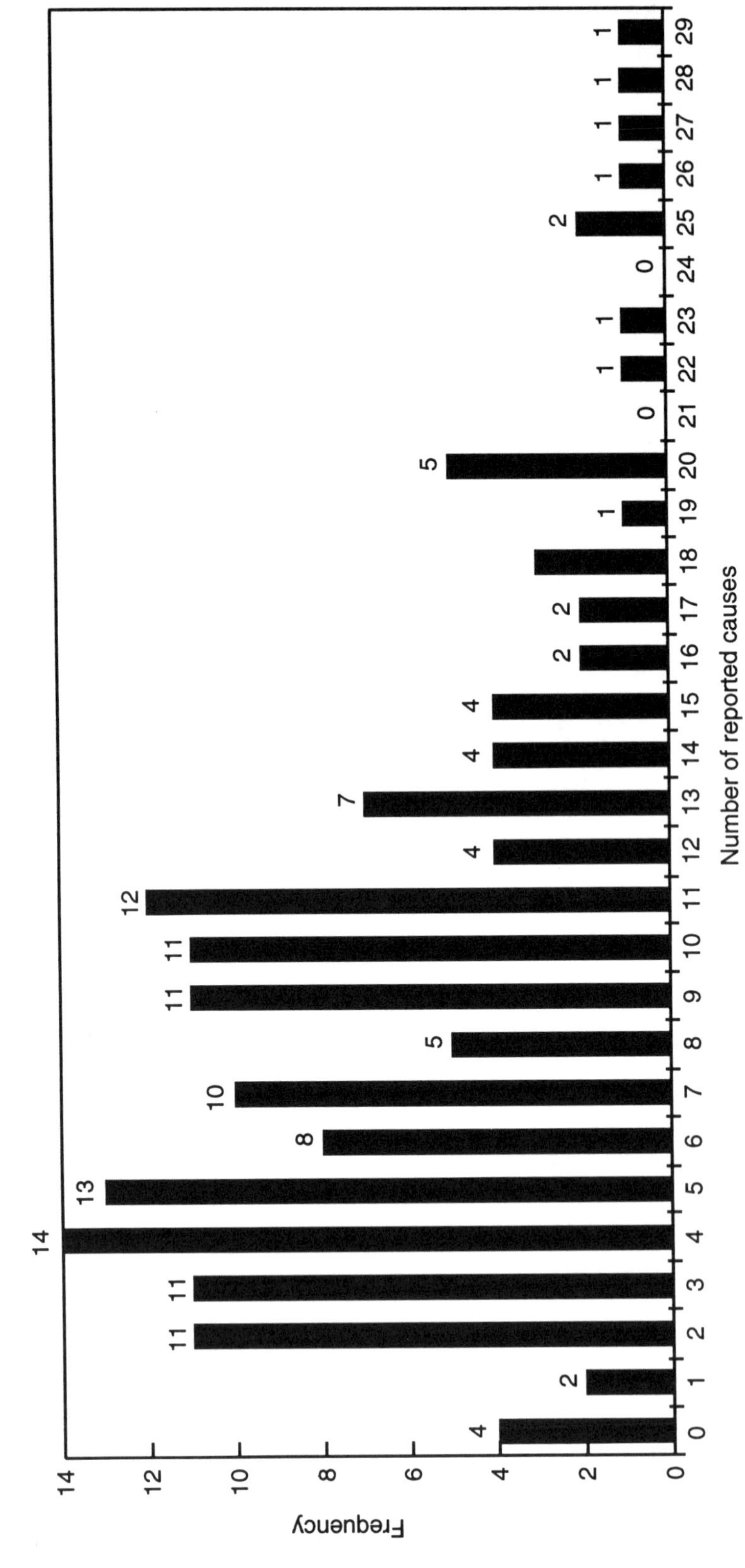

Figure 3.1: Number of reports of N caused.

patterns and whether they occur separately must be considered in any theory and any new hypothesis generation.

We asked women whether these habitual patterns varied at any life phase. For 28%, the reply was 'yes.' For N, almost half report that their N experience did vary with periods of life. These vulnerable periods included pregnancy, injury, illness, dietary changes, and the like, with pregnancy far and above the period most noted; periods of dietary change were ranked second but noted six times less frequently. However, when asked directly about the life stages at which they felt most nauseous, for over 50% it was adulthood, with only 10% recalling most difficulty in childhood and 20% in adolescence. The same trend occurs for V, with a somewhat higher percentage in childhood, and a somewhat reduced adulthood incidence reported (down from 53% to 42%). Contrary to the risk variables typically identified in clinical studies, adulthood, not childhood, is the most risky period. One must distinguish, however, specific risk onsets, for example, operations or cancer chemotherapy where investigators control for age, as opposed to this normal population who report from all sources. As always, there are individual differences, because, in the 20% commenting on particular common lifetime changes, the aging trend is in the direction of less frequent/less painful V for 7%. With regard to typical duration, less than one hour for N is modal (34%) followed by half a day (18%), two hours (15%), one day (11%), several days or more (5%). It is most important in recognizing N as a feature of quality of life that, for about 33% of women, their N spells are long – half a day or more.

These 'normal population' experiences substantiate the clinical and, indeed, the animal study findings of different individual patterns and different NV patterns within the same person, as well as across groups.

Precipitants of NV in a normal population: lifetime prevalence

We asked about perceived causes of NV, presenting a recognition list derived from a pre-test. Beginning with the most prevalent, 'food poisoning' is reported by 65% of the population as a cause of both N and V. This is followed by 'stomach virus,' at 58% for N (52% V). (Public health studies suggest that such self-diagnosis may wrongly overplay the virus.) The other causes are as follows:

- Pregnancy: 54% N, 35% V
- Food tastes and smells: 52% for N but only 17% for V

- Smells as such: 47% N, 16% V
- Automobile motion: 44% N, 20% V
- Anxiety/nervousness: 39% N, but only 9% V
- Headache: 33% N, 15% V
- Fasting/dieting: 32% N, 8% V
- Alcohol: 31% for both N and V
- Stress: 31% N but only 7% V
- Drugs/medications: 31% N, 14% V
- Boat and amusement park ride motion sickness: 27% N, 9% V.

About 20% of the women report surgery, menstrual cramps/discomfort, seeing the unpleasant, medication, pain or pain-causing injury, airplane motion, second trimester PNV, anger, and grief as NV causes. About one-sixth of the population report causes of N as high altitude, third trimester PNV, fear, and fatigue. Less commonly reported, at 10% or less for N, are infections, allergies, excitement, and jealousy. We were surprised when less than 1% of women said that they suffered NV when observing someone else vomit. We proffer the guess that men, less exposed to regurgitating infant care, might be more vulnerable. The foregoing listing shows the great diversity of precipitants, 'systematized' by us as GI, pregnancy, smell/taste, psychological states, dietary change, alcohol and drugs as toxins, pain, motion, disease, and autoimmune reactions.

There are only two instances where V is precipitated as much as N: these are alcohol and 'food poisoning,' with 'stomach virus' close at 58%. Perhaps one may invoke 'mechanisms' and closer approximation to classically defined 'reflexive' V, so favored by pharmacologists, or Darwinian, evolutionarily conserved efforts at toxin expulsion (however failed), particularly for these patterns. But, in contrast to alcohol and what people tend to call 'belly bugs' for all other 'causes,' N is more common, albeit over quite a range, in those cases such as after surgery at 23%, infections at 8%, and allergies at 7%. One notes with interest that, for PNV, V becomes a greater component in distress with increasing gestation length, i.e., last trimester 54%, then second trimester 22%, and third trimester 15%. The lowest ratios of V to N are found in fasting/dieting at 32%, fatigue at 15%, smells for foods at 52%, other unpleasant smells at 47%, and for emotions: seeing the unpleasant, at 21%, anger at 19%, stress at 21%, anxiety/nervousness at 39%, excitement and jealousy both at 6%.

In only a few of all the precipitating conditions is V as common as N. We can see that recognition terms elicit different NV cases from recall, e.g., altitude heights, work, fatigue, etc. The full range of these should be included in any categorical system. One should not make too much of percentages when proportions are measured in small groups; they are often not tested for significance primarily because the power to yield *p* values of less than 0.05 is low when small numbers are involved. Nevertheless, the diversity of precipitants is striking, as is the difference in ranking. It is very obvious that most events are environmentally provoked, although individual differences in susceptibility/propensity are inferred, and substantiated elsewhere. To some extent, at least, pregnancy NV is also 'ecological,' obviously so when it is a response to odor/food.

One assumes that the variety of patterns demonstrated, and of the precipitants systematized, reflects etiological and psychobiological differences, as well as ecological, sensory, neuromessenger, anatomical, biochemical responsiveness, and 'signal processing' differences by event. It is our observation and thesis that molecular, pathway and, also, simultaneous contextual network and 'molar' activities must occur differentially, 'underlying' the different circumstances of discriminant periods of N and V.

If we recap on major life periods (childhood, adolescence, young adulthood and middle years, and later) and recollected N prevalence, adulthood is the period of greatest sensitivity/prevalence with two exceptions: for menstrual cramps there is a very slightly higher recollected incidence in adolescence and for automobile motion this is in childhood.

Distribution of precipitants as individual vulnerabilities/predispositions

We arrayed the sample in terms of the number of 'causes' that, on response to our query, our respondents said had produced N or V in themselves. We limited the array to the 29 most frequently cited, so a few were excluded. Some women who had reported no N experience earlier in the questionnaire/interview nevertheless reported having it when presented with a checklist; likewise, some who had earlier reported N experience did not respond to any of the checklist items as precipitants. These inconsistent cases are noted on Figure 3.1 which shows the distribution of reported N causes, by number, stated by the women to have precipitated N in their lifetime experience.

Figure 3.1 shows a skewed rather than a normal distribution. The average woman indicates that she experiences N from eight sources; the median is 7%. Four per cent here report no lifetime N experience whereas, at the other extreme, one woman had suffered from all 29 of the checklist precipitants.

We see that there are wide individual differences, and that most women will experience N from many different sources. In this sample, NV from iatrogenic interventions – the sort followed in clinical trials – are rare. Only one sample member appears to have had cancer chemotherapy.

But NV do occur quite normally for over half of our group as a 'part of living.' As a research issue one asks if it is only above this 'normal range' of NV responsiveness that one should characterize any iatrogenic procedure as particularly emetogenic. As the checklist procedure seems to yield underreporting, it may well be that iatrogenic procedures (however consequential to physician and patient) are not necessarily productive of higher NV incidence than the perturbations of normal living/illness. The literature does suggest that cisplatin therapies for cancer, bone marrow transplantation, strabismus surgery, fourth ventricle neurosugery, and abdominal surgery may constitute these unusually emetogenic circumstances.

Interrelationships, strength of association, among various N precipitants

We wished to learn which kinds of N 'go together,' i.e., where a woman reporting one cause, or categories of similar 'causes,' would also be likely to report experiencing N from another source. We arbitrarily grouped together precipitants that appeared to us to involve sensory-related stimuli and only presumed processing at similar central nervous system (CNS) levels.

Table 3.1 shows these 10 major groups of N subjectively perceived and the recollected precipitants in cross-tabulated association with one another. Playing with possible markers for different underlying processes, one might take the highest statistical association (gamma values) as presumptive evidence for a specificity of underlying biopsychological process. To illustrate, using the two strongest associations – pain sensitivity and PNV or food N predisposition closely associated with drug/medication/alcohol sensitivity – one may hypothesize that these two strong groups both express a different underlying process (i.e., two phenotypes and one genotype). The notion would lead PNV workers to focus on pain, not hormones, and gastroenterologists to look for other special features with ingestion NV-vulnerable groups.

Table 3.2 presents these same results in a different fashion, ordering all precipitants/perturbations reported in a descending order of strength of association. It is an easy count that 39 specific

Table 3.1: Gamma values for relationships between 10 N categories

	Emotions	Motion	Pregnant	Drug	Sensory	Illness	Surgery	Food	Pain	Fatigue
Emotions										
Motion	0.25									
Pregnant	0.65**	0.55**								
Drug	0.65***	0.52	***0.36							
Sensory	0.67***	0.57***	0.74***	0.60***						
Illness	0.62***	0.78***	0.66***	0.71***	0.61***					
Surgery	0.39	0.40	0.55	0.78***	0.67**	0.70**				
Food	0.60***	0.56***	0.16	0.81***	0.60***	0.67***	0.58**			
Pain	0.71***	0.43**	0.83***	0.54***	0.43	0.66***	0.36	0.50**		
Fatigue	0.78***	0.55**	0.67	0.74***	0.55**	0.73***	0.65***	0.45**	0.76***	

**Significant at 0.01 level.
***Significant at 0.001 level.

Table 3.2: Strength of relationships between 10 N categories in descending order by gamma value (statistically significant relationships only)

Relationship	Gamma value	Relationship	Gamma value
Pregnancy by pain	0.83	Emotions by drug	0.65
Drug by food	0.81	Surgery by fatigue	0.65
Emotions by fatigue	0.78	Emotions by illness	0.62
Motion by illness	0.78	Sensory by illness	0.61
Drug by surgery	0.78	Emotions by food	0.60
Pain by fatigue	0.76	Drug by sensory	0.60
Pregnancy by surgery	0.74	Sensory by food	0.60
Drug by fatigue	0.74	Surgery by food	0.58
Illness by fatigue	0.73	Motion by sensory	0.57
Emotions by pain	0.71	Motion by food	0.56
Drug by illness	0.71	Motion by pregnancy	0.55
Illness by surgery	0.70	Motion by fatigue	0.55
Emotions by sensory	0.67	Sensory by fatigue	0.55
Pregnancy by fatigue	0.67	Drug by pain	0.54
Sensory by surgery	0.67	Motion by drug	0.52
Illness by food	0.67	Food by pain	0.50
Illness by pain	0.67	Food by fatigue	0.45
Pregnancy by illness	0.66	Motion by pain	0.43
Emotions by pregnancy	0.65	Sensory by pain	0.43

cross-tabulated stimuli/conditions are related at least to one other and, generally, to several other N susceptibilities. There is one confounded association, because we included food allergies in two aggregate categories. This effect should be small; only about 9% report food allergies as a N cause. Yet even these predict two-thirds of the other experience categories. Overall, calculating all possible relationships as 45, 39 in Table 3.2 show a significant association and six do not.

Table 3.3 considers all possible categorical relationships. With a total of 10 categories for a woman reporting N from one of these precipitants, there are potentially nine others that she may also have experienced as a 'cause' of N over her recollected lifetime. Dramatically shown, three kinds of N experiences serve as predictors of having experienced N from all other (here aggregated) sources. Thus N induced by fatigue, illness, and sensory experience, if reported by a woman as having been 'causes,' generates the prediction that she will have experienced *all* other causes of N as well. Least

Table 3.3: Number of statistically significant relationships for each of the 10 N categories

Category	Number of significant relationships
Sensory	9
Illness	9
Fatigue	9
Emotions	8
Drug	8
Food	8
Pain	8
Motion	7
Pregnancy	6
Surgery	6

useful for prediction, and thus perhaps indicative of more isolated rather than general biopsychological N processes, are PNV and PONV.

A general predisposition for many women

Importantly, these data suggest that vulnerability to N consists of underlying, general predispositions, i.e., common covariance or dispositional genotype. These may also be restricted to only a few experiential conditions. As this sample has little cancer chemotherapy or radiation experience, we cannot know how generally other 'normal' N precipitants would contribute to this as risk factors for patients about to undergo such treatments. A more refined research question is to ask which of the several patterns of cancer chemotherapy prediction is assisted by knowledge of prior markers for all N risk, i.e., fatigue, illness, sensory experience, and which cancer treatment NV occur as currently unpredictable. The question of research enterprise has considerable clinical importance for assigning risk tracks to patients entering cancer treatment regimens, particularly if the design is multivariant, e.g., environmental, and allows interaction effects to be examined. Findings would be important for theories of NV that rest on highly specific explanations such as enterochromaffin serotonin release, and antagonism. To the extent that predispositions measured by lifetime causal multiplicity predict one or another cancer or PONV pattern, one must also test for reported dose and toxicity whether cytoxin or radiation specific. It is likely that one will find perturbation responses that are more pervasive than can be accounted for by single neurotransmitter actions. In contrast, insofar as general predilection fails to predict the NV outcome for cancer chemotherapy or radiation, then limited explanations using neuropharmacologically activated receptor and pathways would have logical substantiation.

Surgery: a special interest case

Sixty-nine percent of the sample had had experience of surgery, and 7% reported presurgical N and 59% postsurgical N. One notes the much higher surgical N rate reported here, of 59% (we assume that those with stress N before surgery were in the larger group with PONV), than in the earlier response to a checklist of items: 23%. This shows that how one asks about NV affects incidence reports. Here it is a methodological flaw. We inquired particularly about abdominal or pelvic surgery, learning (depending on the accuracy rate of reporting!) that 39% had those areas as operative sites (one suspects probably reproductive); of these 37% were recalled to be 'band aid size,' i.e., for endoscopic incisions. Direct inquiry revealed that 25% of the sample had NV in connection with local, spinal, or dental anesthetic.

Whatever the respective surgery rate for individuals, perhaps half of all those suffering NV had it without having had a general anesthetic.

The fact that most women have NV in response to a number of events, only a small fraction of which may be iatrogenic, implies that N is at least partly a nonspecific predisposition. Figure 3.2 shows the range of N-only causes – because it is the more common phenomenon – reported by women in our sample. To construct that chart we excluded a few causes that were denied on the checklist even though they emerged in our pre-test. The data program does not present the empirical reality.

NV intensity as pain

We now compare evaluations of the two experiences, N compared with V, rating their general pain intensity.

Figure 3.2 shows the ratings on an analogue scale, from least pain 'akin to a skin scratch' at value 1 to 'the most extreme imaginable' at value 10. The mean and modal central tendencies are pain intensity ratings of 6 for N; this is somewhat higher than the central tendency midpoint of a normal distribution of judged painfulness. The distribution might be normalized with large numbers of persons, but its present form promotes speculation that it could be bimodal, because

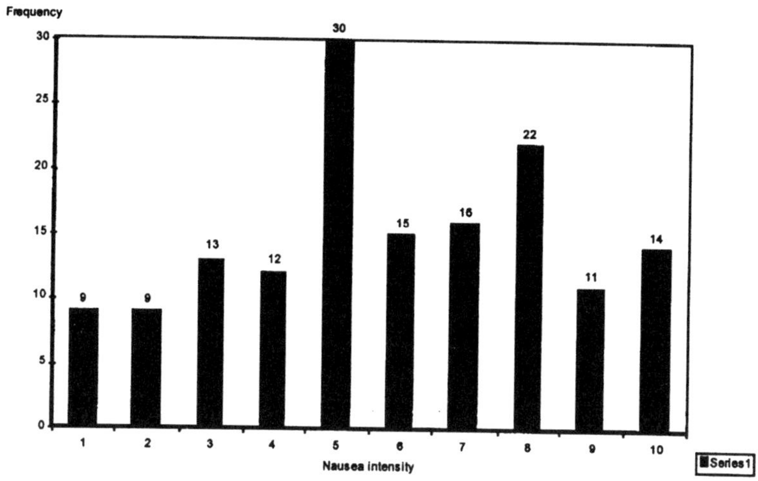

Figure 3.2: NV experience as pain intensity.

we see a concentration of persons for whom N is ranked as quite severe pain indeed. Ratings 8, 9, and 10 constitute almost a third (31%) of our normal population. N is, insofar as the prevention and relief of pain are the primary mission of health practitioners, a matter of consequence. And it may be that populations may be categorized on their N-as-pain sensitivity.

Figure 3.3 shows that, for V, the mean, rounded, and mode as measures of central tendency converge at 7, a one-point higher rating than N pain. This distribution does not forecast a normal bell-shaped curve, but, instead, one of bimodal experience and sensitivity. Here two groups of women emerge, one with low or midpoint pain sensitivities, another for whom V is an extremely high, maximally imaginable pain experience. Combining the 8, 9, and 10 ratings one

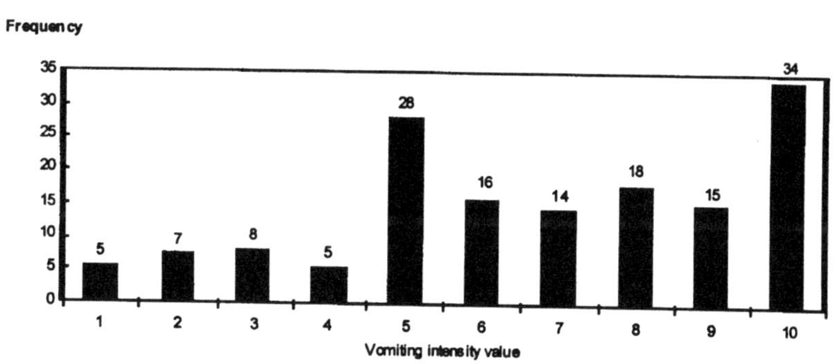

Figure 3.3: Vomiting intensity chart.

finds 45% of the population, with 23% rating V as the maximal intensity of life-experienced pain. This is serious business.

Prior child delivery predicts painful V

Unlike clinical studies which report N as the more extreme, acute and enduring discomfort, these women find V slightly worse, including a large group for whom it is extremely painful.

An obstetrician, mindful of the extreme pain that can be experienced during childbirth, might suggest that, for an otherwise healthy woman, labor pain could be the extreme standard against which other pain would be compared subjectively. If so, one expects that women who had had babies to be more conservative in rating the pain of V. We tested this expectation and were surprised. On a means test averaging V intensity scores, there was no difference between women who had and those who had not been pregnant. On the other hand, when we took those scoring V pain as extreme, rankings 8 and 9, a statistically significant difference was observed in the unexpected direction: more mothers rated V as the most intensely imaginable pain than did nonmothers. Does pregnancy (with or without PNV) sensitize women to V? Puzzled, we proposed that it would not be pregnancy generally, but PNV in particular, that would sensitize to later NV as pain. We tested those mothers with and those without PNV for extreme pain ratings on both V and N, and found no differences.

A puzzling relationship of most painful V to a history of motherhood

We are left with the inexplicable relationship of pregnancy or childbirth itself, or perhaps some correlate relating to age, fertility, maternal empathy, to rated NV pain intensity. Future research, should these findings be replicable, must account for this rather remarkable relationship with pregnancy/motherhood as possibly NV pain sensitizing. Herxheimer, in critiquing our work, remarks that the immediacy and overwhelming subjectivity of the experience of both nausea and pain (which can occur simultaneously and be overlappingly described) contribute to difficulty in objectifying these via recall, i.e. retrospectively, in the reliable, quantifiable ways that research on lifetime prevalence, as here attempted, requires. Thus, data based on their recall can be suspect. Because of their passing nature, not ordinarily leaving measurable external signs as sequelae, these phenomena are more difficult for clinicians/researchers to keep in mind when not immediately present. Comparatively, there is a much greater body of research on pain and its alleviation – consider the common presence of pain clinics – in contrast to NV. As long as NV are viewed as 'normal', having adaptive function or 'just a side effect' there will be insufficient attention paid, including to developing a more astute methodology for measuring N.

The compassionate caregiver dare not be uninformed

Given the data of these chapters on NV prevalence, disability, untreatability, and pain, healers and caregivers should feel compelled by their oath and compassion to attend to NV. Insofar as their own procedures as surgeons, oncologists, prescribers, or attending professionals 'cause' the pain and disability of NV, its prevention and treatment should be preoccupying. It is our own observation, compatible with the research literature and consistent with the rarity of textbook attention to it, that clinicians are underinformed and underattentive to even iatrogenic NV, whereas the NV of ordinary living, except for a commonly recommended over the counter drug (OTC) with no known efficacy, are completely ignored by the professions. At the very least, there is a world of opportunity for better pharmaceutical and alternative products to be better tested and marketed.

Benign NV

We asked the oddball question, were there ever times when N or V was *not* unpleasant? Indeed there were: 15% of women said there had been an occasion(s) when N was not unpleasant, 20% when V was not. Foolishly, the prestructured interview failed to inquire about the frequency or conditions for this 'benign' NV. We wondered if it might be bulimic or anorexic or Roman, but there was only one woman who indicated that her benign NV was self-induced V. However, and this is typical of inconsistencies in interview/questionnaires, a question asked a different way in a different context can yield a different result. Thus when we asked 'when was V not unpleasant?,' three women (2%) said this was the case when it was self-induced; another 2% said that it was not unpleasant when it occurred very suddenly (as can happen normally in motion sickness or rejected food), and need not be a warning of a brain tumor, where projectile V often occurs. Given the semantic clarity with which women discriminate NV from other stomach distress, and the generally high pain ratings for N and V, one is indeed puzzled about the possible descriptions offered by the other 11% reporting the experience of benign V – whatever the frequency – and the 20% reporting benign N. Subjectively we cannot come to terms with any hedonistically neutral 'N.' Someone else must do a better inquiry.

Self-induced V is not unpleasant, or at least it appears that this can be learned. For self-initiated activity, the involvement of higher cognitive centers is required. Motivation should be one distinguishing feature that allows a benign/malign distinction; it also implies, in medical–psychological therapeutic interventions, that 'meanings' and self-control may be tools with which one works for the therapeutic redefinition of pain, just as self-control techniques for delivering analgesics potentiates analgesic protection. Learning the events/mechanisms at work so that NV pain is absent will surely be of interest to the clinical research worker.

Self-treatments

About half (53%) of women have self-treated their N; the things described as helpful are: crackers (12%), OTC antacids (12%), carbonated beverages and hard candy (4%), bread (3%). Tea, ginger, and water are on the list, as are OTC antacids, rarely used (4%) for N, and again crackers and carbonated drinks. We note that, in earlier clinical interviews, women had told us of other home remedies for PNV: spaced eating, bland foods, warm teas, warm milk, gentle stomach rubs, cola drinks, vitamin B_6, ginger (again), and marijuana. Some said that eating to control PNV was also helpful. This contradicts notions of food restriction as being helpful to avert 'crowding' of the stomach, or defines a separate group of women. Further comparison of the group with PNV who were helped by eating with those helped by smaller intakes would be interesting.

When asked if their home treatment efforts for N control had ever failed, 19% noted failures. This implies a successful N treatment rate among 75% of these women.

Only a minority (29%) reported that they had sought to control their V by any treatment. As almost all had suffered it, a curious passivity is inferred. In the face of the high pain/discomfort rating, we distrust the report, and the limits of the prestructured interviews. As to the success of treatment endeavors (here we have only lifetime prevalence, not summary incident counts), at best the data review indicates that most (74%) of those who say that they tried home remedies for N find them successful. Of the fewer numbers who have tried prescription AEs, 77% have had success, and for V control, 80%. These percentage differences are inconsequential.

What is important in conclusion is that only 29% – and recall almost all had suffered V – say that they have ever successfully controlled their V by either a home or prescribed remedy.

Monetary costs

Our student, Craig Thomas (see Chapter 10), provides estimates (in dollars) of the cost of NV nationally. These are consequential and are a further argument for increased attention to NV. His estimates of overall NV costs range, depending on the economic and methodological assumptions made, between $4 billion and $16 billion annually. If one takes the midpoint, $10 billion, this is about 8% (and possibly 10%) of the annual cancer costs. Far more is invested in cancer research than in efforts to alleviate NV. Cancer is, of course, more painful, deadly, and more feared, but even when considered a prosaic 'normal,' 'compulsory,' 'developmental,' or unavoidable iatrogenic condition, NV are far more expensive, measured in dollars as well as suffering, than may previously have been assumed.

NV risk factor overview

Earlier discussion and data presentation have noted NV risk factors. These are important clinically in anticipating whether a patient undergoing a procedure is likely to be at risk of NV. They are also very important theoretically. Any theory of how NV arises – beginning with some external or internal environmental perturbation and going through events in the brain and enteric regions – must eventually be able to account for the processes that a risk factor represents statistically. A risk factor identified demographically or as a personal attribute is only a summary category; it tells us nothing of the relationship between X or Y and what is going on to increase the chances of experiencing NV under conditions A or B. And one keeps in mind that individual risk factors for NV generally appear modest in their ability to contribute to accurate outcome forecasts for groups or individuals. Our finding of differences in general predisposition/vulnerability to NV from a variety of sources may prove to be a weightier predictor. It explains nothing. There is much need for thorough work to allow better weighting for known risk factors under one situation or another and, ignored to date, to seek to identify interactions among them.

From the array of clinical studies offering risk data and the Health

Survey, one can see quite a range of conditions that can be identified as predisposing to NV under conditions of exposure to typical 'causes.' Excluded from this list are the quite specific procedural risks that operate powerfully in surgery and cancer treatments. In surgery, NV are affected by such things as pre-treatments, site of surgery, kind and route of delivery of anesthetics, nitrous oxide adjuncts, oxygen mask provision, etc., whereas chemotherapy NV vary with cytotoxins used and administration schedules, or radiation amounts, sites, and extent, whether the patient is chemotherapy naive or has recurring cancer, etc. These are considered practically in Part V and also methodologically in Chapter 7.

NV risk settings, situations, precipitants: from common to infinite?

All humans (with the exception of a few clinical cases) appear capable of NV. Our limited lifetime prevalence study shows that NV precipitants are immensely varied across environmental, sensory, emotional, disease, pregnancy, pain, stress, and other categories. Given the diversity of settings in which humans experience NV, there may be an almost infinite number of potentially precipitating conditions. We shall propose, and in later chapters elaborate upon, an instability of adaptive response systems that are sensory integrating and which respond to 'alien' and uncontrollable 'perturbation' (one way of defining any NV precipitating context); potentially (although not statistically) any disturbance in the human's controllable steady state could lead to N or, less likely, to V or to both. Table 3.3 shows commonly shared predisposing triggers. Note that most are defined by the reaction (often psychobiological) and are not attri-butes of any apparent particular ecological structure.

NV risk: medically characterized conditions

Many differing disease/disorder states and bodily responses to these increase NV risk so that NV are said to be associated with these conditions as symptom/sign, as 'presenting with,' and the like. We can categorize these grossly in terms of organ systems, typologies of illness, and associated diseases with notable NV risk. Uncertainty is introduced when one asks how it might be that these conditions act separately to produce NV. Yet there is a considerable body of knowledge that elucidates mechanisms and implicates substrate actions known or presumed to be at work in NV of disease processes.

The list below is only a recitation, not an explanation. The list reminds the practitioner that NV can signal illness in almost any organ system, and that NV are a common accompaniment to disease. Indeed, along with malaise, pain, fever, and exaggerated dysfunction, they are one of the common responses expressive of, secondary but not (as best we can tell) intrinsic to, the pathological process itself, unless it is, for example, V that leads to a broken bone, hemorrhage, etc. The list includes major conditions.

- **Acute abdominal site emergencies**: inflammation of viscus as in appendicitis, cholecystitis, intestinal obstruction, acute peritonitis.
- **Disorders of the GI tract**: peptic ulcer, motility disorder and gastric atony, infections including bacterial toxins (food poisoning), parasitic infestations, cancer metastasis.
- **Gastroenterology**: liver: hepatitis, Reye's syndrome, pancreatitis.
- **CNS disorders and injury**: neoplasms, encephalitis, hydrocephalus, pseudoneuroma cerebri.
- **Vestibular disorders**: labyrinthitis, Ménière's disease, motion sickness.
- **Other**: head injury, migraine, acute meningitis, tabetic crisis.
- **Cardiovascular (CVS) disorders**: acute myocardial infarction, (chronic cardiac failure (CCF)).
- **Immune disorders**: AIDS.
- **Metabolic and endocrine disorders**: uremia, diabetic ketoacidosis, hypo- and hyperparathyroidism, hyperthyroid crisis, adrenal insufficiency, arginine vasopressin change as in hyponatremia.
- **Genitourinary disorders**: renal calculi, testicular pathology (pain), cervical pain (e.g., dilatation).
- **Reproductive states**: pregnancy.
- **Psychiatric disorders:** one may or may not wish to include here the common psychophysiological states listed earlier: anxiety, depression, fatigue, stress etc., although to do so is to medicalize most human acute or chronic absence of wellness. Bulimia, anorexia, panic disorder, borderline and antisocial (manipulative), 'psychogenic' V.
- **Other conditions** producing severe pain or arousal of the autonomic nervous system (ANS).
- **In infants and children, supplemental**: Reye's syndrome, congenital diaphragmatic hernia, AIDS, opportunistic

pneumonia, sudden infant death syndrome, congenital duodenal obstruction, pyloric stenosis, cystic fibrosis, Down's syndrome (regurgitation).
- **Epileptic seizure**.

Iatrogenic NV risks

In the course of dealing with a range of disorders, including pain arising from them, physicians and nurses (also sometimes psychologists when granted prescription privileges) give medications. Perhaps any medication, given a theory of infinite capacity among humans to detect, define, and respond adversely to a vast range of perturbations, could precipitate NV, i.e., be an emetic. Some drug classes have an intrinsically high risk. But no chemical molecular commonality has been shown to forecast NV. There are now sets of findings and data that encourage neuropharmacological, and particularly neurotransmitter, work on mechanisms of action. At present few of these have been elucidated to the full even in the best of texts, e.g., Goodman and Gilman's *Pharmacological Basis of Therapeutics* (Gilman et al., 1993)

The list below cannot be complete, given either an almost infinite perturbation possibility theory or the wide range of drugs in use, and the diversity of patient risks and responses. Elucidation of the role of NV in illness is further confused when drug–drug interactions occur.

- Drugs and supplements as NV precipitants, or emetics: aminophylline, anesthetics, antibiotics, bromocriptine, cardiac glycosides, chemotherapy agents, disulfiram, dopamine agonists, histamine, ipecac, mineral supplements, nonsteroidal anti-inflammatories, estrogens, opiates.
- Procedures: chemotherapy, chiropractic, emergency poisoning control, radiotherapy, surgery.

Chemotherapeutic agents and emetogenic risk levels

Table 3.4 illustrates clinical views of NV risk arising from chemotherapeutic agents. There will be some disagreement about risk levels, the test of which will be by observations controlling other risk features.

Overview of adverse effects of NV

Should any risk predisposition, setting, context, disease condition, injury, accompanying stress/pain, reaction, procedure, drug, etc., lead to NV, there may be acute or chronic adverse effects other than

Table 3.4: Risks for different chemotherapeutic agents

High risk	Medium risk	Low risk
Actinomycin D	L-Asparaginase	Androgens
Cisplatin	5-Azacytidine	Busulfan
Cyclophosphamide	Carboplatin	Corticosteroids
Dacarbazine	Daunorubicin	Progestins
Mithramycin	Doxorubicin	
Mitotane	5-Fluorouracil	
Nitrogen mustard	Hexamethylamine	
Procarbazine	Mitomycin C	
Streptozotocin		

For a more detailed list, see Kucharczyk et al. (1991).

the common and serious suffering, emotional–cognitive preoccupation, depression, or physical disability that leads to loss of work and functional capabilities. There are increased costs for nursing care, drugs, and hospital stay as well as loss of work income. We have also emphasized cancer treatment withdrawal as a subjective decision that risks earlier morbidity and mortality. Some other specific adverse effects of NV themselves include:

- acute Mallory–Weiss esophageal tear
- alkalosis
- aspiration pneumonitis (in surgical patients)
- bone fracture
- cachexia (as weight loss, weakness) in cancer patients
- electrolyte imbalance
- exaggerated renal damage risk from chemotherapy
- GI hemorrhage
- interference by AE agents in potency of chemotherapy agents
- loss of tooth enamel
- malnutrition
- metabolic alkalosis
- severe dehydration
- splenic tear
- vitamin deficiencies
- wound dehiscence
- wound disruption/dehiscence
- asphyxiation
- death from aspirated vomitus
- HG: malnutrition, fetal loss.

AE drugs

With so much at stake in the control or reduction of NV there will be strong medical efforts to achieve this control. Primarily employed are AE drugs, most of which can be categorized by their chemical structures/pharmacology and/or known or presumed action on neurotransmitters and selective pathways in the CNS, ANS, or enteric NS. The characterization of an AE compound as such most certainly does not assure that it is effective, nor that it has only the effects desired or ordinarily described. (Indeed, no single AE can be relied on for assured efficacy defined as even short-term control of NV.) A considerable range of individual responses occurs including those that are adverse. 'Assurance' is a statistical concept of a probability of N or V control, but clinically it represents the standard of caregivers and patient as outcome expectation. No doubt these vary considerably. Treatment success will vary with these expectations, with outcome criteria employed as well as risk factors reviewed in this chapter, together with other features as yet unidentified but subsumed as 'individual differences' and setting and population variables. Published efficacy results depend largely on the designs of clinical trials, most of which have been wanting to date.

AE compounds have different probabilities of success depending on the NV initiating condition, drug, procedure, etc. It is exceedingly unlikely that any have only specific effects on one organ, tissue, or receptor, because general CNS or other organ system effects are observed – and experienced by patients. In practice, when NV are severe and in the applications that have been studied most – chemotherapy – initial optimism about single AEs as 'cures' has been replaced in practice by combinations, 'cocktails' of possible AEs, where actual knowledge of 'mechanisms of action' may be absent. Absent too are sufficient studies of drug–drug interactions when cocktails are given.

It is obvious that intrinsic uncertainty faces both patient and clinician; however, currently available compounds will offer at least some relief to most patients even those at high risk, and even for chemotherapy cytogens with high emetogenic potential. 'Relief,' however, must be defined by the kind of NV present, measurements, and the risk factors in that context. We reiterate that N is less likely to be controlled than V. Longer-term N or V is less controllable than immediate fast intervention. Table 3.5 gives AE drug classes with examples.

Table 3.5: AE drugs

Class	Drugs (illustrative only)
Anticholinergics	Atropine Scopolamine (hyoscine) Promethazine
Antihistamines	Promethazine Diphenhydramine Cyclizine Dimenhydrinate Meclizine Tigan (trimethobenzamide)
Phenothiazines	Chlorpromazine Promethazine Perphenazine
Benzodiazepines	Diazepam
THC (tetrahydracannabinol)	Marijuana/cannabis
Butyrophenones	Haloperidol Droperidol
Dopamine antagonists	Metoclopramide Domperidone
Corticosteroids	Dexamethasone Methylprednisone
5HT antagonists	Ondanestron Dolasetron
Tigan (trimethobenzamide)	Granisctron

Overview: typically recommended AEs selected by precipitating risk

Clinical textbook authors differ somewhat in their recommendations about what AEs are best or best suited for use under a particular iatrogenic condition. Clinical trials suggest that clinicians can be quite experimental, sometimes dangerously so. Table 3.6 contains

Table 3.6: AEs recommended for different conditions

Condition	Typically recommended
Motion sickness	Phenothiazines, antihistamines, anticholinergics, piperazines
Vertigo, other labyrinthine GI disorder	Antihistamines, phenothiazines, substituted benzamides
Migraine	Phenothiazines, substituted benzamides
Postoperative	Phenothiazines, anticholinergics, substituted benzamides, benzodiazepines, butyrophenones, substituted butyrophenones, serotonin $5HT_3$ antagonists, benzquinamide, neostigmine
Chemotherapy	Serotonin $5HT_3$ antagonists, corticosteroids, cannabinoids, antihistamines, phenothiazines, butyrophenones, antihistamines, substituted benzamides, benzodiazepines, substituted butyrophenones
Radiotherapy	Antihistamines, corticosteroids, phenothiazines, substituted benzamides, serotonin $5HT_3$ antagonists
Pregnancy NV	Given malpractice suit risk any treatment for PNV as opposed to hyperemesis gravidarum is a legal risk, i.e., a 'litigen'

compounds that are conventionally but rarely used, or sometimes used only in combination. The reader can refer to Part V for practice guidelines, *not* as evidenced-based medicine, recognizing that the clinician has to be the astute and sensitive listener and observer when recommended dosages of compounds do not work and he or she has to suggest alternatives, wisely adding nonpharmacological comforting and diverting nonintrusive interventions. The reader is referred to Hawthorne's (1995) discussion and table, and to Kucharczyk et al. (1991). For evidence from controlled clinical trials on AEs, refer to Chapter 6.

Historically, PNV was usefully treated with doxylamine and dicyclomine as part of Bendectin. Before 1977, Bendectin included vitamin B_6 (pyroxidine). Ginger also seems useful but contains a mutagen component which makes its use inadvisable (Sovak, M., personal communication, 1993).

Obviously individual factors operate here, as elsewhere in the art of patient care. This makes practice and theory uncertain. The multiplicity of 'sometimes' or 'almost' AEs would seem to compel the conclusion that no one linear system operates to 'cause' or to 'cure' N and/or V.

Paradoxical effects

Paradoxical effects are those where an AE is also an emetic. And compounds not ordinarily employed as AEs, but capable of that action as, for example, in sedation, may be found to have similar effects, which in some cases is sufficient reason not to use them. Paradoxical effects do not seem to have occupied research, or even strong clinical attention, although their existence can prompt curiosity. Our list is incomplete but is intended to arouse that curiosity, so leading to research on theories and treatments of NV. Implicated in paradoxical effects are dosage, manner of administration, and NV-suppressing sedation/anesthesia. 'Plasticity' is assumed. Compounds that have been observed to be capable of paradoxical AE and then emetic effects, or experimentally in animals as emetics and then AEs, include: prochlorperazine, ergotamine (used to treat migraine and thus, indirectly, migraine NV), atropine, pyroxidine, benzquinamide, serotonin $5HT_3$ antagonists particularly zacropride, alprazolam, lorazepam, ketorolac, and metoclopramide. The list is no doubt incomplete. Given a postulated possibility of almost infinite precipitants of NV, one presumes that other AE drugs with a CNS enteric action might, in some individuals, induce NV.

Models for NV show that gastric stasis is a necessary prodromal preliminary event in the sequence toward V. This is, however, by no means always the case. Whether looking at acetylcholine as a cholinergic agonist that increases GI motility but yields NV, or at post-abdominal surgical 'dumping' in which faster food transit also produces NV, there are exceptions. These too are paradoxical, unless one abandons the linear model for gastric motility and thence NV. All cholinergic agonists act as parasympathetic agents, e.g., ACTH, muscarine, methylcholine, carbachol probably giving rise to peristaltic enteric activity which can yield NV. Atropine, a belladonna alkaloid, is used to block these effects. It is of interest that belladonna is only of limited effectiveness as an AE; from this it can be concluded that the centrality of enteric action and its effects, in whatever way it is associated with dosage, can give adequate explanation for the AE–emetic or emetic–AE paradox.

AE side effects

Any compound likely to reduce disturbing and explosive phenomena such as NV can be expected to have systemic as well as specific effects, and most AEs do; typically these are on the CNS, ANS, and circulation. Outcome severity ranges from common drowsiness to irreversible Parkinson disease-like symptoms to, happily rare, death. No overview can offer a complete list; indeed new side effects can be reported at any time for compounds in use. Table 3.7 gives common adverse effects.

Table 3.7: Adverse effects of AEs

Drug	Effects
Anticholinergics	Drowsiness, dizziness, blurring of vision, dry mouth
Atropine, scopolamine (hyoscine)	Allergy, lactation suppression, headache, dizziness, difficulty in swallowing, lower threshold for heat prostration, impotence, agitation. For others see PDR
Antihistamines	Sedation, drowsiness
Phenothiazines	Hypotension, dry mouth, extrapyramidal toxicity (chlorpromazine: elevated prolactin level, dystonia, hepatoxic)
Butyrophenones	Sedation, extrapyramidal syndrome, hypotension
Dopamine antagonists	Metoclopramide: hyperprolactinemia, heart failure, atrioventricular block
Domperidone	Cardiac arrest, neuroleptic syndrome
Corticosteroids	Cushingoid features, suppression of immune system with prolonged use, osteoporosis
5HT antagonists	Headache, chest pain, thrombocytopenia, constipation, cardiac arrest
Cannabinol or THC	Euphoria, hallucination, dysphoria

Nonpharmaceutical interventions

Given uncertainty in prescribing AE application and anticipated outcome, the tendency to administer combinations with unknown interactions and multiplied side effect risks, the by definition undesirability of side effects, and the high costs of drugs such as the serotonin $5HT_3$ antagonists, it is not surprising that renewed interest occurs for nonpharmaceutical interventions (see Chapters 17 and 18). It is also sensible to seek positive placebo effects.

NV folk healing practices abound, varying with culture and, for herbals or aromas, local availability. Nursing and family interventions such as comforting all seem consequential although little studied: helpful diet selection, social support, diversion, provision of a pleasant milieu free of environmental risks (offensive odor, anxiety and stress prompters, music). Psychological interventions such as hypnosis, psychotherapy, and deconditioning are employed when NV appears learned or otherwise psychogenic, whereas the new class of behavioral therapies including imaging, relaxation, deep breathing (compare yoga) are reportedly somewhat efficacious. Acupuncture and more recently acupressure and wrist electrical stimulation or magneto therapies have been subject to clinical trials reporting success. We suspect, given a postulated major role for the olfactory organ in some NV, that aromatherapies hold promise as yet untested. Practical comforting, supportive, and self-care remedies are widely employed; Hawthorne (1995) wisely, and almost uniquely in NV medicine, appreciates these approaches.

Part II

Methodological and related conceptual issues

CHAPTER 4

Intended antiemetic drugs: the case for caring, caution, consumerism, and reflection

This chapter looks at what prescription compounds are used to treat nausea and vomiting (NV). The compounds are typically called antiemetics (AEs), which means that they are really only tested, in a very limited way, to see how well they control vomiting. In this chapter we look at the research which purports to describe 'efficacy' or 'control' of these prescription medications so as to get some estimate of how good they are, insofar as this can be inferred from clinical trials. As many clinical trials are not very well done, a 'fact' demonstrated by the data of this chapter, the excellent work of other analysts and reviewers (see, for example, Herxheimer in Chapter 6 and his many consumer-friendly publications), and the existing scientific standards as to how a clinical trial should be done, the chapter's tone is not very optimistic. The 'fact is,' so we believe ('facts' in this field are but opinions of various sorts), that the usefulness of most AEs is difficult to predict in actual care.

As this is a methodological chapter (and in that way regrettably tedious for some readers), we talk about the basics, the logic and care necessary so that what one gets out of a trial of a medication at least has some predictive utility for its use when prescribed in ordinary practice. Ordinary 'practice,' note well, is for iatrogenic NV, i.e., NV arising as a side effect from procedures that doctors do in clinics and hospitals, NV as a side effect of other medications, or, paradoxically, NV that can arise from drugs supposedly given to control NV.

The limits of this current work are implied by what we have just said; trials are almost entirely on pharmaceutical products, i.e., manufactured compounds that are intended for sale, and prescribed for profit. The trials are those on patients already in medical care whose NV arise primarily during treatments such as cancer chemotherapy or radiotherapy, surgery, or other drugs. They are in fact on patients observed for their emesis, V while they are in the hospital or clinic or at best shortly after they leave. The major human problem of such research is that it tends to count emetic episodes, excluding more important N, rather than asking patients how they feel or how NV impinge on their lives, i.e., about their 'quality of life' (QoL) – that ever so important 'Ziggy' factor.

No-one knows about the important set of facts for treating NV across its 'real' range of variously initiated and variously patterned forms, i.e., what do people do by way of taking something, or doing something to feel better, and how does this self-treatment work compared with what doctors give NV patients in hospital. We venture the guess, and it is just that, although we do have some data from our small 'real life' study of women, that NV happening outside are far more extensive than those occurring under immediate care. Thus, the whole focus on prescription compounds, although very important, represents a narrowly 'medical' focus. As the medical model has, until now, tended to be a rather mechanical one in its NV thinking, pharmaceutical research, and simplified clinical trials, there are a lot of possible variables affecting NV onset or NV treatment success that are ignored. This in itself is a fundamental problem in clinical trials.

We have summarized the chapter's themes, but if you want to review the various prescription compounds used for different types of NV, classified by either their chemical basis or the typical initiating condition, or to learn about the range of AE 'control' across a broad number of trials, read on. Likewise, if you are interested to see the degree of consistency when comparing reviews of clinical trials, or to consider how the clinical trial outcome data themselves produce a view of NV as nonlinear and complex, and by implication that 'linear' drugs are insufficient, then again read on.

Best of all, if you as a consumer, whether a physician, nurse, physician's assistant, psychologist, other caregiver, or patient or ordinary NV sufferer, want new standards and more background to allow competence in your own critical evaluation of the information that journals or manufacturers provide about AEs efficacy, read on. The US Food and Drug Administration (FDA) does what it can, and this is a great deal because its standards are high, to assure quality and efficacy, but it cannot guarantee the care and intelligence of those reporting clinical trials, or of doctors prescribing AEs, nor the objective honesty of manufacturers. The wise consumer is an educated critic before he or she becomes an AE user.

Evidence-based medicine

Archie Cochrane, one of the great practical minds in modern medicine, said in 1994: 'It is surely a great criticism of our profession that we have not organized a critical summary . . . adapted periodically, of all relevant randomized controlled trials.'

Our work in this chapter is not that grand an enterprise, but it intends to advise consumers, and to allow simple conclusions about typical clinical trial outcomes and their reporting. Cochrane's own admirable goal is being pursued through the worldwide Cochrane Collaboration (see Chapter 6) in which the literature of randomized clinical trials – there are an estimated one million for all treatments – is being meta-analyzed and summarized as rational guidance to clinicians. A superb example of this approach is found for women's health in Chalmers et al. (1989). Such endeavors are part of a movement called 'evidence-based medicine.' It is an optimistic and potentially massive effort which assumes that good trial data exist, that meta-analyses of multiple trials work, and that guidelines, once established, will be followed. It is a statistical–epidemiological approach to practice, seeking, in David Sackett's words: 'The conscientious, explicit and judicious use of current best evidence'.

This chapter, however, deals with the trial literature as it exists. Most of this – the sort read in ordinary scientific journals – is more haphazard. It is on this kind of trial that ordinary practitioners rely. This chapter shows how uncertain the results can be. What emerges is the need for consumer caution with respect to findings and certainly when reading the advertisements of pharmaceutical firms.

In Chapter 1 we said that physicians do not know enough about NV, and also do not read or care enough about its treatments. One excuse for this is that some caregivers rely on clinical 'instincts' and the 'art' of medicine versus sound methodological empiricism. There is resistance to information, reading it or using it, and in medicine it requires work and change. This is certainly recognized by the Evidence-Based Medicine Working Group (Naylor, 1996a, b). Naylor (1996a), for example, wisely states: 'Publishing recommendations and guidelines on medical practice . . . is no guarantee that anyone will follow them,' because the good trial design requirements are not so diverse as to disallow the careful selection of studies for meta-analysis that should be the standard.

Note that, in this chapter, we do not offer the 'hands-on' precept-or guidance of the clinical section (Part V) – with respect to what expert clinicians, who typically are authoritative textbook writers, recommend. However much support is given, one must recognize the need for evidence-based medicine to use statistical medicine of the sort that is presented by Sackett et al. (1991). For the field of NV treatments, the evidence, although supportive of particular compounds, is woefully incomplete. The physician treating NV will, however, feel the need to do something. It may be trial and error, but it will frequently end up being a 'cocktail' of several AEs, the 'mechanism' and the interaction of which are known. If the patient feels better and no harm is done (and, be warned, some AEs *do* harm) this constitutes the 'art' of NV treatment as it now stands.

How trials begin

Clinical trials are allowed by regulatory agencies such as the FDA only after animal studies have shown the safety of a compound (stage 1 trials). Tests then proceed to detailed observations on very small samples of volunteer humans, patients who could potentially benefit, where attention is paid to a range of tests of safety, side effects, and (crude) efficacy (stage 2 trials). A compound meeting these requirements receives an investigational drug certification (IND) allowing clinical trials using strict protocols, the results of which will be carefully reviewed by the FDA. These stage 3 trials require larger patient samples (100 or more). Typically, these trials will occur in several respected settings/institutions with experienced clinical investigators, and will be paid for by the manufacturer. Incentives for the investigator include a clinical interest in finding better agents, the benefits of publication, and being seen to be active in furthering treatment developments. Until these stage 3 trials are complete, and pending further FDA approval, the manufacturer cannot decide whether the drug is marketable, nor will any but an experimental drug identification be given to it. If the drug is marketed, further post-marketing trials will be paid for, although sometimes only through the provision of free samples to clinicians with a protocol form to follow. At this stage, sample sizes, patient characteristics, and what the compound is compared against will all vary as reported in journals by clinical investigators whose range of methodological skills varies considerably. This hodgepodge is what the practitioner usually sees in print.

Efficacy is a comparative notion, entirely dependent upon the outcome measures used, the period of time and how many of the drugs are used, the inferential statistics employed, and what comparison measure is used for its effect on outcomes. Comparisons are typically stated in terms of a difference in outcome between the tested compound (if new) and a known compound against which the new medicine is compared. Placebos are ideal in designs, but ethical considerations deny their use when patients are likely to suffer and when medications of known usefulness already exist. But be warned, 'usefulness' may be only an assumption based on poor trial data. In rare trials, an active placebo is employed (for example, nicotinic acid which is harmless, but it brings a flush to one's face so that the subject is likely to be aware of a physiological effect). Perhaps the most dramatic NV example of an active 'placebo' was employed by psychosomatic investigator Stewart Wolf (1985) who, upon assuring a PNV woman that the medicine he was giving her would cure her, administered the ordinarily powerful emetic, ipecac. The result was NV control! Barnes (1984) observed that placebo effects could suppress motion sickness. No surprise then that 'inert' placebo effects can be far reaching and powerful, capable of inducing a variety of bodily changes (for reviews and bibliographies, see Blum and Heinrichs, 1988; Chaput de Saintonge and Herxheimer, 1994; Roberts, 1995). Although stage 4 investigators may elect to compare the paid-for compound with competing drugs, it is not in the interest of manufacturers to encourage this, because early on they have no assurance that their compound may not do worse; given the wide range of trial outcomes, there is always the risk that other therapies will outperform. This is not a regulatory concern – efficacy is. Absolute superiority is unlikely to be proven because of free market profit strategies by manufacturers, and fundamentally because the results of clinical trials depend upon conditions so variable in expression and measurement as to disallow a general statement of 'overall best.'

It is also the case that lower dosages (less costly) are not preferred in most studies, nor are those involving drug combinations, although for NV the 'cocktail' is the most likely 'efficacious' approach of practicing oncologists. Antiemetic effects are sufficiently unpredictable to require clinical trial and error, often leading to cocktails. This is the reality that requires the 'art' of medicine.

An exemplary informative study is that of Roila and his colleagues in the Italian Group for Antiemetic Research (1995) which finds in favor of drug combinations. They note that an ideal consumer-conscious (and health maintenance organization) design for beginning studies will use one less expensive compound, e.g., dexamethasone, rather than granisetron (the latter, in any event does not work singly as determined by their and others' trials), to learn whether that cost-saving approach will work for individual patients. This clinical 'art' approach of trying the cheap and simple first, being guided by feedback from the patient, illustrates the difference between efficacy as a more rarefied concept, and effectiveness as the way things work in practice. Warren and Mosteller (1993) also remind us of the profit interests guiding and sometimes biasing drug trials. They wisely, as does Martin (1992), observe that drug trials, for all their exasperating methodological limitations, are done in ideal conditions, compared with the real world of practice. In the latter world, patients may not be cooperative in treatment, comorbidity may diminish efficacy, caregiving personnel make mistakes (including failures to generate compliance through poor instructions, insensitivity, etc.), and, in fact, outcomes good or bad may be entirely missed or misreported. As an important example, recovery can be quite spontaneous but wrongly attributed to a medication.

We should also remember that investigators and journals tend not to publish nil results, and pharmacological manufacturers are not required to release these or other adverse findings. Cheating does occur in reporting results. It is up to the manufacturer to decide, whatever data from a range of trials may be submitted to the FDA, which, if any, comparison study is reported in package inserts, or in that basic commercial reference text, *The Physicians' Desk Reference* (PDR) (1997) (see also Herxheimer, 1995).

What a manufacturer requires for marketing, beyond regulatory approval, is profit. And what manufacturers need from clinical trials is an empirical basis, a marketing platform for later promotion. In the same way, stage 4 clinical trials that involve as many physicians publishing in as many journals as possible are desirable to provide advertising exposure and to habituate clinicians to use of the new drug. Exposure becomes less desirable if some time-lagged adverse effect is reported (see the exchange in *The Lancet* between physicians reporting cardiac failure and death from the AE ondansetron and the response from professionals employed by the manufacturer: Letters, 1992). Such examples suggest what can be left out by way of initial trial findings which are set forth as risk data in package inserts and PDRs.

What the consumers, and physician, pharmacist, patient, or private or governmental insurer, require include at least efficacy, safety, quality defined as reliability, shelf-life, ease of administration, ease of storage and transportation, patient acceptability in terms of taste, vehicle, etc., assured availability from manufacturers, etc., appropriateness for local conditions, etc., acceptable costs, costs relative to alternative treatments, risk–benefit ratios, preferred ratios of nonlethality measured by no lethal dosage (L/D), the fewest side effects, and the like. What the consumer also requires is maximal and accurate information to allow informed decisions, including information for placing drug therapies in the overall context of disease management and the patient's long-term interests. This is a concern that is by no means always shared by manufacturers. Readers interested in these issues may wish to review the periodical *Essential Drugs Monitor* published by the World Health Organization and perhaps also refer to Blum et al. (1981).

Equally important to any drug measure are patients' reports of N, how they feel and how they may be disabled when on and off test medication. But quality of life, 'well days,' is rarely an outcome measure. No wonder patients may not be pleased with their prescription care, or that Haynes (in Warren and Mosteller, 1993) argues for more psychosocial scientific involvement in health care and education. Traditional biomedical trials rely on short-term measures of V. These are easily counted by a nurse and are the most frequently employed measure of AE outcome efficacy. This emphasis on short-term emesis, rather than longer-term N, illustrates how over-simplified clinical trial methodology and clinician inattention may be.

Do clinical trials dominate the NV journal literature to the exclusion of science, methodology, theory, and epidemiology?

To test our impression that clinical trials dominated the entire NV literature, we selected a Medline continuous printout packet of abstracts obtained during our (annual) NV literature search through Medline, Psycho Info, and Cancerline Search; in this instance we searched from one portion of the years 1993 and 1994. Of 372 abstracts in the continuous segment, clinical trials constituted only 35%. These were surely not random, but we do not know what variables influence selection at these three major electronic data sites. In any event, in this literature sampling of unknown but certain bias, clinical trials constitute about one-third of the journal literature on NV. We suggest that fewer and better-designed trials would be welcome, as would more work derived from the interdisciplinary, broader perspective that we advocate throughout this book.

It was our impression that AEs tested for use in cancer treatments dominated the trial literature. Of 130 clinical trials in this packet,

63% were among cancer patients, 12% were among postoperative patients, and 0.08% were among patients with hyperemesis gravidarum (HG) and other pregnancy NV (PNV). The remainder were distributed among other forms of NV, i.e., motion sickness, toxin ingestion, gatsrointestinal (GI) disorder, etc.

Sampling does make a difference, because we selected from another group of 1994 trials under analysis ($n = 80$), where 53% were from cancer treatment patients, 30% postoperative, and the remainder GI disorders, poison, experiments with ipecac emesis induction, comparisons of patient-controlled versus administered (nonparticipatory doctor's decision) AE outcomes, seasickness, and the like. One sees so simply here, as in the clinical trial reports below, that how one comes by a sample does make a difference to outcome figures. Yet, one may conclude that the largest number of AE tests are with cancer AEs followed by postoperative AE studies.

'Ordinary' condition

The above studies are on acute conditions. There is little evidence of researcher interest in 'ordinary' or chronic N – more common than V – conditions. In the sample there were a few motion sickness studies, two on migraine (finding no difference among AEs in their effects), and none on such things as stomach 'flu. PNV is a special case because, except for life-threatening hyperemesis medications, prescribed compounds are forbidden territory for pharmaceutical testing or sales in the USA. For PNV there is a testing taboo. One company research director said to us, as we sought to test the folk remedy ginger as an AE for PNV, that any prescribed AEs for PNV are 'litigens.' In our clinical trial review, the few AE studies on PNV reported were European. Ginger *was* found to be useful, but one of its components is a mutagen. A very recent study has found vitamin B_6 to be useful as well. Fortunately, PNV women can find relief via home remedies; indeed, referring to our own crude epidemiological findings, and consistent with a few other studies, women with PNV report greater relief from folk remedies than from prescribed substances. There is very little reported work on over-the-counter (OTC) remedies.

Trials analyzed and compared

For Table 4.1 we analyzed 364 studies. We excluded most of a smaller set of cocktail-only studies which compared outcomes for different combinations of compounds. We did include a cocktail when a so-called primary AE was shown to do best with one or

Table 4.1: Results of worst, best, and average trials for a range of AEs

Drug	Best TC	Average percentage	Worst TC	Worst side effect
Alizapride	CT V 33%	26%	V 5%	Extrapyramidal syndrome
	PONV 66%	N 5% (with)		Not reported
Batampride	CT V 60%	46%	V 20%	Hypotension
Granisetron	CT V 98%	± 67%	14%	Elevated liver function
	1 day			
	V ± 47%			
	5 days			
	CT N 75%	37%		
Ondansetron	CT V 97%	45–70%	4%	Hypertension*
	'with'			
	N 92%	45–70%		
	N 'with'		30%	
	CT ultra-high-dose chemotherapy	0%		
	CT V 'major control'	100%		
	CT N 'major control'	100%		
	PO V 63%	52%	25%	
	PO N 45%	38%	25%	
Tropisetron	CT C 88%	1 day	20%	Extrapyramidal syndrome
	CT N 77%		37%	

(contd.)

Table 4.1: (contd.)

Drug	Best TC	Average percentage	Worst TC	Worst side effect
Zacopride	CT V 43% High dose with MC (one study only)	Low dose with MC	13%	None reported**
Scopolamine	PO V 89%		V 65%	Urinary retention
Marijuana (THC)	CT 64% decrease NV	50% decrease NV (one study only)		Dysphoria
Prochlorperazine	CT V 86% CT N 71% with	40%	20%	Not reported
Dexamethasone	CT V 76% CT N 76%	48% 42%	20% 27% with	Well-being only
Methylprednisone	PO V 87% PO N 82% CT V 79% CT N 82%	59%	66% 36%	Headache
Diazepam	Results not quantified			
Lorazepam	CT V 85% with	60%	24% with	Amnesia

(contd.)

Table 4.1: (contd.)

Drug	Best TC	Average percentage	Worst TC	Worst side effect
Droperidol	PO V 95%	73%	36%	Neurological damage possible
Metoclopramide	CT V 90% CT NV with 53%	65% 33%	13% 13%	Extrapyramidal syndrome
Ketorolac	PO NV 81%	55%	29%	Not reported**
Domperidone	CT 82%	V 55%	NV 30%	Diarrhea
Cinnazirine	Motions 69% Criteria were 'improvement'; placebo yielded 31%	49%	35%	
Dolasetron	CT 52%	28%	24%	Not reported**

*Compare *The Lancet* nontrial report of deaths.
**The PDR shows ketorolac as producing renal failure, GI hemorrhage, etc., and also N; thus it is one of the paradoxical compounds used to treat NV that induces them as well. Note: a journal report without any observation of adverse effects cannot be taken as evidence of safety, nor indeed can we be sure the PDR is up to date on dangers.
CT, cancer therapy; MC, metoclopramide; PO, postoperative.

several supplemental compounds administered simultaneously. By no means does this provide evidence for the efficacy of the primary compound that is purportedly of interest to the investigator, because their design disallows such conclusions. Given the absence of complex drug interaction studies in NV pharmacology, and design inadequacies, we do not know what observed outcomes should be attributed to. We note at this point that, with an already bulging bibliography, we have not cited the individual studies among the 364.

Drugs tested in this review sample

What appear in Table 4.1 are phase 3 or 4 trials or simply the curiosity of later clinicians. They attend to outcomes for the following which were set forth as primary investigational targets:

- alizapride (a dopamine receptor antagonist)
- alprazolam (a diazepam, benzodiazepine derivative)
- batampride (a serotonin receptor antagonist)
- cinnarizine (an antihistamine)
- dexamethasone (a corticosteroid)
- dolasetron (a serotonin antagonist)
- domperidone (substituted butyrophenone as dopamine antagonist)
- droperidol (possible dopamine antagonist)
- granisetron (serotonin receptor antagonist)
- ketorolac (nonsteroidal anti-inflammatory)
- lorazepam (benzodiazepine, tranquilizer and sedative)
- marijuana (dronabinol, tetrahydrocannabinol, or THC)
- methylprednisone/methylprednisolone (corticosteroids)
- metoclopramide (dopamine antagonist, a benzamide)
- ondansetron (a serotonin receptor antagonist)
- prochlorperazine (tranquilizing anticholinergic, calmodulin inhibitor)
- scopolamine (a belladonna alkaloid)
- tropisetron (a serotonin receptor antagonist)
- zacopride (a serotonin receptor antagonist).

Listed below are drugs used in the studies but reported as either combined in cocktails or, where compared singly, the design disallowed a quantified conclusion. We enter a few of these below to illustrate understudied compounds, but perhaps, being as inconsistent as the investigators, eschew most work disallowing quantified entries in Table 4.1. Sometimes a drug, which was stated to be of primary interest (see above), was nevertheless tested only in combination with the drugs in this secondary list, or with another drug from the primary list.

Additional presumed AE compounds tested in the sample of reports analyzed (1993–94):

- amantadine
- atropine
- betamethasone–dioxyrazine
- biperiden
- cimatidine
- clemestine
- dehydrobenzperidol
- diazepam (benzodiazepine tranquilizer)
- dihydroergotamine (α-adrenergic blocker, possible serotonin antagonism)
- dimenhydrinate
- diphenhydramine
- ephedrine
- ginger (unknown, one claim of serotonin receptor effects)
- haloperidol
- lidocaine (lignocaine)
- lorazepam
- meperidine
- methotrimeprazine
- metopimazine
- neostigmine (anticholinergic)
- promethazine
- retrobulbar bupivacaine
- scopolamine (hyoscine)
- sumatriptan (serotonin $5HT_3$ antagonist)
- tetracosactrin
- thienylpromazine
- timperone
- zatosetron.

This list does not exhaust the current pharmacopoeia with reference to prescribed, or investigational, compounds used or tested as AEs (e.g., cyclizine, a common piperazine antihistamine, was not in the test group reviewed). Again we note our exclusion of AEs, although several studies were of propofol used as if it were an AE. The general classes of AEs are represented:

- phenothiazines (dopamine blockers)
- butyrophenones (dopamine blockers)
- metoclopramide (a substituted benzamide, dopamine antagonist, GI tract motility stimulant)
- cannabinoids (unknown)
- glucocorticosteroids (uncertain), euphoric, proposed as AEs to interfere with prostaglandin synthesis
- antihistamines and antimuscarinic/anticholinergics
- serotonin $5HT_3$ antagonists
- benzodiazepines
- substituted butyrophenones/benzimidazole derivatives as peripheral dopamine blockers, e.g., domperidone
- scopolamine and other belladonna alkaloids
- opiates, antidepressants (e.g., nortriptyline)
- ergotamines (5HT serotonin antagonists in part)
- nonsteroidal anti-inflammatories
- the unusual local anesthetics
- anesthetics themselves.

On uncertainties as to where and how AEs act

Hawthorne (1995) comments on the dopamine (itself a catecholamine, precursor to norepinephrine) activity of many of the AE compound classes. He attributes AE efficacy to the antagonism of dopamine-involved gastric motility (overcoming stasis associated with V), and to the presence of dopamine receptors in medullary/ventricular regions. The chemoreceptor trigger zone (CTZ) and the nucleus tractus solitarius (NTS) are found often, but not always, to be involved in V. Yet one must note that dopamine receptors are widespread throughout the brain, and they are strongly implicated in at least the expression of psychiatric disorders which is why dopamine antagonists such as haloperidol (itself a butyrophenone) are widely prescribed for serious disorders.

Every bit as important as an observed effect of most classes of AEs is tranquilization or sedation. For example, haloperidol is a (butyrophenone) tranquilizer (its actions in this regard are not clear, but note that it is a paradoxical AE capable of inducing NV). We make no claim about the similarity of feelings from one patient to another, but CNS-tranquilizing and sedating effects can be observed with phenothiazines, antihistamines, anticholinergics, benzodiazepines, substituted benzamides (metoclopramide induces drowsiness in 70% of chemotherapy patients advises the PDR, but it can also cause restlessness, severe depression, and lassitude), and cannabinoids (euphoriant for some people, dysphoriant for others). Steroids may easily produce euphoria, whereas serotonin level changes, whether up or down, will show associated sedation; Barnes (1988) found that fenfluramine (an anti-appetite drug), although having sympathetic co-mimetic (resembling amphetamine) action, nevertheless antagonizes cisplatin emesis (in ferrets), with serotonin levels being lowered (in the area postrema and elsewhere in the CNS); general CNS depression occurs as well as a feeling of well-being which is why it is a drug of abuse. Once again it is emphasized that AEs have actions on mood and alertness in the CNS as well as specific local tissue and organ actions, e.g., enterochromaffin GI actions.

Supported by the FDA and formulary approvals, a specificity of prescription recommendations for AEs by precipitating condition has evolved, together with a multiple drug administration/prescription which is far from specific; use of the latter can be clinical in sequences (typically in surgeries with pre- and postoperative treatments), or when the physician or nurse observes that an initial compound is not working or the patient demands greater relief; typically it can be used in cancer treatments, as combined drugs. In any treatment there is a concern about side effects, because no compound that is powerful enough to have a CNS or presumed enteric effect can be considered sufficiently safe to have only the desired effects.

Another illustration of indirect effects, including major general effects of putative AEs with no impact on NV, is given with sumatriptan. Sumatriptan treatment of the NV of migraine is generally indirect, aimed at the migraine itself, which as a perturbation is considered to generate NV as a nonspecific disturbance. Lidocaine, for example, probably acts, when in a nasal spray, on the trigeminal ganglia, which have pathways to the medial raphe nucleus, in turn implicated in NV. This may act to reduce NV associated with migraine. Likewise, as a $5HT_3$ agonist (not antagonist), sumatriptan acts selectively on vascular receptors to produce vasoconstriction and significant relief. It does not appear to have an affinity for other serotonin receptors, and would not be considered paradoxical vis-à-vis $5HT_3$ antagonists used specifically as AEs. Likewise, the postulated parasympathetic migraine involvement via the palatine ganglia, in contrast to enteric and other ANS sympathetic activation of at least V, is not paradoxical in terms of temporal sequencing. These contrasting involvements, 'ordinary' NV versus migraine, do, however, suggest that an overwhelming perturbation such as migraine may activate messenger systems, ordinarily not involved in NV, and yet not negate an NV outcome. Later we shall see evidence for a profound association between migraine and one kind of NV, hyperemesis gravidarum (HG).

Whatever the uncertainties, there are NV conditions for which particular compounds are typically prescribed. Ordinary uses are as follows:

- **Motion sickness**: anticholinergics, antihistamines.
- **Pre- and postoperative**: butyrophenones, substituted butyrophenones, anticholinergics, antihistamines, phenothiazines, substituted benzamides, (new) serotonin antagonists, piperazines.
- **Migraine**: ergotamines, phenothiazines (one would expect work with serotonin antagonists), substituted benzamides, lidocaine nose drops, sumatriptan.
- **Anticancer treatment reactions**: serotonin antagonists, steroids, benzodiazepines, cannabinoids, substituted benzamides, antihistamines and anticholinergics in combinations, piperazines.
- **GI disorders**: substituted benzamides (e.g. omeprazole), phenothiazines, benzodiazepines. For acid reflux, histamine H_2-receptor blockers (cimetidine, ranitidine, famotidine, dramamine) or antacids and stomachics (earlier from the Latin 'carminatives') including sodium citrate, calcium carbonate, magnesium trisilicate, sodium bicarbonate, bismuth (whether albuminate, bitannate, carbonate, oxybromide, salicylate, subsalicylate), dextrose, levulose and phosphoric acid (as in RX Emetrol).
- **Vertigo**: phenothiazines, antihistamines, anticholinergics.

Placebo studies

Placebo controls are surprisingly absent in many studies (where ethical considerations, including patient consent, allow this) This is important because placebo effects are powerful, so placebo effects and trial designs must be considered, especially in self-limiting conditions such as NV, against spontaneous recovery. Consider Roberts (1995) citing Moerman in controlled drug trials for ulcers, in which there is no difference between placebo and active compound in 60% of these trials and when, generalizing across studies, effectiveness can range from 10% to 90%, with an average of 35% (Beecher, 1955). In sham surgery for angina pectoris, Roberts (citing

Turner et al., 1994) showed improvement that ranged from 52% to 100%. Roberts' general estimate of the impact of placebo is for an improvement of about 33%, against which all trial results should be considered. For those placebos in which there is a clear expectation of success on the part of the healer, then the impact of the placebo may affect two-thirds of the patients, particularly where psychosocial influences are at play. The finding of Calamandrei (1994) was striking: they found that, when comparing ondansetron and metoclopramide with placebo, V was greater in the metoclopramide than in the placebo group (ondansetron, on the other hand, outperformed placebo). One notes, of course, that the absence of NV is not proof of a placebo effect, because not everyone experiencing the same surgical procedure will suffer NV and, even in randomized small groups, other individual differences will affect outcomes. In any event, it is not surprising if, in AE trials, placebo can be found to be outperforming manufactured compounds. This is especially true if the preferred blind design does not allow the administering doctor or nurse, patient, and outcome rater (usually a nurse, but in N studies the suffering patient) to know, so they cannot communicate expectations or the unconscious reporting of the expected better results from the prescribed AE compound.

One expresses a fundamental attitudinal concern here. Healers heal and expect it to work; treatments are expected to work, even though quite frequently they do not, or success is misattributed to recovery processes innate to the ill person, or to placebo effects that impact illness. This point is fundamental to 'evidence-based medicine' and the Cochrane Centre randomized trial that summarizes effort. A difference should be recognized between the person, patient 'doin' stuff' à la 'Ziggy' – which is being alive, happy, and functioning – and healers carrying out treatments that may be grounded in cultural, psychosocial processes not recognized by the partics to it. One must raise the question: Should we, as consumers, be ever more skeptical when a great success is claimed initially? Probably yes. Remember the aphorism: 'Use a new treatment when it first comes out, before it loses its efficacy!' But to balance this, we must keep in mind how old theories are adhered to long after there is evidence for their inadequacy. Open-mindedness, plus well-educated criticism would appear to be the mix for the reader of NV clinical trials.

In real experimental life, investigators may overanalyze subgroup differences, publishing because of the hopes that they would come up with a positive finding at some time. This is not too hard to accomplish if sufficient variables and groups are studies because five of 100 such statistical tests will, on a theoretical (expanded binomial) average, be 'significant' by chance. It could be that no patient who fails to complete a treatment is included in the outcome analysis – the investigator or pharmaceutical company may argue it is not 'fair' to count as failures people who did not complete, or perhaps even begin, treatment. Statisticians argue that one of the hidden variables here is the attractiveness/repulsiveness of a treatment. For AEs, one must be aware that failure to complete treatment can never be a reason for exclusion from an outcome analysis. Failure to monitor patient cooperation when medications are self-administered is another supervisory failing, because it is not only well known that people are not good at compliance – the general figure is 50% failure (see Blum and Heinrichs, 1988, for a review) – but noncompliance could arise from patient observations of side effects that could lead to nonuse, and communication with the physician is inadequate. There is the intriguing finding that patients in the Continuous Coronary Drug Project, who faithfully took their placebos, also lived longer than patients who were noncompliant with their placebo (work by Canner, and continuing studies by this group).

At the very least, groups that are noncompliant differ from others; it is an illustration of a larger psychological principle that people who deviate from a norm in one important matter are likely to deviate from the norm in a number of ways. This suggests that there is some general factor in individual differences that affects not simply compliance, but, as in the work by Canner, also morbidity and, by implication, individual risks. The *Science* (Cohen, 1995) review reports that investigators either systematically err in favor of a hypothesis or downright cheat in their data analysis and reporting. 'Surrogate markers' of outcome are a particular problem. A surrogate marker in a cardiac medication study may be irregular heart beat rather than morbidity outcome, but in AE research, as a measure of emesis is taken at the same time to be a measure of N, V as a surrogate marker is by far the most common outcome measure; it is one that leaves us almost entirely in the dark about AE effects on the more widespread and painful N.

An all too common failing is that the population entering a study is not the same one observed at the end, i.e., attenuation occurs. This is a particular problem when severe emetogenic risk is high, as with cytotoxins in cancer treatments, where some quit and the efficacy measure is made only on those who remain, thus maximizing reports of efficacy. The same artifact occurs, whether judged as sample continuity, panel, or outcome duration, when populations are followed for arbitrarily brief periods – for example, for acute cancer chemotherapy only – rather than until all patients report no further NV. This will inevitably require home observation, and may be extended for some. Strenuous efforts must be made to retain sample members: to insure that all observers specified in the design (typically the family of the patient) continue to cooperate in reporting, and that inducements are certain. One is reminded that the curves for NV over time may not be smooth and downhill, because patterns of later emergent V can occur and, indeed, may be extended to anticipatory NV (ANV), over repeat cancer chemotherapy or radiation cycles. In such a case, one may study NV over a period of several years (we are not aware of such a study), where the sampling method becomes that of a 'panel' of committed patients.

Outcome measures are of critical importance, and as we have seen are usually those V ones that are most easily measured rather than N of at least equal duration; for clinical populations patient pain and disability are of greater importance. Who the outcome observer is, whether he or she is 'blind,' how he or she is trained, where observations are made, how long such observations continue, what instruments for N are selected (and N may not be a unitary variable), and what their reliability is are all matters of consequence. Record keeping by observers must be supervised. Multiple measures may be preferred, as these are quantifiable. Observers do differ consistently, for example, child patients will report their V as more severe and frequent than will the observing parent. Franklin (1994) found that there are differences, and therefore rating unreliability, among nurses, doctors, and patients in GI distress ratings ('toxicity' is the Dutch term) and that these differences, in turn, vary in degree of reliability for each of the reporting measures used. Of course, differences are a function of where people are and when, what their criteria are, how good communication is, and who keeps what records according to which standard and how well supervised. Cohen et al. (1994) examined hospital records for N and compared them with patient interview and reports; they showed very poor correspondence, ranging in kappa values from only 0.19 to 0.60. For example, in one hospital, 38% of patients interviewed said that they had N, but charts recorded only 8%, a ratio of almost 5:1.

Bonneterre et al. (1991), who earlier referred to using a diary method that included QoL, appetite, and N intensity, found no differences in V incidents, but patients and physicians disagreed as to which was the more important; patients stated that N was more important, and patient concern lasted much longer. When rating for preference, even with no overt V incident differences, patients significantly preferred one AE over another. Similarly, Findlay (1993), in a well-designed study sensitive to reliability among outcome measures, found that observer-rated V, which would report differences in AE efficacy, differed from patient self-ratings for both V and N. It appears that patients found no appetite differences or V ones but, nevertheless, they did express preferences which in fact mirrored the V ratings by staff. Such findings need exploration but suggest that V *per se* may not be the measure, aside from N, of subjective experience that is most important to patients. Perhaps one should bear in mind, as one possibility, our epidemiological study findings in Chapter 3 of NV occurring without feelings of unpleasantness.

Some basics of clinical trial research

These include the random assignment of patients to however many treatment groups are set up, and when possible comparison with controls on other AEs, and also with those who receive placebo. There is an ethical problem here, however, because, if patients are known to be at risk of, or undergoing, suffering, and if there is an intervention of known efficacy with low risks, or one known and acceptable to the patient, and if a patient has not given full consent to be in a trial in which unknown patients will receive placebo, then one may not deny palliation. For an example of a debate about this point when testing AEs, see Citron (1993) who comments on Beck et al. (1993). It is for this reason that new medications being tested are normally compared with existing compounds, although existing compounds, which are presumed to be efficacious on the grounds of some earlier, badly designed, clinical trials, may in fact be no better than a placebo. One can seek to persuade patients, under fully informed consent and perhaps with payment, to participate in a study in which some, although no-one knows who, do receive placebo. And if a placebo subject suffers or calls for a remedy, a rescue medication – again of presumed potential efficacy – is employed. There is a signal case of an ethical failure in reverse, when patients were given drugs (encainide, flecainide) for irregular heart rhythms that were shown to be capable of suppressing them. When there was a challenge about whether the drugs made a difference to actual mortality, many doctors refused, on ethical grounds, because the folk beliefs of the medical community linked such control to an assumption of reduced mortality. The study was, however, started and stopped mid-course, not because of increased deaths among those not receiving the drug, but because there was a three times greater death rate among those receiving it! Nothing so dramatic is likely to occur for AEs, but one can show – those paradoxical effects we discussed earlier – that drugs assumed to be AEs in fact produce NV, as well as paralyzing (dystonias) and sometimes fatal side effects. At this point we observe the obvious caution – calling a drug an 'antiemetic' does not necessarily have anything to do with its effects. We do not wish to be hypnotized or seduced, by claims, nomenclature, or even hospital formularies. Folk medications are also anti-N and anti-V, and their placebo effects, as for those from AEs manufactured by 'real' drug companies, are also 'real.'

In the 'one can do nothing about it' realm, the realm of the ethicolegal, one assures bias by requirements of human subject-informed consent. Those who cooperate and volunteer in any study are likely to be different from those who do not – just as those in blind studies who take their placebo as scheduled have better outcomes than refusniks and regimen delinquents. But another very human problem arises if the doctor biases the informed consent from embarrassment over any admission that he or she (or the whole field of medicine, for that matter) cannot rationalize the use of random control trials as a result of the desire that the patient think highly of treatments. This is probably a feature of placebo confidence in any event (see Silverman, 1995).

Another 'must' feature is that the experiment be blind, i.e., to control expectations and unconscious errors in favor of a hypothesis that can be readily communicated and can have powerful effects requires that the patient, the person giving the possible remedy, and any person judging outcomes must not be aware of which patient receives which possible remedy. In a thoroughly careful study, the person who hands out the drugs, or otherwise allocates interventions, will also not know which is which. This requires delivery in similar guise. 'Controls' is a word wisely used; it usually implies a comparison group(s) which is necessary for any statistical trial. As with most things, exceptions occur, as, for example, in 'natural laboratory' studies where real life populations are observed. Examples include: those exposed to Chernobyl radiation, clouds of drifting Paraquat pesticide, or salmonella epidemics; where an available public health intervention of only one on-site AE may have results analyzed retrospectively for predictors to be found in population characteristics; or where on-site personnel may be ethically involved because of uncertainty about dosage, frequency of AE administration, and the like.

'Controls' is also used when speaking of how one deals with factors, variables that may affect an NV outcome. If one knows that women are more at risk (and they are consistently so for every known type of NV, given the exposure to a potential precipitant) then, when testing the effect of an AE compound B at dosage C in group I compared with compound F at dosage G in group II, one must insure that there is not a preponderance of women in group I and of men in group II. This is a kind of control by population characteristic/trait allocation or matching, in cases where one knows that a predictor variable affects NV and could therefore predict AE response (an assumption that must in fact be tested). Another kind of control is by manipulation of factors in a more experimental situation in nature; for example, when testing the effect of a behavioral intervention, such as hypnosis or music, or a dietary one, to see how it interacts with a constant (and so controlled) administration of AE X at dosage Y for a sample suffering from, say, PNV (in such a case, because of the risk of a lawsuit, it may be best to test a folk remedy used by women, such as a cola drink and rest).

An important practical point to watch for is, as fatigue is a self-reported variable that affects NV, that the women in the trial should be equally rested (i.e., not some with seven children to look after and others sufficiently well-off to have a maid or home help); to insure this, they should all be put on the same 'resting' regimen for a day or two. We know from some studies that anxiety may play a role; we can therefore elect to match all women in the sample on anxiety (state and trait) test scores, i.e., an allocated risk control. For the intervention, this can be music, hypnosis, guided imagery, crackers, or no crackers with everyone receiving their 'I do it anyway' cola drink and rest. We manipulate variables by allowing some women to listen to music or to have hypnosis or guided imagery or crackers and various combinations of these. If one finds, for example, that music plus rest quintuples the number of women with N control, but with anything else N reduction is simply additive, one may have an 'interaction' effect. This means, just as in drug–drug potentiation, that 1 and 1 do not make 2 , they make 5 or 6. The foregoing is, by the way, not just a silly experiment; much more needs to be done to test folk uses and behavioral interventions and, given the ubiquity of side effects, to be educated when prescribing AEs.

Another feature that is important to clinical trials, and to their evaluation, is that there should be adequate population selection and sample size. Such variables that are known, from the literature, to be risk characteristics of populations should be set out, and whenever possible be included by means of subgroup and interaction testing in outcome analyses. Adequacy of population size may be defined as sizes necessary for making statistical inference, or large enough presumably to include that immense variety of known and unknown variables which constitutes risk and individual difference. Small sample studies are usually discouraged unless we are testing for expected specificity of outcomes in homogeneous samples which have characteristics important to the hypothesis. Large sample studies, although preferred statistically and providing the opportunity for small but important variables to be identified, may, on the other hand, have a problem when conducted as cooperative or multicenter enterprises unless supervision is exceedingly strict, including training in the protocol and constant quality control.

When control appears to be defined as less than zero, for example, the 'best' and 'worst' percentages are not reported. Table 4.1 presents the calculation of the average total control (TC), and the V and N in all studies of the drug reviewed. The worst side effect of each drug is also listed. A particular problem exists when investigators, although purporting to test the efficacy of a compound, do not in fact give it on its own, but add it to other compounds in several different presentations or 'cocktails,' and test these against another cocktail. Thus the only study of alizapride purporting to measure impact on N combines alizapride with dexamethasone and is tested against metoclopramide and dexamethasone; this gives the curious outcome of exactly the same control over each. A few studies compare different dosages, but not all report the dosages. Some clinical trial papers concern themselves with anesthetics, each of which is a risk factor that can vary depending on its nature and the operation, comparing these for NV outcomes with or without particular AEs. Anesthetics may also be compared with or without pretreatments, oxygen masks, various administrative methods, and in combinations, for example, with or without nitrous oxide. We consider these to be studies of risk factors in the emetic situation rather than of AEs, although the literature of anesthesiology leads to some confusion.

Reported side effects can be multiple, and agreement among studies is not assured. Our choice of 'worst' in Table 4.1 is arbitrary and, as we see with clinical trials, reports may be more benign than the later letter warnings in journals. This last is a reminder that studies carried out after marketing do not insure the detection of severe adverse effects which may occur over longer periods of time, with longer periods of administration, in special patient populations, etc.

The random nature of the designs and presentations of the trials confounds simple tabular presentation. When a 'best' or 'worst' outcome involves an additional AE, we have added 'with.' Some studies were reported so poorly that one could make neither head nor tail of them; typically they failed to report sample size, to use any quantified outcome measure, etc. We have occasionally entered such a finding, typically when it was the only study. And 'worst' or 'best' control may well mean 'sometimes' or 'under this limited condition of dosage, type of chemotherapy, and period of observation.' When there have been several 'best' results, depending on these or other variables controlled (or otherwise) in the same study, we have taken the highest reported total control of N and V, or, when not differentiated (which tells us even more about the state of the trial art), we indicated 'NV' problems. When attempting to review clinical trial data with the aim of a sophisticated meta-analysis (hardly our goal here), there will be far fewer studies that qualify for inclusion than are actually published in the literature. This gives the reader an idea of the problems facing the doctor or patient when it comes to assessing a drug's probable impact. Table 4.1 speaks for itself when it comes to outcome reliabilities.

Do clinical trial outcomes currently distribute themselves in a normal distribution (anchored at 0 and 100)? Should this turn out to be the case, one might in the future wish to demonstrate, when any extremely successful initial drug trial outcome is observed, that it is only a random effect. Of course the body of literature on AEs has previously been taken much more positively, and we will not play more than the devil's advocate here. Certainly we would not wish to massage the numbers in Table 4.1 as though they had profound importance, but for what they obviously suggest.

One wishes that there had been more N control studies, and that all had separated N from V. As it is, the best–worst cases are too few to pretend to fancy calculation. We did do one simple thing: average the difference between the eight N and V 'best' controls shown. It came to a bit less than 10 points, with only one instance of 3% where N control results are said to be better than those for V. The foregoing crude discrimination allows a somewhat more optimistic view about V control, and reflects the general thrust of the literature that N is more poorly controlled. Before we applaud the control claimed, we should be reminded that studies relying on nurses underreport nausea, and that good measures of patient reporting require some rigor by application of carefully developed scales, and that they are time-consuming.

Does reliance on large sample studies make a difference?

It is generally held that large sample studies for clinical trials yield more trustworthy results than small ones. There is an assumption of greater population heterogeneity with respect to NV risk distribution in the larger patient population, although we know of no NV study where populations were representative. There is the more trustworthy feature that, insofar as comparisons are made of drug effects (possibly varying procedures, risk, etc.), the larger sample sizes are likely to be sufficient to insure the power to detect, using tests of statistical inference, small 'real' differences, thus showing that one or another variable is making a contribution in that study (at least to observed outcomes).

We drew, from the sample of 372 studies taken from Medline, etc., those that had over 275 patients (an arbitrary figure) and quantified results. There were 17 studies on the serotonin $5HT_3$ antagonists ondansetron, granisetron, and tropisetron. The largest had an impressive number of participants (n = 2673). Variables that were not constant across studies included: dosages, days of post-conditioned taste aversion observation, results with other drugs, e.g., patient sex (a risk factor), cycle of chemotherapy (a risk factor), and whether N was included. The best and worst results for V control only were 76% and 21% for ondansetron, 78% and 37% for granisetron, and 65% and 52% for tropisetron only, for NV combined (in one study). The overall outcomes for combined antagonist V control range from 21% to 78%, a rather narrower set of results than shown in Table 4.1, where smaller samples were included. As one presumes that the percentage total control is, in each study, an averaged outcome, rather than identifying a single peak patient, the function of the larger number would seem to be the typical statistical sampling one of reducing extremes.

At this point we add one other large study, carried out on metoclopramide and dexamethasone (n = 357). It observed a combined NV control of 52%. Once again we do not sum the different features, but in doing so would find an average 'best' V control with serotonin antagonists, under all conditions, to be 53% and, for N, excluding 'with' combinations, 59%. The metoclopramide/dexamethasone combination, although less specific, yields about the same efficacy as these other drugs.

These central tendency measures above are close to the midpoint of Table 4.1. It is unusual that N control reported here is higher. For us it is a reminder of the variation in study outcomes when one always keeps in mind the larger literature. Across studies it would suggest the possibility of a pattern of NV where there is, for anti-cancer therapies, V without N. Ordinarily this is not reported.

Our foregoing large sample review leads to the clinical expectation, based on central tendencies, that about half of the patients taking serotonin antagonists (here combined) will enjoy complete control of V, or the NV that immediately follow cancer chemotherapy. Presumably fewer would enjoy that same control if taking a placebo. The conclusion from the review of the large samples is hardly different, although for a wider range (sigma differences) than the results in Table 4.1. There is some confounding here because Table 4.1 includes those large sample studies that included these studies, none of which were weighted for sample size. Once again the question arises about whether the distribution of efficacy outcomes will approximate a normal distribution for NV drugs, and if, with the expansion of numbers of studies, it will approximate a bell curve with a remarkably conventional midpoint, on a scale of 0–100, of about 50% as an averaged best control outcome. If this were the case, and if risk factors did not operate to allow better individual forecasts (we have seen no study that actually tests this), and clinicians were relying on the dictum that the best individual forecast is the group statistical one (as Meehl proposed many decades ago), they would essentially be flipping a coin every time they forecast control of immediate V after cancer chemotherapy. We trust that the situation is much better than that, with feedback and drug combinations constituting the 'art' of oncological care, but these kinds of data are not entirely reassuring.

Later we shall look at nonpharmacological interventions for NV, but at this point we must notice the rather good results of a small N study mentioned here to prompt reflection on placebo, neurotransmitters, and where we stand on NV theory; this study reports on acupuncture/acupressure studies in NV conditions such as postsurgical NV or PNV. An early study by Ghaly et al. (1987) used Chinese acupuncture, finding it equivalent to cyclizine, a histamine receptor antagonist used to control postoperative NV.

Some sophisticated illustrations of these trial designs are in Tarkkila and Isola (1992), Hursti et al. (1993), Edwards et al. (1989), Andrykowski et al. (1992), and Troesch (1993) (we take these almost at random from a range of well-done studies). Read Aapro (1993) and Marty et al. (1993) to find examples of excellence in straightforward clinical trial design, against which you could compare other evaluative, rather than interactive, studies.

Among the variables that sophisticated clinical trial investigators must be aware of are discrete patterns of N and V, separate or together; these affect, depending on the precipitant, contexts and AE medication outcomes. The work of Marty et al. (1993) is illustrative, showing one patient group with a sequence of NV (measured by the 'surrogate' V) who were responsive to AEs and which, in turn, predicted greater control on later cancer chemotherapy courses. In contrast patients who did not respond earlier had a greater increased risk. This contradicts more general data showing increased risk over repeated cancer chemotherapy cycles, which is arrived at by analyzing heterogeneous populations with no awareness of the patterns that describe AE response predisposition. What appears to be the case is that this subset of NV events can be partialled out, with several subsets differing in their NV observed after cancer chemotherapy and under AE medication. There are those who respond early and those whose later NV from their medication continue to be even more responsive with lower NV rates. Another subset are those with no NV at all (this may include two groups if AEs are routinely given, so that it is impossible to know who does not suffer in the absence of medication) and another is those with NV who do not respond early on, or respond well ('refractory') to AEs – or at least to AEs used in this study.

Of similar relevance are the findings of the Italian Group for Antiemetic Research (1994), which were arrived at with a careful multifactorial design. We have alluded to their identification of differing patterns before.

In a comparative test clinical trials rarely include a variety of interventions such as OTC medications, behavioral or other nonpharmacological factors, or complementary/comforting efforts. In later chapters we encounter a few studies of acupressure or of electrical stimulation of acupressure/puncture sites. To communicate the findings from well-done British studies, they can be more effective than placebo and are in the range of outcomes for prescribed preparations.

For the most part, as a subject for research the NV treatment world is strictly pharmacological; it is the commercial domain of manufacturers who are counting on physicians doing what they have traditionally been trained to do. Yet, even for NV, and as we have suggested, tradition and the very best intent are insufficient; at least they are sometimes misguided. To draw an analogy with internal medicine, and referring to the splendid work of Alan Barbour, in his *Caring for Patients: a Critique of the Medical Model* (1995), roughly one-third of general medicine patients will be misdiagnosed and mistreated through the application of the medical model. We make no estimate here, for no research tells us yet, but a proportion of NV patients will require other or additional interventions, attention to and evidence of which will not be found in journal reports of AE clinical trials. Insofar as stress and environmental perturbations are major sources of NV, again psychosocial and emotional processes are at work.

Efficacy findings determine outcome measures, as well as the compound kind of NV in terms of its initiating conditions (surgery, chemotherapy, administration of an emetic, etc.) and risk distribution in the sample. By definition, an AE is tested by impact on V, i.e., in retching episodes. N and V are often linked. A drug test should concern itself with N that is the more common, enduring, and uncomfortable experience, and may be the physiological state that initiates V as relief. Most studies, whether animal or human, speak in terms of 'control' of V, but even when that is qualified as 'total' it may meet a definition that is, say, three episodes or less over a time period X. Sometimes this is stated as 'major control.' And obviously, the period specified and observed matters. We commented that there is disagreement about the clinical epidemiology, whether, for example, immediate or delayed NV are more common after cancer treatment. Most say immediate, but 'immediate' may be defined at will. We shall attend more specifically to the experimental design of protocol factors affecting outcome reporting, and also consumer information.

Range of outcomes by major drug studied

The question is one of reliability and (implicitly) of validity. How much consistency is there among efficacy studies, even without attending to the important matter of side effects? If there is wide disagreement among outcome studies of the same drug, one must question the accuracy ('validity' as defined as the drug doing what the manufacturer says it does) of drug impact characterizations. To be sure, there are means of patient and doctor self-protection; the best is when the methodologically trained clinician selects the best-designed studies. These will meet the Cochrane Collaboration criteria. What we, in fact, find across the range of ordinary studies is massive disagreement.

Quite a range

In sum the 'efficacy' outcome figures in Table 4.1 range across the board, for ondansetron alone from 0 to 100%. This is not the 'fault' of the drug or of the investigators; it does suggest different chemotherapies, different periods of observation, different outcome measures (N or V), different doses, different patient populations, and different environments, and of course when cocktails are used all drug interactions contribute to trial unreliability.

A 50/50 chance midpoint, i.e., a normal distribution for all phase 4 trials?

One sees, calculating the average of the sum of effects across all 372 studies, that it comes very close to 50% (46%) for N and V 'control' with extreme anchors at 0 and 100%. If one relies on the placebo findings cited by A. H. Roberts (1995), where placebo healing of ulcer occurred in 48% or as discussed by Roberts, an inventive study of therapies believed to be efficacious but which, on follow-up, found only nonspecific effects with 40% 'excellent' outcomes (equal to total NV control?) and 30% 'good,' there is almost 70% efficacy where doctor and patient are both expecting positive outcomes. Insofar as there is reason to suspect placebo 'control' in other situations of up to 50%, there is a tantalizing worry given the distribution in Table 4.1. The outcomes with less than 50% control are chance occurrences, i.e., these are what a placebo could also accomplish. Indeed should one consider interpreting the distribution in Table 4.1 as suggesting that these mostly ill-designed trials do not allow the conclusion that AEs 'work' much better than placebo or, as a hypothesis, are relatively more specific?

Setting, placebo, and distribution midpoints

It is not simply placebo effects (whatever these may be) that need to be borne in mind when one seeks to attribute drug outcomes to drugs as independent variables; variations across settings and persons should also be considered. We discussed earlier the largest study that we have found (Cohen et al., 1994; n = 16 000). Comparing four hospitals and keeping NV outcome data on individual anesthesiologist's patients, the range of average NV control was 39–70% for the *same* compounds, dosages, and operations. As collaborative studies suffer from distance effects (i.e., things do not go as presumed on paper), one should allow for variations in these protocol-defined dosage controls and perhaps other deviations as well. It is likely that placebo and setting effects interact. By inference, these may account for placebo levels of 33% up to 73%. That is something to think about when looking at clinical trials.

The 'worst' aspect to be borne in mind was mentioned earlier and will be reiterated later; it is N that is ordinarily worse for patients, so what one achieves by way of V control, which is measured comparatively easily by nurses, is not what a 'best' medication should primarily aim to achieve ('best' as defined by patients). Quite simply, not only are the results of arraying clinical trials capable of discouraging notions of efficacy, single or any mechanism, they also show continuing inattention to what should matter most: how the patient feels. Based on what is in Table 4.1, there is a long way to go before patient NV suffering can be predictably relieved.

A more positive view

The results in Table 4.1 might be said to confirm traditional clinical wisdom that different drugs are more and less effective depending upon NV-initiating conditions. The 'best' results of Table 4.1 could then be argued to show that good outcomes do come from drug treatments and that these appear to have at least some of the specificity that textbooks and clinicians take for granted. If one abandons the 'total control' criterion, it may be that large numbers of patients enjoy at least some relief from NV. There is no study that tells us what percentage this might be across a range of trials, but 'some improvement' is probably common. It is complicated of course by spontaneous recovery and the downhill NV slide that occurs after a few days of chemotherapy when delayed NV appears, or even later when, on a return visit, ANV appears, neither of which, the trials agree, is readily controlled by current medication.

One does not dismiss rough conclusions arising from less than ideal trials, for example the AE failures to control V in half of all chemotherapy. One very much wishes not only that better trial designs were practiced, but that one by now knew the range of contributing variables as, for example, that data showing that – reasonably enough – milder chemotherapy cytotoxins produce less NV. But in what patient does that not hold? And is NV severity and duration ever to be routinely measured as part of such work? Indeed, does a patient history of prior NV severity predict to less AE efficacy? We are introducing caution and clinical skepticism, not nihilism. Understatement is preferable regarding claims from trials about any single neurotransmitter playing a total role in NV-generating signals/information transmission. The caution about specificity in neurotransmitter function, i.e., with antagonistic AEs, is appropriate. Consider the not infrequent equivalent clinical effects of quite diverse transmitters, the generally better effects of cocktails including AEs with unknown 'mechanisms,' the paradoxical effects of AEs that are likely to induce NV as emetics, and the multivalent nature of many synaptic receptors as responsive to different neurotransmitters. Further, such responsivity is itself, whether in vitro or in vivo, quite varied depending on neuromodulators, network conductance, baseline states, oscillations/rhythmicity in network and neuron, neuronal learning, etc. Once this caution is allowed, one then reaches the important conclusion that linearity as such and 'mechanisms' as models are not the only way to view brain function in NV and its control.

Further constraints on the concept of linearity

Even with an apparently clear temporal stimulus–response, dare one assume, in the case of humans, simple pharmacological causality, i.e., linearity? Dopamine, for example, which is now implicated in many psychiatric disorders, is itself a catecholamine, a precursor of norepinephrine, and a neurotransmitter in ANS pathways; it is used medically for treating shock, and its antagonists are used as AEs. In the PDR it is described as producing N and V as side effects. Yet these may result as shock components, general sequelae, or interactions with the diffuse and powerful effects of dopamine on muscle and vascular tissue including heart and kidney, or other downstream effects of norepinephrine release. More complex explanations must be kept in mind for apparent emetic or AE effects. For all this, the importance of pharmacological work within the confines of the traditional medical model must not be denied or considered exhausted in the search for better prevention and control of NV. There is no question that some neuropharmacological mechanisms are quite clearly delineated, particularly in V and in AE treatments constituting, at least for the carefully controlled outcomes of iatrogenic interventions, the 'best' AEs available. In general clinical use, however, for average outcomes with their large range of efficacy, however narrowly defined, complexity is the normal condition leading to 'average' AE clinical outcomes.

An argument for more research on drug–drug interactions, as well as expanded clinical trials, is compelling. Consider, when adding compounds to treatment regimens, i.e., making cocktails, that NV control is usually improved albeit quite differently; quite unknown 'transmission mechanisms' are frequently at work. The study of Roila and the Italian Group for Antiemetic Research (1995) is a heartening instance of excellent designs leading to 'best' results; these workers showed that, for chemotherapy patients receiving moderate cytotoxin cocktails of dexamethasone and granisetron, there was 93% total V control, 72% N protection, and also protection against delayed N. Wisely cost-conscious, the research group found that the corticosteroid alone yielded good outcomes at low cost. In contrast, the expensive serotonin $5HT_3$ antagonist did not prove itself worthy of use.

Is the control of NV even less predictable in women?

In an earlier discussion, we have seen how many control variables may influence AE efficacy, however measured, but here comes a whopper:

Murakawa (1994), in a little noted but potentially most important study, given the much greater vulnerability of women to NV, found that clinical trial findings had less predictive power for women than for men. We have not seen a replication of the study. The variability that is seen in PNV prevalence rates, the inconsistency, and the risk factors would be identified as being a failure in any clinical trials that have not identified the range and statistical weights; quite possibly they could interact with situation, predisposition, and one another, which would be best suited to clinical trials. There must be clinical trials that use larger female populations. Why are women more at risk of NV? And if these results prove to be replicable, how are women less responsive to conventional AEs? Such research could well change the direction of women's health care.

The data in Table 4.1 and the following raise questions about neuropharmacological specificity for NV. As noted, the most strongly argued case (except for histamine transmitters for motion sickness) for specificity is for the action of a chemotherapy-elevated serotonin activity in the stomach wall (enterochromaffin cells in the gut are replete with serotonin receptors, although studies there do not find increased serotonin levels corresponding to V); this implies a specificity of particular $5HT_3$ antagonists that act there to reduce that activity and bring NV relief. But not so with the work of Roila and the Italian Group for Antiemetic Research (1995). It appears that some simultaneous actions, as yet not identified for dexamethasone, granisetron, and ondansetron, are required for NV protection. One would appear to be in the stage of empirical (i.e., trial and error rather than theoretically rational) therapies for NV.

Nevertheless, in research and treatment in areas of medicine other than NV, it has been well demonstrated that action specificity exists. It may be that granisetron, ondansetron, etc., act specifically and 'best' in their interaction with corticosteroids (or the other AE groups). This possibility, which contradicts earlier more optimistic claims for sole treatment by ondansetron/granisetron, etc., strongly suggests the need to identify drug–drug interactions and their loci.

Further comment: non-specificity again

One must escape from the sole premise that a locus for NV must be in only one place, that 'center' that varies as groups of cells in several neuronal networks. Keep in mind that, logically and inferentially (for the full anatomical study of NV is only just beginning), 'loci' need to be not only in paraventricular, medullary reticular, or enterochromaffin tissue, but also in other more or less well-defined tissue. They may also be conceived of as multiple, changeable regions that are involved in information transfers. There are pattern transformations in the brain. For NV these may be thought of as perturbation-induced cascades which characterize broadly involved regions whose actions are not only neuronal and pathway responsive, but provide definitions of the state of 'ingredients' widely distributed in a milieu. Some writers characterize this as a brain chemical 'soup' (Sivilotti and Colquhoun, 1995). Even in an area that is as well charted and with such a high cell response pattern specificity as the visual cortex, network conductance is demonstrated (Douglas et al., 1995), leading investigators to conclude that populations of neurons cooperate in pattern formation/restoration which is latent in connectivities, that these characteristics are likely to occur in other sensory areas, and thus that 'receptive field properties are not so much determined by the specific patterns of [here] thalamic inputs but are shaped by the collective behavior of large populations of cortical cells.' One can conceive that this connectivity, collectivity, and relative nonspecificity, compared with earlier linear notions, may apply to new 'best' searches for and definitions of loci as well.

When considering theories of 'mechanism of transmission' as applied to AEs, one keeps in mind that synaptic receptors are responsive to multiple neurotransmitters. Specificity of bonding varies remarkably and is subject to many neuromodulating features, including varying protein behavior within the neuron. In the case of serotonin $5HT_3$ antagonists, one cannot rule out their effects on other messenger system receptors elsewhere in the brain. These include the very powerful 'general' effects summarized by the terms 'depression,' 'inhibition,' and 'suppression;' these can lead to decreased arousal via the reticular system, sedation via effects on sleep or diurnal cycle regions, sedation as a local or general anesthetic, or, as with tranquilizers and steroids, some suppression, via inhibition of stimulation such as anxiety or pain-enhancing depression; all generate an improved feeling of well-being. When 'stress' is an NV component, corticosteroids may have this general remedial capacity.

The foregoing are quite general descriptors of assumed actions that are inferred in global terms. They tell us little except that AE effects are not likely to be as specific as the 'mechanisms' imply (at least in those cases in which quite different compounds contribute to effects and specific drugs do not achieve total NV control). The brain does appear to act quite specifically and yet simultaneously across and/or sequentially through multiple regions. The 'where' and 'how' of action are functions of the preferred observation methods and theoretical orientation intrinsic to the worker. NV are obviously 'localized' for any activity shown in the DNA, in G-protein activity, at synapses, via single neuron modulators or multiple neuron transmitters, affected by neuropeptides, hormones, regional 'volume,' and rhythmic patterns. Obviously 'local' becomes 'widespread' with many locales. For NV processing, we believe these to be usefully conceived at this stage of knowledge – as 'alien' precipitated perturbing interactions whether seen as perceptual, olfactory processing, enteric chemical, or spontaneous CNS activity (including whatever underresearched baroreceptors are found to be perturbation responsive in the future). A variety of initial conditions leads to final common pathway processes in NV.

So conceived, dynamic pattern formulations and interactive milieu conceptions can also work as ways of thinking about NV. If one allows simultaneous multi-level activity, as specific as any particular microbiological study can get, or as focused on collaborating regional networks as one can be, and the immense mix of media chemistry conceived as a delicately responsive, regulatory, brain 'soup' (Sivilotti and Colquhoun, 1995), then the dynamic language of chaos theory adds a critical tool for thinking about the scattered and unpredictable clinical trial results.

Even for the exact corticovisual system (and where connectivities are limited), it is in order to have a principle of multiple hierarchies and descriptions in terms of degrees of freedom that allow intrinsic indeterminacy (Hilgetag et al., 1996). How localized a locus is depends on what it is connected to, what its intrinsic pattern and pattern flow potentials are, how replicative these are (as attractants), and which, of many or any, hierarchical systems are in play affecting what is being observed. We shall discuss such principles again but, here, just as in encountering contrary experimental data, when the array of clinical trial outcomes suggests that, for a given patient, setting, drug, or initiating condition variables may be considered individually as setting degrees of freedom that can be tested by replication of treatment or trial whenever the specific mechanism theory fails, it should encourage at least two trains of thought. One is to entertain simultaneous specificity and nonspecificity as likely occurrences in the precipitation and treatment of NV; the other is to encourage trials of multiple engagements – patient with healer and her environment, as, for example, the range of placebo proposed by Chaput de Saintonge and Herxheimer (1994). This brings us back to the clinician's art of 'seasoning to taste,' guided initially by the research and clinical literature and local formularies for dosage, administration, and the best mix, but to which have been added the complementary, psychosocial/milieu, and comforting therapies. And it should produce more interesting clinical trials and, one hopes, more replicable 'best' outcomes and conceptually expanded experimental work as well.

Clinical, experimental, and theoretical observations in NV are not disparate arenas. They point in the same directions. These directions are informed by work in associated neuroscience which is not really that far afield. Pharmacology must certainly continue its efforts in messenger identification. We should be mindful of Martin's assessment that the clinical trial is the best case test, because most patients in normal settings fare less well. We conclude that NV represents a therapeutic, methodological, experimental, and conceptual field that is very much in need of further endeavor.

Checking consistency and problems: a review of reviews

When we compared the distribution of trials by kinds of patient and procedure, in the Medline and Cancerline output for the same years, we saw many variables. These were reflected in different AE efficacy figures, depending upon the sample of studies drawn upon. What the prescribing consumer enjoys by way of review conclusions will depend on which journal is read, which meeting is attended, or, worse, which drug salesman is persuasive. In our own case, you see that our summaries of AE clinical trials are certainly more pessimistic than narrower reviews. So let us see how NV trial study reviewers themselves (those selecting an array of clinical trials) may have differed in their conclusions from one another. As we saw here in our own review, the major difficulty for reviewers is likely to be that, unless imposing the strict standards of a systematic review, reviewers are challenged to integrate a melange of differing designs with varying levels of adequacy. The review process itself has generated comment about methodology. Mulrow (1987) was the first to draw attention to inadequacies in the review processes, and pointed out that reviewing clinical trials is hard work and complicated.

Marcus Torrey, our student, has undertaken a review of reviews (n = 30). Torrey's purpose was not to evaluate which medications were superior but to arrive at insights about the review process, the underlying studies, and from these to make statements about the state of the art, proposals for future work, and further guidance for the healer and patient as consumers.

Torrey found that most reviews shared a common problem: the inability to conduct sophisticated meta-analyses because of the inconsistency of design and reporting in the trials themselves.

Most clinical trials were found to rely on inadequate N episodes. Reviewers were cautious enough not to make weak inferences from weakly powered work. A particular problem lay in sample attenuation: patient drop-out from chemotherapy that makes control of NV so consequential; clinical trial investigators began with samples that were too small to compensate for this sometimes large effect. But withdrawal is also a problem when investigators report their efficacy findings just on the remaining patients, so that the 'worst cases' of drop-out escape inclusion in outcome statistics. Also, with regard to sampling, a large sample (as we have seen) does not in itself guarantee easy generalization when demographics, risk factors, NV-precipitating conditions, patterns of NV, etc., differ from the population studied – if and when its characteristics are that faithfully reported – and other patient populations being treated in other settings.

A failure to follow up on the drop-out group also disallows a very much needed study of patients at greatest risk of dropping out. No follow-up means that there can be no feedback received as a reflection on their experience and withdrawal decision, as opposed to clinic-based exit interviews (in this instance with overtones of doom) from these patients. In a very early quality of care study (Blum, 1958), it was found that what patients told the doctor or nurse as they left the hospital could differ markedly from what they had to say when at home. Such NV drop-out probing might learn what patients believe to be unnoticed side effects that can be corrected, or psychosocial interventions that might assist them in completion of their chemo- or radiotherapy (or combined therapies). In such a long-term follow-up, information on the setting variable, found by Cohen (1995) to be so consequential, might emerge as a criticism of care, or folk remedies that are useful in controlling their N at home. Some comment, too, might arise about new procedures for informed consent for cancer patients whose treatment is of dubious outcome, thus allowing more focus on the wisdom of the decision to terminate, to die with dignity; patient and family wishes often seem to be disregarded in this regard, because the physician is hell bent on doing what he knows best how to do. It may be easier to give chemotherapy than to spend compassionate time with a dying patient.

Inconsistency in trial designs was the plague of reviewers, from randomized crossover to parallel to placebo control to nonrandomized sequential, to the almost, 'Well, I need a promotion to associate clinical professor, so I think I will watch some patients today and publish.' The method using crossover with own control can use only those patients who have lived from one chemotherapy cycle to another, but they have a demonstrated risk of being more ill, and less responsive to AEs, including the development of anticipatory NV (ANV). The usual problems of counting can occur when one asks who counts what? Are they blind with regard to the drug employed? And how is continuous V or N quantified except by infrequently applied incident duration measures? And how are these combined to arrive at a generalization? And to what extent is pre-treatment food intake controlled which affects the capacity to vomit? Or once counted, quantified as aggregate numbers, what means are used for statistical inference for significance, if any? It is also the case, as noted earlier, that delayed chemotherapy NV is less often measured and, in most studies, this occurs when the findings increase pessimism about efficacy. Similarly, in the studies available to reviewers, N was less often observed and, here we make reasonable speculation, itself measured in different ways by different instruments.

Even with these stark difficulties, some reviewers were simultaneously able to be thorough, critical and informative: Kris (1997), Roila and others in the Italian Group, and Stevens, to name but a few. Stevens (1991) and Mitchelson (1992, Parts I and II) stand as models. Wise reviewers delimit their work, or portions of their review, to sectors such as chemotherapy noncisplatin versus (the more toxic) cisplatin regimens, for pediatric work, or one serotonin antagonist versus another. There were then fewer apples mixed with oranges than in our Table 4.1 overview. Even with narrowed focus, Torrey finds that reviewers emerged with dramatically different conclusions about the efficacy of those newer serotonin $5HT_3$ antagonist compounds, which occupied the greatest proportion of study and reviewer attention in 1997 in the situation in which NV is most life threatening: anticancer treatment reactions.

Characterizing serotonin $5HT_3$ antagonists: the details of differing findings

Characterizations of serotonin antagonist effects, based on the studies available to reviewers (we did not compare their sampling of reviews, although this is in order), are set forth below. We do not include the fewer reviews not including serotonin antagonists. When several $5HT_3$ antagonists are compared, the list selects the highest control value for the least toxic (thus noncisplatin) regimen. We are less rigorous than the best reviewers in not listing separately treated outcomes from dosage, administration, population (pediatric versus adult), etc., variables which were controlled by reviewers whenever possible.

Reviewing differing conclusions about serotonin antagonist effects

Serotonin antagonists:

- are equal to other regimens, e.g., metoclopramide
- have better side effect profiles
- are not helpful in controlling delayed or multiple-day regimens or show (minor) adverse effects in 45% of patients
- produce cardiovascular distress
- are a major clinical advance
- with cocktails, increase control
- are more expensive, with a need for cost–benefit research to balance efficacy, side effects, costs
- by consensus, are more efficacious than cocktails or metoclopramide
- have major differences, children versus adults vis-à-vis chemotherapy with naivety as risk

- in chemotherapy versus radiotherapy onset: differences demand attention
- show 'best':
  - 60–90% major V control
  - 60–80% major V control
  - 72–100% major V control
  - 58–95% major N control
  - 76% major V control
  - 64% major V cisplatin control
  - 68% major V control
  - 92% major V control
  - 66% major V control
  - 100% major V control
  - 0% major V control with placebo
  - 32% major V control in 'worst group'
- patients' preference: prefer ondansetron over metoclopramide
- a confounding effect in studies (failure to attend to pattern differences with V absent or present with N)
- concealed actual solo serotonin antagonist effects compared with metoclopramide, dexamethasone, diphenhydramine in N control.

As N measures receive no attention, we are indebted to Andrews and Sanger (1993) for their thorough review of up to 478 published reports of N assessments. They observe that the variable measured most after chemotherapy is frequency, then intensity, then duration.

In the list above we see important differences between our own overall Table 4.1 and subordinate large N sample of reviews compared with the detailed work of 'best' reviewers. Foremost is the preponderance of conclusions that serotonin antagonists provide total V control for a majority of patients. Our earlier observation of a 50% efficacy would be discarded. Only two reviews, each reporting two subsets of studies, offered efficacy for total V control for less than a majority of chemotherapy patients. We do not know the source of bias here, but optimistically we ask whether reviewers, in selecting studies more readily susceptible to analysis, thereby found that selecting better designed studies led to findings of better control outcomes. If reviews that show little difference between serotonin antagonists and metoclopramide, dexamethasone, etc., were included here, outcome efficacy estimates would drop. Nevertheless, careful reviewers in the field (stated in terms of a preponderance of evidence available to them as probability statements, not certainties) conclude in favor of serotonin antagonists for use in anticancer treatments. In doing so they offer support to the optimistic view of a more than likely chance to control immediate (not delayed or anticipatory) NV; further, this constitutes evidence of the partial, sometimes dominating, utility of linear, conventional, neuropharmacological work and its premise regarding mechanisms of NV. Patient preference is also addressed in a few studies and commented on by a few reviewers. Medication, another treatment preference, is an ideal measure because patient comfort is the goal and patients should be considered as guides. It remains remarkable that so few studies use preference measures.

A 0% control finding for cisplatin-induced V control by placebo in one study/review is important for discussion purposes. This can be contrasted with the 92% control by an AE. If this were a consumer's conclusion, one would have accepted it with no other reference or requirement for replication or further confirmation, as would be done in a meta-analysis. If it were found that there is *no* placebo effect for chemotherapy, with severe cytotoxins, a theoretical limit would have been put on placebo effects. Psychosomatics would have met its match in extreme NV. Were such a 0 placebo 'standard' confirmed, the reading consumer, turned investigator, would then be justified, in the case of a failure, to include a placebo control in an efficacy trial.

The problem with this arises from those findings on NV chemotherapy incidence discussed earlier in Chapter 2. These, like Table 4.1, the normalized distribution from the larger studies, and other reviews above, are a reminder that not only are most findings not so extreme, although perhaps 3 sigmas from the mean 0 and 100 anchor, but that, when examining the incidence of NV resulting from chemotherapy, a lot have no control, whether AE or placebo. Bleiberg (1992) found that 33% were entirely uncontrollable immediately after chemotherapy (with 0 control for delayed NV). This figure is close to that of Graves (1992) – 30% uncontrollable NV – and of Tonato et al. (1994) – 30–40%; it was Bleiberg who wondered whether or not all immediate chemotherapy NV control was a placebo effect of short duration yielding to NV emergence in uncontrolled delayed NV. More pessimistic are those earlier findings of del Favero (1992), which showed 86% uncontrolled chemotherapy NV, or those of Kaiser (1992) at 78%. As usual, dependent on the cytotoxin and the day measured, there is a range of outcomes, from bad to worse control in studies focusing on incidence – whatever the drugs employed – rather than clinical trials.

There appears to be a difference in the level of optimism or pessimism about efficacy depending on the selection of the reviewer as well as on the focus of the research worker. We do not know, but ask: Do clinical trials have a 'demand quality' such that all concerned have expectations which yield generally better control outcomes? Contrariwise, do workers with a more epidemiological bent, and doing studies not financed by manufacturers – for almost all clinical trial work is so financed – fail to impart expectations of success which might, as placebo and setting variables, yield more NV control? The argument here may go beyond double-blind to the famous triple-blind study of Joyce and Weldon (1965), and even then may fail at expectation control if anyone knows that a clinical trial versus an epidemiological study, or a paid versus a voluntary or grant effort, is at stake.

The finding of Edwards et al. (1989) (reviewed by Morell, 1996), that single neuron synapse studies in crayfish show that neurotransmitter responses to serotonin 'differ dramatically depending on the animal's social status,' is provocative (indeed, astonishing and compelling). In dominant animals, serotonin's impact on neuronal firing is excitatory; in dependent animals, it suppresses firing. If this is so in the lowly but socially sensitive crayfish, one may not be entirely mad to raise the possibility that psychosocial factors may also be expressed in whatever serotonin levels (in chemotherapy) are related to NV and to serotonin antagonist actions in humans.

Do status impositions (doctor vs patient in one setting) affect humans as they do in crayfish, in regard to serotonin antagonist effects of $5HT_3$ medications? This is unlikely from crayfish extrapolation, of course, but nevertheless sensibly conceived for more experimentation in self-controlled versus physician-controlled administrations of chemical agents and AEs. Kaufmann (1994) appears to have found that, when patients were in charge, controlling their own postoperative dosage of AEs, greater NV control was achieved than when they were passive recipients of what the doctor ordered. This may well be a matter of feedback and timing sensitivity as well as that felt confidence that is so well demonstrated in health psychological studies as favoring feelings and outcomes. Much more of this work is required. And also in order are more studies of placebo in NV as carefully controlled as the best of AE work, mindful of the interdisciplinary comparative literature.

Death: surveillance to report outlying dire effects

There is another important review that brings attention to cardiovascular risk of the ondansetron which has not been observed elsewhere. This outlying risk of death as a rare departure from the generally good effect profile of ondansetron reminds us of a sampling observational problem: How do we insure that the consequential rare event is detected and reported? With ondansetron we may say that it has been reported, albeit relying on *The Lancet*, after several deaths. Post-marketing surveillance is a necessity, requiring attentive clinicians and efficient government notifications and, when etiology is questionable, immediate investigation. We have seen here the role of the review that brings attention to the rare adverse outcome that generated fatalities. Thus the attention given to adverse effects in reviews is of particular value, as a warning for surveillance.

Conclusion

The value of well-designed clinical trials as the basis for evidence-based medicine has been established. The inadequacy of trials that do not follow a randomized assignment design using controls and, wherever possible, placebo and large samples is evident. One is convinced, with Torrey and the best of reviewers, that much that is published should not be in print. Underlying this is the fact that much that seems simple about NV is wrong.

Design is more difficult as a result of the complexity of NV itself and the many variables known to affect its patterning, course, and measurement. Perhaps, more importantly, given a fundamental absence of knowledge about NV as a process, there are no doubt many variables that are unknown and which therefore contribute to unreliability of clinical trial outcomes. It is this that, with patient, setting and variability in drug interactions, sets limits on 'evidence-based' medical practice. The 'art' of medicine is necessary, but comes into play when the caregiver is fully informed about what is known. That is not the ordinary situation.

There is much to be desired about the outcome measures typically used, i.e., emetic episodes in hospital. Too often measures are missing much more widespread, enduring N, NV occurring outside the medical treatments that have induced them, of which cancer treatments are the most commonly studied, and quality of life as a measure.

The tremendous variability in outcome reported compels caution, especially as a well-designed trial situation is 'ideal' compared with practice realities. One does not take much by way of reporting 'on trust.' Variability in outcome reporting not only reminds us of methodological difficulties, but also tells us how very complex NV are in terms of what can induce, affect, or terminate them, how they are experienced and reported, and how important basic research is for any hope of improvement in existing treatments.

For the reader who would like a more thorough presentation of NV-pertinent clinical trial methodology, we recommend reading any or all of the following: Aapro (1993); Andrews and Sanger (1993); Christensen et al. (1998); Krasnow (1989); Oliver (1992); Silverman (1995); Tedeschi and Tedeschi (1968).

CHAPTER 5

Consumers' corner and clinical trials: what does the consumer get to read?

Our intent in this chapter is to assist the consumer, whether doctor, nurse, physician assistant, or patient, to judge the adequacy of one of their major information sources: the package insert. For the most part these will mirror the major practical medicines' reference work, the *Physicians' Desk Reference* (PDR). At the outset be warned. The information presented is often limited, and can be a biased selection, with respect to clinical trial data reported.

Our student, Sarina Behara, compiled package inserts against some of the array of clinical trial data described in this chapter. Her disclaimer, in comparing package inserts with trials in which the large trial is the criterion of excellence against which the insert has been judged, is clear from what we have seen in the foregoing: trials themselves may be flawed and, irrespective of design excellence, can yield differing outcomes.

But Behara examined whether or not clinical trial data were presented at all and, when presented, whether the manufacturer provided what we could consider a fair range of outcomes, or an average outcome for efficacy, as opposed to the advertising temptation to select a most favorable study.

The package inserts shown in Table 5.1 were examined.

Alprazolam

No clinical trials with alprazolam were found in the Medline search of nausea and vomiting (NV) from 1992 to 1994. This may be the result of alprazolam's primary use in the treatment of anxiety disorders (including panic disorder), of which N is one symptom of many.

This insert was detailed in its description of an anxiety disorder, the antiemetic's (AE's) clinical pharmacology, precautions, side

Table 5.1: Package inserts

AE	Pharmaceutical brand name and administration method
Alprazolam	Xanax tablets
Dexamethasone	Dexamethasone tablets, USP, Dexamethasone oral solution, and Dexamethozone Intensol
Dronabinol	Marinol capsules
Droperidol	Droperidol injection, USP
Granisetron	Kytril granisetron hydrochloride injection
Lorazepam	Ativan tablets
Methylprednisolone	Solu-Medrol sterile powder
Metoclopramide	Reglan tablets
Prochlorperazine	Compazine tablets
Promethazine	Phenergan tablet and suppositories
Scopolamine	Transderm Scop system

effects, and dosage. It cautioned against over-long use and reminded that: 'The physician should periodically reassess the usefulness of the drug for the individual patient.' Of patients in a study, 16.5% (n = 641) reported NV as a side effect. One again meets the paradox that a drug used to alleviate N causes N as well. The insert clearly advised patients to weigh the risks of taking the drug, because some patients experience dependence and withdrawal symptoms.

Trial efficacy findings were not presented until the last paragraph. Although the insert appears to be fully disclosing to the consumer in discussion of adverse reactions and dependence, it is likely that benefits remain unclear, because the 'clinical studies' paragraph does not offer exact efficacy results. Instead it states that 'Xanax was significantly better than placebo.' The efficacy with respect to treatment of specific symptoms (N) of anxiety/panic disorders is not mentioned. We consider the clinical trial information to be grossly deficient. Alprazolam is, however, not important as an AE, so one presumes that few doctors and patients are at risk from their efficacy ignorance.

Dexamethasone

There is a long list of disorders that dexamethasone is used to treat in the package insert. It is surprising that NV are not included, because dexamethasone is widely used as an AE. There is also a list of adverse reactions. The insert lacked specificity in discussing its uses and adverse reactions. The conscientious physician unfamiliar with the clinical trial data could not rely on the material to justify or guide NV prescribing.

The problem is that no company has applied for a license to market dexamethasone as an AE, and that package inserts are not allowed to include information on unlicensed uses. Where new unpatented uses are developed for old drugs, this rule works against the public interest.

Dronabinol

No clinical trials with dronabinol were found in one Medline search of NV from 1992 to 1994. Some data addressing dronabinol's efficacy as an AE were presented in one study of 454 patients in chemotherapy-induced emesis, reporting 33–36% with complete control of V and 31–32% with partial control. The absence of placebo control data disallow a conclusion about the drug's efficacy. One is glad for the large sample size.

Unlike dexamethasone's presentation, there is a discussion of cocktails: 'Combination antiemetic therapy with dronabinol and prochlorperazine may result in synergistic or additive antiemetic effects.' The dosage section advises: 'Administration of dronabinol with phenothiazines, such as prochlorperazine, has resulted in improved efficacy as compared to either drug alone, without additional toxicity.' One would have welcomed clinical trial data on efficacy of the cocktail combination compared, for example, with the range of individual AEs. The data here do not support the insert conclusion about the combination's greater value.

Unlike some other inserts, the adverse reactions given were also based on the same clinical trial data. In general, the dronabinol insert was judged to be useful but not fully satisfactory.

Droperidol

Droperidol (injectable) is offered as a tranquilizer and to reduce NV postoperatively. No clinical trial data were given in the insert, and no citation or quotation was offered. 'Droperidol produces an antiemetic effect as evidenced by the antagonism of apomorphine in dogs. It lowers the incidence of NV during surgical procedures and provides antiemetic protection in the postoperative period.' Our limited comparative search of 1992–94 found only a few trials, one of which gave efficacy results: 82% control of V in a postoperative study of 120 patients.

Little information was given in regard to precautions, adverse reactions, and dosage. No specific information was presented on efficacy. One judges it inadequate.

Granisetron

Granisetron is used primarily as a post cancer treatment AE. Extensive clinical trial data are offered in the insert in relation to differing outcomes for doses of cisplatin therapy. The insert data present four trials, as follows.

Trial 1(*n*=28)

Too small a sample to allow confidence in the conclusions; 93% were found to have no V in this single-day cisplatin therapy study. We found no comparable study in Medline. See Table 4.1 and our view of reviews to learn that serotonin $5HT_3$ antagonists do not average 93% control.

Trial 2

In a study of single-day high-dose cisplatin therapy of 157 patients, 31–68% had complete control of NV, the range being attributed to different dosage administrations. The study in the insert was also found in our Medline search (Riviere, 1994). The data were accurately presented in the insert. This too-rare insert practice of full citation to a trial is welcome and necessary.

A similar trial, found on our search, reported 49% complete control of V. This result fits into the range presented in Trial 2. Another trial (*n* = 100 patients) resulted in 39% control of V. This range, 31–68%, is compatible with the trial literature under different chemotherapy and dose conditions.

Trial 3

Results from a study of 353 patients receiving single-day high-dose and low-dose cisplatin therapy were also presented, with control of NV ranging from 15% to 43%, depending on AE and cisplatin therapy dosages.

We found a trial in 496 patients receiving low-dose cisplatin therapy of whom 56% had complete control of V, a higher percentage than Trial 3 in the insert (Rudd and Nayiro, 1992).

Trial 4

This was a study of single-day, moderately emetogenic chemotherapy with 266 patients, where 68% had control of NV. A similar trial in our search had a sample size of 164 patients, in which 36% had control of NV. As is so often the case, the results differ markedly. Do note that the manufacturer has chosen to include a much more favorable report.

Compared with the other inserts, the granisetron insert presented extensive data on efficacy of granisetron depending on AE and cisplatin therapy dosages. The trial of 28 patients should not have been included because of its exceptional claim for control and low sample size, and inconsistency with the well-presented, large trials. One sees again the range of clinical trial results. Which results are most accurate? For granisetron at least, the manufacturer's insert selection showed higher and lower efficacy when compared with the insert data. The material provides an interesting range of control, defined by dosages, from 15% to 93%. As the consumer can appreciate from the chemotherapy and AE dose contributions, an education in AE variation is implicit. Such instruction should always be included in insert material. A problem does arise even so: the presentation may be difficult for the patient to understand. A larger review of trials, more discussion, and specific conclusions would be helpful to the consumer.

In regard to other subsections, the insert was less comprehensive. This is the opposite case from most other package inserts reviewed here. However, clinical trial data were referred to in the discussions of adverse reactions, pregnancy teratogenic effects, geriatric use, and carcinogenesis in rats. The insert substantiates its assertions with reference to clinical trial data. The granisetron insert served well.

Lorazepam

No clinical trial data on lorazepam as an individual AE were found in the Medline search, although several included lorazepam in cocktails. The insert included no clinical trial data on lorazepam's efficacy as an AE, presumably because this is not a licensed use. All that was mentioned in terms of efficacy was that long-term studies over a period of more than 4 months have not been done to assess long-term efficacy – presumably in the management of anxiety disorders, for which lorazepam is used. There is no mention of N or V in the insert, except that N is, again, paradoxical – a rare adverse reaction to lorazepam.

The insert was comprehensive with respect to lorazepam except for its AE role in NV.

Methylprednisolone

In our 2-year review, one clinical trial with methylprednisolone was found, which was for a cocktail. No clinical trial data were presented in the insert. Here again is a compound that is used to treat a variety of disorders. The only place NV are mentioned in the insert is in the 'adverse reactions' subsection. Methylprednisolone's use as an AE, which is not licensed, is not discussed.

The insert generally was insufficiently thorough and specific in giving warnings and indications. Clinical trial data are needed in reference to its efficacy in the treatment of disorders. We are again struck by the failure of manufacturers to note and advise upon this product as an AE.

Metoclopramide

No clinical trial data on the efficacy of metoclopramide are included in the insert. The only data mentioned are in relation to a carcinogenesis study of rats and to adverse reactions. Some clinical trials found in the Medline search give some description of adverse reactions, but not enough to compare specifically with the insert's information. Most metoclopramide clinical trials found in our review either included metoclopramide only as a cocktail or provided no outcome statistics on NV control. One study on 120 postoperative patients reported 73% control of NV.

The insert does include a good discussion of the clinical pharmacology of metoclopramide and goes so far as to discuss a possible mechanism for the drug's AE action. However, there is little mention beyond that of the use of metoclopramide to treat NV. And paradoxically, with metoclopramide, N is an adverse reaction. There is adequate information on warnings and indications.

Prochlorperazine

'Severe nausea and vomiting' is the first condition listed on the insert for treatment with prochlorperazine, an anxiolytic tranquilizer. The insert presents detailed information regarding the use of prochlorperazine to treat NV in pregnancy, chemotherapy, and postoperative patients. However, no discussion or data of efficacy were included. Various studies of prochlorperazine were in our comparative review (see also Table 4.1). In one study of 136 patients undergoing chemotherapy, prochlorperazine resulted in 86% control of V (Oliver et al., 1994). It would have been valuable to include such data on the insert.

The insert was one of the most detailed in giving information regarding precautions, adverse reactions, and dosage in reference to various conditions. Yet because of the severe danger associated – neuroleptic malignant syndrome and tardive dyskinesia – this drug is not one of choice except for severe NV and is specifically advised against for pregnancy NV (PNV); where hyperemesis gravidarum is 'intractable' (teratogenicity is also reported), the cautions are wise and welcome.

Promethazine

According to the insert, promethazine is used for its antihistamine, sedative, and AE effects. Specifically, promethazine is used in prevention and control of postoperative NV (PONV). No clinical data regarding promethazine's efficacy were included in the insert. The only study mentioned was in respect of teratogenic studies in rats. Our review uncovered only cocktail trials for promethazine with small sample sizes. These did not give outcome statistics on control of NV.

Scopolamine

The transdermal scopolamine disk described in the insert is used to help prevent NV of motion sickness for up to 3 days. One clinical trial is described in the insert, in which 195 patients had a 75% reduction of V in the incidence of motion-induced NV. The data are unclear about what reduction refers to: complete control or partial control of V. No results regarding control of N are given; it is surprising because it is an NV treatment. A scopolamine trial was found in our review – a transdermal scopolamine patch – for emesis induced by chemotherapy (Khojasteh, 1993) with 71% control of NV but the sample size was not indicated. One notes that the trial used scopolamine in the treatment of a condition not discussed in the insert, presumably because it is not an officially approved use.

Summary: caveat emptor!

Behara's work shows that inserts differed in detail and adequacy. Trials may not refer to proposed treatment uses. In contrast, four of eleven inserts did not mention NV as a condition for which the medication may actually be used. In general, few trials were cited or data shown in relation to efficacy in treatment of NV. Possible adverse outcomes go unnoted; the conclusion of this package insert study is that the doctor and concerned patient may not be advised as to risks, particularly of serious adverse reactions. The absence of an educational and balanced approach does not facilitate compliance. Nor does it support the medical argument that doctors know best, or that patients should always comply or cooperate with care.

Few inserts had sufficient efficacy data to allow comparison with our own limited trial review. Only one, the granisetron insert, gave data from more than one trial. Every insert examined was found lacking in some respect on its presentation of clinical trials and none discussed the inconsistency of AE trial outcomes as a characteristic of the field.

From the consumer point of view, the inserts are not user-friendly; a health professional would have to explain many of the terms and concepts to the patient and many laypeople for whom the insert is presumed – but obviously not actually – written. Given studies of caregiver time constraints and limited information exchange with patients, one doubts that prescribing physicians take the time to explain or to warn the patient. One fears that NV patients on these AEs may remain uninformed. As some side effects are mortal, others permanently disabling, and there are the risks of any AE failing to be efficacious, any deficiencies in information are to be regretted.

The ideal insert would provide extensive information in each subsection and give clinical data wherever necessary to substantiate claims, whether about efficacy, adverse reactions, or carcinogenesis. A compilation of efficacy results obtained from an array of only excellent clinical trials would be the most helpful. Cocktail combination possibilities must be set forth with particular sophistication that would presumably help the physician unfamiliar with the literature. Inserts in general, including the PDR and NV AE inserts, require substantial improvement.

Further non-technical guidelines to clinical trials

Ideally, every health caregiver would be highly trained in research methodology, familiar with the practical problems of doing such research, and thus able to assess what he or she reads with a critical or, when appropriate, appreciative eye. Yet clinicians are rarely trained in research and, even in highly reputed research medical schools (our own, for example), we may find little by way of formal training in the philosophy, logic, design, best models, and appropriate statistics for such trials. In our view much clinical research that is done is wasted because the conclusions reached are not warranted, and yet these may be generalized to become accepted practice. Furthermore, serious problems of ethics and commercial interest can arise to bias findings. The Nobel Prize winner Harold Varmus, Director of the National Institutes of Health, discussed, in an address (in 1994) on clinical trials, the intertwined relationship between ethical and institutional supervisional failures, and those of methodological education. 'The best solution is to teach young doctors how clinical studies should be done.' One may also quote Oxford epidemiologist, Richard Peto, 'Ignorance is the biggest form of misconduct' (cited by Kish in *Science*, 1994, July 29).

For our presumed readership of, primarily, nonspecialists, we can at this point only expand upon the general remarks already made in our review of clinical trials, point to some of the 'must' standards, encourage all of us to be mindful of the complexity and the ease by which unrecognized error in method or logic can occur, give a few examples of currently sophisticated work, and offer some suggested reading.

The American Association for Advancement of Science magazine, *Science,* finds no 'quality assurance' in clinical trial monitoring. *Science* conducted a study of clinical trial monitoring and found that there was no overall monitoring system for trials funded by the National Institutes of Health (NIH). The Special News Report of 1994 is a troubling one and should serve as a continuing reminder of problem areas even when studies are quite well designed, as one would expect from NIH-funded work. The problems are human failings. For example, randomization fails when physicians bias assignment to treatment groups, again mostly as a result of ignorance of the logic of random assignment. The failure to assure this by making all participants blind (i.e., not letting those assigning know what the treatments are and by whom they will be received) led to a finding by Schulz et al. (1994), who observed, on examining a large group of perinatal studies, that efficacy differences between treatment and control groups were greater when patient assignment to these groups was not blind; i.e., the expectations of doctor, patient, or data analyst were biased by knowing which patients were in the treatment group and thus expected to do better.

Are trial designers indifferent to quality of life?

Quality of life and functional competence measures, that 'Ziggy' ability to 'do stuff,' must be paramount in evaluating treatments – pharmacotherapeutic and otherwise – for NV. That advocacy is by no means new, but has yet to be fully persuasive. Goodwin's (1994) provocative proposal that American medicine's values rest on Puritanism suggests that it disapproves of good living, encourages self-discipline – as we know for certain it does not take full measures to alleviate terminal pain – and thus may consider as trivial how content or happy patients feel. 'What does it matter if a woman suffers from nausea? Life is hard! Pain builds character.' Or some such. There are good questionnaires and rating scales, some of which are carefully standardized – if one would only use them. There are also dozens of measures of variables likely to affect NV; some are of the sort already noted in these chapters, such as demographics, personal history, personality, anxiety; others are possible physiological baseline variables such as responsivity of the autonomic nervous system, related cortisol levels, and of course those parts of the precipitating situation, including iatrogenic ones, that are the often dominant determinants of kinds and duration of surgery, anesthetics used, kind, dosage, and cycle of cancer chemo- or radiotherapy, the interaction between anesthesiologist and patient, comfort given, diet, etc. The list is not yet endless because there is insufficient research to define major sources of individual difference by setting and precipitating context, and their likely interactions which have not been demonstrated, statistically, except for in a few experiments.

Conclusion for consumers

Our goal here is to be persuasive about NV complexity and to let consumers know that much of the clinical trial work is not sophisticated. There is as yet no study (or it may never be possible) that tries to put all known variables into the hopper and make observations on thousands of cases because these are systematically (1) controlled as identified and (2) manipulated, including interaction observations.

There are a few research groups, e.g., the Italian Group, which appear to have in mind a program of studies. We hope for more such endeavors. In the meantime, the consumer who reads clinical trial reports, whether those presented in advertisements or those in run-of-the-mill journals, is advised to be critical, cautious, skeptical, and self-tracking. Our bodies belong to us; science as a way of knowing belongs to us all. We had best all learn it well enough to practice good healing or good self-protection as patients.

The findings in this chapter constitute a recommendation to those not well trained in research methodology to avoid taking primary responsibility for clinical trials. All of us must take responsibility for whatever treatments we employ: pharmacological, behavioral, dynamic psychological, nursing and other comforting, nutritional, or alternative. And unless engaged in approved experimental work, or knowingly exploiting placebo or general effects, the treatments employed will have been tested by clinical trials meeting standards of excellence that the consumer, who reads report, either applies directly in judgment, or by depending upon teachers, textbook writers, and reviewers who exercise these judgmental standards.

CHAPTER 6

Drugs to prevent and control nausea and vomiting: a survey of trial reports published since 1950

This chapter describes in outline what clinical trials have been published on the effectiveness of various methods of preventing or controlling nausea and vomiting (NV). The trials are presented in three dimensions: (1) the different conditions and circumstances in which NV occur; (2) the various drugs that have been used; and (3) the years in which they were published in medical journals.

First, some brief background about clinical trials: they are necessary to determine how effective a treatment is, and to do that one has to compare that treatment with what would have happened if it had not been used. We thus need a comparison group, called the control group. To make sure that any differences in outcome between the test group and the control group can be attributed to the test treatment, everything else about the groups should as nearly as possible be the same – the severity and duration of the illness or symptoms, the staff and lay carers looking after the patients, their food, and so on. The best way of making sure that the participants in the treatment and control groups are as similar as possible is to randomize them – that is to determine by chance which group each trial participant will be in. Then, the larger the groups, the more alike they are likely to be in all their characteristics. Randomization is the most effective way of minimizing bias, i.e., of allowing an objective assessment of the effect of a treatment. It is the single most important feature of a trial; evidence from randomized trials carries far more weight than information from studies in which participants were not randomly allocated to either a treatment or a control group.

Some general points about NV are important in relation to trials. One is that the likelihood of NV in a particular context is influenced by many factors (discussed in more detail in other chapters), notably the patient's previous experiences, feelings and expectations, and the drugs used – for example, analgesics, anesthetics, oxytocics. This is another important reason for the use of control groups: to assess the 'baseline risk' that NV will occur. Prevention of NV thus encompasses far more than the administration of antiemetics (AEs): it includes informing the patient about what to expect, allaying anxiety, explaining what she or he can do to minimize risk or the intensity of NV. Research on these aspects is not included in the survey described in this chapter, and is only briefly noted here. Controlled studies of the effects of psychoeducational interventions on recovery, postsurgical pain, and psychological distress in surgical patients are briefly reviewed by Devine (1992). The interventions were in three cat-egories: (1) information relevant to health care, e.g., about what was going to happen, who would do what, on self-care; (2) exercises to perform; and (3) psychosocial support, e.g., identifying and alleviating patients' concerns, encouraging questions, helping their problem-solving skills. Five randomized studies assessed N, V, or patients' use of AEs. A later review of the effects of psychoeducational interventions in patients with cancer (Devine and Westlake, 1995) found 19 randomized trials of various forms of behavior therapy, relaxation training, desensitization, or distraction to reduce the NV caused by cancer chemotherapy, including anticipatory V.

Suggestion can control as well as induce NV, as is graphically illustrated by the case of a woman with severe pregnancy V who obtained relief by taking ipecacuanha, a notorious emetic (Wolf, 1959). Placebo effects on NV can thus be powerful and must be allowed for in the design and evaluation of trials. A review of acupuncture did this (Vickers, 1996). It included 33 trials of stimulation of point P6 (on the wrist) for the control of NV in early pregnancy (seven), after surgery (21), or after cancer chemotherapy (five). The methodological quality of all the trials was debatable but 11 were judged of good quality. The point was stimulated manually or electrically, by acupressure applied manually or by an elasticated wristband, by transcutaneous nerve stimulation, or by injection. In four trials where stimulation was done under anesthesia, the effect was equal or inferior to that of the control. In 27 of the other 29 trials acupuncture was statistically more effective. The results for the different types of V were not analyzed separately.

Prevention also includes the avoidance where possible of emetic drugs and procedures. This is illustrated by three important recent reviews examining the influence of different anesthetic agents on postoperative NV (PONV):

1. The omission of nitrous oxide, a commonly used anesthetic gas, in general anesthesia (Tramèr et al., 1996)
2 The use of propofol used for induction or maintenance (with other agents), compared with other anesthetics (Tramèr et al., 1997a)
3. The comparison of those two with propofol-only anesthesia, so-called 'total intravenous anesthesia with propofol.'

In these reviews the results are expressed not only in terms of the reduction in incidence of V but also as the number-needed-to-treat (NNT) (Tramèr et al., 1997b). This is the number of patients who on average need to be treated for one of them to benefit, i.e., not to vomit.

Omitting nitrous oxide on average reduces V by between 12% and 60%, depending on the baseline risk (measured in the control group); the NNT for studies with a high baseline risk was five. When the baseline risk is thought to be low it is not worth omitting nitrous oxide. The second review showed that, when propofol was used for induction, the NNT was more than nine and when used for maintenance it was at best six, a modest and short-lived effect in preventing PONV. The third review found the trials of total intravenous anesthesia too poorly documented to permit appropriate comparisons with the other treatments.

It is also worth noting that the mechanism by which NV are produced determines their responsiveness to drugs. Drugs may prevent NV by acting at a variety of sites in the brain (see Chapters 7, 8, 9, and 25), or by blocking emetic stimuli from the periphery (e.g., the gut or the heart) from reaching the center. What a drug can achieve depends partly on its pharmacological action and partly on its ability to reach its target: drugs differ in the extent to which they enter the brain and various parts of it. A further complication is that the mechanism of NV may not be the same at different stages of an illness and its treatment. This seems to be the case with severely emetic cancer chemotherapy, where NV during the first 2 days of treatment ('early' NV) may respond to AEs differently from NV occurring later.

Method of the survey

As data from uncontrolled studies are unreliable and often misleading, this chapter summarizes only evidence from randomized clinical trials (RCTs), i.e., trials in which the participants were randomly assigned to the treatments that were being compared. Trials have also been included if it is uncertain whether randomization was performed. The trials were identified by searching the Cochrane Library, 1997, issue 3. This includes the Cochrane Database of Systematic Reviews (CDSR), other systematic reviews assembled by the York Centre for Reviews and Dissemination (CRD), and the Cochrane Controlled Trials Register (CCTR), containing over 130 000 references to RCTs published up to 1996, most with abstracts. Some additional reviews were found through personal contact with authors. The search strategy, summarized in the Addendum, aimed to categorize the trials by (1) the cause or context of the NV and (2) the drugs/treatments tested. It employed both standard Medical Subject Headings (MeSH) as used for indexing articles in Medline (the database of the US National Library of Medicine) and ordinary text words. As it was not possible to verify for every report retrieved that it primarily concerned the prevention or treatment of N/V (P/T of NV), it was decided to include all those where this remained uncertain. The number of trials may thus have been overestimated by inclusion of reports that mention P/T of NV incidentally. On the other hand, some relevant journals have not yet been systematically hand-searched by participants in the Cochrane Collaboration and will very likely be found to contain additional reports.

The titles and, where possible, the abstracts of the trials were examined to ascertain what questions each had addressed. When an abstract mentioned a drug X that was not being tested in the trial but was either given to all participants or used as 'rescue medication' when a test treatment was insufficient, that trial was omitted from the list of trials of drug X. As every RCT compares two or more treatments (i.e., one or more active treatments and a control), each trial appears several times in the detailed tables – e.g., a trial comparing ondansetron, granisetron, and tropisetron will be listed under each of the drugs.

Results

Of trials reported between 1961 and 1996, 1035 were found. In each decade the number published has increased strikingly (Table 6.1). Table 6.2 shows their distribution among the main categories of causes of NV. The great majority were performed in patients undergoing cancer chemotherapy or surgery; in most the treatments were intended to prevent or alleviate NV. Fewer trials concerned motion sickness, early pregnancy, migraine, or NV associated with gastrointestinal disease.

Table 6.1: Number of trials published, by 5-year periods, 1961–96

Years	Number	Years	Number
1961–65	2	1981–85	94
1966–70	47	1986–90	229
1971–75	33	1991–95	481
1976–80	48	[1996	101]

Table 6.2: Number of trials by type of NV

Cancer therapy	500
Palliative care in cancer	4
Postoperative/anesthesia	425
Gastrointestinal disorder	24
Early pregnancy	23
Motion sickness/labyrinthine	18
Migraine	13
Pharmacology of AEs	22
Others (e.g., mountain sickness)	6

The drugs tested

Table 6.3 shows the sequence in which drugs used in order to control NV were introduced into medical practice. It also shows, separately for each main therapeutic category in which the drug was tested, for which year the Cochrane Controlled Trials Register records the first trial.

Atropine and scopolamine (hyoscine), the belladonna alkaloids, have been used in anesthesia for over 100 years, but not primarily to prevent N or V. In fact atropine has no useful effect on V, but scopolamine is a strong sedative and also prevents motion sickness. It was the first drug shown to do this and continues to be useful for the purpose. The sedative effect makes it unsuitable for use against pregnancy sickness.

The antihistamines were developed and used first to treat allergic conditions, but their effect against motion sickness was discovered quite early, in the 1950s and 1960s, especially with the compounds listed, which resemble scopolamine in having central anticholinergic activity. Trials in postoperative care and in oncology came much later, were few, and gave unimpressive results.

All the other drugs in Table 6.3 are too 'heavy' for use in pregnancy sickness or motion sickness. The phenothiazines were quickly

Table 6.3: Drugs used in control of NV

Drug class	Main members	Year when introduced	Year of 1st trial in: PONV	Chemo	Motn	Prg
Anticholinergics	atropine	(19th century)	60	–	–	–
	scopolamine (hyoscine)	(19th century)	61	–	51	–
Antihistamines (H_1-receptor blockers)	promethazine	1949	67	82	51	55
	dimenhydrinate	1950	71	90	50	–
	hydroxyzine	1957	63	93	–	–
	cyclizine	1958	66	76	67	–
	meclizine	1962	–	–	66	62
	cinnarizine	1968	–	91	94	–
Phenothiazines	chlorpromazine	1954	55	83	–	–
	perphenazine	1958	58	–	–	–
	prochlorperazine	1958	66	59	66	–
	thiethylperazine	1964	65	83	66	–
Butyrophenones	haloperidol	1960	–	–	–	62
	droperidol	1968	70	83	–	–
Dopamine antagonists	metoclopramide	1966	67	79	73	–
	domperidone	1977	78	79	–	–

Table 6.3: (contd)

Drug class	Main members	Year when introduced	Year of 1st trial in: PONV	Chemo	Motn	Prg
Corticosteroids	dexamethasone	1959	91	83	–	–
	methylprednisolone	1962	–	83	–	–
Cannabinoids	dronabinol	1975	–	75		
	nabilone	1978	94	79	–	–
Anesthetics	propofol	1985	85	–	–	–
$5HT_3$ antagonists	ondansetron	1989	91	89	89	–
	granisetron	1990	94	90	–	–
	tropisetron	1991	94	90		

Notes: PONV = postoperative NV; Chemo = chemotherapy; Motn = motion sickness; Prg = early pregnancy.

tested against PONV and mostly much later in oncology. Droperidol is related to them and shares this pattern.

With nabilone, on the other hand, trials in oncology came first, and this also happened with the serotonin $5HT_3$ antagonists, but, with these, studies on PONV followed within 2–4 years.

Successive waves of clinical research

Motion sickness

Trials in motion sickness came first, but there have been few. They were led by large studies on sailors at sea. Then laboratory studies predominated, because they made it possible to control the stimuli precisely. In the 1960s the drugs studied were scopolamine and the antihistamines. In 1973 metoclopramide was tried. An adhesive skin patch delivering scopolamine over 72 hours was tested from 1979 to 1986, and found effective and convenient. In 1989 ondansetron was found to be no better than placebo, suggesting that the structures in the brain on which this class of drug acts play no part in motion sickness. In the same year, the control of neither balance, nor the eye movements associated with posture, was found to be affected by powdered ginger. In 1994 cinnarizine was found to be effective both in the laboratory and at sea. In 1995 P6 acupuncture was tested, and in 1996 scopolamine was found to diminish unpleasant symptoms induced by exposure to virtual reality. The sponsorship for motion sickness research has come mainly from military and space exploration programs.

Early pregnancy

Jewell and Young (1996) systematically reviewed 21 trials that met their inclusion criteria. Of these, 17 tested drug treatments, among them the following nine antihistamines: buclizine (in one trial), dimenhydrinate (one), doxylamine in Debendox/Bendectin (three), hydroxyzine (one), meclozine (three), mepyramine (one), pro-methazine (two), thiethylperazine (one), and trimethobenzamide (one). Nine of the 12 antihistamine trials were published between 1951 and 1964, the heyday of this group of drugs, the other three in the 1970s. Two trials compared pyridoxine (vitamin B_6) with placebo; in six of the antihistamine trials pyridoxine was either given as part of the test drug or used as a control. Antihistamines can clearly reduce the incidence of NV, and pyridoxine may do so. The first-generation antihistamines commonly cause sedation, however, and this limits their usefulness. Two other medications tested in single trials were adrenocorticotropin (ACTH) injection, which had no apparent effect, and powdered ginger root, which weak evidence suggests may have helped. Four trials of P6 acupressure (at the wrist) in pregnancy were published between 1988 and 1996; the results were equivocal. The Cochrane Controlled Trials Register lists two further trials: an *n*-of-1 trial for treatment of hyperemesis gravidarum (Magee and Redman, 1996), and a trial of sensory afferent stimulation at the wrist (Evans et al., 1993).

PONV

Work on the NV that often follow surgery PONV began with the study of various drugs used before or after surgery, and of different anesthetic regimens. Table 6.4 shows when trials testing each drug appeared. Two drugs, metoclopramide and droperidol, have regularly featured in trials for around 30 years and seem to have become the standard drugs against which new ones are compared.

The oldest drugs, scopolamine, atropine, and promethazine, continue to pop up in trials repeatedly, presumably because they are deeply rooted in traditional anesthetic practice.

Prochlorperazine may also belong to this group. The effects on PONV of chlorpromazine, hydroxyzine, thiethylperazine, and domperidone have aroused only passing interest. Propofol has intrigued investigators because it may be the first anesthetic that helps to reduce the risk of PONV. Dexamethasone remains a mystery: it has turned out to be a valuable component of combin ation AE therapy in cancer chemotherapy, and this led to trials for PONV.

Two reviews have examined published trials of ondansetron for PONV. Tramèr et al. (1997c) examined its effectiveness given intravenously in established PONV early (0–6 hours) and late (6–24 hours) after administration. They found nine trials in eight reports, five comparing different doses of ondansetron with placebo, two comparing it with droperidol, and one with metoclopramide. The three doses of ondansetron tested (1, 4, and 8 mg) were similarly effective; no evidence was found that droperidol or metoclopramide differed. During the preparation of the review, it was discovered that one multicenter trial had been published three times, with different titles and by different authors. This raised a general question about the impact of duplicate publication on reviews, which the authors

Table 6.4: PONV: reports of trials of AEs. Numbers by drug tested and year of publication

Drug	<65	65/9	70/4	75/9	80/4	85/6	87/8	89/90	91/2	93	94	95	96
chlorpromazine	1	1											
perphenazine	2	2	3		1	1						1	
atropine	1	2				1				2	1	1	
scopolamine	2	6		2	2								
hydroxyzine	1	1	3		1	4	4	8	5	1	4	5	1
thiethylperazine		3	1										
prochlorperazine		1		1				3		1		1	1
promethazine		1	4	2		1			2	1	1	2	1
metoclopramide		4	6	2	4	5	3	6	12	5	11	8	7
droperidol			1	2	4	6	7	11	14	9	8	25	15
domperidone				5	2	2							
propofol							1	1	5	4	9	12	17
dexamethasone									1		2	1	4
ondansetron									11	10	16	15	21
granisetron											1	3	6
tropisetron											2	1	5

Total no. of trials categorized = 425.

tackled next (Tramèr et al., 1997d). They examined 84 trials of ondansetron for PONV, published between 1991 and September 1996, and found that 17% of published full reports and 28% of the patient data were duplicated. Trials reporting greater treatment effects were much more likely to be duplicated. Inclusion of duplicated data in their meta-analysis led to a 23% overestimation of ondansetron's AE efficacy. GlaxoWellcome, the manufacturers of ondansetron (Zofran), have not responded to the analysis in the *British Medical Journal*. However, when pressed by a journalist, they acknowledged the duplicate publications but 'denied taking part in any attempt to exaggerate the efficacy or safety of Zofran,' putting the responsibility for the misleading publications on their investigators (Matthews, 1997).

The explosive ondansetron trials program has the hallmarks of a strategic marketing battle plan, and it will be difficult for the makers of the competing drugs granisetron and tropisetron to amass a database of comparable size, even though they have made a prompt start. However, the extensive duplicate publication of data uncovered by Tramèr et al. (1997d) shows that bulk may be deceptive, and that reliable conclusions will require detailed analyses.

Children were studied in 90 of the 425 trials of PONV: they deserve separate detailed review. Forty of them concern squint surgery, in which the risk of V is particularly high. Tramèr et al. (1995) reviewed 24 of these 40 trials, with 38 treatment arms. The drugs studied were droperidol, metoclopramide, atropine, scopolamine, dixyrazine, ondansetron, lorazepam, lidocaine (lignocaine), and propofol. For droperidol only the highest of four doses given (0.75 μg/kg) reduced the proportion of patients who developed V, by about two-thirds. Metoclopramide (0.15 or 0.25 mg/kg) was similarly effective. Propofol was not very effective and often undesirably slowed the heart; the authors conclude that it should not be used in strabismus surgery. The effectiveness of the other drugs was found to be poorly documented. The authors end with an important point:

> Preventing vomiting in these children is clearly desirable and would also reduce enforced overnight stay and re-admission. What is striking is that rates of vomiting in the control groups varied widely across the studies . . . Postoperative vomiting has many causes. At what point is prophylaxis a sledgehammer used to crack a nut? If on average 50% of children vomit without treatment, and the best studied regimen prevents vomiting in 75%, then the real 'yield' is 25%. This begs the question as to whether it would be better to wait and see who vomits and then treat. That is the pragmatic question that needs to be answered and perhaps defines the research agenda.

Cancer treatment

The prevention and control of V caused by cancer chemotherapy and radiotherapy became an increasing challenge as more and more combination chemotherapy regimens came into use. Almost all cytotoxic drugs used to treat cancer are emetic. Even those referred to as 'moderately emetic' are very unpleasant for most patients receiving them, but the 'severely emetic' cisplatin compounds are worse. Effective AE prophylaxis and therapy are therefore an essential component of modern cancer treatments. This is the one category of NV that is often a matter of life and death, because it may be so bad that the patient is unwilling to accept a treatment that offers some chance of a cure. Great efforts are being made to find practical solutions to the problem. Several complementary strategies are being followed:

1. A search for effective anti-cancer drugs that cause less NV, preferably none
2. A search for new effective AE drugs
3. Working out the best ways of using the existing drugs, in terms of dosage, timing, and combination of drugs with differing pharmacological actions.

The second of these led to the development of the $5HT_3$ receptor antagonists, the third to the realization that the initially recommended doses of some drugs, e.g., ondansetron, were higher than necessary, and that it is often worth combining a dopaminergic drug such as metoclopramide or a $5HT_3$ antagonist with lorazepam and dexamethasone.

Table 6.5 shows, in chronological order, when trials testing each drug appeared (drugs used in fewer than five trials are not shown). The drugs at the top of the table were tested and came into use first. It is worth noting that cisplatin, which causes far worse NV than other cytotoxic drugs, became widely used in cancer chemotherapy in the early 1980s, and dramatically moved the goal posts for AE therapy. A little over half of the 500 trials in cancer chemotherapy involved patients receiving cisplatin. Children were included in only 28 trials of NV in cancer therapy.

In the first period, up to the mid-1980s, the two cannabinoids dronabinol and nabilone were tested, but then faded away. The most widely and continuously tested drugs since their introduction into cancer therapy have been metoclopramide and dexamethasone. Domperidone was tested concurrently: it has a similar action to

Table 6.5: AEs in cancer chemotherapy: reports of trials. Numbers of reports by drug tested and year of publication

Drug Years	70/4	75/9	80/4	85/6	87/8	89/90	91/2	93	94	95	96
prochlorperazine	1	2	6	7	3	4	3	6	2	2	2
dronabinol		4	11	9	4	1	1		1	1	
domperidone		3		4	4	1	1		1	1	
metoclopramide		2	16	34	35	33	40	19	15	16	13
nabilone		1	3	6	3						
thiethylperazine			2	2	2	1	1	2			
chlorpromazine			5	4	3	6	2	3		1	
lorazepam			4		5	11	8	6	4	3	1
dexamethasone			5	16	21	19	32	17	19	18	12
methylprednisolone			4	9	9	8	10	4	2	3	3
droperidol			1		1		2	1		1	
ondansetron						6	35	21	21	23	19
granisetron						6	9	12	8	21	8
tropisetron							4	3	10	5	6

Total no. of trials categorized = 500.

metoclopramide but unlike the latter has little effect on the brain. This is probably a disadvantage, because cytotoxic drugs cause V through a mechanism in the brain.

Methylprednisolone is closely related to dexamethasone and has similar effects; the main differences are that it causes some sodium retention, acts for a shorter time, and is perhaps less convenient to inject. These modest differences may account for the wider use of dexamethasone in trials and in practice.

The neuroleptic AEs prochlorperazine, thiethylperazine, chlorpromazine, and droperidol have played a minor and steadily diminishing role. Their AE effects are accompanied by severe drowsiness and a range of other effects which may be more disturbing in cancer chemotherapy than in postoperative care. The rise of lorazepam began in the early years of cisplatin therapy, and it is now widely used in AE regimens. Its special contribution is to wipe out the memory for the NV. A patient who does not remember how awful the last cycle of therapy was is much more able and willing to accept the next.

The $5HT_3$ antagonists, a new class of drug, represent the latest wave of AEs. They have been and are being tested in many trials. As in PONV, the research field is led by ondansetron, followed by granisetron and tropisetron. Perez (1995) has compared the pharmacology and efficacy of these three $5HT_3$ antagonists in preventing chemotherapy-induced NV in seven large trials, five of them in patients treated with the highly emetic cisplatin. Each drug completely controlled V in similar proportions of patients, ranging from 44 % to 89%. In patients receiving moderately emetic therapy, comparisons of granisetron 3 mg i.v., ondansetron 8 mg i.v. or 24 mg orally, and tropisetron 5 mg i.v. have not detected any differential effects. In three of the four crossover trials patients preferred granisetron.

Finally it is interesting to compare Tables 6.4 and 6.5. Some drugs were first tested in oncology, later in PONV; with others the reverse happened.

Discussion

Devine's reviews (Devine, 1992; Devine and Westlake, 1995) underline the importance of what patients are told and understand about what will happen to them when they undergo surgery or any other treatment. Patients' beliefs and expectations, and the quality of their aftercare, can greatly affect the symptoms they experience and the intensity of these symptoms, which include NV. It has also been found in a pilot study that patients given a restricted diet while receiving cisplatin chemotherapy eat more and suffer less NV than patients who chose their own meals (Menashian et al., 1992). The design of most trials concerned with prevention and control of NV does not take account of such basic context factors, and this probably explains some of the huge variation in the incidence of NV in groups of patients who have had the same sort of operation. These aspects need to be examined and described in reports of future trials.

The reviews by Tramèr and his colleagues concerned with anesthesia and PONV fall into two groups: those examining the effects of AEs, drugs given specifically to prevent or control V (1995, 1997c, 1997d), and those examining the propensity of anesthetic agents themselves to cause PONV (1996, 1997a, 1997b). The two are complementary. This difference is even more important in cancer chemotherapy: the incidence and intensity of NV vary greatly for different treatment regimens, but with all of them AEs are needed. A point to be noted for both types of trials is that early V (in the first 6 hours after a procedure) and late V may differ in important ways, both in their relationship to the emetic stimuli and in their responsiveness to AE drugs. Data on early and late vomiting may therefore need separate analysis.

The same group of reviewers was the first in this area to introduce the notion of the number-needed-to-treat (NNT) as a means of briefly summarizing how useful a treatment is. The decision on whether or not to use prophylaxis should be related to the NNT, and this depends critically on the expected frequency of symptoms, e.g., NV, without drug prophylaxis. If the likelihood of V is small then routine use of an AE is not justified, and V or N should be treated when it occurs.

The review of ondansetron, granisetron, and tropisetron in the prevention of chemotherapy-induced NV calls attention to the need to examine separately the different doses and different routes of administration of the same drug.

Only when it has not been possible to distinguish differential effects is it appropriate to synthesize the results in a quantitative summary.

The reviews cited and discussed in this chapter are thorough, conscientious, and helpful, although some of them may not have addressed important issues that they could have included. The moral is that reviews should not be regarded as static: they are almost always in some respects incomplete and anyway quickly go out of date. Their readers should help the authors to improve and update them, as is beginning to happen with the reviews in the Cochrane Database of Systematic Reviews. The Cochrane Library includes a facility which enables readers to send comments or criticisms directly to the editors and authors of a Cochrane review by e-mail or fax. They respond and, where appropriate, incorporate or act on the points in the next revision that will replace the current version of the review in the Cochrane Library.

Finally, the reviews of trials of the effects of ondansetron on PONV reveal a serious practical problem: duplicate reporting of the same data. After they had identified the reports of the relevant studies in the literature, it took Tramèr's group many months to discover that a substantial number were duplicates. The scientific community must guard against covert duplicate publication in the future, and meanwhile reviewers must look out for it.

It seems quite likely that there is duplication among the trials surveyed for this chapter, so the numbers of trials, particularly in oncology, may not accurately indicate the extent of the research effort and should not be taken at face value. They need detailed verification which was not possible during the preparation of this chapter.

Concluding remarks

This descriptive historical survey of a broad area of clinical research is merely a beginning. But this beginning would not have been possible without the Cochrane Controlled Trials Register, laboriously assembled by people all over the world who have searched journals by hand. That work continues, and anyone can join in – contact your nearest Cochrane Centre if it might interest you.

Implications for practice

The baseline risk of NV should be considered before using drug prophylaxis; where it appears to be low, drug prophylaxis is inappropriate. It is always desirable to explain to the patient what is likely to happen and how NV will be managed should it occur. Non-drug measures are worth trying first, especially for NV in early pregnancy and often for motion sickness. Drugs known to cause NV, such as morphine and codeine, should if possible be avoided in susceptible people.

Relatively few of the drugs that have been used to prevent or treat NV have been extensively studied in controlled trials. The choice of AE treatment must be based not only on the results of good trials but also on other considerations, including the pharmacological properties of the drugs, their adverse effects, their convenience and cost. For motion sickness scopolamine hydrobromide, promethazine, and cyclizine are effective and well established. They are all sedative. If a drug is needed for NV in early pregnancy, short-term use of promethazine is a reasonable choice.

For prevention and treatment of postoperative NV metoclopramide is effective, but it is liable to cause alarming extrapyramidal reactions in young people. Droperidol is an alternative, but can be strongly sedating.

In highly and moderately emetic cancer chemotherapy prophylaxis appears to be most successful with a combined drug regimen that includes dexamethasone and lorazepam, with either metoclopramide or a $5HT_3$ antagonist or perhaps both. The best dosage, route, timing, and duration of treatment with each drug in the combination remain to be worked out for the various forms of chemotherapy.

Implications for research

Many important questions remain to be explored, among them the following, concerning:

1. The methods used in trials need to be developed and standardized, for example, the measurement of N. Del Favero and his colleagues (1992) have found that more detailed assessment of the various dimensions of N – e.g., maximal intensity, duration, and quantity – may increase sensitivity in detecting differences between treatments.

   Comparisons of assessments of endpoints made by patients and by nurses have shown differences in some important respects (Oliver et al., 1994). For example, in two crossover studies the patients recorded more V episodes, whereas the nurses recorded more anxiety and sedation than the patients. This resulted in the patients detecting a difference between the side effects of the AEs being compared that was not apparent from the nurses' forms. Some such differences reflect differences in the timing and frequency of data collection: nurses collected data regularly during the assessment period, whereas patients reported their experiences only at the end of 24 hours. Both assessments are useful.
2. The use of placebo controls: In what types of NV trials is it essential to include a placebo group of patients who receive no AE treatment? Conversely, in what types of trial is it unethical to leave some patients untreated in this way? In situations where the risk of NV is relatively low, variable, and unpredictable, it is

necessary to use a placebo; where the risk is high and predictable, and an effective treatment exists, use of a placebo cannot be justified. In between there is a gray area where the arguments seem evenly balanced.

3. Informing participants: What are the participants in a trial told about it before they are asked to take part? Reports of trials virtually never describe this, but until they do we have no means of improving what we do.
4. How are research priorities decided? How do the scientific interests of individual investigators, the interests of organizations providing health care, of pharmaceutical companies, of charities interact? To what extent and in what ways do the needs of the funding organization determine what questions a trial addresses?
5. What sorts of trials and which particular ones can in retrospect be considered to have been a waste of time and resources? At what earlier point might this conclusion have been reached? How might such mistakes be avoided in future?

Acknowledgments

I thank Iain Chalmers, Trisha Greenhalgh and Alain Li Wan Po for valuable suggestions, and Elizabeth C. Devine for additional information about the studies included in her meta-analyses.

Appendix: The search strategy

The Cochrane Library was searched using the following terms:

1.	nausea-pre* OR vomiting-pre*	[prevention]
2.	nausea-dr* OR vomiting-dr	[drug therapy]
3.	nausea-th* OR vomiting-th*	[therapy]
4.	antieme* OR anti-eme*	[antiemetic, antiemesis]
5.	1 OR 2 OR 3 OR 4	
6.	anaesthes* OR anaesthetic*	
7.	anesthes* OR anesthetic*	
8.	pre-anest* OR pre-anaesthe* OR preanaesthe*	
9.	postop* OR post-op* OR peri-op*	
10.	analgesia* OR analgesic*	
11.	6 OR 7 OR 8 OR 9 OR 10	[all to do with surgery]
12.	5 AND 11	
13.	nausea-che* OR vomiting-che*	[chemically induced]
14.	antineopl* OR neoplasms-dr*	[drug treatment]
15.	cancer-che*	[chemotherapy]

16. bone-marro* OR bonemarro*
17. irradiatio* OR radiotherap*
18. whole-body* OR hemibody*
19. 13 OR 14 OR 15 OR 16 [all cancer chemotherapy]
20. 17 OR 18 [all radiotherapy]
21. 5 AND 19
22. 5 AND 20
23. 21 OR 22 [all N or V in 13 to 18]
24. cisplatin* OR CSDD* [all cisplatin treatment]
25. 24 NOT non-cisplatin [excluding non-cisplatin]
26. ondanse* AND 23
27. tropise* AND 23
28. granise* AND 23
29. dexamet* AND 23
30. methylpred* AND 23
33. chlorprom* AND 23
32. prochl* AND 23
33. thiethylpera* AND 23
34. perphenaz* AND 23
35. metoclop* AND 23
36. domper* AND 23
37. lorazep* AND 23
38. hydroxyzine AND 23
39. cyclizine AND 23
40. nabilone AND 23
43. tetrahydroca* OR dronabinol [tetrahydrocannabinol]
42. 37 AND 23
43 -59. repeat drug searches 26 to 40, and 42 substituting 'AND 12' for 'AND 23' [use related to surgery]
60. hyoscine* OR scopolam*
61. 60 AND 12
62. 60 AND 5
63. atrop* AND 12
63. cinnariz* AND 5
64. flunariz* AND 5
65. dimenhydrinate AND 5
66. motion-sickness* AND 5
67. pregnan* and 5 [all N or V in pregnancy]
68. 61 NOT 12 [excl. postsurgical N/V]
69. meclizine* AND 5
70. migraine-dr* AND 5 [drug-treatment]
71. apomorph* AND 5
72. dose-re* AND 5 [dose–response]
73. acup* AND 5 [acupressure, -puncture, etc.]
74. child* AND 12 [surgery in children]
75. child* AND 23 [cancer treatment in children]
76. strabismus AND 74

CHAPTER 7

Puzzles and possibilities confronted in experimental neuroendocrine/ pharmacoanatomical work

In this chapter we provide illustrations from experimental studies, primarily animal preparations but also studies of humans, which illustrate the difficulties facing those who would find a neat predictable (and thus relatively closed system – 'mechanisms' and 'centers') explanation to account for the phenomena of nausea and vomiting (NV). Both Chapters 2 and 4 allowed the conclusion that experimental work done to date has not identified mechanisms – whether neurotransmitters or other – whose role in NV would lead to the development of compounds constituting an entirely reliable pharmacotherapeutic armamentarium.

In this chapter we show how perplexing findings at basic levels of research can be. These findings demonstrate the difficulty that faces mechanism- and derived theory-based treatment development. However, a perplexing outcome from one or a set of experiments does not justify abandonment of mechanistic methods which have been the foundation, in fields other than NV and to some extent also in NV therapeutics, for the great advances in medicine. But a perplexing outcome does set a limiting condition on a theory underlying the generative hypothesis. And the outcome, if from good and replicable work, must be accounted for in any revised theory of processes leading to NV. As most studies are neuropharmacological, their perplexing outcomes in some ways define what other neuropharmacological messenger information-exchange system functions must be capable of. In response to this, some researchers will develop either descriptive terminology ('plasticity' is the most commonly encountered term) or new theories whereby to encompass such neuronal activities.

Specificity is one of the characteristics of NV action at the synaptic receptor, molecular level; in terms of the actions of compounds, whether as emetics or antiemetics (AEs), and specifically, which antiemetic in an animal experiment may reduce the emesis that is induced by one or another emetic. This specificity in animal studies, for example, is in remarkable contrast to the nonspecificity of clinical action defined in terms of whether or not X% of NV control can be consistently achieved in humans by using compound Y, or the definition of disability/disease targets for a compound.

But consider that a compound such as the serotonin $5HT_3$ antagonist ondansetron is now clinically employed for a *range* of NV, even though it was developed on the basis of a theory, and also the finding of *specific* serotonin receptor responses to emetogenic cytotoxins used in cancer treatment. Originally it was the serotonin receptor sensitivity, consequential as a gastrointestinal (GI) tract sensory apparatus, to cytotoxins that was invoked as an explanation of AE effectiveness. Indeed, AE specificity, measured as affinity to binding sites, can be compared for neurotransmitters acting in various transmitter systems. For example, among $5HT_3$ antagonists such as ondansetron, its affinity is 1000 times greater for its receptors than metoclopramide on those same receptors. Serotonin is known to interact with at least 14 different transmitter receptor-binding sites (Hen, 1993). Again, metoclopramide is 50 times more potent on its dopamine D_2-receptors than on its $5HT_3$ ones (Tyers, 1992).

Nevertheless, as NV treatment difficulties continue, the tendency is to apply a belief about an AE that is specific to a proposed 'neurotransmitter mechanism' for a particular kind of V to other types of N and V as well. Thus, treatment moves clinically from reliance on a neuropharmacological theory of exactness to a clinical effort to override specificity in the hope for palliation. The specificity of AE antagonists pharmacologically led Michaloudis et al. (1993) to expect a summation effect for AE drugs, such that lower doses of drugs acting on diverse sites, obviously some with high or low specific affinities, would, when combined, be more effective than any one single specific compound. Implicit to this is the important theoretical premise that NV constitute a multiple pathway phenomenon. Their results were positive. Yet the experimental literature suggests exquisite specificities in the isolated preparation. Hikasa (1992) examined α-adrenoceptor agonist subtype emetic action in the dog (clonidine, epinephrine, phenylephrine) with tests of known α-blocking agents. Yohimbine was found to be most effective against emesis, showing that only α_2-adrenoceptors appeared to be involved, with β-adrenergic, cholinergic, dopaminergic, histaminergic, serotinergic, and opiate receptors not being active. Thus when using agonists and antagonists that are known to the transmitter system, this study showed other transmitter systems not to be at work in 'the emetic pathway' of this surgically 'disconnected' and reablated animal. The problem is that, in the intact animal, there is a final common pathway that involves multiple medullary regions, parallel activity (see Hickok and Morrow, 1993), and plasticity which may include α-adrenoceptor action.

The clinical and theoretical aspects cannot be separated by the thoughtful student, when that student seeks and finds crossover NV effects using different AEs. The problem is not only that drug–drug interaction effects are unknown, but that neuropharmacological specificity as a theory must at least coexist with evidence of diffuse and diverse subsystem pathways. Given the large number of brain regions involved in precipitating and processing NV final common motor pathways, we are quite unable to state, in the case of complex human NV, where or how the full range of processes is occurring.

Serotonin antagonists in treatment of non-NV disorders

Consider that ondansetron, for example, is now employed to treat not only NV induced by cancer radiotherapy and chemotherapy and postoperative NV, but also to treat antibiotic-induced NV in pneumonia patients (Roarty and McCallum, 1995, citing Gompels et al.), pruritus, theophylline poisoning, projectile V as a result of head trauma, gastroparesis (delayed stomach emptying, mostly among younger women, often with no known cause), and also NV arising in diabetes, lupus erythematosus, and resulting from opiates and other medications, and to treat irritable bowel syndrome (the last being a nondisease according to some scholars).

Much research has been done on serotonin antagonists, all of which is important because of their widespread use in seeking to alleviate iatrogenically induced V.

Serotonin is probably the most widely studied transmitter for NV pertinency because of its extensive distribution in the GI tract, and serotonin antagonists are useful in the treatment of NV after cancer treatment. Serotonin is usually produced in response, increasing in enterochromaffin (EC) cells, under the specific influence of cytotoxins, e.g., cisplatin. Our review of experiments, many of which are also considered in the excellent discussions by Hawthorne (1995) and Roarty and McCallum (1995), yields inconsistent and challenging findings.

Gastric stasis?

Most studies report that V is preceded by gastric slowing, or stasis. We have already noted that patients with more V than N experience this static sequence, and it is also seen with the use of some pharmacological agents, which speed food transit, as AEs. We rely here on careful studies from small samples; thus again there is no epidemiology. N may occur without evidence of altered stomach activity; in the dog a great deal of gastric distention may be produced experimentally without V or signs of discomfort (as indeed can be found after a well-fed dinner) (Abbot et al., 1952; Storm et al., 1987).

Serotonin antagonists, which are the compounds used most optimistically as AEs, may not affect or can even reduce stomach motility (and do not reduce intestinal transit time) (Steadman et al., 1992), which is contrary to expectations of a linear sequence notion of mechanisms. The work of Del Beccaro et al. (1991) is pertinent, which shows that, even when stasis leads to gastric distension, V may not occur – even though death may (in this sample of cerebral palsy children). Adding to the inconsistency, Davidson and Andrews (1993) found that the highly emetogenic cytotoxin, cisplatin, induces stomach motility and yet may lead to V. The autonomy of this effect is suggested by the failure of vagotomy to abolish cisplatin motility, an effect that is not impacted at all by ondansetron.

As a further demonstration of the considerable range and variability of gastric activities, particularly for N, reference should be made to Koch (1990) who studied N of 32 pregnant women, 'most' of whom had PNV and 16 non-PNV controls; the subjects rated their PNV while undergoing gastric motility (ECG) observation. One of the non-PNV controls had an abnormal ECG. Among PNV women, most had dysrhythmias, about half had tachygastrias (this is paradoxical, given any expectation of stasis) whereas 6 of 32 had entirely normal ECGs. Self-rated N intensity scores were lower for the tachygastric group. Among dysrhythmias distributed by degree, there were no corresponding subjective associations of the intensity of discomfort. The reader concludes that subjective intensity of PNV was unrelated to the ECG, that a woman may have NV without GI abnormality, and, rarely, abnormality may be seen on the ECG without subjective discomfort.

Serotonin itself has paradoxical effects, as do other drugs acting as emetics and AEs. Antagonists are likewise paradoxical; for example, in regions found (sometimes) to be involved in V motor triggering, such as the area postrema (AP) and nucleus tractus solitarius (NTS), $5HT_3$ may be inhibitory or facilitatory. For example, Sancilio et al. (1991) found that zacopride, a serotonin $5HT_3$ antagonist, 'blocks its own emetic action.' This appears to vary at least with route of administration, dosage, individual animal, emetic source, and feeding state. Understandably, Hawthorn considers serotonin (we would add other $5HT_3$ blockers) a 'capricious' modulator which, acting on various organ systems, can initiate or reverse processes, such as heart rate. It is important in psychiatric work because it may increase anxiety. One knows that anxiety may generate or enhance NV, and one allows that the spread of its actions might in theory have a reverberating effect on NV thresholds.

Gastroenterologists who are aware of the autonomous, reflexive nature of the enteric nervous system (ENS), the GI tract, may acknowledge, when considering NV, that higher centers could receive projections activating processes there (see Davis et al., 1986), but tend to state that V itself proceeds independently as a 'reflex.' However, it is the autonomous GI reflex that appears to require afferent/efferent paths to various medullary motor centers, where this output affects respiratory, cardiovascular, and other autonomic nervous system (ANS) activities. This activates V, and projections to the cerebral cortex activate awareness of V where cerebrocortically mediated events can suppress the response. Roarty and McCallum (1995) suggest that these lead to large-scale serotonin release from the small intestine, thus becoming 'overloaded' with serotonin circulating to receptor-rich areas such as the AP, chemoreceptor trigger zone (CTZ), and NTS, or in parallel, activating the vagus.

A definitive study in dogs by Fukai et al. (1993) showed that, on treatment with intravenous cisplatin, the rise in 5HT was up to three times the basal levels within 100–180 minutes, with V beginning at 115 minutes. Blood plasma 5HT levels rose more dramatically to 20 times basal levels also within this time period. It is proposed that either intestinal contractions or the absorption of blood platelets overloaded with 5HT into paraventricular or medullary regions (and thence motor pattern triggering) accounted for emesis (see also Leslie et al., 1990).

The current limitations in understanding NV activity, even when attention is restricted to the GI tract and ENS, are demonstrated when its relationship to the central nervous system (CNS) is studied, typically with respect to neuropeptides and neurotransmitters involved in overall control of GI activities. (Their characterization may be dependent upon a glandular origin or synaptic origin, on whether specific to circulating or nerve pathway, and whether neuron self-modulating or specific to axonal–dendritic synaptic activity.) Such work has been extensive and is typically carefully restricted, as has NV work to date on the medullary–vagal–GI axis.

Krowicki and Hornby in Gaginella (1995) have provided a thorough description of neuroactive substances presumed to control or interact with other information carriers involved in GI function. There are at least 21 compounds identified; these are presumably active in linking various motor nuclei of the medulla. (The research emphasizes connection via the vagus but one is now aware that the vagal connection is not essential or exclusive.) The studies specify that the medullary areas of the dorsal motor nucleus of the vagus (DMV) and nucleus ambiguus (NA) as well as the NTS are of consequence, and the group is termed 'the dorsal vagal complex' or DVC. These authors are confident that the basic organization of the vagal nuclei is understood, although again the work of Lawes (1990) and of Miller and colleagues (Miller et al., 1994; Miller, 1995) indicates that small and varying regional connectivities are a necessary conceptual tool for consideration of activities within larger regions. Microinjection and microstimulation studies reveal that particular sets of cells topically arrayed (geographically and specifically located) engage in activities also specific for spatially specific sectors of the GI tract. This is known as 'viscerotopic' organization, and is best known from visuocortical research. One is reminded from this cell- and column-specific topography that there is also a self-organizing regional activity that is not found in the much simpler medullary–enteric axis, although dendritic fields are more widely innervated. In any event, Krowicki and Hornby (in Gaginella, 1995) conclude that the DMV is the main source of preganglionic fibers to the GI tract. For those with NV interests, one is again reminded that NV may occur with a sectioned vagus, that splanchnic nerves may also be involved, and that one should not rule out circulating compounds as also being active.

Research to date, however, reveals that the nuclei of interest, and associated multiple information carriers, interact primarily with the esophagus and stomach (and from the NA to the pharynx and smooth muscle of the cardia as well), rather than with the lower region. For those of us with an NV interest only, this is pertinent knowledge – providing one considers testing the assumption that these regions are involved in NV as dysregulation as well. As it is, NV appear excluded as an interest area for those doing work on neuroactive compounds in the primary hindbrain because this deals with GI regulation. If it were shown that the regulatory and NV excitatory/disruptive activities were in some way reciprocal, with the

DMV being considered pertinent, then the NA would be added to the already implicated NTS as 'way' stations for V if not NV. We note that the area postrema is one of the medullary regions considered, although, in practice there are disagreements among anatomists working on cats as to the exact identification of this area. Differences between experimental animals, typically for studies such as those of rats and cats (as opposed to the NV requirement for V animals leading to the use of shrews, ferrets, dogs, cats, etc.), are also a problem both in definition of and thus reliability of specification of anatomical regions, and in generalizing across species to humans. Of course individual differences occur within species, some of which are quite dramatic at both anatomical levels and genetically or functionally. These make it more difficult to control variables easily.

One measure of the excellence of an experimental method is its ability to generate agreement among those using it about what is being measured and what those observed quantities/qualities are. The methods employed to date (Krowicki and Hornby, in Gaginella, 1995) have not generated the feasibility of fields acting as possible conductance networks, as opposed to study of adjacent or chain synaptic neuronal afferent connections. For general methodology providing for definition of connections in the hindbrain–GI axis, these authors describe reliance on dye and enzyme injection tracing methods for adjacent retrograde neuron identification and of pseudorabies virus tracing to allow multiple synaptic portrayal. We see from this and from other work that ablation (functional or physical), experimental innervation, c-fos tracers, various imaging methods (positron emission tomography [PET], single proton emission computed tomography [SPECT], functional magnetic resonance imaging [fMRI], magnetometry, superconducting quantum interference device [SQUID]), and potentially EEGs when higher brain level interactions are sought, may all have application. As a general issue, however, one must keep in mind that even at the level of the most controlled and detailed work, methods define what is observed, just as interventions alter what is being observed (the well-known Heisenberg effect), and contain within themselves error sources.

Many neurotransmitters have yet to be shown to carry NV processing information, but again there is disagreement. Perhaps a category of regulatory transmitter systems and molecules will yield insight. With respect to the 21 neurotransmitters reviewed by Krowicki and Hornby as bearing information on the interaction between the DVC (also hypothalamic nuclei) and enteric regions, they have not been identified by other research as possibly being involved in NV. Whether this is a discrepancy requiring further attention, or a sign of NV specificity apart from regulatory functions, has not yet been concluded. Regulatory carriers implicated in NV functions are: the catecholamines; serotonin; acetylcholine; gamma-aminobutyric acid (GABA); cholecystokinin (CCK); nitric oxide; opiates; oxytocin; vasopressin; prostaglandins (proposed in PNV); although not shown, so we suspect to be unlikely, substance P; and (probably minor) vasoactive intestinal polypeptide (VIP).

One sees that at least 12 of 21 regulatory compounds narrowly identified by the dorsal nuclei of the vagus have elsewhere been at least suggested as playing an NV role. Krowicki and Hornby themselves allow that several compounds, including *mu* opiate agonists, may not operate in the dorsal nuclei but via the ANS sympathetic pathways.

Selectivity is not specificity

Metoclopramide is a dopamine antagonist, and is widely used in high doses as an AE. As those dosages are so high, beyond receptor saturation levels, it was demonstrated that metoclopramide may be a $5HT_3$ antagonist as well. Current psychiatric pharmacology focuses on the role of serotonin–dopamine interactions as central to schizophrenia, or at least its treatments (Kapur and Remington, 1996). Psychiatric pharmacotherapies involve $5HT_{1A}$ and $5HT_2$ receptors, not $5HT_3$ whose antagonists are the AEs. ($5HT_3$ differs from these in how signals are carried. For $5HT_3$ only they are transduced by ion-gated channels; however, there are multiple 5HT receptor subtypes in the bowel.) One understands how delineation of precise roles for 5HT has so far eluded researchers. Even so, molecular selectivity, as opposed to specificity, is such that, in higher doses (just as with dopamine), agonists and antagonists may have diffused their multi-receptor spread of effect.

A question arising for NV is the possibility not simply of a mixture of transmitters as the mode of neuronal receptor site activity, each being presumed to have a stable synaptic pattern, but also of effects resulting from information interactions induced subsequently via new pathways and in heretofore uninvolved regions. For example, when both vagus and splanchnic nerves are sectioned, both can play roles in V with the vagus presumed to be foremost, and novel, i.e., unattributable, V activity can occur (Andrews et al., 1990). It is the emergence of novel, unexpected V, when presumed essential paths, regions, and messengers are absent or when novel time sequences are experimentally imposed, that has led some of the foremost workers so strongly to call attention to 'plasticity.' It is this general characterization, coupled with paradox, puzzle, and inconsistency, that at the level of the experimental study appears to parallel clinical trial and NV prevalence findings as set forth in Chapters 3 and 4.

Even at the level of specific sensory cells in the gut, it is the case that single neurotransmitter theories (as with single motor ones) must be modified by acknowledging multiple messengers. Nor, for example, is synaptic activity itself all or none, simple or without intrinsic determination, because synapses are themselves remarkably complex multigradient information exchange centers. But, even when one is dealing with a single subset of actors, as with $5HT_3$ antagonists, subtle molecular differences can make major differences in AE efficacy. Ondansetron and granisetron are commonly used AEs, whereas zacopride, which experimentally also blocks serotonin receptors, is observed to be an emetic as well as an AE; for example, 'in ferret ZCP and its antinomers both cause and prevent emesis and defecation with different doses.' However, one learns from another study that the emetic effect of zacopride was blocked by zacopride and tropisetron (another $5HT_3$ antagonist) in ferrets depending upon manner of administration and prior feeding.

There is a very important receptor density variable. This varies with estrus cycle and may well be involved in female NV. Odor sensitivity is an item of interest along with cyclical cerebral cortical changes. It is not simply what the receptor affinities are as defined by binding, but how many receptors there are. The work of Dorries, discussed by Arnholdt (Serby and Chobar, 1992), finds that the density of serotonin receptors in rat olfactory bulb glomeruli varies with estrus cycle stage. As olfaction does vary with female hormonal levels, i.e., there is a pituitary–olfactory and thence an amygdala–cerebral cortical integration, the question arises as to whether this factor of estrus receptor density may be operating for any NV process involving olfaction and/or cerebral awareness. The same question applies to cholinergic ANS involvement. As females are more sensitive to NV, whether from cancer chemotherapy or postoperative NV (PONV), and women's PONV is shown to be a dependent on menstrual cycle status (Lindblad, 1989; Hokavaara, 1991), it appears that research is in order. Allowing that the pituitary hormones/neuropeptides are active, and knowing that increases in vasopressin level can induce as well as be induced by NV, one may wish to look for NV sex variation determinants beyond the GI tract. If there is no accounting for female risk within the ENS as a self-contained system, one puts the degree of such autonomy for NV in question.

Quite importantly, as odor sensitivity may be learned not only as a function of general exposure and enhanced discriminatory efforts (as in perfumiers), but also sexually from endocrine sensitization, there may be proliferation of receptors that are specifically odor sensitive, particularly with respect to steroids (Dorries in Serby and Chobar, 1992). So it appears not only that cyclic modulation of receptors for sensitivity is driven by sex hormones, but also that short- or longer-term, learned receptivity then occurs as density, area of glomeruli, cell size, and sensory neuronal organization all become more competent at steroidal odor molecule recognition. (This is true for others as well; see discussion in Chapter 12 on the major histocompatibility complex HLA trait sensitivity that determines women's preferences for men, which changes with progesterone levels.)

Yet there may be a slender clue to sex difference, because Rao (1992) studied the benzamides in rabbits (which do not vomit) and found a greater gastroprokinetic bioavailability. The problem was that these should be associated with greater gastric stasis, so there is reduced V risk. Indeed, one might expect (if human bioavailability is the same) substituted benzamides to be thus less effective as AEs in females. Their bioavailability, however, would be a matter of bioavailability of any combination of neuroactive or kinetic compounds. This would seem to be in question within the confines of hormone thinking. One is forced to entertain the most complex subsystem notions, for example, interacting expansions. Think about those neuropeptide/endocrine flows shown in Chapter 9. Given the reminder by Dowling (1979) that there are hundreds of billions of neurons in the brain, most of which are capable of thousands of connections using graded and alternative actions, with (in 1989) at least 40 synaptic modulators, and that cells send, receive, or modulate information, then one must continue to assume that it is the definition of subsystems and their interactions under perturbed (and thus probabilist) circumstances that is a conceptual requirement. And at this point, one entertains the recollection that perhaps differing basic variables such as widely distributed estrogen receptors exist.

Gastric function is shown to be sensitive to olfaction, and NV, related to conditioned taste aversion, are postulated by McLean and Shipley (1992) to occur through a system based on anatomical evidence of main olfactory bulb (MOB) projections to (mouse) insular cortex. Estrogen levels have an influence.

Possibly the medial frontal cortex integrates these MOB signals, where visceral and olfactory information converges and from which there are projections to the NTS and ventral medulla. (It is also the case that odor messengers go to the medial preoptic nucleus of the amygdala.) This region, in turn, is influenced by estrogen levels affecting mRNA, as well as by cells containing cholecystokinin (CCK) (also produced by intestinal mucosa). With pituitary involvement, one may assume that these affect all mammalian sexual behavior. Given the density of serotonin receptors in the NTS, the question must again be asked as to the extent of reflexive NV's autonomous integrity within the ENS-medullary axis, for connectivities here allow interactions at the olfactory and hormone levels as an NV process route that is influenced by estrogen levels, CCK, and, for olfaction and NTS, serotonin. Olfactory pathways also project to the hypothalamus and other aspects of the limbic system (wherein lies the amygdala), which is in turn of consequence because the hypothalamus via the ANS, and including pituitary functions, is a homeostatic regulator, as are downstream medullary nuclei, with regulating 'way stations' also found in the GI tract.

Further complexity, which could eventually yield explanations, come into it when it is realized that $5HT_3$ receptor antagonists can inhibit skin pain, including that in visceral organs; whereas granisetron appears to have this effect in duodenal inflammation, ondansetron does not. The effects of granisetron depend on the route of administration; intravenous administration is effective, but intracerebroventricular administration is not. Similarly surprising differences are seen in AE effects, depending on the manner and locale of administration. In this instance one would exclude a CTZ ventricular site for granisetron – at least with respect to GI pain. Contrariwise, ondansetron is found to reduce upper GI pain such as heartburn with no effect on abdominal pain.

Interestingly, one hypothalamic projection extends to the suprachiasmic nucleus controlling circadian rhythms. This rhythmic function is considered with respect to PNV as 'morning sickness'. Mitchelson (1992), in a fine review of emetic drugs, observes that, at least in cancer treatments, N risk appears to be inversely related to urinary cortisol excretion which is not simply a stress variable. One might expect a direct N to cortisol relationship (see Grundberg and Singer in Caccioppo and Tassinary, 1990), but this may vary with circadian rhythm. Corticosteroids of course have major physiological functions, including, generally, resistance to many noxious stimuli, anti-inflammatory action, facilitating some adaptation, and effects on mood; under acute administration mood elevation is found (see Haynes, in Gilman et al., 1993).

Levels of cortisol are also involved and can become measurable risk factors. What generates cortisol increase other than 'stress' or 'emotion'? The answer could be biorhythms as well as the crucial cyclicity of the reproductive woman.

The work of Hursti et al. (1993) affirms that lower endogenous cortisol levels predict greater NV risk for cancer chemotherapy. These investigators link this effect to corticosteroids, which act as AEs, and propose that higher endogenous levels that are shown to protect against NV are equivalent to the AE effects of exogenous cortisol. In a welcome demonstration of a theoretical test affecting drug efficacy, it was shown that ondansetron–corticosteroid (dexamethasone) treatment cocktails work best on patients with low urinary cortisol levels. One may infer that whatever variable is determining baseline cortisol levels is also an NV threshold variable. One wonders, for example, whether cognitive memory processes may themselves contribute to acute cortisol level changes. Ask, for example, whether the 80% of anticipatory nausea and vomiting (ANV) patients in Kvale et al's (1991) study who were asked to imagine earlier cancer treatments and who reported N upon thinking about it (compared with no NV when 'imagining' other medical procedures) had acute cortisol changes or, alternatively, lower cortisol levels? Boakes et al. (1993) also found that thoughts could provoke ANV, as could odors, whereas Andrykowski and colleagues (Andrykowski and Redd, 1987; Andrykowski, 1990) found that state (chronic) anxiety was an ANV predictor. Obvious contradictions exist because higher stress, itself ordinarily predictive of acute cortisol rise, also predicts ANV. Just as multisystem plasticity is invoked for neuroanatomical uncertainty in V, so too are there complex relationships in psychoendocrinological investigations.

In considering cortisol–NV relationships, one must not exclude attention to biorhythms as an underlying covariance. In consideration of PONV, we shall see that the menstrual cycle phase strongly affects NV operative risk. What is the role of daily rhythms in these situations, excluding sleep, as baseline or subsystem variables in the suprachiasmic or other systems.

Is the PNV that is 'morning sickness' indeed dependent (presuming CNS and enteric coordination) on diurnal rhythm controls? In the same way one may ask whether what appears to be the pulsating release of vasoactive intestinal polypeptide (VIP) to such structures as the raphe nucleus may in any way contribute to or participate in the rhythmicity, indeed the pulsating spasticity, of V itself. Indeed is the GI tract ever 'autonomous' in NV? Investigators must ask about sensory linkages and 'downward' controls.

In any event the 'autonomy' and intrinsic reflexive control of the GI tract is by no means agreed upon, with functional anatomists in conflict with pharmacological gastroenterologists. It is our view that the evidence is stronger for 'override' capabilities from ANS, sympathetic and parasympathetic, to ENS sources as diverse as the cerebral cortex, hippocampus, thalamus, and reticular arousal system; most of this occurs via the hypothalamus which, in turn, activates endocrine messenger systems and smaller control centers in the brain stem, including the NTS.

Linkages of NV activation with simultaneously operative sensory apparatus are not excluded as NV influences. For example, olfaction can be powerfully affected by cancer chemotherapy. The olfactory tubercle itself projects to the thalamus (medial dorsal nucleus) and the orbitofrontal cortex is presumably active in sensory integration and contributes to awareness of smell and, as shown by lesions, it is shown to be necessary for odor discrimination.

At the very least we propose the presence of potential olfactory–neuropeptide/hormonal–amygdala–NTS 'downward' controls, which are capable of being affected by AEs for any class of messengers contained in such structures/regions cited above. How could this input, which is demonstrated in animal anatomical studies, not be active when there is strong clinical and epidemiological evidence that odors affect NV, not simply in the supersensitive PNV woman, but in other humans as well.

Multiple, 'timely,' and diminishing

Chapter 4 (and this chapter as well) discuss why a number of purported AE compounds have dual and opposing effects. In animal and human studies, dosage is considered to be the likely variable, which in turn allows speculation about altered receptor impact. For example, a dopamine antagonist molecule at a higher saturation occupies other neurotransmitter system receptors. There are, however, data showing that time variables are essential for neuronal learning and synaptic action, i.e., when information arrives and how it is paired with other information. These are predicted by Stein and Meredith (1993b) and the Haaken–Kelso theory of space–time as a definition for the self-organizing pattern of energy flows in the CNS. Thus, we can ask whether increasing attention to time sequence rhythmicity would reveal that more than simple dosage effects are involved.

An investigation by Makale and King (1992) bears on these matters. They found that, by employing laparotomy, then radiation, and varying the time of intrusion, conscious ferrets always vomited; the unconscious others did not. In the same way, V in anesthetized ferrets was reduced by splanchnectomy, but sectioning did not reduce it in conscious animals. If the interval between vagotomy and irradiation was 4–9 hours, the vagotomy group showed reduced V. If the interval was 7 days, vagotomy did not reduce V. We see that V is dependent on consciousness, so its effect in reducing V is only on the unanesthetized preparation, and that the vagotomy effect is both consciousness and temporally dependent, i.e., interactive. One may use terms such as 'plasticity,' 'redundancy', or 'adaptation' as descriptions of the processes themselves. We may accept that consciousness is a profound variable at least in mammals. For V induced by constant dosages of an emetic compound, it was found that, when there was vagotomy followed by splanchnectomy, or when there was only the latter, thresholds were higher than when splanchnectomy was the initial procedure followed by vagotomy. In this case, thresholds dropped by 40%. The sequential variable is identified by Miller's group (1994) in another study showing plasticity and combination of visceral nerve sectioning when serotonin agonists were employed to lower thresholds.

Characterizing any compound or situation as 'emetic' is simply a statement, because we see that whether N or V occurs depends on a host of variables identified or unknown interactions. The emetic trait is putative. It cannot be applied in species that do not vomit and in those clinical cases in humans also found to be incapable of V. Variables that investigators may believe account for results may not take into account uncontrolled variables, and the process of NV is such that, even under the most controlled of animal experimental conditions, completely accurate predictions are not expected.

Biederman and Davey (1993), who aimed to suggest a method for ultimately avoiding V in humans, based their work on rats. In this study of the association of V induced by a rotating platform it was found that the emetic (in this case, pentobarbital) could lose its initial emetogenic trait as a result of being paired with benign food or flavor. What is purportedly shown is that a particular precipitating emetic condition can be prevented by use of a clue associated with the earlier experimental desensitization, whereas the thrust of their thinking is on the use of such a design for food/flavors, e.g., saccharine paired with lithium to be employed as a cue to act as a preventive with people before chemotherapy. The claim is that the timing, pairing, and comparative awareness of prior emetic experience, including its diminution, is an experiment that can be applied to treatments. Given the unreliable association between conditioned taste aversion and NV, we suspect not. But if the basic data about rat desensitization to pentobarbital are replicable, this allows at least a further complexity and qualification of variables in animal studies.

For humans, the risk forecast is hardly of desensitization over the short term when highly probable emetic circumstances are employed. One may find that the reported experience and aging reduction of motion sickness provide evidence of desensitization. Consider that patients in cancer chemotherapy treatments who repeat chemotherapy cycles are more at risk of NV than naïve patients when the same AEs are given; in the case of metoclopramide used for control of variceal bleeding, initial control is 80% but on administration for rebleeding it drops to 60%. Such figures are not, however, written in stone. One may wish to contemplate whether time is an intrinsic mediating variable, possibly termed a 'modulator' itself. If so, the failure of most AEs to control chemotherapy-delayed NV is not simply because delayed NV have a different pattern expressed by different processes, but because time may be conceived in terms of attenuation or sensitization to NV perturbations interacting with AE compounds and dosage. Should Biederman and Davey be on target, one adds, as possible variables, conditioning or other learning.

At the animal level, in the cat, abdominal vagotomy and splanchnectomy slow the appearance of V upon cisplatin administration. Neither the afferent signal to medullary regions, nuclei such as the AP, the NTS, nor the motor afferent pattern that triggers V via the vagus can be accounted for in this instance. And when there is either vagotomy or splanchnic nerve section, it has the only effect that it takes a higher dosage of this emetic, but it is not abolished. One does not rule out that the threshold here may have a time component as well. When one reads the work of Miller and Nonaka (1992), describing combined vagal and splanchnic lesions, one learns that again dose thresholds for emesis were raised, but V was not abolished.

In these studies time is a dosage variable, and there is possible evidence of several V pathways; however, reduction in V is not elimination and individual differences within species can be dramatic. Koga and Fukuda (1990) concluded, using inference from muscle recordings in decerebrate animals, that the 'activity of arterial and/or central chemoreceptor afferents must exceed some (CO_2) critical level to induce transition from retching . . . to V.'

A major experimental contribution demonstrating 'plasticity'

In the same way, again with a major experimental contribution to the demonstration of plasticity, Miller and Nonaka (1992) found using the cat: (1) individual variation in emetic response to the serotonin $5HT_3$ agonist phenylbiguanide (PBG) with regard to its occurrence at all, i.e., for some animals it was not an emetic; (2) a range of thresholds for V from 2 to 8 mg/kg; but (3) that lesions of the AP, the nucleus to which motor pattern generation is so often attributed, had no effect on V incidence whether from PBG or from electrical stimulation of the vagus; and further (4) that thresholds, not the capacity for emesis, did increase through supradiaphragmatic vagotomy, with (5) greater threshold increase with splanchnic nerve section, although in other work the role of the splanchnic may be found to be of no consequence. Their conclusion emphasizes that, with serotonin agonists, visceral afferents play a (differential) role but the AP as medullary generator does not. In a complementary study, Jovanovic et al. (1989) found in cats that abolition of the AP abolished V induced by some but not all presumed emetics, and that individual variation was such that not all cases of AP ablation in cats affected the emetic response, again varying with intended emetic stimulus.

We call attention in the findings of these studies to differences among animals in their individual emetic dispositions, to inconsistency in the role of medullary centers as a function of the transmitter system proximally stimulated, and to the fact that even vagotomy does not eliminate emesis. Other regions and pathways are at work and the plasticity so beautifully documented experimentally by Miller and Nonaka must conceptually lay to rest simple medullary–enteric, hardwired, reflex circuitry notions.

It is useful to entertain plasticity as a general function. Lashley's famous work in the 1930s on higher cerebral function in the brain-injured or operated human showing substitutability is repeated here, apparently with regard to the ENS and medullary motor regions. This plasticity is complemented by the specificity in animals when it is found that V control depends upon which emetic is administered. The clinical studies in humans also suggest specificity for AEs such as the serotonin $5HT_3$ antagonists. On the other hand, corticosteroids with no known immediate gastric V effect may have a more general AE action. Some suggest that producing a sense of well-being, inhibiting anxiety, or at least reducing that experience of pain arising from NV perturbations may otherwise intensify those nociceptive afferent impulses.

For an overview discussion of pain, see Jessel and Kelly in Kandel et al. (1991). As one considers how awareness of pain is not the same as the 'raw' impulse, keep in mind the statement, 'The relationship between the perception of pain and the activation of nociceptors is a good example of the principle: All perception involves an abstraction and elaboration of sensory inputs' (page 385). Note that nociception as an afferent impulse is enhanced by neuropeptides and neurotransmitters of which serotonin is one, in addition to prostaglandins and substance P, and this is of potential relevance in considering future work on NV at levels beyond the GI tract. In so far as NV and pain overlap, antagonists of serotonin, such as histamine, may inhibit nociception. Pain is also reduced endogenously by opiate peptides, some of which may also be involved in NV by direct cortical analgesic stimulation, by descending pathways, and by spinal level stimulation of non-nociceptive tracts. This could be a kind of neural distraction or interference, which Melzack and Wall (1994) discovered and have continued to characterize as 'gating.' Extreme stress/emotion may also inhibit nociception, but whether any AE acting centrally may produce similar neurochemical effects is unknown.

Conditioning V, learning immunosuppression

Hollis (1997) analyzes pioneering work on learned immunosuppression by Ader and Cohen (1981, see also Ader et al., 1991). They used cyclophosphamide as an immunosuppressant in conditioning studies where it produced V in animals and then was paired with saccharin water (and where the cyclophosphamide produced fatalities, thus a methodological problem). Because of the Pavlovian taste–V pairing, saccharin became an effective immunosuppressant on its own. But one may ask if once paired it might also be learned V. In any event, an immunosuppressant which is also emetic can be, in animals when paired, conditioned to alter immune system function. But since we later ask if NV in humans may also have an immunomodulating impact, may not some of the immunosuppression have been at least a partial NV effect? If that were one day shown, the design of animal experiments would be compelled to consider, as Pavlov did, the learning, and as with Pavlov, individual animal difference (here fatal or non-fatal response) variables.

Fear and helplessness operating?

One is allowed the presumption that an experiment which invokes NV, and such severe physiological toxic impact that death may result, will early on generate ANS stressor response, including fear. And further, that compounds used as immunosuppressors, emetic agents may be ones to which animals are, or learn to be, odor sensitive. Odor may be in humans a powerful N and V agent, and whilst ill studies, should be capable of similar effects in sensitized, thus learned, conditioned animals. Hollis reminds us, following the work of Overmier and Seligman, and of Minor, Dess and Overmier whom she cites, that learned helplessness – 'conspecific defeat' – can be induced through conditioning. We later ask if in humans such learned helplessness, (perhaps described as 'fatigue', that so common self-attributed cause of women's NV) may not therefore be a determinant and expression of NV. In the meantime, in considering the role of conditioning, odor sensitivity to V, and then quite possibly conditioned paired stimuli (e.g. in the foregoing, a sweet flavoured water) one expects not simply the need for new controls in V studies, including environmental cues capable of being accidentally paired, thence learned, but also the likely greater complexity, possibly an experimental environment producing NV for the unanesthetized animal, subject, as we know, to individual differences in same species animals. The upshot of these questions is to suggest new variables accounting for inconsistency and plasticity in animal studies, and again to suggest that the conscious animal 'preparation' is, like us, a creature responsive at many levels to multiple stimuli.

A different source of experimental challenge: China, the South Seas, and Germany's Hegel

A different set of experiments, not carried out on animals, offers instead simple findings. They also provide intellectual challenge to theories of mechanism, specificity, and traditional medical models. They are made up of studies on NV using acupressure and analogous electrical wrist stimulation. Most were carried out by Dundee's group, but other workers (some with quite poor methodology) have brought inconsistent findings (Stannard, 1989; Dundee, 1990a, b, 1991a, b).

This is illustrated with one study (Dundee, 1990a) on chemotherapy-induced NV. Sixty-six per cent of patients were said to have full control over a 24-hour period (one infers no control over delayed NV) with only 6% not improved. There was no placebo control group, but one recognizes the findings to be within the range of acceptable clinical outcomes using data in Chapter 4 as a comparison. With respect to an expected placebo effect, we should rely on Kanigel's review (1983). This is overall about 33%; relying on Beecher's pioneering work on 1082 patients, the value is about 35%. More unusual studies lacking a theoretical and major empirical research base require greater controls in their design. This should certainly be the case if work on acupressure is to be persuasive, but one must hold all clinical trials to such a standard, and not simply unconventional approaches.

Belluomini (1994) employed as a placebo a sham acupressure point that was not consistent with the proper theory of placement, and further employed a welcome randomized and blind design. Women in the authentic (our term) placebo acupressure point group showed a significant reduction in N compared with the control group. However, neither group experienced less V. Age was an interacting variable with older women being less responsive to acupressure.

In a demanding trial design, one of excellence rarely encountered in Western trials, magnetotherapy was used; Schaoxiang et al. (1991) found total relief in about 64% of patients among a sample restricted to patients with severe NV from chemotherapy who were not responsive to pharmacological AEs. Only about 11% found no relief, compared with controls of whom 78% experienced NV. Furthermore, the Niguen point magnetic disk was applied before cisplatin administration so that the results reported are of complete prevention. A study of such consequence must be replicated in other populations, again assuring most careful controls.

A second set of challenges, which we will consider again in Chapter 12, comes from anthropologists: foremost, Margaret Mead's observations among the New Guinea Arapest, although her results are supported by other observations in nonliterate societies. As we all know, PNV is common. Ask most any physician or pregnant woman what accounts for it and these days at least one or another version of the endocrinology of being pregnant emerges. Seven anthropological studies tell us that this cannot be, because women in their studies do not have PNV. Shall all of the conflicting studies reviewed in Chapters 3, 4, and 7 be jettisoned? Not because there are non-replicable findings (which is the case), but because whole societies of women can be pregnant without experiencing NV. What kind of endocrinological etiology is this? Perhaps one should go back to the earlier psychosomatic emphasis in obstetrics (Fairweather, 1968) that PNV is all 'psychological.' Such an explanation of such cultural differences shows either a remarkable heterogeneity or inadequate observer methodology.

In this chapter, we have considered inconsistency, contradiction, surprise, and, finally, the failure of narrowly focused studies to give satisfactory illumination. As for human NV, we have seen interesting questions arise which may suggest other approaches to the exclusive singular, linear one. From a Hegelian philosophical point of view, this is inconsequential. One expects higher resolution to arise out of contradiction, i.e , synthesis to a higher form through reflective examination of apparent externalities and intuitive integration. Reconciling contradictory scientific data or integrating diversity from several levels of focus does not find such synthesis an alien process in acquiring knowledge. And we believe that it can be useful, when confronted with contradictions in data, to move to philosophic-al grounds. In Hegel's case, he would hold that it was impossible to expect rational observation of the world as a whole (here it would be of biological processes external to us) when all that the mind can comprehend of subject–object relationships is, ultimately, its own operations. It is these which, he held, shape definitions of reality, although the modern reader may be more optimistic about knowing.

As we consider the immense differences reported to this point, we suspect that, for the field of NV as it now stands, consensual scientific closure is not close at hand. We trust that going about the process of knowing in the spirit of science will eventually allow greater agreement, but a requirement is that broader perspective suggested by work and commentary, which includes work other than studies of tissue levels and counts of retching. To date there is very little work in NV beyond animal experiments and clinical trials. We forecast the interplay of levels of foci, the definition of closed systems where mechanisms exist, of relatively open systems where regional connectivities and pattern flows are dominant, and the inclusiveness of new variables for attention such as cultural or ecopsychological ones. Exact prediction at this point seems an unreasonable goal. We need new conceptual approaches, for example, those that would apply if NV were characterizable, as in Thom's chapter in *Complexity, Language and Life* (1988). In this, the terms are of a set of limited subsystems conceived as assuring regulatory homeostasis, the functions of which 'perform correctly to insure canalization of the metabolic state of the system around a specific attractor.' If one takes NV as a response to sensory, ideational, emotional perturbations beyond the design capacities of body and mind, then one faces a set of processes 'on the loose,' not canalized. Is it not difficult to write canonical equations for a 'loose cannon' perturbation?

Part III

Expanding upon the basics

CHAPTER 8

Brain–enteric regions and messengers: the latest picture in pictures

A number of brain structures have been identified as associated with nausea and vomiting (NV). The following is a summary of those findings with maps and charts to illustrate the complexity of NV (Figures 8.1–8.10; Table 8.1). Their striking feature is the obvious involvement of the brain-stem areas and the important role of higher brain regions in the NV phenomena. By no means are NV a simple reflex; they are characterized by many possible origins, mechanisms, pathways, and networks.

Our material was compiled by a search through the existing literature. Brain structures that appeared repeatedly are those mapped here. The role(s) of those structures should be included in any comprehensive theoretical work on the mechanisms and origins of NV. This map is not the final word. Future studies will undoubtedly clarify, redefine, and discover new roles for these and other structures

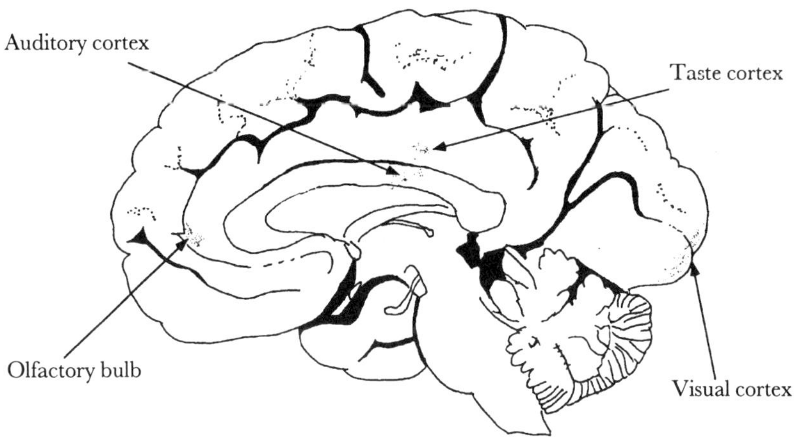

Figure 8.1: Sensory areas of the cerebral cortex.

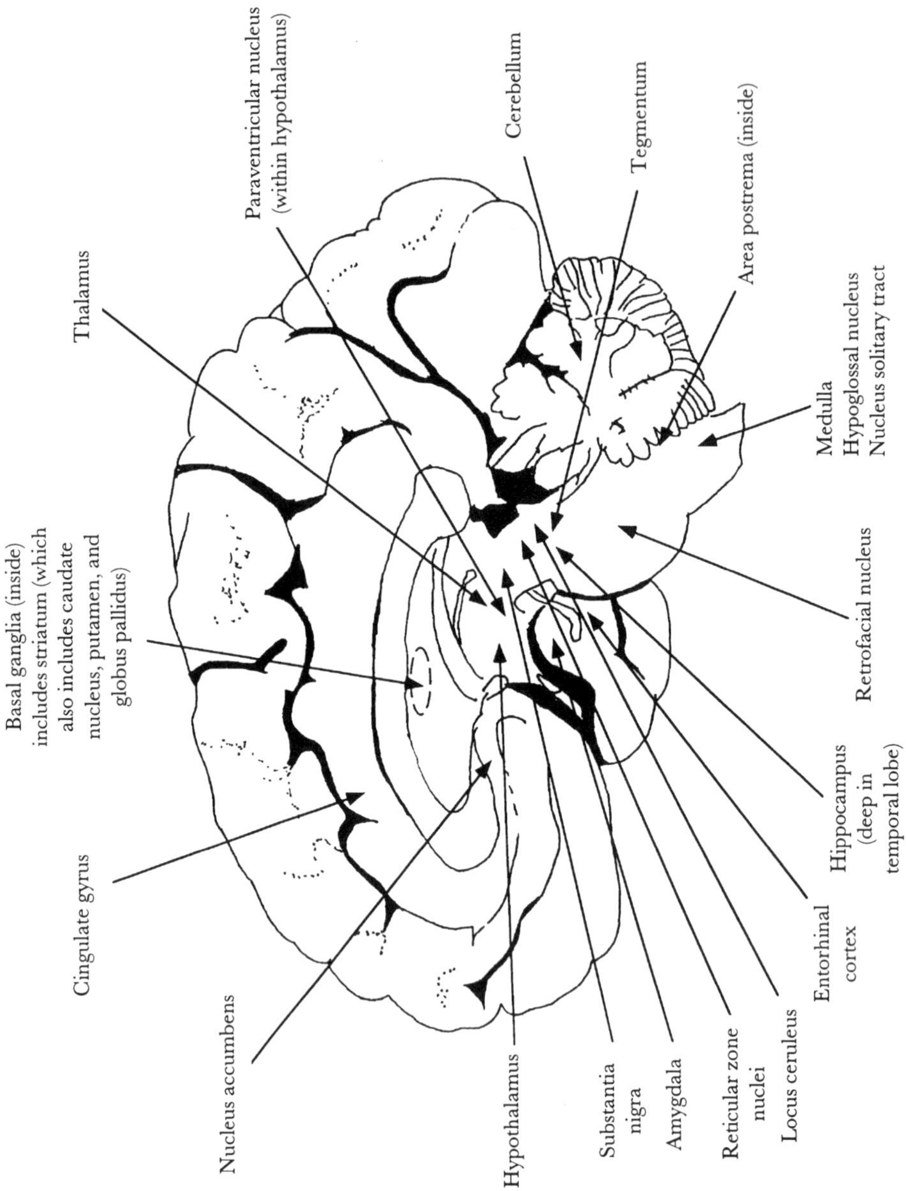

Figure 8.2: Some major brain areas implicated in NV

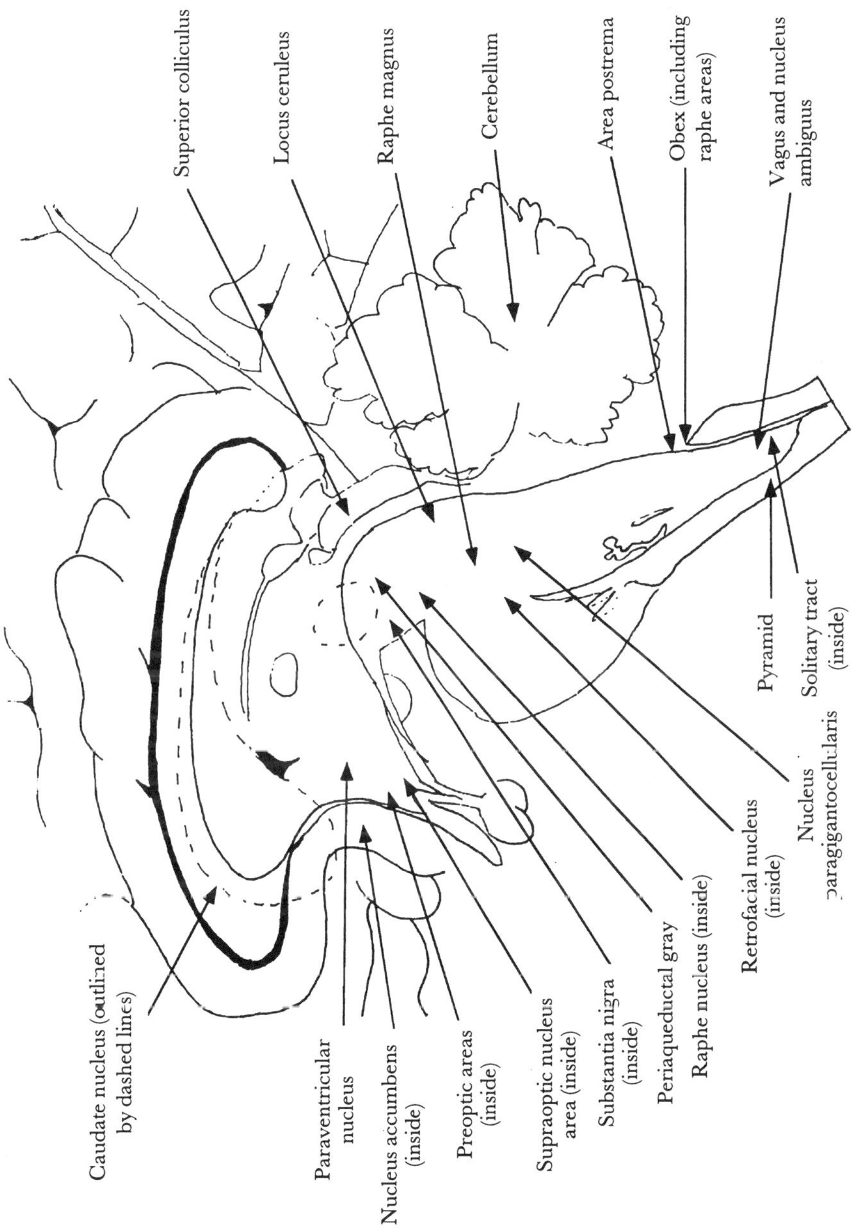

Figure 8.3: Brain stem view.

previously thought inactive. A word of caution: anatomical studies are conducted on animals; their applicability to humans is debatable.

Some NV-implicated brain structures and their functions

Accumbens nucleus

This is one of the nuclei of the precommissural septum and a part of the ventral striatum. It is located ventromedial to the anterior horn of the lateral ventricle and is continuous laterally under the lateral ventricle with the head of the caudate nucleus. It has dopaminergic input and is implicated in schizophrenia.

Amygdala

This is part of the limbic system and a subdivision of the basal ganglia. Located in the temporal lobe, anterior to the inferior horn of the lateral ventricle and partly beneath the uncus. Its two main parts are a corticomedial nuclear group (anterior amygdaloid area, nucleus of the lateral olfactory tract, and the medial cortical and central amygdaloid nuclei) with olfactory and subcortical connections, and a basolateral nuclear group (basal, lateral, and accessory basal amygdaloid nuclei) connected primarily to the overlying cortex. It connects to the hypothalamus and is associated with the olfactory cortex. It has a role in emotion and the affective components of odors.

Area postrema (medulla)

This ventricular organ receives fibers directly for the vagal and glossopharyngeal nerves. Its efferent fibers go directly to the nucleus solitarius and the parabrachial nuclei and indirectly to other areas. It has been shown to be related to NV.

Basal ganglia (cerebrum)

These are subcortical masses of gray matter of the cerebrum, classically comprising the caudate nucleus, putamen, globus pallidus, amygdala, and claustrum. It receives input from the motor cortex, substantia nigra, subthalamic nucleus, and centromedial nuclei of the thalamus. There is output to the same nuclei and to the motor cortex through the thalamus.

Caudate nucleus (cerebrum)

This is part of the basal ganglia, and is made up of a head which forms the lateral wall of the anterior horn of the lateral ventricle, a body overlying the lateral part of the dorsal thalamus, and a tail located above the inferior horn of the lateral ventricle. The caudate nucleus and the putamen, together, constitute the striatum or neostriatum. They respond to strong mechanical stimuli related to pain.

Cerebellum

This is concerned with equilibrium, coordination, and the regulation of muscle tone.

Dorsal horn

This is a dorsal gray column, containing the following cell groups: substantia gelatinosa, nucleus proprius, thoracic nucleus, and secondary visceral gray. It has a role in taste and cardiovascular control.

Entorhinal area (cerebrum)

This is the anterior part of the parahippocampal gyrus, comprising most of the gyrus. It is along the amygdala and is believed to be involved in affective components of odors.

Globus pallidus (cerebrum)

One of the basal ganglia (see Basal ganglia for function).

Hippocampus (cerebrum)

This projects into the inferior horn of the lateral ventricle. Its function includes long-term memory and it is associated with olfactory pathways.

Hypothalamus

A subdivision of the diencephalon located on either side of the third ventricle, just ventral to the hypothalamus sulcus. It is divided into medial and lateral areas by a sagittal plane through the column of the fornix. Its function is in the regulation of various visceral functions.

Lateral reticular nucleus (medulla)

This nucleus is located in the medulla oblongata, dorsolateral to the inferior olivary nucleus. Its caudal portion is a somewhat compact cluster of cells. Its afferent connection comes from the cerebral cortex, red nucleus, fastigial nucleus, and spinal cord. Probably all its efferent fibers pass through the inferior cerebellar peduncle to end in the homolateral half of the cerebellum.

Locus ceruleus (pons)

This is a bluish area on the floor of the fourth ventricle. The neurons are rich in norepinephrine, and have fibers that distribute widely throughout the central nervous system (CNS), from the cerebral cortex to the spinal cord. Functions include control of blood vessels, within the CNS, regulation of respiration, and rapid eye movement (REM) sleep. It may also play a part in arousal and response to stress. These neurons have a role in orienting and attending to sudden contrasting or aversive sensory input.

Medulla oblongata

A caudal subdivision of the hindbrain interposed between the spinal cord and the pons. Its functions include digestion, breathing, and heart rate control.

Nodose ganglion

The visceral afferent ganglion of the vagus nerve, located in the jugular foramen below the superior ganglion of the vagus. It contains the unipolar cell bodies of fibers from the pharynx, larynx, trachea, and esophagus, and all the organs in the thorax and abdomen that receive vagal autonomic fibers. It also contains the cell bodies of some taste fibers from the region of the epiglottis. It has a function in taste.

Nucleus ambiguus

This slender, intermittent column of special visceral motor cells is present in all but the most caudal part of the medulla. It is located in the ventrolateral part of the medulla, about halfway between the spinal nuclei of the V and the dorsomedial corner of the inferior olivary complex. It supplies motor fibers to skeletal musculature derived from the third and fourth visceral arches, the stylopharyngeus, and most muscles of the pharynx, larynx, and upper esophagus. Neurons of the ventrolateral nucleus ambiguus provide the principal parasympathetic innervation of cardiac ganglion which innervates the heart.

Nucleus solitary tract or nucleus tractus solitarius (NTS) (mainly medulla)

This fiber tract is composed of descending visceral afferent fibers of the facial, glossopharyngeal, and vagus nerves. Most fibers terminate in the adjoining nucleus parasolitarius. Some fibers (for taste) descend only a short distance to end in the dorsal visceral gray. It controls the output of the autonomic nervous system and receives sensory information from most major organs.

Obex (medulla)

A small transverse fold overlying the caudal tip of the fourth ventricle at its junction with the central canal of the closed medulla.

Parabrachial nucleus

This consists of noradrenergic cells adjacent to the superior cerebellar peduncle in the region of the pons–midbrain junction. Among their connections they appear to receive afferent fibers from the nucleus raphe dorsalis and the area postrema, and to be connected with the hypothalamus. It functions in taste.

Paraventricular nucleus

This is in the dorsal thalamus, a small nucleus of the median cell group, close to the ventricular surface near the stria medullaris. Fibcrs from this nuclcus have been traced to the amygdala. It has a role in feeding behavior. Along with the supraoptic nuclei, it contains magnocellular neurons that release oxytocin and vasopressin.

Periaqueductal gray (midbrain)

The cellular area surrounding the cerebral aqueduct of the midbrain. The area, rich in enkephalins and opiate receptors, is concerned with pain inhibition. Lesions are known to result in akinetic mutism. It functions in pain perception.

Preoptic (hypothalamus)

This pertains to the area adjoining the part of the third ventricle immediately anterior to the optic chiasma. It also has steroid receptors. Its function is primarily related to the visual system.

Putamen (cerebrum)

This is part of the basal ganglion, the lateral part of the lentiform nucleus. One of the basal ganglia, it is continuous anteriorly, around the anterior limb of the internal capsule, with the head of the caudate nucleus. (See Basal ganglion for function.)

Raphe magnus nucleus (medulla)

The major nucleus in the caudal part of the raphe. Its descending, serotoninergic fibers project mainly to the spinal nucleus of the trigeminal nerve in the medulla and the dorsal horn of the spinal cord, and appear to inhibit the discharge of neurons related to the transmission of pain; it also appears to be a part of the endogenous opiate system.

Raphe nuclei

In the brain stem, these are a series of cell groups along the raphe. It has a role in REM sleep, sleep induction, and serotoninergic pathways, and it modulates the general behavioral state, perception of pain, and the sleep–wake cycle.

Reticular nucleus (dorsal thalamus)

A narrow layer of cells between the external medullary lamina of the dorsal thalamus and the internal capsule; it is continuous ventrally with the zona inserta. Although considered to be a part of the dorsal thalamus, it is said to be derived from the ventral thalamus. Its cells resemble those of adjoining thalamic nuclei. It is connected with other thalamic nuclei, particularly in the intralaminar group. It may be a 'way' station in the multisynaptic ascending reticular system and diffuse thalamocortical projection system.

Retrofacial nucleus

In the pons and medulla, this is a cluster of nerve cells interposed between the facial nucleus rostrally and the nucleus ambiguus caudally.

Striatum

This is composed of caudate nucleus and putamen (see Caudate nucleus and Putamen).

Substantia nigra

Connected with the basal ganglia, this is a nucleus of pigmented nerve cells in the dorsal part of the basis pedunculi of the midbrain and in the caudal part of the ventral thalamus. It consists of: a pars reticulata composed of scattered cells separated by fiber strands (a pars compacta) more dorsally placed, whose cells are closely packed and significantly larger than those in other parts; and a small pars lateralis, the oldest part, in the rostral lateral part of the nucleus. It is involved in Parkinson's disease (dopaminergic projections).

Superior colliculus

A rounded elevation on the dorsal surface of the midbrain, on either side of the median plane in the rostral part of the tectum. Its main function is in vision and is related to the oculomotor system.

Supraoptic nucleus (hypothalamus)

One of the magnocellular hypothalamic nuclei, consisting of large, deeply staining cells located over the lateral border of the optic tract in the anterior hypothalamic area. The cells elaborate mainly antidiuretic hormone (ADH). Other cells, to a lesser extent, produce oxytocin. These neuroendocrines are carried to the neurohypophysis along the supraopticohypophyseal tract.

Tegmentum (midbrain, pons)

The dorsal part of the cerebral peduncle of the midbrain between the cerebral aqueduct and tectum dorsally and the basis pedunculi ventrally, and the dorsal part of the pons between the fourth ventricle dorsally and the basis pontis ventrally. It is connected to the olfactory cortex.

Thalamus (diencephalon)

This is located on either side of the third ventricle just above the hypothalamic sulcus and bounded laterally by the posterior limb of the internal capsule. Its function includes perception of smell.

Vagus (nerve)

This provides preganglionic parasympathetic fibers and visceral afferent fibers for thoracic and most abdominal viscera. It also supplies the musculature of the palate, pharynx, and larynx, and carries taste fibers from the epiglottis and some fibers for cutaneous sensibility from the external ear.

Regions not included in the brain map

The cranial nerves are not included in the brain map; these include the vagus and the glossopharyngeal nerves. Another region not included in this map is globus tympanicum, a paraganglion of the middle ear which arises from the glossopharyngeal nerve, innervating the oropharynx.

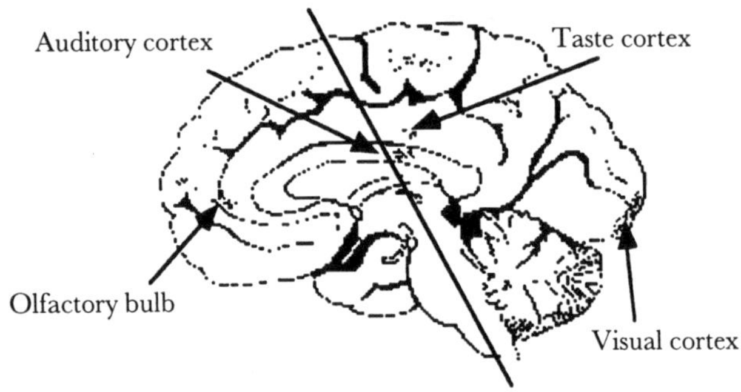

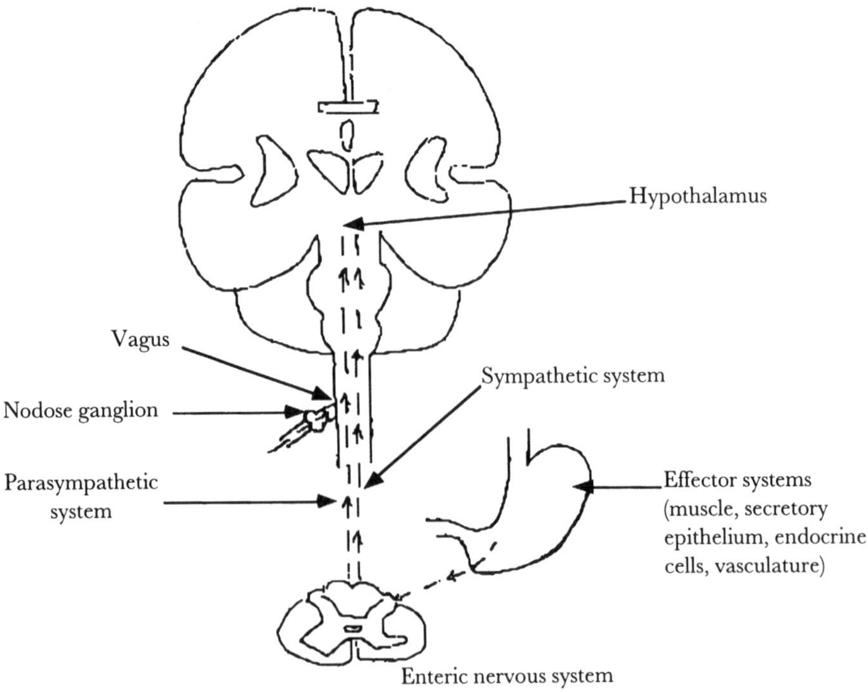

Figure 8.4: Enteric pathway.

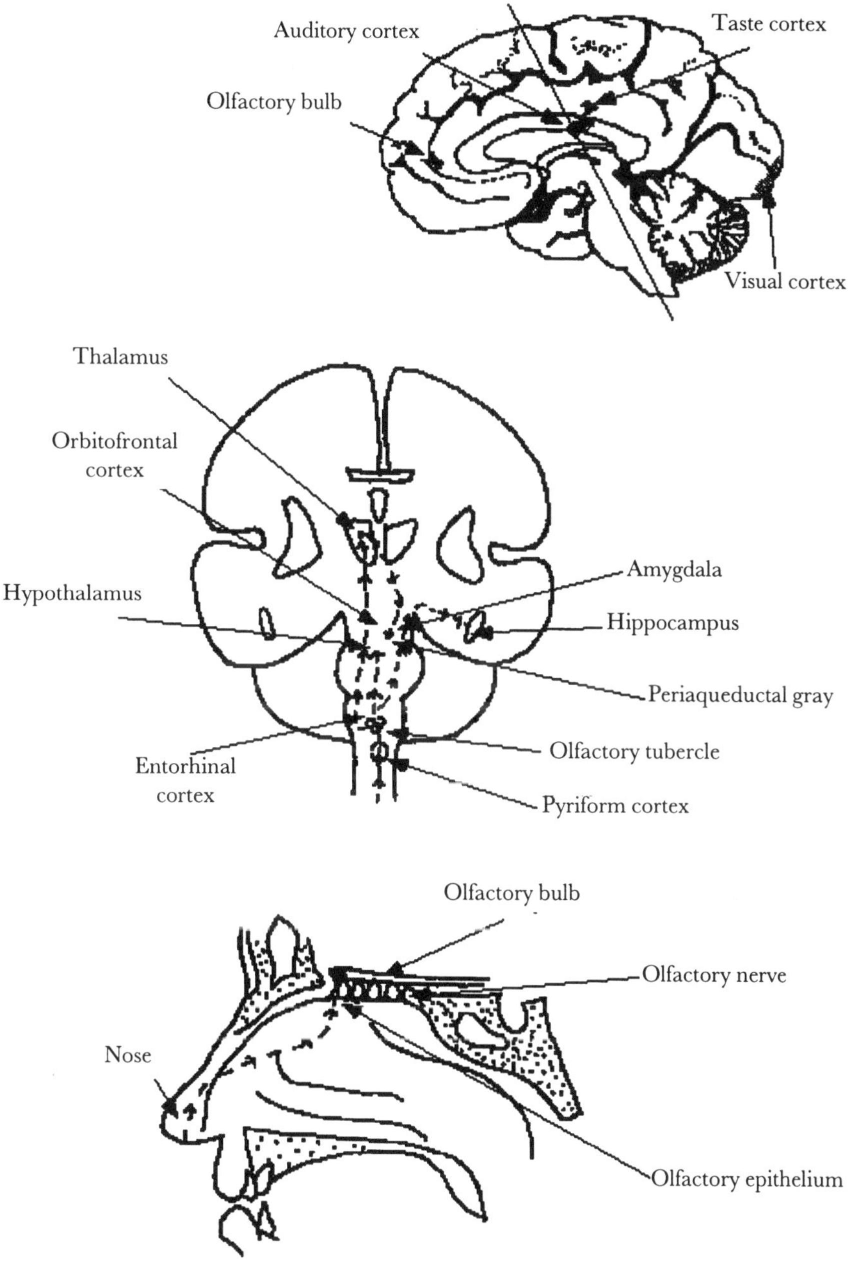

Figure 8.5: Olfactory pathway.

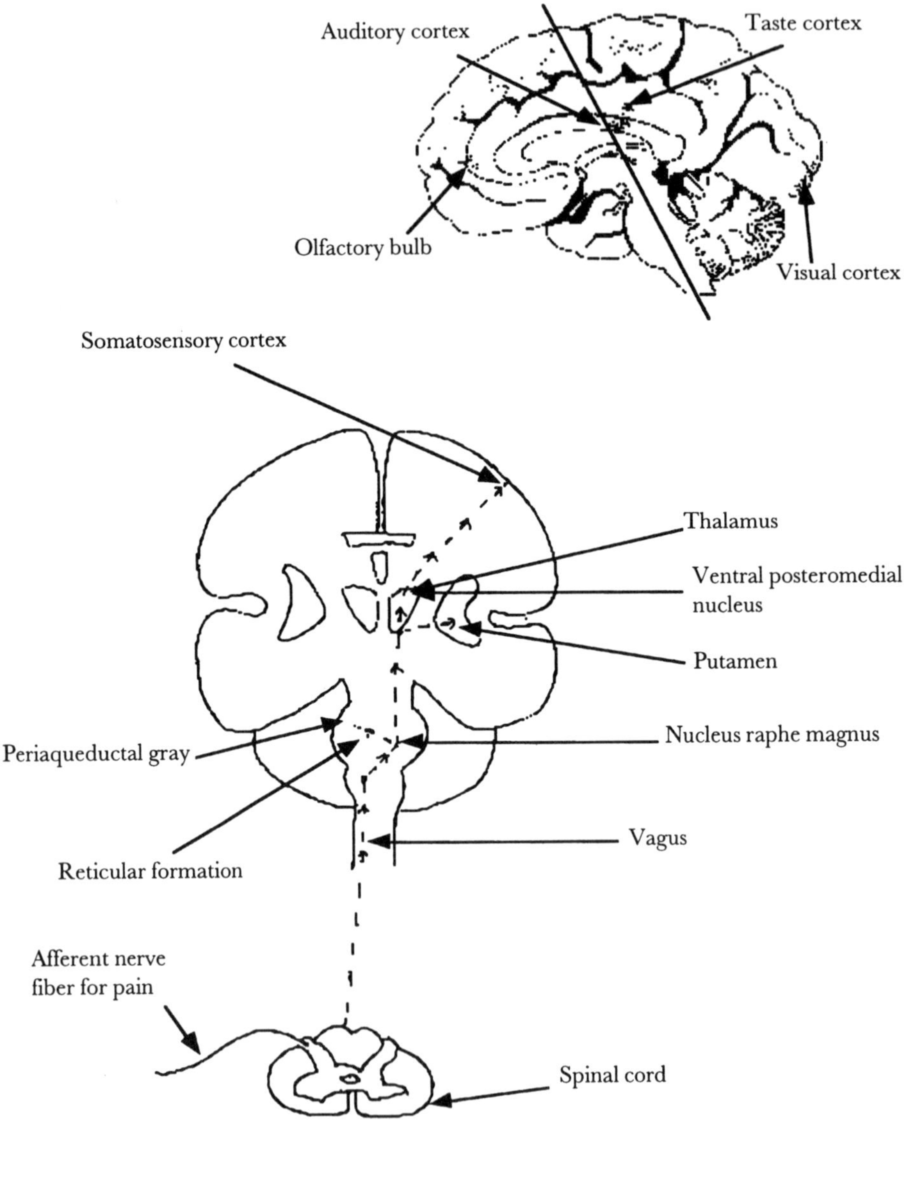

Figure 8.6: Pain pathway.

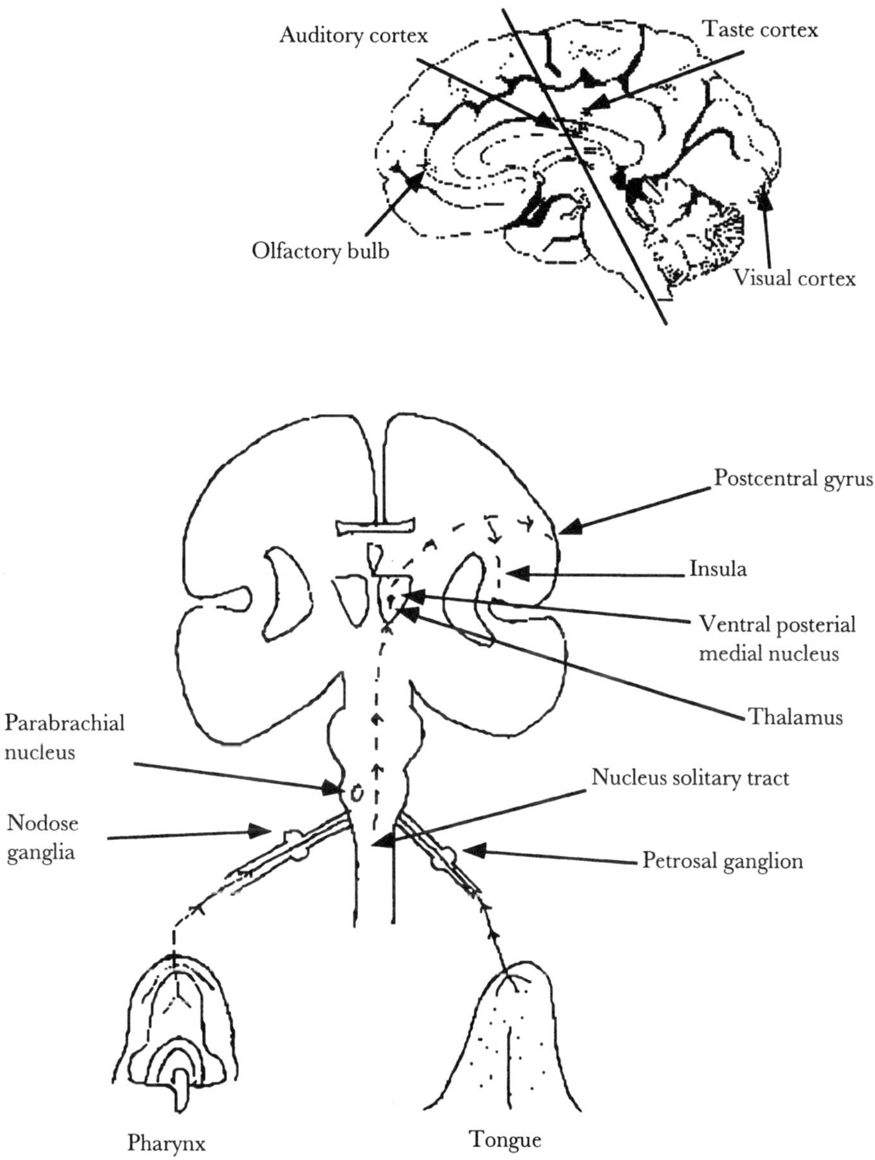

Figure 8.7: Taste pathway.

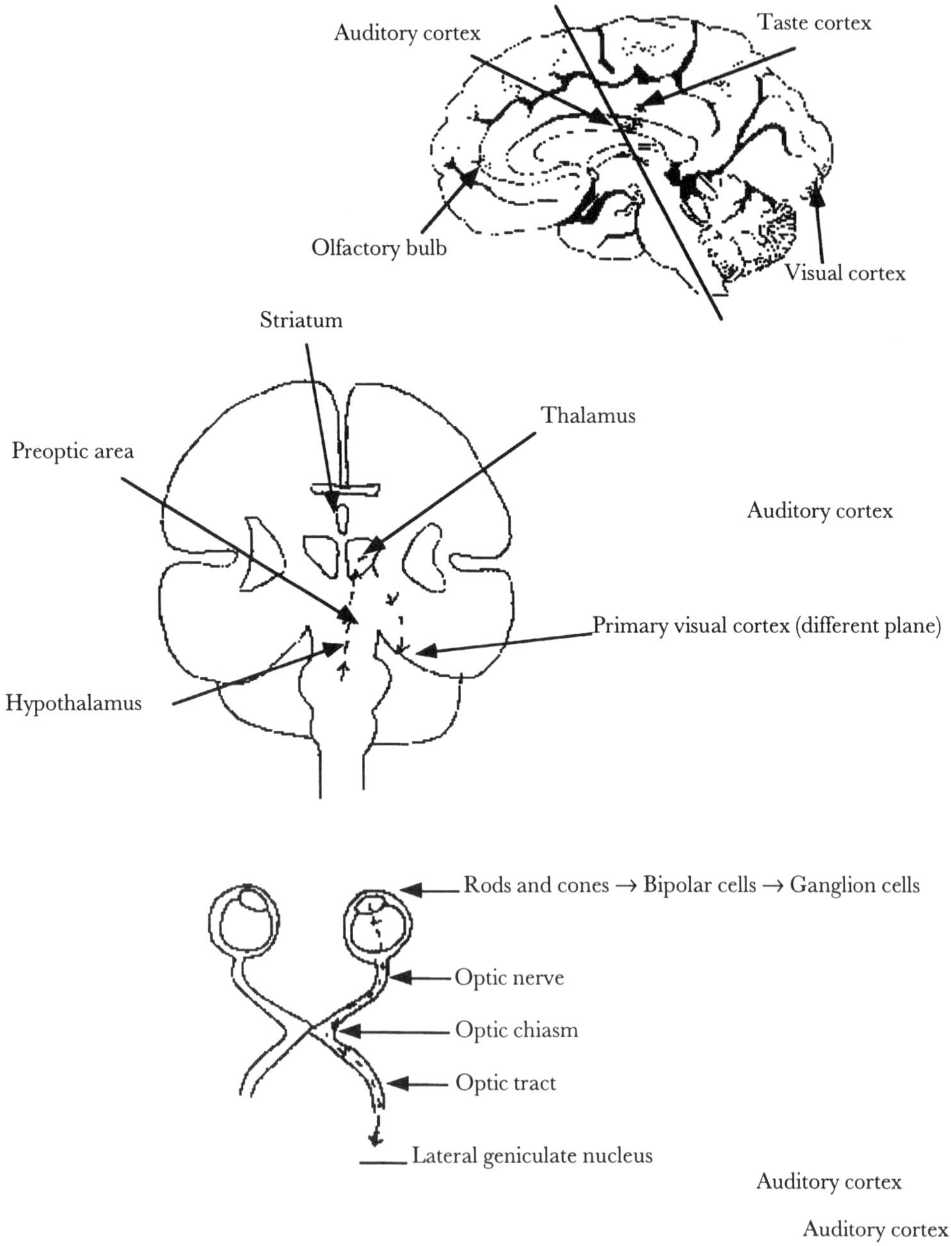

Figure 8.8: Visual pathway.

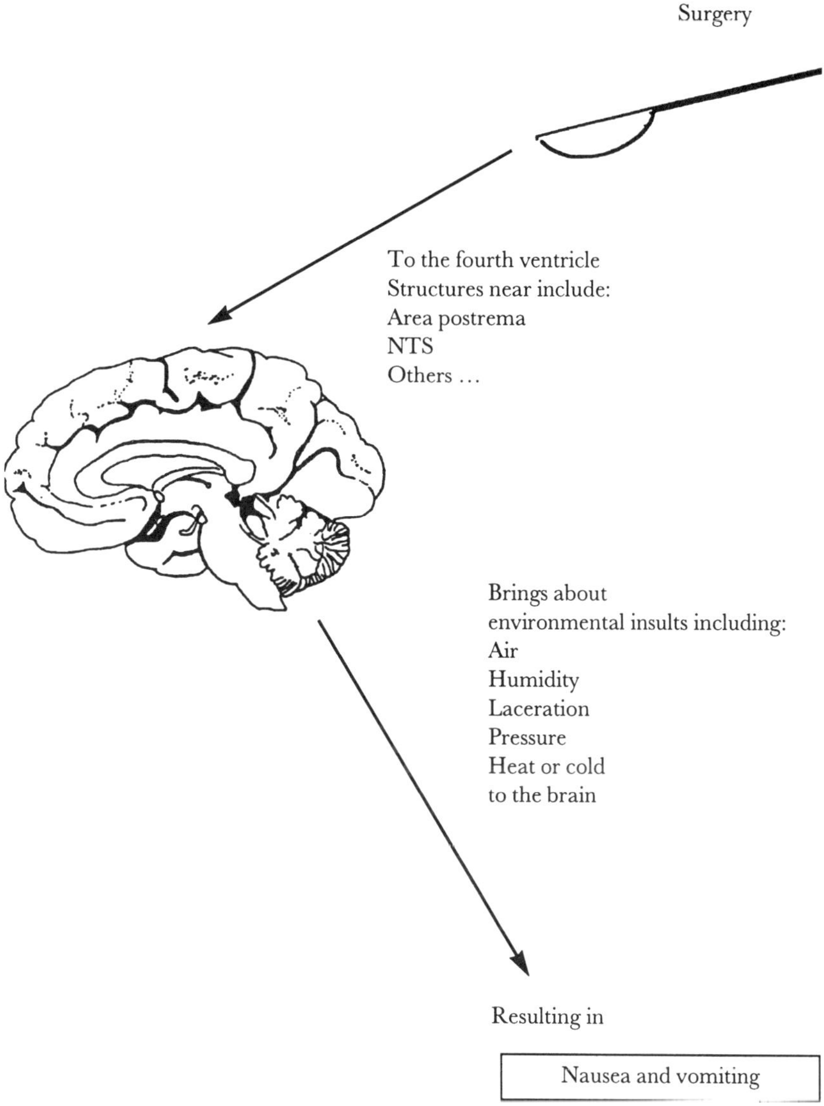

Figure 8.9: Stimulating NV by surgery.

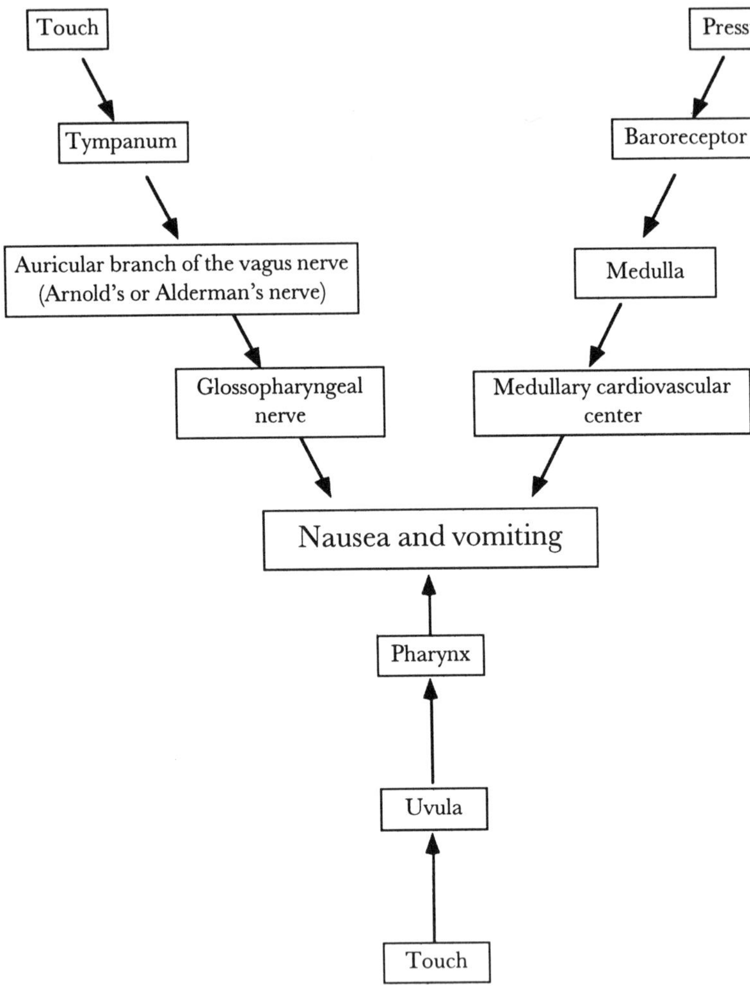

Figure 8.10: Other ways of stimulating NV.

CHAPTER 9

Neuropeptides and some neurotransmitters

Of the few things known concretely about nausea and vomiting (NV), one fact is that they are mediated and controlled in the nervous system. This fact alone is reason enough for neuropeptides and neurotransmitters to be the focus of intense attention in the fields of NV research. In fact, through various studies using immunocytochemical staining and retrograde labeling techniques, many researchers have been able to identify specific relations between certain peptides or transmitters and brain regions known to be involved in the NV response. (To determine whether a region is implicated in NV, most techniques usually involve destroying the specific area in an animal's brain, and determining if the desired effect still exists afterwards.) Using a large reserve of accumulated data on neurotransmitter and peptide pathways, brain maps augmented by chemical pathway schematics for some of the more involved neurotransmitters in the brain related to NV are provided. The pattern the schematics follow is as follows: a box represents a brain region, an arrow outside a box is an efferent axon, and the name indicated at the terminal of the axon is the main transmitting chemical of the neuron. The chemical within the box, for example, 'c-fos,' is simply the implicated releasing factor which stimulates the next efferent neuron from that region. Therefore, in the case of c-fos in a vasopressinergic system, the box containing c-fos holds vasopressin-filled nuclei. These nuclei, when activated, synthesize the c-fos protein, which then stimulates the release of vasopressin upon the efferent axon. Finally, the arrows within each region serve to show where the released chemicals go to stimulate further pathways within the chemical schematic (Figure 9.1).

Table 9.1: Neuropeptides involved with particular areas of the brain and the sensory systems affected

Brain structure	Method	Reference	Neuropeptide	Sensory system
Brain stem	Areas infused with HRP or WGA-HRP	Strominger et al., 1994	ACTH, VP, OT, CCK, c-fos, AT, VIP	Pain
Rostral ventrolateral medulla	in 30 ferrets that were perfused transcardially			
Parabrachial nuclei	after 24–72 hours			Taste
Amygdala			VP, NE, AT, GRP, SS, VIP	Olfactory
Paraventricular nucleus			c-fos, ACTH, AT (hypothalamic)	
Medulla	Fictive vomiting was induced by	Miller et al., 1994	GABA, CCK, VIP, Enk, 5HT, NE, AT, Met-enk, SS	Pain
Retrofacial nucleus	a combination of emetic drugs and electrical			
Obex	stimulation of abdominal vagal efferents		VIP?	
Solitary tract nucleus	in decerebrated paralyzed cats		NE, CCK, c-fos, ACTH, AT, GRP, VP, VIP	Taste
Ambiguus nucleus	Antibodies against c-fos protein used to map	Yousfi-Malki, 1994		
Lateral reticular nucleus	first- and higher-order neurons in the rabbit		AT	
Area postrema	medulla after electrical stimulation of vagus		NE, CCK, c-fos, AT, VIP	
Nodose ganglia	Emetic drugs (cisplatin, labeline, naloxone	Miller and Ruggiero, 1994	c-fos	Taste
Tegmentum	and apomorphine) administered in cats.		VIP	
Raphe magnus	Brain stem and spinal cord examined using		c-fos, VIP	Pain
Spinal dorsal horn	fos-like immunoreactivity as a monitor		ACTH?, NE	
Striatum	Measure dopamine receptor activation at	Cenci et, 1992	AT	Visual
Globus pallidus	the cellular level after dopaminergic			
Caudate putamen	denervation and reinnervation by fetal		Enk, CCK, GRP (basal), VP, OT, SS, VIP	
Nucleus accumbens	nigral transplants in rats			
Preoptic area	No method cited (review article)	Lawes, 1990		Visual
Periaqueductal gray matter				Pain
Supraoptic nuclei			NE, VP, AT, GRP, VIP	Visual
Locus ceruleus			NE, c-fos, AT, GRP, VP, SS, VIP	

Table 9.1: (contd)

Brain structure	Method	Reference	Neuropeptide	Sensory system
Vagus	An autoradiographic study of the binding of [³H]DAGO to the brain stem of the ferret	Barnes et al., 1991		Auditory, pain
				Tactile
Reticular nuclei	was done to indicate high density μ recognition sites		NE, VP, OT	
Thalamus	Ten patients receiving ≥ 350 cGy in a single fraction of radiosurgery to the area postrema received ondansetron i.v. 1 hour before treatment; it was the most effective	Bodis et al., 1994	NE, 5HT, GRP, VIP (midline)	Taste, face sensations, pain
Hypothalamus			c-fos, NE, 5HT, VIP, AT, GRP, OT, SS, Enk	Vision
Hippocampus			NE, 5HT, AT (CA3 field), GRP (CA3), OT, SS, VIP	
Cerebellum			NE, 5HT	Motion
Caudate nucleus	Distribution of [³H]granisetron-labeled $5HT_3$ receptors found in these receptors	Burton, 1993	Met-enk (trigeminal)	
Entorhinal cortex	No methods cited	Kupferman, 1991		Olfactory
Basal ganglia			NE, AT (subthalamic)	
Substantia nigra	Examined effect of $5HT_3$ receptor antagonists, Ly27735 and granisetron on the suppressant action of the dopamine agonist, apomorphine on active dopamine cells in the substantia nigra and ventral tegmentum area	Minabe, 1991	SS, VIP (pars compacta)	Motor control
Superior colliculus	Psychological methods used to examine pattern of imports from different sensory cortices and individual superior colliculus neurons	Stein and Meredith, 1993b	AT, VIP	Visual

ACTH, adrenocorticotropic hormone; AT, angiotensin; CCK, cholecystokinin; c-fos, ????????????; DAGO, ?????????; Enk, enkephalin; GRP, growth-regulatory peptide; 5HT, serotonin; Met-enk, methionine-enkephalin; NE, norepinephrine; OT, oxytocin; SS, somatostatin; VIP, vasoactive intestinal peptide; VP, vasopressin; WGA-HRP, ????????????????.

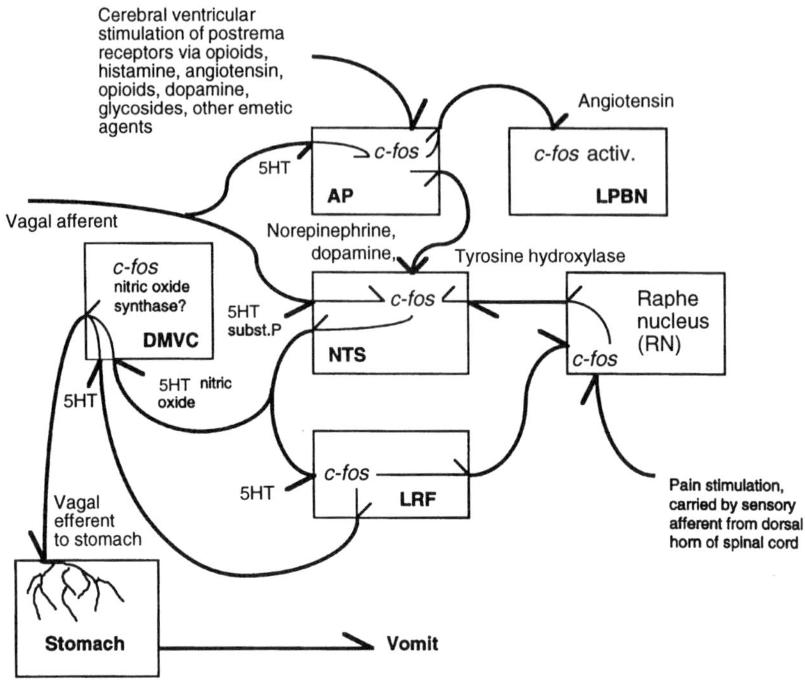

Figure 9.1: Some pathway relationships in emesis, including motor pattern generation areas and transmitters involved.

Angiotensin

Angiotensin is a hormone/neurotransmitter usually circulating in its highest concentrations in response to low blood pressure. It is released as a result of stretch receptor activation in the great arteries in cases of hypotension and bradycardia. It is important to note that implicating angiotensin encompasses the entire angiotensin family. In some cases, such as activity in the paraventricular nucleus, it is mostly angiotensin II that is active. In other sites, it may be simply angiotensin that stimulates activity. The material used in constructing the schema for angiotensin contained many inconsistencies in labeling which version of the chemical was used, so the present author has opted to use only the generic term angiotensin to indicate stimulation in a brain region by an angiotensin-related chemical (in most cases, though, it can be expected to be angiotensin II that is involved).

Most angiotensin stimulation occurs through the cerebral ventricles, activating the area postrema. The pathway from the area postrema is not large, yet it is important because it serves somewhat

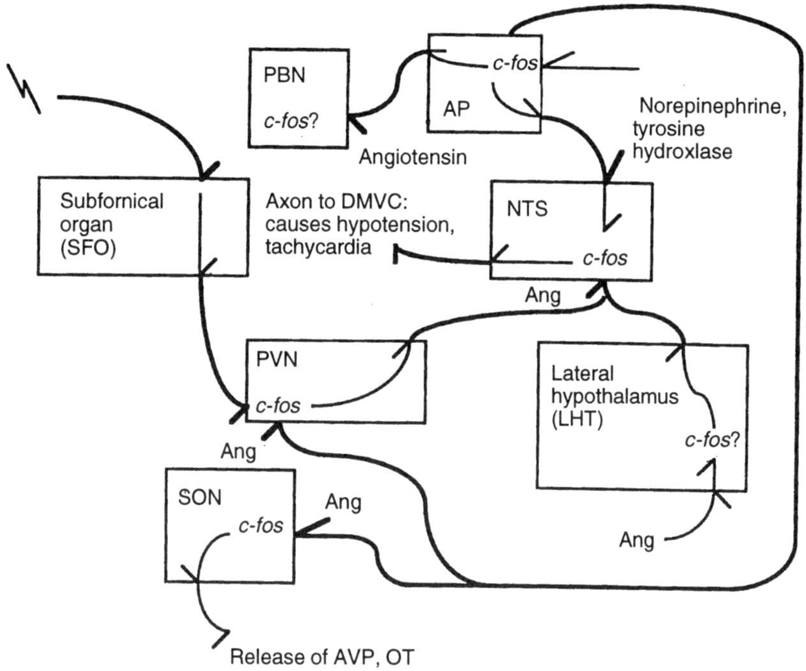

Figure 9.2: Angiotensin II (ATII).

like a second-messenger system, stimulating the release of vasopressin and oxytocin. These two chemicals are highly involved. Worthy of note is that the only pathway which did not demonstrate a strong correlation between the sites of angiotensin receptor binding and that of angiotensin-responsive neuronal activity was that of the nucleus of the solitary tract (nucleus solitarius or NTS). This could be because of the NTS's strong involvement in other pathways, and therefore it may have adapted a nonspecific axonal 'trigger' stimulating general emetic activity, in this case adrenergic-active efferent neurons. Also, a slight anomaly: angiotensin has been reported to cause activity in the complex of the dorsal motor nucleus of the vagus nerve (DMVC), which supposedly increases the beating of the heart. This is inconsistent with the normal inhibiting parasympathetic action on cardiac muscle. Perhaps angiotensin inhibits a certain area of the DMVC, decreasing the vagal output to the heart, while stimulating the esophageal projections from the DMVC to facilitate vomiting.

Cholecystokinin

Cholecystokinin (CCK) is unique in this group of chemical schematics in that its main stimulating center is on afferent vagal projections to the area postrema and the NTS. Also unique is that this is very much the limit of CCK's role within the motor pattern generator for emesis within the medulla. CCK mainly serves to stimulate c-fos-immunoreactive cells within various brain regions, which tend to use serotonin (5HT) as a neurotransmitter. Axons implicated in this system serve to activate N1 and M1 receptors on the supraoptic (SON) and paraventricular (PVN) nuclei, respectively. Interestingly, nicotine, a highly emetic agent, follows this same pathway of stimulation from the area postrema to the SON, and therefore to the release of vasopressin and oxytocin, via numerous nicotinic receptors on the area postrema. In addition, for CCK, however, ACTH is released from the PVN, and the nucleus accumbens is activated (independent of the ACTH release), via oxytocin or vasopressin transmission. Unfortunately, the result of the latter has not been consistently determined. However, the release of ACTH is postulated to be connected

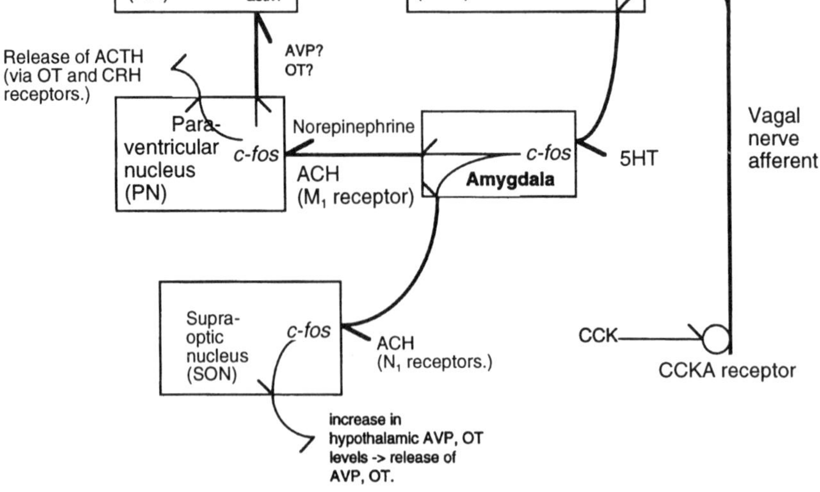

Figure 9.3: Cholecystokinin (CCK).

to emesis, whether enhancing or inhibiting, as a result of its close correlation with vasopressin and vasoactive intestinal polypeptide.

Vasopressin

Vasopressin is a highly studied chemical previously thought to display only hormonal properties. As studies progressed, however, evidence was gathered that implicated vasopressin as a widely used neurotransmitter, especially in the pathways involved in emesis. It is also involved in learning and memory, as its presence in Broca's and surrounding areas shows. Interestingly, this may provide future researchers with a connection between NV and memory recall, for example, how the remembrance of a specific past experience or event can produce NV.

According to most research, it is the stimulation of the vagal efferent to the abdominal area that seems to be the vasopressinergic contribution to NV. Again, 5HT is highly useful in the perpetuation of this system, as is c-fos immunoreactivity. There has been little research in determining whether the c-fos activity in the amygdala

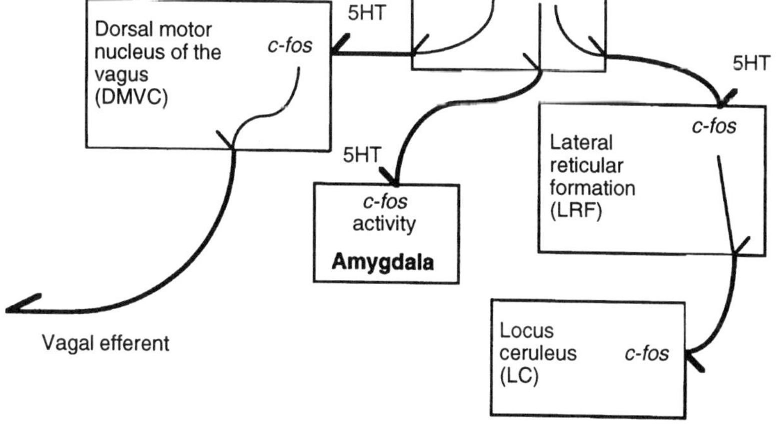

Figure 9.4: Vasopressin (AVP).

results in efferent projections to the PVN or SON and therefore release of more vasopressin, possibly implicating a vasopressin positive-feedback loop.

Oxytocin

Oxytocin is another neurotransmitter which, to most of the scientific world, displays prominent hormonal tendencies. It is frequently implicated as the main agent for histamine-induced emesis, through stimulation of postrema receptors via the cerebral ventricular system. In addition, oxytocin release is especially enhanced during the pregnancy period, adding evidence to oxytocin's involvement in NV as a result of the high level of NV during pregnancy.

A significant difference in the oxytocin and vasopressin schematics, which has a very important effect on NV study, is that oxytocin receptor binding to the area postrema eventually leads to release of ACTH from the PVN and oxytocin and vasopressin from the SON. This indicates the presence of a positive-feedback loop for oxytocin and is a very important concept, considering that there is a definite pattern in NV of continuous, long-lasting cases of sickness, and this example of self and vasopressin-enhancing oxytocin behavior may be a cause for this pattern. Also of note is the activation of the bed

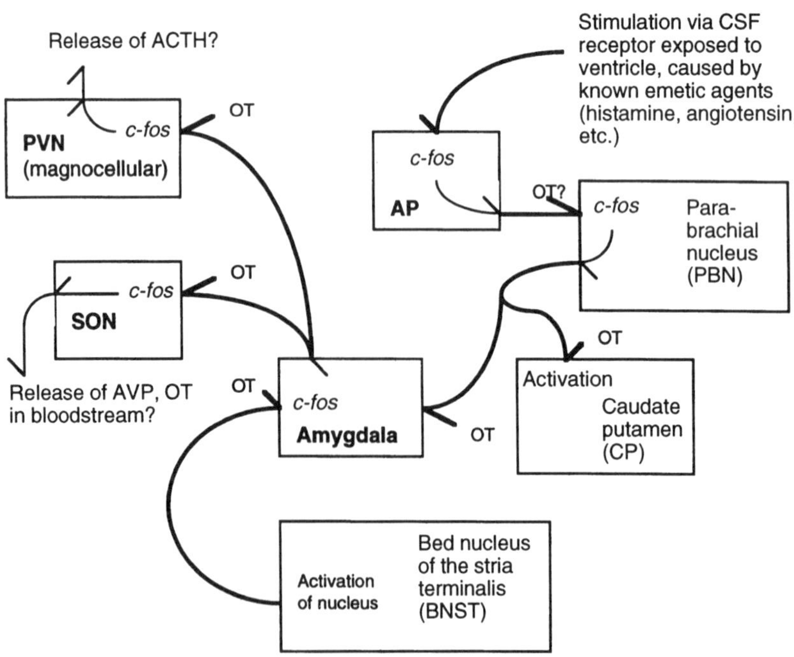

Figure 9.5: Oxytocin (OT).

nucleus of the stria terminalis, which is known to be connected to olfaction, and adds to the oxytocin, vasopressin, and ACTH release in the SON and PVN, respectively (Figure 9.5).

Interleukin-1

Interleukin-1 (IL-1) is a unique case, included because of demonstrated high levels of activity and stimulation along the proposed emetic pathway, but with little outside evidence of implication in NV causation. The pathway of IL-1 is centered around 5HT transmission, with two different sites of initial stimulation. There are many receptors along the afferent vagal nerve which can bind to IL-1, leading to expression of c-fos activity in the NTS. Also, however, the area postrema can be activated, although the levels of IL-1 must be increased in concentration to a level that is more than that needed in the vagal receptor stimulation. This may be because of IL-1's difficulty in crossing the blood–brain barrier, but this is only a hypothesis. Again, as in oxytocin's case, the BNTS can be activated, leading to an already prominent pathway from the amygdala to the PVN and SON, although the results of this stimulation are not as concrete as in the case of oxytocin, where vasopressin, oxytocin, and ACTH are all released.

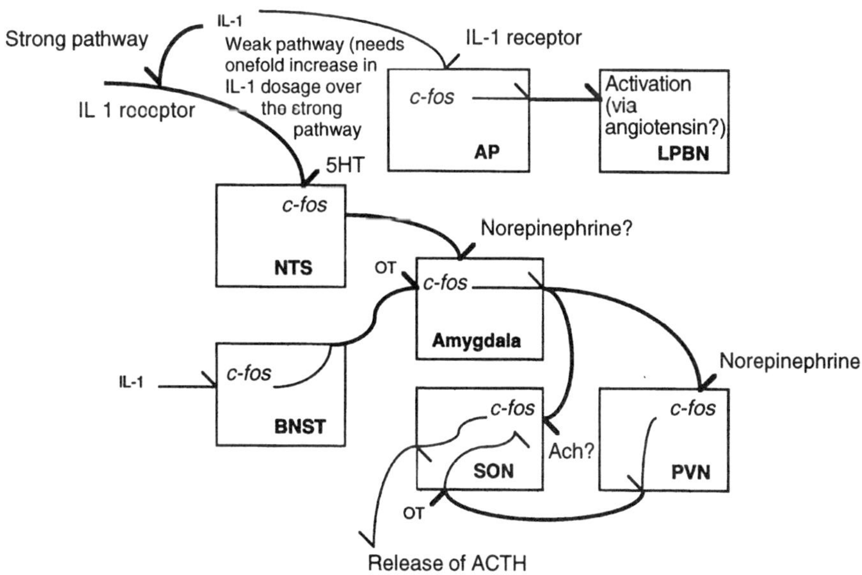

Figure 9.6: Interleukin 1 (IL-1).

Nitric oxide

Nitric oxide (NO) was the last of any of these chemicals to be recognized as a neurotransmitter in the emetic pathway, or, for that matter, as a neurotransmitter at all. As a result of this, little is known about the actual chemical interactions of NO within the central nervous system (CNS). However, enough has been studied to gather data for a basic schematic on the pathways of NO, and its emetic consequences. NO differs from the other involved neurotransmitters in an important way: it is not c-fos that is the expressed factor within an NO-stimulated brain region. It is a protein called nitric oxide synthase (NOS), and its immunoreactivity to specific NOS-binding radiological ligands is the very way most researchers have been able to identify NO's presence and patterns within the brain. NOS is the factor which, when activated by an afferent NO axon terminal, begins the transcription process of more NO within the nucleus or region involved.

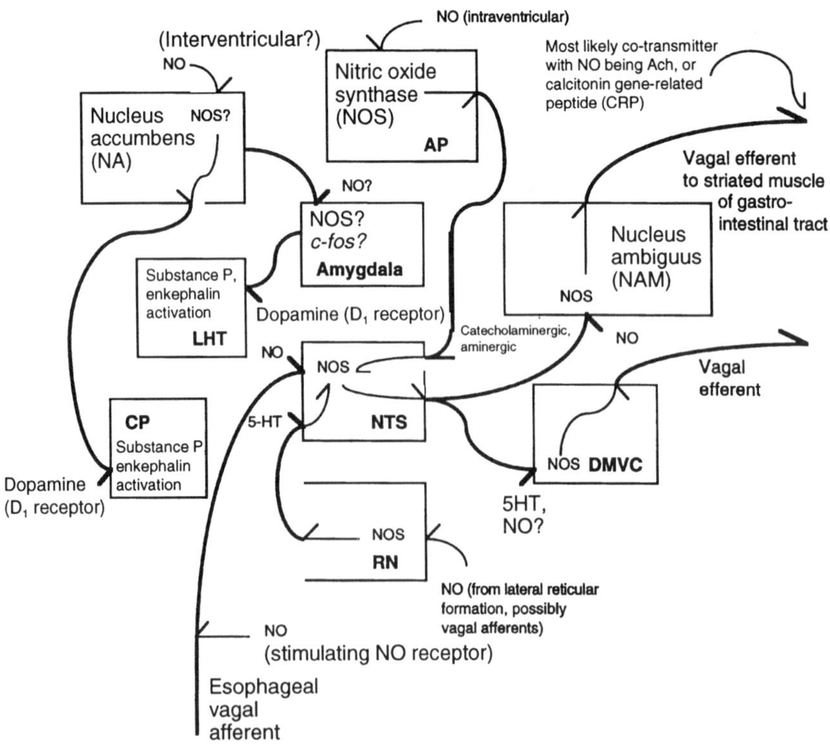

Figure 9.7: Nitric oxide (NO).

Another important aspect of NO is that it serves as one of the only, if not the only, single-chemical neurotransmitting connection between vagal afferent and efferent activity. NO stimulates many portions of the emetic pathway, but in this case it is the vagal afferent that holds major receptors for NO, possibly all within the nodose ganglion. This sends NO to the NTS terminal of the vagal projection, stimulating NOS expression. This then activates axonal projection from the NTS to the nucleus ambiguus, where further NOS expression stimulates a specific efferent to the vagal esophageal plexus. This efferent utilizes NO, and possibly acetylcholine, as a co-neurotransmitter. There is some documentation, although scarce, implicating calcitonin gene-related peptide (CGRP) in the efferent as well. In addition, the NTS, via stimulation from the afferent along with the raphe nuclei and area postrema, sends projections to the DMVC (via 5HT), which then stimulates further vagal activity within the gastrointestinal tract.

Vasoactive intestinal peptide

Vasoactive intestinal peptide (VIP) is by far the most involved gastroactive chemical in this group, because its stimulation and binding sites have been extensively mapped throughout the gastrointestinal tract. In the brain, however, most research involving VIP is connected to sensory information processing. However, there have been many studies linking VIP to the emetic complex, specifically, to the motor pattern generator of the V act itself. VIP, being almost 85% co-localized with acetylcholine, has led researchers to believe that it is a neuropeptide involved in the parasympathetic division of the autonomic nervous system (as a result of acetylcholine's known strong presence there). Because of its link to V, it is the vagus and the DMVC that have received the most attention in NV-related VIP research. However, from Figure 9.8, it is apparent that many other systems are also affected, and possibly linked to emesis.

The area postrema is the main target of VIP, and its stimulation causes a pathway of activation through the NTS that is all too well known (at least after reading this chapter), leading to the DMVC, and terminating in the vagal efferent to the esophagus and stomach, which causes increased gastric secretion and retching. Additional to that is the nucleus ambiguus (NAb) and the suprachiasmatic nuclei (SCN) which are also sensitive to VIP concentration, resulting in a number of interesting pathways. The axonal pathway leading to the BNST may be hypothesized to be connected in some way to the

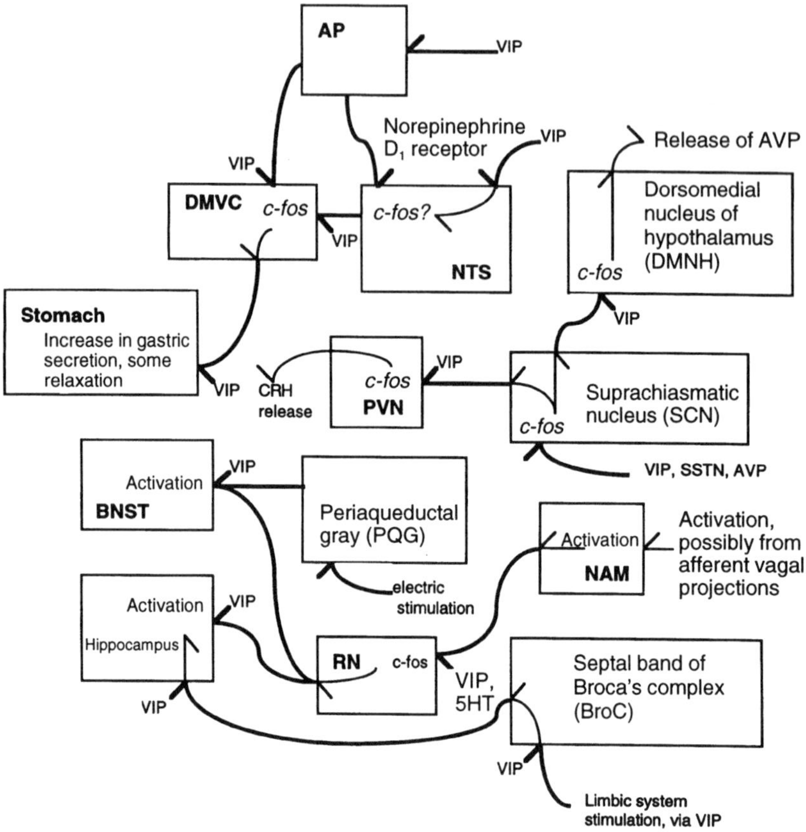

Figure 9.8: Vasoactive intestinal peptide (VIP).

oxytocin schematic, although the author has chosen to leave the two separate to limit the level of abstraction. Also, activity resulting in the hippocampus, a prominent portion of the limbic complex, from VIP stimulation in the SCN and NAb may be a cause for the feeling of anxiety and general emotional imbalance preceding the V action.

VIP stimulation also serves to release other important factors in emesis, such as CGRP and, more importantly, vasopressin. It has also been found to increase in concentration in the presence of potassium (K^+). This is a similar trait to the one followed by angiotensin, possible linking the two during emetic activity. However, the location and duration of K^+ release during NV are beyond the scope of this chapter. In addition, there is a consistent connection between ACTH and VIP levels in the brain. As VIP concentration rises, so do ACTH levels. However, even though there are relatively few studies on ACTH and its relationship to NV, there is documentation proving that ACTH is involved in decreasing NV incidence. As a result of the lack of plausible studies and concrete data, ACTH has not been included in the schematic charts. Finally, if there is only one indisputable fact about VIP and NV, it is this: as VIP levels rise, so does the incidence of NV. This fact has made VIP very popular in the NV research field.

Somatostatin

Somatostatin is a neuroendocrine regulator. Its behavior is much like that of a hormone, such as vasopressin (although we now know that vasopressin also functions as a neurotransmitter). Somatostatin's main areas of activation related to NV are concentrated within the limbic system, with the pathway of activation running from the circumventricular organs (area postrema) to regions such as the hippocampus and amygdala. Somatostatin also poses a paradox in that it can prevent the secretion of ACTH, which is antiemetic in some cases, whereas VIP and angiotensin, two of the most emetic compounds known, are also reduced in concentration. Vasopressin levels have been shown to rise in certain regions of the brain, such as the SCN, when somatostatin is added. The great inconsistencies that somatostatin causes in NV research have demonstrated two things: it is without a doubt implicated in the NV process, and it will be a long time before anyone figures out how. As a result of these realizations, we include some of the more relevant facts about somatostatin, yet do not include a schematic, as it would probably make little sense.

In exploring these charts and descriptions (Figures 9.1–9.8) the reader should be reminded that these schematics are the result of intense field research, not lab research. Therefore, because the actual connections for each graph are derived from many different sources, they should be used only as a point of departure for further research and should by no means be regarded as exact and unfailing. However, the author has taken great lengths to certify the reliability of each resource, leaving out other pertinent compounds and pathways that have displayed inconsistent results. Therefore the information represented in this section can still be regarded with a high level of confidence as a strong representation and thorough culmination of the current scientific position on neuroactive NV research.

CHAPTER 10

The economic impact of nausea and vomiting

Health care expenditures are projected to resume their rise as a proportion, of the gross domestic product (GDP) of the USA, increasing from the recent 14%. Part of the sharp increase in the industry's market share is significantly related to the exponential price growth of some of the larger components of health care costs: drugs, physicians' fees, hospital stays, and the more high-technology intensive treatment methods. Major changes in the US health care system, to managed care, health maintenance organizations (HMOs), preferred provider plans, and efforts to change Medicare and Medicaid are a (now inadequate) response to the unacceptable growth in costs. One hitherto unrecognized high cost is that of nausea and vomiting (NV).

As the costs rise, there need to be more ways to make the system more efficient. However, there is a limit to how many days can be cut off an average length of stay (LOS) as illustrated by the fact that, in 1995, the average LOS in hospitals rose for the first time in 13 years. The focus for health economics moves beyond counting the number of syringes used and staffing hours. One area for rationalization is the appropriate distribution, where there are chances, for advance research funding as priorities for more costly afflictions. NV are costly phenomena. Our research demonstrates that the commonly occurring condition of NV costs the US economy between $4 and $16 billion per year. Cancer costs average nearly $104 billion per year. However, were more resources dedicated to NV, an affliction that absorbs at least 4% and perhaps 10% of the dollar cost of cancer, its prevention and control would be improved. The prevailing unsupportive attitude is summarized as 'What's a little nausea and vomiting – everybody gets it, and you too'll get over it, soon!'

We focus on four elements in determining the costs of NV to the US economy. The first, hospital formularies, shows how hospitals can over-prescribe marginally effective antiemetics at great cost. The second, absenteeism and NV, determines the total cost to the economy of people who miss work as a result of this phenomenon. The third element, postoperative NV (PONV), describes costs endured by patients and for health care facilities and programs. The fourth deals with costs associated with cancer radiation and chemotherapy and the resulting serious NV. We then discuss consumer economics and indicate areas requiring additional study.

Hospital formularies and drug choice analysis

A variety of antiemetic (AE) compounds exist; so does popularity of their prescription. The serotonin $5HT_3$ antagonists are the current 'darlings' in AE drug therapy. The major $5HT_3$ antagonist is ondansetron. It has been the focus of many cost-effectiveness studies. Its use is reviewed by the University Hospital Consortium (UHC) to set up appropriate guidelines for its dosages and indications for use. For us, two issues are foremost: prescription predilection and cost-effectiveness of ondansetron.

Prescription predilection

First, the rate of prescribing, and over-prescribing, of ondansetron in AE drug therapy will be assessed using the standard UHC guidelines. We address formularies for chemotherapy patients because there are few studies that evaluate the excessive prescription of the drug in PONV settings. Furthermore, the recommended doses for oral ondansetron use in the PONV setting have only recently been published and there has been too little time to allow trials comparing prescribing patterns for outcome efficacy.

Cost-effectiveness

Much work concludes that ondansetron is not a cost-effective AE and that the administration of metoclopramide has a much lower than preferred cost/utility ratio.

Indications

In 1995, Glaxo Wellcome, the producer of ondansetron, received \$618 million (£386 m) in worldwide sales from the drug. Although data were unavailable on individual US sales of the drug, a study by Vermeulen et al. (1994) reviewed records of patients who received ondansetron at various US academic medical centers. In the study, 641 cancer chemotherapy patients' data were analyzed using the UHC hospital formulary. Of these patients, 583 (91%) were found to satisfy at least one indication for the drug's use.

Ondansetron has been approved only for use in short-term emesis patterns. For example, the continuation of treatment is considered inappropriate in emesis cases that last more than 24 hours. Nine percent of the cancer patients did not present with NV appropriate for ondansetron use during chemotherapy. Upon further review, 25 of the patients receiving ondansetron were deemed not to have met UHC guidelines for ondansetron prescription.

Dosage

The US Food and Drug Administration has approved ondansetron to be prescribed at 0.15 mg/kg every 4 hours for a total of three doses. The Vermeulen study showed that in excess of 17.5% (9147 mg) of the total amount of ondansetron administered in the study was above dosage requirements. At the estimated cost of $5 per mg, the excess cost was $68.27 per patient.

Furthermore, of the 53 260 mg used, 16 185 mg did not meet the requirements for dosage, indication, or both. This is 31% of the total quantity prescribed and involves 62% (417) of the patient pool. The total cost per patient for the over-prescription of ondansetron was $121. Relying on Vermeulen's work, we calculate that, if a hospital treating 10 patients per week with ondansetron adhered to the prescribing guidelines set forth by the UHC, it would save $62 000 each year.

Consider the implications, realizing first that the study was carried out at 23 US academic medical centers: the same consortium responsible for drafting the UHC guidelines! If physicians in these same academic centers failed to adhere to the prescribing guidelines in 62% of the cases, imagine the abuses that are probably occurring in non-academic hospitals. Inpatients and outpatients receiving emetogenic chemotherapy across the country are being given the wrong medication for their NV, if we accept UHC guidelines. At a derived cost of $121 per patient per treatment, ondansetron consumes as much as 3% of hospital drug budgets for inpatients (Zbrozek et al., 1994). Note that, when heavier doses of ondansetron are prescribed, there are no conclusive studies that show a consistent dose–response relationship in the literature. More is not better. What is occurring is that physicians have been prescribing ondansetron in doses ranging from 0.10 to 0.18 mg/kg, ignorant of the utility/efficacy for increased units of the drug. In addition, with the recent approval of oral ondansetron, 16 mg one hour before the induction of operative anesthesia, more abuses are likely to become apparent, for hospitals as norm-setting groups, and for individual physicians who develop their own idiosyncratic prescription-writing styles.

Examine the cost-effectiveness of ondansetron compared with metoclopramide. In the Zbrozek et al. study (1994), patients treated with ondansetron experienced on average 2.03 incidents of acute emesis that were cisplatin induced. Patients treated with metoclopramide experienced 2.66 cases of emesis on average. Other chapters warn us of the limitations of measuring only retching episode counts, or the typical short duration of counting, for ondansetron is ineffective for delayed NV, usually 24–36+ hours after intervention. The study estimated the total costs (drugs, materials, labor) for two sample groups: people weighing 40 kg and 70 kg. The 40-kg group was designed to represent women and the 70-kg group represented men. On average, the ondansetron group were protected from 0.66 cases of emesis more than the metoclopramide group.

The marginal benefits of the ondansetron treatment were placed into quality adjusted life year (QALY) units. On this scale 0 is death and 1 is a year of perfect health. Zbrozek et al. estimated the value of 0.66 fewer cases of emesis, reduced N, and the avoidance of extrapyramidal symptoms – a risk of metoclopramide – to be 0.05 over 24 hours. Extrapolating to 1 year, one arrives at 0.00014 QALYs, suggesting that treatment with ondansetron adds 0.00014 years of healthy life to each person who receives the treatment.

Can one determine a dollar amount that each QALY would cost with ondansetron treatment? The average cost of treatment for a 40-kg person was $139.38 ($133.96–148.66) and $116.35 ($108.58–129.07) in the ondansetron and metoclopramide groups respectively (95% confidence interval). The total cost of treatment for a 70-kg person was determined to be $211.00 ($205.58–220.28) and $154.56 ($146.78–167.28). Taking the average differences between the mean costs, the difference for the 40-kg group was $23 and for the 70-kg group $56. Dividing the average differences by the QALYs obtained from the treatment with ondansetron yields $168 391 per QALY for the 40-kg group and $407 667 per QALY for the 70-kg group. According to Zbrozek, both costs exceed the acceptable $50 000–100 000 range for new technologies established by Laupacis et al. (1992).

Rubenstein (1994) comments on the Zbrozek study, questioning the accuracy of the findings. They call for a more ‘compassionate’ assessment. It is proposed that gains in QALYs will vary by the type of cancer each patient has. For example, a patient with lung cancer whose life expectancy is only 2 years will receive much more value from the gained QALYs in comparison to a patient experiencing testicular cancer with the average life expectancy of 45 years after early diagnosis. They argue that the economics of ondansetron depend upon whose perspective is employed. Perhaps, but in a world in which health care costs continue to rise and financing resources are limited, it is the people paying the bills who will have the final say. HMO profits are also a 'bottom line' prescription policy determinant. Governments and insurance companies are likely to be less tolerant of marginally beneficial treatments such as ondansetron, particularly if overused, and will wisely limit its use to UHC-like provisions. For example, ondansetron has not been demonstrated to reduce inpatient chemotherapy LOS days and its cost per QALY is above an actuarially acceptable level.

In a cost-burdened system, over-prescription of ondansetron becomes increasingly intolerable. As third party or consumer dollars are more carefully watched, doctors will be required to remain within prescription guidelines, or else face the consequence of sanctions introduced by their managed care or other hospital employers, or dropped from PPO lists. One understands that patients would prefer to restrict their V by 0.66 incidence, but 'ideal health' is a social and economic as well as a personal standard. 'Ideal' competes for other resources. Patients may have become resigned to receiving the slightly less-effective care, for example, metoclopramide, the cost-effective alternative.

If it can be termed an 'optimistic' note, V is of less concern to patients than is their N. And N is much less controlled by ondansetron or any AE drug than is V. Thus, the next generation of studies should be measuring QALYs with respect to drug efficacy on N, using refined measures for NV combined. The standards for assessing ondansetron and metoclopramide will change.

Absenteeism from work because of NV

NV produce direct and indirect costs, for example, when people miss work. According to the Department of Labor Statistics, average hourly earnings in 1993 were $10.96. For ease of calculation, assume men's and women's wages are equal, acknowledging real sex differences in some industries. Here, absenteeism after surgery and chemotherapy will not be considered.

The 1993 Vital and Health Statistics estimates from the National

Health Interview Survey give figures about NV in absenteeism. Men missed 5 708 000 days of work as a result of illnesses in the category 'Indigestion, nausea, and vomiting.' Women missed a total of 14 207 000 days of work in the same category. In addition, two other categories are of interest. Assume that, in the group suffering 'Intestinal virus, unspecified,' 10–50% of the days missed were predominately the result of typical symptoms of an intestinal virus, with symptoms of NV. Others had diarrhea. Make the same assumption of 'Viral infections, unspecified;' some portion of these will suffer NV.

For men, this yields an additional 20 323 000 work days missed as a result of NV. For women, an estimated 27 326 500 additional absent days are added. The sum of total days of work missed as a result of NV is 67 564 500. In an average work day of 8 hours at $10.96 per hour, the total loss to the economy approximates $6 billion (in 1993) ($5,924 055 360). Table 10.1 estimates the direct cost of absenteeism as a result of NV for varying estimates, 10–50% of the viral infections having NV as a disabling (work loss causing) symptom.

Table 10.1: The range of dollar costs to the US economy in relation to the incidence of viral infection producing NV

Percentage of viral group having NV as major symptom	Additional days of absenteeism involved	Total cost of all work days missed due to NV ($US)
10	9 529 800	2,581 720 064
20	19 059 600	3,417 292 928
30	28 589 400	4,252 865 792
40	38 119 200	5,088 438 656
50	47 649 000	5,924 011 520

Many uncertainties exist when one bases cost figures on assumptions and convenience of calculations. The costs calculated do not specify whether money was paid to the people who missed work (representing 'sick leave') or represents lost productivity. A 'real' figure is most likely a blend of both. In any event, a $6 billion cost is a genuine and substantial loss to the economy as a whole.

Putting that figure into perspective, the 1996 annual US GDP was approximately $7 trillion. The losses in productivity and income from NV amount to a little less than 1% of total output for the largest estimates. On the other hand, the costs of cancer in the USA are $104 billion per year, representing over 9% of the annual GNP. The midrange of estimated NV costs at $10 billion are 10% of those of cancer, not an insignificant proportion.

Economic impacts of PONV

PONV attracts studies attending to health care costs. Medical management seeking to reduce PONV can reduce hospital and patient expenses. In addition, the psychological toll of suffering for patients experiencing PONV is large. In two separate studies, the morbidity 'costs' as a result of PONV were examined. In the Netherlands, about 23% of pre-surgical patients feared PONV. In another group, 50% of those patients who had outpatient gynecological surgery did experience PONV. Of that group, 54% considered the PONV to be more debilitating than the effects of the original surgery.

Management and prevention of PONV have improved in recent years with the advent of propofol and other new anesthetics. On the other hand, surgical frequency rates also rise for some conditions. Note that many of the factors contributing to NV's presence are outside a physician's control. For instance, women are between two and four times, depending on the study done, more likely to experience PONV than men. Children are two times more likely to experience PONV than adults. Spinal anesthesia produces fewer occurrences of PONV than does general anesthesia. People with a history of PONV and motion sickness are at greater risk to experience it again. Specific types of surgery and anesthetics are more likely to induce PONV than others. The anesthesiologist, hospital, and nursing care contribute to varying levels. In Table 10.2, the incidence of PONV after several types of surgery is estimated.

Table 10.2: Estimated incidence of PONV in adults

Type of surgery	Incidence of PONV (%)
Intra-abdominal (laparotomy)	70
Major gynecological (laparotomy)	58
Laparoscopy	40–77
Orthopedic	40
Ear, nose, and throat (ENT)	71
Strabismus (children)	85
Adenotonsillectomy (children)	58

In many cases, pre-treatment with the recommended 16 mg ondansetron can lower the prevalence of PONV, as well as limiting the amount of post-surgical pain and movement of the patient. Some of the direct and indirect costs of PONV must be assessed in an attempt to determine whether use of ondansetron – an illustrative drug in the high-risk groups – is cost-effective.

There are six major reasons to avoid PONV (Table 10.3). Each ties in with either a direct or indirect cost of PONV.

Table 10.3: Importance of avoiding PONV

1. Dehydration and electrolyte imbalance may result
2. Vomiting may lead to internal bleeding and intracranial pressure that may rupture the surgical wound
3. There is significant patient morbidity/anxiety with PONV
4. Cases may disrupt the flow of outpatients into the recovery room and, if severe, lead to hospital admission
5. Cases take up staff and professional time in NV management efforts
6. Occurrence results in the use of AE treatment and requires more supplies such as bed linens, juices, crackers, and janitorial services

Direct, indirect, and total costs

A direct cost will be defined as a cost arising because of an illness and is billed directly to the patient or hospital. An example of a direct cost would be the cost to a patient of being admitted to the hospital for overnight observation as a result of NV. Indirect costs, that is, those affecting the economy as a whole, may result from PONV. Lost productivity and absence from work are indirect costs.

For PONV both hospitals and patients bear specific costs. The health care establishment – or any third party payer including the Government – as a whole, especially insurance companies and HMOs, may be responsible for covering many of these costs. Their particular role is beyond the scope of this analysis. Costs will be assigned to two groups: patients and hospitals. Keep in mind that what the patient is billed does not necessarily accurately represent the cost to the hospital.

Excess time in the post-anesthesia room

PONV may begin in patient anxiety and predisposition before surgery, in the operating room, but the recovery room is the major site for its evolution and resolution. Patients with PONV will spend, on average, 47–61 minutes extra in the recovery room (Hirsch, 1994). This time, in terms of nursing labor costs, equates to an additional $2.28 per patient experiencing only N and $6.12 per patient experiencing NV. Further physician attention may be required, adding to the costs for the patient, either directly or indirectly.

Decreased throughput

A second element of the cost structure of PONV is an indirect cost to the hospital: the loss of the use of recovery facilities; thus other surgery, which might otherwise have been performed at a profit for managed care industries, could have been carried out if the additional time in the recovery room as a result of PONV had not occurred. Inefficient use is also a cause for non-profit. In the time that it takes to treat one patient experiencing PONV, an average hospital could have performed an additional 0.40 procedures in an outpatient setting. Thus, the opportunity cost for a typical setting fell within the range of $253 270–1 519 617 per year, or an additional 96–576 more procedures per year. Multiply this figure by the number of outpatient institutions in the USA and one gets a huge figure as an indirect cost to the hospital for NV.

The Dexter et al. (1995) study contradicts a finding of major loss, claiming that eliminating PONV would only reduce 4.8% of all recovery room time. Dexter et al. estimate that this gain in recovery room time poses no additional labor costs to the hospital because outpatient schedules were drafted to compensate for PONV. (Alternatively, larger facilities must be built and staffed to erase this source of costs.) The argument fails to recognize the indirect cost of the foregone surgical procedures that might have been performed within this time period. No figure acknowledging loss is provided. Indeed, arguing most conservatively, and holding the type of surgical procedures constant, revenues might increase by 4.8% if there were an absence of PONV.

A related but unassessed cost for which data are unavailable is the decreased operating room throughput that stems from treating a high-risk patient postoperatively: the unavailability of the anesthesiologist whose participation with patient assessment and treatment in the post-anesthesia room (PAR) prompts delays in resuming the surgical schedule. This factor aggravates the capacity of the surgical suite to function efficiently, and reduces the professional fees of physicians. Large surgical facilities hire a stand-by medical consultant to monitor and assist with PAR medicine, again adding another unassessed, indirect cost.

AE drugs and nursing /patient care supplies

PONV adds to the cost of surgery because its management often requires AE therapy. Ondansetron may be one component of this treatment post-surgery, with its average recommended dose of 4 mg intravenously. At $5 per mg, an additional $20 is required to use ondansetron to treat the patient. And, 'cocktails,' any, and all treatments may be ineffective! Including ondansetron. Also, patients may require the 'soda cracker or iced, carbonated beverage' supplement after taking ondansetron, adding a small, additional, usually indirect factor to the total cost of management.

The critical participation by PAR nurses in the diagnosis, treatment, and reassurance of nauseous patients cannot be slighted. A major portion of the nursing staff's effort is dedicated to control of PONV. Projections have not been made evaluating the potential reduction of PAR nurse staffing if PONV was diminished.

Bed linen contamination increases laundry costs, and bathroom mishaps, V on the floor, anywhere but the basin, requires janitorial attendance that add to the overall cost of PONV. Maintenance of suction equipment and disposable supplies (catheters, mouth pieces, etc.) contribute to these additional costs estimated at $7. Problems with possible contagion control (TB, AIDS) also arise, but are not calculated. And there is a rare death risk from aspirated vomitus. That *is* expensive.

Unscheduled admissions

Currently, in the USA, 60% of all procedures are performed on an outpatient basis. In these 'same-day' procedures, PONV occurs in from 8% to 45% of the cases depending on the type of procedure, risk factors, and study methodology. If a patient undergoes violent PONV, she or he must often be admitted to the hospital for overnight observation. This becomes a direct cost of PONV because the patient would otherwise have been at home. A one-night stay in the hospital at our Stanford University with normal nursing care ranges (1996) from $851 to $884 depending on the choice of a private or semi-private room. Some outpatient surgical centers are now introducing innovative ways to eliminate this added cost. For example, a patient, accompanied by a family member, can check into a hotel close to the hospital where a physician will come and visit them in the event PONV becomes more severe. In addition, hospitals are also using this hotel alternative to eliminate inpatient stays for procedures that usually required a 1–2 day inpatient stay. Many endoscopic surgical procedures, such as anterior cruciate knee ligament, reconstructive surgery, laparoscopic hysterectomy, and prostate gland resections lead to 23-hour admissions or short stays at 'hoptels.'

According to conservative estimates at Stanford University Hospital, 1% of all 'outpatient' procedures end up as unexpected inpatient stays as a result of NV. In the USA, the National Hospital Discharge Survey estimates that, in 1992, 20 426 000 outpatient procedures were conducted. At a 1% transfer rate, NV will compromise an additional 204 260 hospital days required for the severe cases. At the Stanford rate of $860 per hospital day (now higher!), $176 million is required to pay nationwide for outpatients experiencing NV who must remain in the hospital for a single night.

Home care costs

The final cost attributable to PONV is the cost of continuing therapy at home after outpatient surgery. One estimates that 30% of postoperative outpatients experience NV at home. Follow-up studies are limited. It may be more. NV require time from both the individual afflicted and nearby friends or family members. Costs include missing time from work and any over-the-counter medication that might be purchased in the at home rescue therapy. Sixteen percent of people afflicted with PONV at home miss an average of a half day of work. In addition, 22% of their at home caregivers miss on average a half day of work as well. Using the numbers from the NHIS, 980 448 of the patients miss a half day of work and 1348 116 of the caregivers for these patients miss a half day of work as well. Assuming that a half day of work is 4 hours and the average wage for men and women is $10.96, PONV at home cost the US economy $51 million in 1993.

Cancer chemotherapy and NV

Cancer accounts for 10% of the total cost of disease in the USA. For 1993, the National Cancer Institute estimated that cancer cost the US economy $104 billion. Of this amount, $12 billion was for morbidity or lost productivity, and $57 billion was estimated for the mortality cost or cost of premature death (American Cancer Society). How much of the $69 billion in morbidity and mortality costs can be attributed to the adverse patient reaction to chemotherapy-induced NV? We examine the direct and indirect costs of managing chemotherapy-induced NV. Second, we look at the effects of unbearable NV after chemotherapy and how the NV-spurred avoidance of this procedure leads to a shorter than expected lifespan and additional mortality costs.

The cost

Several studies examine the effects of chemotherapy-induced NV. The study of O'Brien (1993) is relevant to this analysis. In their study, 78% of the patients who underwent cancer chemotherapy experienced at least one episode of NV. The average cost of N and emesis for patients experiencing these symptoms was $Can184 which is about $US129. Of this figure, $US85 are indirect costs of NV and $US44 are direct costs of managing only V. On average, in this study, each actual chemotherapy procedure results in an additional cost of $US104 to the Canadian economy ($US37 for direct costs and $US67 for indirect costs). (Dollars for the rest of this analysis will remain in the US denomination unless otherwise specified. The exchange rate is assumed to be 0.7 $US/$Can.)

Applying the results to the US economy, the direct cost of 42 additional hours of nursing time is incurred by patients experiencing emesis. The total number of patients in the Canadian study was 92. Of that number, 38 (41%) of the patients experienced emesis with or without N and 72 had at least one occurrence of N and/or V. The mean cost of the extra nursing time was $Can17.80 for each of the 72 patients experiencing NV. This presumes a $21.60 per hour wage rate for nurses. Assume that the wage rate in the USA is on a par with that of Canada for nurses and that, for every chemotherapy procedure performed, an extra $11.55 is spent on nursing labor costs as a result of NV.

A serious problem with the Canadian study in its direct costs is that it greatly underestimates the current US average cost per procedure for unexpected hospital admissions caused by N and/or V. With 72 patients involved and an estimated cost of $Can 31.90, for the nine hospital admission days in the study, this works out to be approximately $Can 2300 for the hospital admissions or $Can 260 per night. In US terms, this figure approximates $179 per night. This is well below the mean cost in the USA for a night in a hospital: at Stanford Medical Center, recall that the 1995 mean cost for a night with regular observation in the hospital was approximately $860, or almost five times higher! Nine nights in the hospital would cost $7 740 with an average of $84 ($7 740/92) per patient involved in the study.

In the O'Brien study, patients did not receive the ondansetron now so widely prescribed (and overused). The approved UHC formulary permits up to 15 mg ondansetron to be used to treat chemotherapy-induced NV. Ondansetron is not used for anticipatory NV (ANV) which occurs in an estimated quarter of the cases or in delayed emesis (> 24 hours). At $5 per mg, it is estimated that the cost of using ondansetron is approximately $75 per patient in each chemotherapy procedure, whereas in the Canadian study, estimating 78% of people experiencing at least one instance of emesis after a chemotherapy procedure, an average of only $58.90 is spent on AE drugs per chemotherapy procedure. Current costs in the USA are much greater than in Canada for stays and drugs.

Regarding the direct costs category, assume that the other O'Brien figures approximate costs in the USA. That study estimates that $Can6 is spent on miscellaneous items at home after a chemotherapy treatment such as over-the-counter drugs and additional medical contacts. This figure is calculated to be $4.20 per patient per chemotherapy procedure.

Increased morbidity and decreased lifespan

In the Canadian study, of the 72 patients experiencing NV, 198 hours of paid employment and 409 hours of unpaid employment were lost. In addition, 186 hours of profitable employment opportunity were lost by caregivers of these patients. If it is assumed that all unpaid employment is valued at the cost of paid employment and that the caregivers' time is also valued at the same rate, then the study yields a $7.56 per hour wage rate in the USA. The wage rate for absentees was higher, $10.80 per hour in the USA. The results should be adjusted to reflect this factor. Thus, in US terms, the cost of lost productivity per chemotherapy procedure is $93.10, which, coincidentally, is the same figure determined in Canadian dollars by the study.

A quick recap of all of the costs per chemotherapy procedure is reviewed in Table 10.4. In addition, the patients' out-of-pocket

Table 10.4: Cost of NV per chemotherapy procedure (n = 92)

Health care cost	Mean cost per patient ($US)
Direct costs	
Nursing	11.55
Drugs to prevent/treat emesis	58.90
Hospital admissions	84.00
Miscellaneous expenses	4.20
Indirect costs	
Patients' out-of-pocket expenses	1.40
Value of lost production	93.10
Total cost per procedure	254.55

expenses in the study are assumed accurately to reflect costs in the USA.

Another assumption required is that the sample size and analytical methods accurately reflect the average costs on the US economy per chemotherapy procedure. Assume that the average of $254.55 per procedure may be generalized to all patients.

In 1992, according to the National Health Discharge Survey, 438 000 procedures of 'Injection or infusion of cancer chemotherapeutic substance' were carried out. With a cost of $254.55 per chemotherapy procedure, NV costs the US economy approximately $111.5 million ($111 492 900) every year for direct and indirect costs related to its occurrence after chemotherapy. Additional indirect costs come about as patients who experience severe NV drop out of treatment altogether because of intolerable NV suffering.

Cessation of therapy as a result of NV

Patients who do not continue chemotherapy treatment because of NV are expected to live shorter lives than patients who continue with the treatment. It is difficult to place a dollar cost on this earlier mortality for those who drop out of chemotherapy treatment, because the life expectancy of distinct cancers varies substantially. One may employ the overall cost estimate of $57 billion, for early mortality cost (Cancer Facts and Figures).

Stewart, in Kurcharczyk et al. (1991), estimates that 20% of chemotherapy patients quit treatment as a result of NV. The figures vary. That study took place before the advent of presumably more effective serotonin antagonists such as ondansetron. We shall assume that the chemotherapy drop-out rate from NV ranges between 10% and 20%. The mortality cost associated with leaving chemotherapy is calculated by multiplying the drop-out rate by the total mortality cost associated with all types of cancer. Thus, a 10% drop-out rate contributes $5.7 billion as premature death costs. At drop-out rates of 15% and 20%, leaving chemotherapy treatment has a mortality cost of $8.6 billion and $11.4 billion, respectively.

This method of calculation has been selected for several reasons. The three most predominant cancers – lung, prostate, and breast – all have very low life expectancies if diagnosed in some middle stage. With the exception of breast cancer, chemotherapy treatment adds marginal life expectation to patients somewhere in the middle stages of the disease. Yet, if caught in an extremely early stage breast cancer can be completely conquered and life expectancy returned to near normal. In addition, a significant number of years can be added to the lives of lung cancer patients after appropriate surgical intervention and chemotherapy treatment. Assume, optimistically, that all cancer cases are diagnosed at an early stage of development and the combination of chemotherapy, radiotherapy, and surgery is able to restore full life expectancy of the average US male, for instance, to 76 years.

Such figures are problematic insofar as they assume that all other cancers are caught in their early stages of development and that chemotherapy completely restores life expectancy to its maximum value. The data are to the contrary. In the future, it would be appropriate to develop a cancer cost constant that predicts the success of chemotherapy treatment for the different forms of cancer, calculating how many years chemotherapy 'restores' to patients' lives. Let this be constant k. Assume a k value of 1.0 for all forms of cancer in early stages of development. However, the average of all k values will rest somewhere between 0 and 1, thus these figures are much in need of data-based actuarial correction. A revised chemotherapy mortality cost function will look something like: \$ cost $= k \times$ (drop-out ratio) $\times$ (estimated total mortality costs). Table 10.5 demonstrates the estimated mortality costs of leaving chemotherapy during 1995, using different k values and drop-out ratios.

This model assumes that the \$57 billion dollar figure estimated by the National Cancer Institute is correct and that k values are acceptable approximations. By the conservative estimate that 10% of patients drop out of chemotherapy and $k = 0.1$, dropping out of

Table 10.5: Mortality costs of early exit from cancer chemotherapy (in \$billion), 1995 data

k	10% CDOR (\$)	15% CDOR (\$)	20% CDOR (\$)
0.1	0.57	0.855	1.14
0.2	1.14	1.71	2.28
0.3	1.71	2.57	3.42
0.4	2.28	3.42	4.56
0.5	2.85	4.28	5.70
0.6	3.42	5.13	6.84
0.7	3.99	5.99	7.98
0.8	4.56	6.84	9.12
0.9	5.13	7.70	10.26
1.0	5.70	8.55	11.40

k, chemotherapy mortality cost constant.
CDOR, chemotherapy drop-out rate.

chemotherapy treatment cost the US economy at least $0.57 billion in 1995 in mortality costs. The upper cost estimate is $11.4 billion.

Consumer economics

Consumers bear many costs of NV. Other than pain and disability are higher health insurance premiums and higher minimum insurance deductibles. In addition, some of the lost productivity in the economy manifests itself in the form of higher prices for consumer goods and services.

Further study

The costs of NV related to economic crime or slippery practices have not been studied. However, there have been many recent examples of how pharmaceutical firms have either suppressed or falsified data in relation to their products. One recent example is the controversy surrounding Upjohn's sleeping drug Halcion (triazolam, a benzodiazepine hypnotic agent). Upjohn has been accused of not releasing research results that highlight some of the harmful side effects of halcion. And Boots, a major 'chemists/drug store' in the UK, was convicted of suppressing research data showing the efficacy of lower cost compounds that could be made competitively available (1996). In 1997 Glaxo, manufacturer of ondansetron, was accused of biasing publication of positive clinical trial data.

One fairly presumes that pharmaceutical companies may distort research on publicly available information on their AE products (see Chapter 4 on self-favoring selectivity in PDR reports).

One must also allow, as an economic crime, falsified billing related to NV. If a patient spends only one hour in the recovery room with NV and is billed for one hour and fifteen minutes, a loss has occurred. Imprecision in hospital billings is notorious, as is defrauding Medicaid. Actual costs cannot be determined without support for research on unintentional misappropriation of charges, and of 'economic crime' in health care. One must pessimistically assume that it costs us many millions of dollars every year.

Conclusion

NV constitute an important and expensive aspect of human suffering. Initial cost estimates offered herein are inexact, but are in the low billions of dollars annually. Insofar as drug research is supported only by pharmaceutical companies expecting greater profits from better, and usually more expensive, therapeutic agents, one can obtain few research data focused on lower cost alternatives. Nor is there a lobby, as for cancer, advocating research for what might yield both economic and compassionate gains.

PART IV

NEW PERSPECTIVES: THEORY

CHAPTER 11

Pregnancy nausea and vomiting: empirical but enigmatic

This chapter attends to those quite different expressions of nausea and vomiting which are pregnancy nausea and vomiting (PNV) or 'morning sickness' and hyperemesis gravidarum (HG). In journals one may find these terms used interchangeably and without definition as to trimester occurrence, severity, and treatments. Clear differentiation can be difficult. Gynecology textbooks do not consider NV in any detail. All 'explanations' rely on one or another mechanistic model. None of these, nor any other theory of etiology, is adequately demonstrated.

Fairweather (1968), the first to do a major review and synthesis, tells us that PNV was described in Egypt circa 2000 BC, and was referred to by Hippocrates and by Soranus of Ephesus, early second century AD, who wrote on midwifery, and women's and children's disorders. His remedies for PNV included fasting, rest, massage, easily digested food, weak wine, passive exercise, aromatics, and herbs.

Modern textbooks, insofar as they venture anything at all on etiology, propose competing gastrointestinal, endocrinological, toxicological, and psychogenic possibilities. The last tends to be admitted to medicine when all else fails. Psychogenic PNV dynamics or functions are not considered in psychiatric or psychological texts. There, as in obstetrics and gynecology, it is a stepchild.

There are good reasons for this. One is that no theory of PNV 'works;' findings continue to be contradictory, and PNV seems to do no permanent harm – as differentiated from the real risk from hyperemesis. The practitioner needs to know what to do and not to do 'right now.' What not to do in pregnancy for PNV, not HG, comes first: neither prescribe nor even recommend any but the most homely folk treatments, because interventions are 'litigens,' that is, likely to cause lawsuits should a pre-, peri-, or postnatal, typically teratogenic, problem arise. PNV in litigious America is known to be dangerous, not for the woman (except for her pain and disability which is taken to be her compulsory fate and hardy lot), but for the practitioner.

Hyperemesis treatments are of a different class, because HG threatens both fetus and mother; HG demands treatments and, on failure of these, hospital admission. Antiemetics as well as intravenous nutrients can be prescribed because the alternative is far worse (the new PNV/HG cocktails are often recommended, e.g. a combination of dopamine antagonist and antihistamine).

The conventional obstetric and gynecology text writer, pressed for a list of 'mechanisms' for PNV, can do little beyond listing those chemical messengers shown or believed to be involved in other NV, but with special emphasis on pregnancy-altered intestinal mechanics ('pressure') or 'exaggerated' levels, interactions of estrogen/progesterone/oxytocin, and the like. By way of reminder, the chemical messengers for biologically activating information implicated in one or other NV, and thus possibly for PNV, include: serotonin, angiotensin, glycosides, endogenous opiates, histamine, dopamine, muscarinic, cholinergic messengers, or no messengers, plus neuropeptide/endocrines such as vasopressin, oxytocin, peptide Y, cholecystokinin (CCK), somatostatin, interleukin-1, vasoactive intestinal polypeptide (VIP), and immunoreactive prolactin as well, because it is a target for estrogen regulation of gene expression in the hypothalamus (see Shivers et al., 1989). Nor dare one discard interest in adrenocorticosteroids, atrial natriuretic peptide (ANP) (little noted since Gibson et al., 1986), prostaglandins, adenosine triphosphate (ATP), glutamate, gamma-aminobutyric acid (GABA), immunoreactivated c-fos, or, within cells, polyphosphoinositide lipids (the PI system) and G-protein cell messengers. (As a note, see Marx, 1987; Jarnfelt-Samsioe, 1987: PNV women are reported to differ from non-PNV mothers in serum lipids and lipoproteins throughout pregnancy.)

In the case of a current set of findings (Jordan et al., 1998; Goodwin, 1994), a provocative recent observation is the finding of a significant increase in total human chorionic gonadotropin (hCG) (159 770 vs 86 420 IU/l; $p < 0.001$) appearing in the serum of 20 women with HG, compared with 20 pregnant controls; Samoan women (10 per group) had higher values than European women (10 per group). The hCG present in the most acidic quartile of the eluates of sera from the HG women was 29 540 IU/l, compared with 8744 IU/l in the control sera, and both groups with HG had additional hCG peaks in the second most acidic quartile.

Related works continue to call our attention to the relationship between HG, hCG and hyperthyroidism, the latter a particular HG pregnancy risk (Tsurata, 1995; Yoshimura, 1995; Tareen et al., 1995; Goodwin et al., 1997). Asian women appear to be at higher risk of thyrotoxicosis (Price et al., 1996). Differences in isoform profile may be genetic, but the mechanism(s) by which acidic hCG isoforms provoke N remains undefined. When considered with the excess acidic isoforms observed in patients with hydatidiform molar pregnancies, which are also associated with elevated levels of hCG and excess N, compared with normal pregnancies, one becomes hopeful that a pathoendocrinological tag for N in pregnancy may at last be in view. If additional studies confirm this preliminary finding, studies can then be designed for understanding this highly morbid form of NV, and perhaps for PNV in general.

Except for the specialized worker, such listings are not helpful. The danger is that the listing of 'we believe' may convey the sense to the student, primary care worker, or psychosocial scientist reader that specialized neuropharmacological research workers 'have the matter in hand.' The medical textbook writer does well to leave presumptive PNV 'mechanisms' alone, as with 'centers' for too easy accounting.

It is the intention of this chapter to provoke reflection, so as to broaden the base of disciplines concerned with PNV in women's health, and to incite new research.

Prevalence

Estimates of how many women suffer PNV depends upon the study one reads. Reported rates for NV in the first trimester range from 30% to 90%. We suspect a reasonable figure of the 'it seems right' sort will be akin to the estimate of the American College of Obstetrics and Gynecology, a cultural normalizing one, that is, 'half and half seems fair' both coinciding at 50%. There is no 'is' there; the figure is satisfactory when employed to indicate that, at least in technological societies where the research is done, there is 'much' PNV, 'consequential to women,' and 'likely to be painful and disabling,' and surprising inexplicable. Tierson et al. (1986), in an earlier broad review, locate a modal point somewhat higher than 50%.

The very range of findings tells us that we are in trouble with respect to any theory of NV which relies on an assumption of a 'normal' endocrinological, gastrointestinal, toxicological, and psychogenic one-source etiology for PNV. Most pregnancies proceed, in well-fed and cared-for populations, nonpathologically.

PNV is statistically 'normal' because PNV appears to be any phenomenon that varies so much, depending on the populations studied (30–90%), as to be surprisingly unstable after all. Phenomena that distribute themselves widely in otherwise normal populations, or unpredictably in the 50% figure, are likely multivariably and individualistically determined. That same variability in the broader picture of NV applies now in etiological searches regarding PNV.

What influences symptom reporting will influence PNV prevalence statistics.

Reporting of N varies with the woman's own self-sensitivity, her awareness or definition of a threshold of distress worthy of reporting, and her cultural standard for reporting, whether 'stiff upper lip' or otherwise. This is a methodological issue which all clinicians should bear in mind. Zbrowski, in 1952, demonstrated that pain reporting varied by ethnic/religious group, with an implied geographical gradient for more pain admission as one moved from northern European to southern European origins. Zola (1973) provided the added empirical insight that complaints occurred, and doctor's visits were initiated, more often among people whose condition interfered with functions that were important to them. Pain or disability by itself need not be enough to precipitate reporting.

One speculates that some pregnant women will consider PNV part of their self-identification as an expectant mother and would be more prone to discuss it should their familiar/cultural origins place a greater emphasis on being a mother. Clark (1952) shows how reporting is linked, among Hispanic Americans, to the 'meanings' of a condition, where pain and symptoms can be used to blame, exonerate, etc., as, for example, in mobilizing social support or at least to generate concern and assistance (if not guilt or pity) from the family; it is thus a means of altering styles of relating (who does what for whom, etc.). And insofar as N is sometimes 'somatization,' that is, a psychosomatic expression of other stress, fatigue, 'copelessness,' nonverbalized need for help and sympathy, it will vary culturally and within cultures. For example, the work shows Chinese women more likely to somatize, when compared with Anglos, but particularly when they were poor, had great household responsibilities, spoke English poorly, and the like.

Downs and Blum (1993) found novel – to the West, not Cambodia – symptoms of psychosomatization, as expressive, manipulative, and culturally defined, among south-east Asian immigrants. Symptoms have uses as well as meaning and stress functions. Barsky (1979) found somatization to be greater in those people who were poor, rural, and either untrained in verbalizing felt distress or trained culturally/familiarly not to speak of personal anguish or stress. For further research on symptoms as to when, where, and their meanings, read Pennebaker's superb work (Pennebaker, 1982, 1984). It is likely that autonomic self-awareness, of pregnancy plus gastrointestinal motility, plays a part if arousal of the autonomic nervous system (ANS) is itself a variable, and also one that is stress related. The psychosomatics expert knows that the body does 'speak,' expresses in its symptoms and movements the situation of the person, including interpersonal difficulties, emotional distress, and the how of interpreting inner states. Variation in PNV prevalence rates will reflect these factors.

There is no 'normalcy' for HG. It is life threatening and limited to about 1% of populations studied, perhaps less. Fairweather (1968) proposes 0.01% and Swedish hospital data give values as low as 0.001% (K'all, 1987). The future will probably show PNV and much NV as a final common pathway for multiple precipitants, although these are quite specific for the situation in pregnancy as an altered state of the internal environment. Viewed in this way, it is an ecological interaction in which NV are a measure of the subject's reaction. As a parallel, think of that block to pregnancy in rodents in which the smell of a male other than the sire will induce early spontaneous abortion in the female (Brennan et al., 1990; Doty and Muller-Schwarze, 1992).

HG is best defined by NV and nutritional threat. The sufficient and serious standard (reliable in wealthy countries for insured mothers) is of intravenous nutrients given at home or admission to hospital, lest fetus and mother become malnourished, suffer related deficiencies and risks, and, if untreated, die. The intractable acute V of a mother has itself led to death. Obviously, occurrence varies with population characteristics of an unfortunately unknown nature. Alternative definitions contribute to some rate variations. PNV of a nonmorbid nature can continue through pregnancy.

Conferring risk advantage?

PNV risk may be considered in several ways: reporting the risks for PNV, or the examination of the risk that PNV poses – and here one thinks of advantage possibly conferred as well as morbidity or other difficulties that are estimated at rates other than expected. For PNV there has been limited consideration of obstetric, perinatal, teratogenic, or even a 'special child' (as in our pediatric mothers' sample?) focus or delayed offspring morbidity.

There would be no reason to expect PNV to lead to either greater or lesser perinatal or teratogenic risk unless the events of PNV itself were physiologically consequential for the fetus, or for maternal capabilities with respect to placental nutrition, birth capabilities, later abilities to care. This does not rule out severe PNV as a marker of problems in the uterine environment. But any consistently replicable finding of PNV as advantageous or adverse must be linked, in theory now and demonstrated later, with intrauterine or perinatal events. And were such to be shown, in contrast to an acute but embryologically indifferent set of events, these would be, in evolutionary terms, highly selective. To date, including the years since Galen or Avicenna, and all folk and scientific observation, nothing suggests PNV as anything but a response to an outer or inner perturbation, that is, nothing but our own unreplicated and untrustworthy finding that the most severe PNV pregnancies may confer obstetric risk.

Recall that women in our own sample did attribute particularly unusual outcomes to their worst, and their best, NV episodes among their multiple pregnancies. Provocative, but not consequential. We have noted that there are other work data suggesting that PNV can confer obstetric risk advantage, that is, women with PNV may – and only 'may' – have somewhat lower risks of lower gestational age, spontaneous abortion, and perinatal morbidity. The literature is contradictory and the logic must be examined. The major studies are by Klebanoff et al. (1985), and Weigel and Weigel (1988). The number of subjects in Klebanoff's study ($n = 9098$) is impressive, although that of Weigel and Weigel ($n = 825$) is not deficient. Yerushalmy and Milkovich (1965), in an earlier study ($n = 3853$), report that women found a significantly lower spontaneous abortion rate: 3.8% among PNV women vs 10.4%, and fewer teratogenic outcomes. Weigel and Weigel, using the same measure, obtained figures of 1% for V women versus 7.25% without N or V. Klebanoff found spontaneous abortion (although somewhat differing weeks were employed in the studies) to be 3.4% for V women versus 7.2% for no PNV. Work by Jarnfelt-Samsioe (1985b) found no risk advantage conferred; Medalie (1957) carried out a pioneering study which, in a small sample ($n = 100$), obtained differences of 0% vs 23%. The sample size here, and the extent of the discrepancy from other studies, make one cautious. Little is immediately relevant. And if it is necessary to differentiate between severe and less severe PNV, then all of the work to date is confounded by samples with mixed predictive traits.

One problem with reliance upon spontaneous abortion rates is the knowledge that the expected population spontaneous abortion rates ordinarily reported vary from 10% to 20% depending on a number of population and environmental variables. Although some studies do enjoy large samples, the natural fluctuation in rates does not allow one a steady base for expected rates against which to compare outcomes. As miscarriage rates are not reliably reported, and older women report fewer earlier losses than younger women, the reliability of abortion counts is in itself a problem. The most careful studies suggest that early loss may be as great as 50%, obviously most of which are not known (or at least not readily noticed) by older and (an assumption) multiparous women. (For a macabre medical science fiction story about that, read G.P. Hosman's tale in *The Medical School*, Claycomb Press.) There is no work to tell us accurately about the sensitivity of women as a variable contributing to their reporting accuracy.

The Klebanoff study would be persuasive about conferred obstetric risk from PNV were it not also contradicted in its specifics by the study of Brandes (1967) whose findings differed in birthweight, generally by that of Jarnfelt-Samsioe (1985b) and, paradoxically arguable because Weigel and Weigel (in whose sample 71% experienced PNV) also found advantage conferred, from the factor analysis of specificity. In Klebanoff's group white had advantage over black, and parity was a risk predictor but more for V in whites than in blacks. Their quite differing sets of women's characteristics were found to predict lower obstetric risk: the first factor was being white, professional, and not drinking. Other factors, as related traits for prediction, were being over 35, and having no history of infertility; a third, unrelated to the others, was no prior history of N during pregnancy. In the first factor, white women were older, Hispanics were younger. Unlike Klebanoff et al., Weigel and Weigel found parity not to be a predictor of obstetric risk, nor was the interval between births. Weigel and Weigel found no difference in predictors of N and V, and therefore none of the 'patterning' that we have come to look for. There was only one consistent trait which predicted higher obstetric risk in their sample: being a housewife. In seeking to link PNV morbidity outcomes to PNV itself, one naturally refers to, or may endorse, one or other of the proposals for NV itself.

Weigel and Weigel, for instance, proposed disturbed hepatic function or estrogen levels high enough to stimulate emetic centers in the brain. Jarnfelt-Samsioe (1986) has observed, in women seeking abortion, differences in the size and placement of the corpus luteum – greater on the right for PNV; she thus suggested that this *might* account for the differences between pregnancies for a woman. She proposed that, as right ovarian veins drain into the inferior vena cava, with impaired drainage these might concentrate steroids in the portal venous system giving rise to a hormonal load on the liver, and leading to hepatic-initiated PNV. That hepatic routes may be involved in PNV induction has been suggested elsewhere, although no consistent observations yield evidence of an impact in PNV mothers of hepatic malfunction. Of course less adequate liver capacity may produce NV and PNV and a potential adverse risk. That hepatic routes may be involved in V induction has also been suggested, and is not unreasonable, although no consistent observations yield evidence of an impact of hepatic malfunction on PNV mothers.

There are many studies identifying one or other PNV risk factor; were this a chronic maternal feature – including environmental – affecting fetal growth or health, perinatal, and postnatal events, the factor might be proposed as adverse rather than apparently conferring advantage. Weigel and Weigel (1988) in their factor analysis sought such 'risk rational' data. They are elusive. The Weigel and Weigel factor analysis yields factors that make no apparent sense. The higher risk among housewives can be accounted for in terms of Pennebaker's symptom sensitivity among housewives, or other women not enjoying as much social stimulation. This suggests that housewives may be more likely to be self-attentive in the absence of richly diversified sensory environments. The rest of the Weigel and Weigel factors do not cohere.

The implications of a conferred PNV advantage are both puzzling and consequential. Epidemiological studies are notorious for their capacity to reverse findings over the years. Yet for all of the methodological problems, one cautiously accepts that obstetric advantage is present in some populations, although, apart from spontaneous abortion, there is inconsistency about what advantage. One then asks whether such advantage for fertility, and for the presumed well-being of the woman who does not have to face the possible psychological trauma of fetal or neonatal loss has any further health or evolutionary selective implications. Data are lacking on reproductive lifetime conceptus viability for these populations. We assume that the aborted conceptus is Nature's wise decision, because pregnancy loss can be attributed to many problems including malformation (particularly congenital heart syndrome), chromosomal abnormality (predominantly autosomal trisomy), gynecological pathology, antigen–antibody ABO blood group response, progesterone deficiency, infectious disease, IUDs, gamete aging, noxious environmental features, anesthetics, smoking, alcohol, radiation, age of the woman, etc. It has not been established from the research data that loss of one conceptus predicts greater lifetime reproductive hazard for the women in these samples. But if sampling is as random as reproductive age, it may well exist.

We could infer from any of the reproductive loss risks mentioned above that they are more likely to be absent during pregnancies in the PNV than in the non-PNV group. We cannot conclude yet that the PNV health of the mother is enhanced, or that the loss is anything but Nature's decision (discounting the PNV teratological risk). There are, however (see Chapter 12), studies that refer to immune factors, specifically odor-mediated selection of mate based on diversity of HLA (human leukocyte antigen) type. Fertility is compromised and abortion risk raised when there is similarity of HLAs between mates.

PNV as a nonspecific response

The simplest explanation for PNV is consistent with the extensive data which tell us that women are generally vulnerable to N and, to a lesser extent, to V. Multiple external and internal environmental events trigger their NV; insofar as V may have an N 'curative' function, V is of less consequence etiologically; N is demonstrated to be the greater response to perturbations as a threat or insult. However much it signals sensory awareness, it is a nonadaptive response as well as a nonspecific one. The tables in Chapter 3 showed the interrelationships of NV dispositions. There are groups of women who are at general risk.

To date PNV appears to be most singularly responsive to odor. A woman's aversive odor response is functional, not shown to be in terms of chemically 'toxic' environments (although this could be the case), but in terms of mating for immunological selection of offspring.

Culture

There are no thorough studies although anthropological work is important for PNV: Mead (1935) reported that, among the Arapesh, there was no PNV. Modern ethnographers, who are more methodologically oriented, consider Mead's work to be generally unsound. However, Minturn et al. (1984), relying on the Human Relations Area Files, identified eight societies in which ethnographers report no PNV. Some were studies of nonliterate, small, integrated societies, and others described general groups such as Egyptian peasant fellahin. Mead was not the first observer of such local differences. Fairweather (1968) tells us that Horowitz, in 1883, found HG to vary by country, and Fairweather himself found it to vary by city, and also that the incidence was lower in the UK in wartime. All research is subject to error. Reliance on a few mischievous informants, men reporting on women in a culture of distance, or perhaps of fear (after all in Egypt and Malaysia clitorectomy and suturing of the female child's labia are still widely practiced), and quite probably a failure to inquire or, if asking, a failure to detect a cultural norm that prohibits a woman from expressing her N pain or V to a stranger. Were PNV to vary with malnutrition and a study were done in a time of near starvation, all these factors would influence findings. But as levels of inquiry go, and with recognition of the careful quantifying methods in ethnographic use (including formal interviews and observations regarding health in each family in a village, as public health workers do) the work of Blum and Blum (1965, 1970) should be looked at; one must conclude that it is indeed quite possible that there are societies in which there is no, or very much less, PNV. Whether ethnographers see HG as a separate condition is not known.

The PNV-free cultural possibility throws a great many explanations out of the window, unless gastroenterology and endocrinology are culture dependent. One then looks to see how the select sample of observed societies without PNV might differ. One can imagine remarkable local herbal medicines that are effective in suppressing NV. Minturn et al. (1984) did ask whether climate, altitude, women's status/work roles as a 'precursor' to neurotic symptoms, or food taboos were different. They were not.

They did, however, find that fats were eaten more often and also green vegetables; eating of corn or maize was found to be significantly different, as none of the PNV societies ate maize as a staple, but seven of eight of those without PNV did. Interesting! They cite Rienken and Gant as having proposed that morning sickness reflected a vitamin B_6 deficiency. We have seen that vitamin B_6 (pyridoxine) is among the PNV treatments. Minturn et al. posit that corn has high vitamin B_6 content that would not be destroyed by brief cooking. But they also found that rice has vitamin B_6 and some of their non-PNV societies *did* cook their corn. Their careful conclusion could only be that the green vegetables – which also include vitamin B_6 (Whohl and Goodhart, 1984, cited in Minturn et al., 1984) – and the high fat all point to diet as a PNV element. But their emphasis on corn/maize overlooks the fact that corn and maize are staples world wide. Some African and Latin countries in the western hemisphere rely on it for about half of their energy intake. The nutritional questions appear to add to the PNV complexity.

Contemplate the issues. Foremost is an evolutionary one. If, for any period of time since modern humans evolved, PNV conferred a genuine teratological advantage (reduced morbidity; earlier or later reproductive survival advantage linked to teratological conditions be they malformation, fetal loss, reduced birthweight, and subsequent peri- and postnatal morbidity or mortality), there would be few, if any (except for mendelian regression), women without PNV.

Ornstein (1993) offers some general calculations, for example, from a survival advantage of only one in 10 000 for each generation from the Pleistocene and early humans (subject to debate over definitions of emergence) over the past million years. Generational expectations vary; these are short at first and grow longer only by very recent times. Ornstein proposes a very short 5 years which yields a population proportion, advantaged over disadvantaged, of 484 million. Be much more conservative: allow 15-year generations (fitting for Rome or the Middle Ages but of course with a high mortality) and 250 000 years (about 16 000 generations), and the proportion, by our exponential arithmetic, would have an advantage ratio of about 50. However much PNV studies of prevalence vary, we do not find, except for cultural exceptions, 98 PNV cases for every two non-PNV mothers. One might conclude that, if PNV confers an evolutionary, naturally selective advantage, it is of a low order indeed.

Alternatively, let us say that PNV is of recent origin, that it is a response to modernity. Let us make some playful assumptions. Assume that, whatever variations have occurred as a function of worldwide fertility/mortality ratio change, the lifetime viability of newborns (defined as staying alive and healthy enough to become reproductive and to confer sufficient advantage upon their offspring to assure similar survival rates) has averaged three per family (discount all real variability). (Barron and Thomson, 1983, display population pyramids and their change with modern demographic transitions.) Assume that PNV confers an advantage of 3% greater live births per 100 women. Assume further that HLA odor sensitivity, as a hypothesized trait expressing this advantage, yields a further evolutionary benefit via odor-mediated mate selection for HLA diversity, which means greater immune competence on the part of the offspring. Speculatively, assume further that severe PNV constitutes a separate group with higher obstetric risk, but that this group is much smaller, and that the 3% includes the exaggerated conceptus loss so derived. Rely on the careful estimates of Abramson (1973) cited by Gray and Doyle (1983); see also the work of Roman and Stevenson in Barron and Thompson (1983) which demonstrates a great but specifically unknown prevalence of spontaneous abortion: 25–75% across populations. We shall fix on 50% of all concepti lost. An actual live birth advantage of 3% per reproductive lifetime per 100 women, as a 47% conceptus loss, all other matters being held equal, would become a major population selectivity impact.

Other 'explanations'

The trend in PNV, and its embedded NV research on women, has been to identify ever more possible biochemical systems as 'the' process, and new brain regions as 'centers.' Psychogenic explanations beginning in the 1960s, and expanding in the 1970s, paralleled reductionist animal, endocrinological, and neuropharmacological studies, the twain never meeting. Mind and body elements were separate particularities. Contradictions within these areas, study by study as well as conceptually, continue. New research by pharmaceutical companies continues to look for 'the' magic bullet. NK1 (natural killer 1) receptor antagonists are the new focus (see Naylor, 1996a, b). No one seriously funds PNV work because there is no money to be made from litigens. Contradictions among disciplines are unresolved, but one now may hope for a Hegelian resolution out of 'higher' integration; for PNV as an exceptional instance of NV, it will mean embracing multi-level schema that incorporate a willingness to be radical in thinking about PNV as an exceedingly important aspect of women's reproductive lives.

More risk variables: incorporating NV risk and implication for PNV

Risk variables became of interest in the 1980s, or indeed considering 'neurosis,' then in the late 1800s. Women, of course, then and now, are more likely to be labeled as 'neurotic,' and by age 16 begin to receive far more prescriptions of tranquilizers than do men. Factors identified for PNV were to include prior dysmenorrhea (Bertling, 1948), postmenstrual syndrome (Vellacott, 1988), prior susceptibility to motion sickness, primigravida status, youth, less education, nonsmoking, (over)weight, and previous pregnancy V. Some of these predict, with low weight, HG as well (Depue et al., 1987; K'all, 1987). But, again, contradictions emerged with reference, for example, to smoking, parity, and age.

Cookson (1986), attending to PONV not PNV, observed that postoperative hypotension, when untreated, increases NV risk from

10% to 66% in both sexes. As hypotension is a normal condition of pregnancy, one asks – but is not answered by any studies of further work – what relationship might exist between PNV and hypotension. Certainly the statistic was an impressive one. The role of arginine vasopressin (AVP) was (and is) to be considered, because subsequent chemotherapy NV yields massive AVP level increases after induced NV (Edwards et al., 1989). Now it appears that other NV may increase AVP levels. Paradoxically, vasopressin injection may also induce NV. Emetics, such as apomorphine and ipecacuanha, increase AVP levels as well as those of oxytocin (Nussey et al., 1988). Thus it has been proposed that NV may activate the hypothalamoneurohypophyseal system to produce these AVP and oxytocin increases. NV are shown to release pancreatic polypeptides as well (Feldman et al., 1988). (N does not appear to induce substance P elevation.)

About half (to be optimistic about it) of otherwise unexplained patient NV is found (Geldof et al., 1986) to be accompanied by abnormal gastric pacemaking, tachygastria, and delayed stomach emptying of solids. This occurs during illness but also on later follow-up. It has been asked whether this more unstable chronic myogastric state provides a more excitable neuromuscular substrate for multiple, possibly perturbing stimuli, that is, as one might now put it, whether abnormal gastric conditions, whatever their origins, are a baseline NV varying possibly with individual autonomic awareness. If this were the case, one might expect one subset of PNV women to show, preconception and post partum, such myoelectrical instability, whereas another subset might demonstrate it as an acute first trimester state only. These earlier 'general' findings allowed the concept of a destabilized substrate as faulty inbuilt regulation akin to unstable or 'hot reactor' psychophysiological ANS baselines. Had Haaken–Kelso's language of critical instabilities in chaos theory been available, it would have been a 'natural' for such a description then as it is now. It allows that one does not search for only one single perturbing endocrine, sensory, or learned/symbolic PNV, or other NV-initiating condition, without taking into account spontaneous substrate activity (Llimas, 1988). The variety of substrate condition becomes not simply levels but are conceived of as interacting through contextual events.

V is generally age related, with a decreasing risk with age – although not in the recollection of our epidemiological sample – so that younger women and thus those of child-bearing age will be more susceptible than older women. The higher risk of primigravidas PNV, had it consistently appeared, could then be attributable to acute state factors superimposed on genetically programmed, or learned adaptive aging ones. Klebanoff et al. (1985) did show the age effect when comparing younger with older pregnant women in their large sample. Obesity is also a general NV risk factor, as may be simply the speed of eating. Obesity as pregnancy weight gain should then be a PNV risk.

Women suffer an incidence of perhaps three times more NV postoperatively. Women's NV is also found to be more severe than men's. Sex differences in PONV are greatest for abdominal surgery, independent of surgical site within the abdomen. Abdominal sensitivity to insult is general beyond surgery, because up to 33% of adverse drug reactions across a range of pharmaceuticals are reported at that site (Bruppacher et al., 1988). The sex-linked postoperative male–female differences in NV prevalence emerge at about age 11, strongly suggesting an NV, PNV reproductive system developmental association. In this sense PNV is abdominal sensitivity, whereas pregnancy is an abdominally centered process. But one should also consider the developmental feminizing sex role with the individual differences in abdominal awareness, body image centering, and subsequent abdominal vulnerability in association with threat and anxiety, or indeed possible sexuality as a cognitive–emotional part of a woman's being.

When Nerenz et al. (1986), among others, found that anxiety and stress were cancer chemotherapy NV predictors, this was consistent with a psychogenic notion of PNV origins, but not of displaced 'mind.' As MacLean (1949) said the old brain's limbic system is 'where the unconscious resides,' and is one of the areas engaged in inconsistent and hierarchically disharmonious fluctuating organization activity; as Ornstein (1993) would have it, mind including 'mind not all of one mind' remains central to the NV picture of PNV. And, again, for PNV it is olfaction, and olfaction is limbic. In the Cohen et al. (1994) study of risk factors (n = 16 000 women), they were youth, being healthy, having an elective procedure, being premenstrual, being a nonsmoker, and having a surgical resident present. (Obesity was not a predictor.) Health and environmental sensitivity were both risks for PNV. It seems that, in general, they are a risk for (more severe) PNV as well.

Typically, for surgery, inhaled anesthetics yielded somewhat more N, as did intraoperative opiate administration, and tracheal intubation. These were unimpressive in forecasting NV – except for minor gynecological surgery yielding more N than V (with N twice as common as V) than, it appears, major surgery (although ophthalmological and otological surgery were also higher-risk procedures), because the greatest variation was attributable to the anesthesiologist and hospital, not to traits or anesthetic interventions. And Cohen et al. introduced their conclusion with the observation of the great importance of NV to the woman in the lengths to which they were willing to go to avoid NV. This suggests that notions of PNV as consciously manipulative are wrong.

When we consider that it is often healthy young women, electing for surgery that is of a minor gynecological rather than intraabdominal nature, together with the skill/embarrassment/awkwardness of a resident's presence, the milieu of the hospital, with all risk factors controlled for this analysis, one is compelled to credit psychosocial factors as being one of the dominant ones in women's PONV. Women's sensitivities emerged as formidable variables in this careful study, which is the largest ever. One would believe that such findings could not help but call attention to where the woman patient's attention was calling the observant clinician, and Cohen and *her* colleagues. Odd, in no text or review have we found reference to this blockbuster – this assumption busting investigation. It was led by a woman.

Kunz-Kostokomanolakis et al. (1987) found, among women referred for inexplicably low serum potassium levels, that surreptitious self-induced V was the predominant cause. Bulimia is now considered a psychiatric disease which, like anorexia, is not unrelated to fashions and self-image for ideal weight. Self-induced V may have, in humans, as one presumes it does for regurgitating wolves feeding their young, a neurophysiologically rewarding, that is, hypothalamic and maternal 'reinforcing,' function (see Kupferman, 1991a, b). That NV have particular interpersonally communicative functions was reported, in a very small psychiatric sample, by Clarke et al. (1988). We have noted that Sartre earlier realized it was a cultural, philosophical, and by no means necessarily a psychiatric phenomenon. As a communicator of distress it is normal.

What we see now in etiological work, in broader conception, as for example in the great investigator Alan Miller's progression from medullary 'preparation' to c-fos and brain imaging, are conceptual configurations of an increasingly complex nature capable of being subsumed under integrating schemata. Such conceptions of configurations of events at several levels are compatible with John's (1980) earlier statistical configuration theory of regionally, neuronally relative, fluid brain activity. John's work was the predecessor to today's work in volume transmission, interneuronal space modulation, and

Haaken–Kelso's dynamic critical instabilities as self-organizing predictors of patterning. It is consistent with a schema for examining PNV allowing individual, environmental, genetic, and of course multiple internal biological events as part of PNV.

CHAPTER 12

Pregnancy nausea and vomiting: some new explanatory hypotheses

For enigmatic pregnancy nausea and vomiting (PNV) four theories of action have been partially demonstrated: psychogenic, gastrointestinal, endocrinological, and toxin sensitivity. The anthropological data, pending validation, also force consideration of a 'cultural/historical' theory. Recall that PNV varies in prevalence by place and population, but also with historical situations (i.e., war reduces PNV risk). The estrogen level is the quick explanation by the ordinary doctor. But there are recent data and theories (some from other disciplines) which provide possible sets of variables that might also contribute to PNV.

The remarkable range in epidemiological findings with respect to prevalence yields figures ranging from 0% allowing the anthropological studies to 90% for specific populations. This baffling variation is typically clinically approached by noting known risk variables such as smoking, work status, etc. Even these are unreliable – obesity, for instance. Nevertheless, individual differences within populations and within the life history of the individual must be considered. The multiparous woman is herself an instance of variability, because, of several pregnancies, only one may be with PNV. The first pregnancy seems to have a slight edge, but the data here are also contradictory.

The eclectic will presume that processes within the domain of each of the extant theories – which are themselves a function of the discipline of the observer – may account for some PNV. A diverse and multiple etiology is allowed. Given the likelihood that PNV confers some obstetric risk advantage, one is interested in absent PNV, not simply as a matter of research and clinical care, but as a general maternal health issue. This would be even more the case if our own unreplicated finding of severe PNV poses obstetric risk as well. PNV is obviously a response to a variety of perturbations and does seem to mark reproductive risk and the evolutionary adaptive advantage. For evolutionary biology, totally absent PNV is also a dramatic question.

An overview of arguments for nonspecificity or reproductive advantage must not divert the clinician from the obvious and immediate; for example, that common psychobiological situational features, such as fatigue (van Lier, 1993) or stress, induce or augment women's NV and PNV. Interpersonal functions may be present for PNV, e.g. eliciting care and attention as social support. More hypothetically, the smell of vomitus repels the stranger/enemy. The fact that, for PNV, odors or odors combined with foods are primary precipitants directs attention to olfaction and its triune brain placement and connections, although genetics, the immune system, and the biology of esthetics are not to be ignored. Multi-level and multidisciplinary data, and a conceptually broad approach, are demanded. Call it 'informed and hard-headed holism.' This is one definition of the new kind of psychosomatics that women's health and, more broadly, medicine and psychology require.

Toxin expulsion revisited: Profet, Pleistocene, and PNV evolutionary emergence

PNV occurs in no other animal than the human, not even the chimpanzee with whom we hold so much in common. Profet has proposed that PNV emerged in humans in the Pleistocene as humans were evolving and as part of our evolution as hunter–gatherers, in the search for new foods. Profet points out that, when trying new plants as possible foods, there would be exposure to teratogens and immediate poisons. PNV could have emerged as an adaptive evolution for the woman. An initial NV experience would also be aversive learning, inducing conditioned taste aversion (CTA). This CTA would be an individual not an 'inherited' learning unless one becomes Lamarkian. Profet does not argue for it, but we note that CTA widely experienced in a tribal group would become folk knowledge: 'Don't eat it.' Human food taboos are indeed widespread: pork, or tomatoes as poisonous 'night apples.' But, although a tribe will easily learn that a plant makes one sick, or kills, tribal folk would not have learned about teratogenicity. We have not yet learned enough about that field ourselves! Profet cites contemporaneous cases studied in which hunter–gatherer tribeswomen recognize that the risk of abortion can be plant induced, and indeed use such plants to induce an abortion. An instance, which is argued as evidence of new plant exposure dangers, is offered by Profet based on a Zambian resettlement program where 60 of 600 newly resettled tribespeople died of the 'Lusitu condition.' She attributes this to plant poisoning but does not cite corroborating data. No evidence for poisoning or abortifacient as folk knowledge of genuine teratogenicity is offered.

Profet proposes further that human allergies, as autoimmune responses, emerged as a defense against environmental toxins or animal venom. She differentiates between the nonallergic immune response, in which immune defense against foreign antigens proliferates to defend, potentially successfully, human survival against pathogens, and the allergic response to a nonpathological antigen (but likewise 'foreign' as in food or pollen), in which the response itself is likely to induce a self-damaging response that is uncomfortable if not tissue pathological. (If one examines Selye's classic stress response, the defensive reaction is not so clearly separated, e.g. fever and inflammation.) The entire class of IgE antibodies has, she writes, as its 'sole . . . purpose' to trigger the symptoms of allergy.

She rejects the possibility commonly held of immunological error as inappropriate recognition/discrimination. Hers is instead a creative Darwinian optimism where IgE symptoms are protective adaptive behaviors. When describing most biochemical release from cells as an immune response to the array of coherent rejecting behaviors – V, diarrhea, tearing, sneezing, scratching, or coughing – she argues that these are the functional and implicitly efficient expulsion of toxins.

The immediacy of the IgE allergic response, its behavioral severity, its prevalence including the response to metals, venoms, pollens, its 'cross-reactivities' to unrelated botanical families (i.e., it is the allergen not the botanical source that requires focus), even the apparent 'capriciousness' of the human allergic symptomatology make sense, she believes, when viewed as massively protective in biological intent (our term) and as a 'last line of defense.' The latter characterization alludes to general rather than to specific mechanisms of human toxin defense: the taste of bitterness (which she holds is toxin sensitive), shedding of epithelial surfaces of exposed organs, skin, DNA repair and antioxidants, and detoxifying enzymes produced by the liver are, she states, not molecularly specific but ongoing (chronic) and diffuse protective action. Allergic responses, including as we have said V and, by implication, PNV, occur when, she claims, these fail.

Looking at the evidence, allergic responses can be represented in the gut by NV (Bogardus et al., 1995). However, most of the 40% of a modern population, who report reliably on adverse reactions to specific foods and believe these to be 'allergic' (i.e., self-diagnosis), will be incorrect. Given the human lifetime processing of about 100 tonnes of food, it is the rarity of real allergies that is noteworthy. True food allergies are the classic IgE-mediated hypersensitivities (which can include skin, respiratory, and anaphylactic responses as well as NV). Bogardus and Kraft describe infant cows' milk sensitivity as the most common, present in 0.3–7% of babies, but prevalence of other true allergies does not rise above 2% of a population. If PNV was an allergic reaction, this figure would rise massively and would constitute a radical revision in gastric immunological thinking. Nor would one expect that a current low 'actual' rate of a maximum 2% could represent the evolutionary selection out of a response that Profet claims exists as PNV because it is a residual of a Pleistocene adaptation. Tangentially, Bogardus and Kraft presume that these IgE mast cell reactions are transmitted to the enteric nervous system (ENS) via histamine pathways. This, as with other 'favorite messenger system' proposals, is probably oversimplified. In any event, Bogardus and Kraft conclude that the etiology of these specific adverse reactions is unknown.

Profet proposes that allergies are more prevalent in industrial than in foraging societies. She attributes this distribution (which is not in fact well established) to failures of women in industrial societies to breast-feed, and so developmentally failing to suppress IgE-activating compounds. She also proposes that respiratory allergies will be more prevalent as a result of pollution and dust mites, and that higher (proposed, not demonstrated) rates for infant respiratory disorder predispose, as a function of population density and diversity, to later respiratory allergy. She does offer data finding reduced blood pressure in allergic response, which leads her to conclude a slower rate of circulation (and therefore toxin dissemination) when toxins have been ingested, injected, or otherwise encountered. In further proposing that substances which bind covalently to serum proteins are acutely toxic as a class, and also bind covalently to DNA, she incorporates carcinogenicity and mutagenicity as actions of the directly acting plant poisons and placenta-permeable teratogens, which she describes as widespread in the vegetable kingdom. The proposed defense in humans is this evolved general allergic response, but particularly PNV.

Profet's thoughtful theses seem to be unsupported. One cannot rely on PNV toxin expulsion, because it is a rare accomplishment in human NV. Her thesis overlooks that NV are unpredictably, and therefore essentially not, correlated with CTA. The learned food avoidances of pregnancy are widespread and, if defined as CTA, they cover a range of normal foods that are obviously not teratogenic. In her Lusita case if it had been plant poisoning rather than typical resettlement starvation and mayhem, the fact that folks died (no observer describes vomiting) would have shown protective failure, not success. In the same way, and after her own work with Ames and colleagues (Ames et al., 1987, 1990), one finds that 'toxin' represents a rubric of a mostly unrealized potential. Humans eat endogenous pesticides, such as toxins, mutagens, carcinogens, of plants – a melange of adverse possibilities – with rare immediately harmful effects, and probably rare long-range ones too. And for Profet's thesis, it is immediacy of aversion, with the wisdom of gestational teratogenicity known by hominids, to which she assigns PNV's function in which CTA to N is also supposed to exist and be functional.

Genetics: an initial inquiry into migraine forecasts of hyperemesis gravidarum

Given our data suggesting the general propensity for NV for some women, which is provoked by a wide range of stimuli, and our inference about major individual differences in the distribution of this 'G' (for general) factor for 'normal' NV, one would expect some identifiable major variables to be associated with and underlie or to co-vary with the 'G' propensity for NV. Unfortunately, the risk factors cited in the literature are most frequently for iatrogenic NV, and ordinarily in small samples. To demonstrate that a risk factor commonly observed, such as being overweight or age, is in fact a general one, observations would have to be made across the range of NV including those of normal everyday life. In our sample, younger age was not a higher risk factor. Being female is the most consistent NV risk factor that we find. It is in that sense 'genetic,' but differentiated by 'G' propensity. One has no idea what aspects of being female contribute, and one cannot exclude social role or environmental variables. One does know that women are more vulnerable generally to dysfunction and pain than men, as measured by more doctor's visits and reported symptoms, but the yin/yang of it is that they live longer, being 'hardy but hazarded' (see Blum and Heinrichs, 1988).

Insofar as one addresses a genetic variable, in the past before DNA and other direct chromosomal methods became available, typically one carried out family studies for reports of similar experience within families, compared with outsiders, or studies of monozygotic twins rather than of dizygotic ones. No twin studies were found in our literature search and only the most casual family NV similarity. Family members readily see one another as alike, but such validity in these reports may arise from similar sociological situations, family learning, mimicked psychosomatic expressive styles, similar experiences (one expects that there will be more early and less later motion sickness in companion children of day sailors than in landlubbers), or the genome. We could not find independent observations controlled for potential bias sources. NV have not been important enough to generate such obviously interesting work.

We can report on findings derived from a somewhat more rigorous inquiry, although it too is limited. Our colleague, Peroutka, is working on the identification of genes predisposing to migraine. His is a dopamine neurotransmitter theory of migraine, postulating that the migraine sufferer is hypersensitive to dopamine. Peroutka also attributes N as such to dopamine activity/sensitivity through the autonomic nervous system (ANS). One major symptom of and diagnostic criterion for migraine in N. Peroutka's recent work asserts a specific genome location and a definitive dopamine–N–V–gastrointestinal (GI) motility–migraine sequence and syndrome for individuals whose dopamine adaptive capabilities are abnormal. In his view, this abnormality embraces other forms of NV, it is to this dopamine function that Peroutka attributes the usefulness of dopamine antagonist compounds in the parenteral treatment of migraine, such as haloperidol, chlorpromazine, prochlorperazine, metoclopramide, and a drug not approved in the USA, flunarizine. One notes that all of these, except for flunarizine (about which we have no knowledge), have been used with varying success – and always with dyskinesia risk if chronically administered – for other NV. Migraine treatment success rates are cited in these studies from 100%, only six subjects, for haloperidol to 60% for metoclopramide. The range of quoted success for dopamine antagonists in migraine appears, impressionistically and without analysis of trial methodology, to be somewhat higher than for NV.

Although our interpretation of the literature allows a less confident role to be assigned to dopamine, we do propose and test the relationship between migraine and NV, specifically hyperemesis gravidarum (HG). A genetic component, with widespread agreement on a genetic basis for migraine (which unless one accepts Peroutka's thesis in itself tells one nothing of process), may then be inferred for some NV, but particularly for HG. By way of introduction to migraine, and as sources for the general statements below, one may wish to refer to Burks (1995), Davidoff (1995), Sandler (1990), and Spierings (1995).

Migraine prevalence occurs at a rate that is about four times greater in females than in males. As always, rates vary with the characteristics of populations selected and the care in diagnostic criteria. Remember that, in Chapter 3, 36% of our sample reported 'migraine' or 'severe headache.' One realizes that 'migraine' is popularly applied to any severe headache. The much greater risk of women themselves allows a gender inference, although not specific because so many psychobiological features of being a woman might contribute to headache per se, and migraine in particular. For example, high estrogen levels are proposed as protective in otherwise susceptible persons and estrogen therapy may reduce severity. Migraine discussion and research require the term to be used restrictively based on careful diagnostic criteria including aura, scotoma, N itself, light sensitivity, throbbing, localization on one side of the head, long duration, and extreme disabling pain. Sometimes, a clinical diagnosis proceeds backwards, inferred from responsiveness to particular drugs such as ergotamines, β-blockers, antidepressants, metoclopramide, buspirone, or, among the many recently recommended (Cameron, 1995), intravenous phenothiazine (a dopamine and α-adrenergic blocker, with widespread side effects including dyskinesias; as a class, phenothiazines are ordinarily used to treat anxiety).

Carefully diagnosed migraine occurs in 17.5% of the population (Stewart et al., 1992). However, refinements to the decimal from prevalence studies of complex conditions, whatever database is used, are misleading if taken too seriously; there is a range of rates. For example, Stewart et al. (1992), in their large Baltimore study, found that white European women had greater prevalence than African or Asian women. In this sample migraine among whites occurred in 20.4% of women and 8.6% of men, a smaller difference than others have found. The proportion was roughly the same in each race. Stewart et al. thereby attribute migraine to genetic factors which are racially correlated.

A variety of theories about migraine have been proposed. The literature can be murky. Migraine is a condition that bears similarities to NV as triggered by multiple events, and it is no surprise that a 'multifactorial' explanation is required, where numerous precipitants ('triggers' in the migraine literature) are identified, a range of drugs including 'cocktail' equivalents is clinically employed, and individual baseline conditions are involved, such as depression and anxiety (which assumes ANS activity). Lifestyle, diet, stress, and light glare are major features that influence incidence. It is of special interest that in children motion sickness sets off their migraine, and presumably N from both, and further that children and adults who suffer migraines also have a reported higher incidence, up to 60%, of motion sickness. Children with motion sickness are at greater risk of migraine, and most adult migraine sufferers have a history of childhood motion sickness (Davidoff, 1995). It is of major interest that migraine sufferers, like PNV women, are particularly sensitive to odors as migraine triggers (Blau and Solomon, 1985).

We conclude that a cross-linking predisposition between migraine and some NV, perhaps particularly PNV and HG, does exist as a personal precipitant.

With respect to personal features indicating NV, or migraine risk one may also wish to attend to personality attributes – not simply those earlier identified risk features of stress and fatigue vulnerability, but moods as such. Depression, for example, of which fatigue is one expression, is a risk for more women than men, at about the same ratio as NV (excluding PNV) and migraine – a factor of 3 to 4 times greater (Culbertson, 1997). And as with Stewart's work on migraine, racial, and thus presumably genetic-environmental factors contribute. The future psychosomatic student of NV, and today's clinician, may wish to attend further to depression or the more general 'negative affect' (anxiety, anger, stress, depression). Do recall our brief exploration in Chapter 7 of the possible role of fear and related 'learned helplessness' as factors perhaps operating in animal NV. For humans, particularly women, we propose a likely contributing role.

Importantly, most studies show that migraine varies with menstrual cycle and reproductive age cycles. Burks (1995) proposes that hormonal changes are the greatest source of variation in migraine incidence, with menstruation being a notable trigger. Most important, and quite generally for our findings and discussion, a common undisputed observation is that atonic migraine sufferers experience relief during the second and third trimesters of pregnancy. It is in these trimesters that HG appears.

You should be experiencing *déjà vu* as you read about migraine, because its situation conceptually and clinically has much in common with 'normal' NV. This is not simply because of its commonality as primarily a woman's condition and related to the reproductive cycle, but because it is precipitated by a variety of situational as well as biochemical factors and where pharmacological agents used for its treatment may paradoxically induce headache or

N, and explanations of mechanisms range widely and include several that occur in the NV literature, e.g. reproductive hormones, serotonin, prostaglandins, allergy (Profet), foods, etc. One is surprised not to see the ubiquitous 'toxin' explanation as well. Obviously N is triggered by migraine in which it is considered to be a by-product of some central state change. Both are disabling and painful, both are conditions that are not considered to be diseases, both need not arise from pathogens or tissue abnormalities, and both are a matter of scientific ignorance and considerable self-management efforts on the part of the sensible patient/person.

But is this all? We thought not and were led to examine a particular hypothesis that arose from our interest in the commonalities noted above, but particularly from the critical temporal relationship between the two trimesters in which both HG and migraine occur. We found no literature of association, although there is one clinical case (Triggs et al., 1992) of a multiply disordered woman having 'atypical' migraine, HG, seizures, psychosis, valproic acid-induced coma, etc., who was cured by the vitamin riboflavin.

Consider a hypothesized migraine to HG association derived from our study data in Chapter 3; having had a baby, independent of PNV, significantly predisposes a woman to being more sensitive to NV as a severe pain than her nonmaternal peers. Is it possible that a pain-sensitizing process in the second and/or third trimester, which eliminates migraine endocrinologically, replaces it with HG? Is there a common process with altered expression? Is HG a 'migraine equivalent'?

Table 12.1 shows that there is a highly significant relationship ($p = 0.001$) for PNV women as such, and for first trimester PNV where N is perceived to be induced by or experienced in connection with headache. 'Migraine' that is self-diagnosed is, in turn, recalled as related ($p = 0.05$) with first and second trimester but not third trimester pregnancy. This is consistent with the migraine literature. To this point, we are aware that PNV is rarer in the second and third trimesters (although in our sample it occurs among 25% and 15% compared with > 50% in the first trimester); there are simply fewer women who might report any second or third trimester relationships with any variable, headache included. We do not know if any woman in this sample had HG. If an expected 1% rate had been obtained in this population, then one woman in our sample 'should' have had HG and 'could' have been reporting not on PNV but HG in the third trimester. This is hardly the stuff of statistical inference.

What is evident is that PNV, excluding HG (i.e., PNV with no nutritional/fluid/electrolyte or mortal threat, and no weight loss), in

Table 12.1: Strength of relationships of headache-related N and migraine experience to pregnancy-related N

Relationship	Gamma value
N from headache by:	
First trimester pregnancy N	0.55***
Second trimester pregnancy N	0.25
Third trimester pregnancy N	0.19
N by pregnancy[a]	0.75***
Experienced migraines by:	
First trimester pregnancy N	0.39*
Second trimester pregnancy N	0.42*
Third trimester pregnancy N	0.29
N by pregnancy[a]	0.20

[a]Nausea by pregnancy includes only those women who had experienced at least one pregnancy.
*Significant at 0.05 level. **Significant at 0.01 level. ***Significant at 0.001 level.

the third trimester (where HG typically occurs) has no self-reported relationship to headache-induced or associated N. Nor does possibly self-diagnosed migraine itself have any significant association with third trimester PNV. Thus headache and N in the third trimester, if occurring at all, do not have any significant relationship. The finding of migraine and PNV in the earlier two trimesters, but not the third, is entirely compatible with other consistent reports that migraine sufferers experience this headache earlier but not later during pregnancy. Headache associated with first trimester N as PNV should be considered as distinct from the N and V of HG in the third trimester. They are different syndromes.

A variety of 'migraine equivalents,' all 'acephalgic,' occur without the pain experience, but with a range of migraine-correlated syndromes, such as scintillating bright spots in front of the eyes (scotomata), visual distortion including partial blindness (bilateral hemianopsia), vertigo, tingling skin (paresthesia), stammering (dysarthria), or inability to find words (aphasia), and muscle weakness. Profound short-term memory loss with retrograde amnesia can occur, as can benign recurrent vertigo with V, sweating, and pallor. These are symptoms that can also be ANS correlates of any NV itself. Vertigo with NV as a syndrome, which is considered to be equivalent to migraine, occurs more often in women. Like migraine itself, it may be triggered by menstruation, so one may presume a hormonal role. Most of the 'equivalents' pose problems for differential diagnosis. 'Abdominal migraine,' for example, as a controversial diagnosis in adults includes very severe upper abdominal pain, N, and V. Whatever it is lasts for some hours, or even days.

Given the range of symptoms experienced with NV, one might look again at HG for its association with migraine, or possibly as something far more dangerous and disabling than migraine itself. Attentive to our finding of enhanced NV pain sensitivity among women who had been pregnant, does migraine as exquisite pain sensitivity predispose to enhanced sensitivity in the pregnant woman so that her NV becomes HG as a 'pain consequence?' Implied in this referentially cloudy concept is that, with NV already being experienced as exquisite pain (the self-rating has still to be done among HG patients), HG emerges from this experience as a short-circuited pain pathway. In cybernetics or system theory, one would propose that, given any 'equivalent' status for HG, a reverberating or feed-forward positive feedback would exist, amplifying the circuit. This is V seeking to 'cure' N again, but becoming 'status vomitus,' rather like the irreversible kindling and spread of effect of epilepsy. Note that migraine and epilepsy were once thought to be associated: seizures may occur during migraine and migraine (basilar) appears after seizures. Davidoff (1995) considers this relationship to be mostly fortuitous. But we wonder about EEGs of HG women.

Out of empiricism, rather than good evidence of 'mechanism,' we asked whether there would be a relationship between carefully defined migraine and equally carefully diagnosed HG. Whether one entertains the pain sensitivity predisposition theory for HG, or simply acknowledges that most migraine appears in childhood or by early adulthood, the life-time developmental time line would be migraine first, HG second; thus prediction will be for HG to migraine, not vice versa. Given the dominant gender, hormonal, and particular reproductive cycle features of both PNV and migraine, it is not unreasonable that HG and migraine may be inferred to have – if not Peroutka's optimistic one-gene base – a multi-gene protein-building block base capable, as one of its developmental propensities, of generating painful vulnerabilities. This loose notion at least allows for the range of pain, visual, and gastric abnormalities that emerge as migraine and thence HG. One would expect commonalities and intercorrelations with respect to NV, vertigo, motion sickness, and odor sensitivity.

Our students, led by Bella Shen and including Craig Thomas and Kate Harding, undertook to test the specific hypothesis that migraine sufferers would be at greater risk of HG than a normal population. Contrariwise, compatible with presuming a common genetic and NV process with a presumed role for estrogen/progesterone or HG, sufferers would be expected to be at greater than expected migraine risk. Note that these are only reciprocal relationships, because population sizes at risk differ markedly. The findings are striking, but require replication.

HG and sample inaccessibility: what traits are implied?

HG patients were harder to locate than migraine patients. We tested the difference between migraine and HG patients who could be reached. HG patients were significantly ($p = 0.001$) less accessible than migraine patients. We do not know what illness, mortality, mobility, time constraint, or cooperativeness factors may have contributed to this. As 'deviance' can be a general feature, i.e., one implying other traits, one allows that HG women differ in other, unknown ways which affect their availability – the 'psychogenic' theory revisited. One suspects that such a finding might well imply personality and sociological differences which, in turn, might reflect HG risk components. Other work might pursue this.

Migraine and HG mortality risk?: a significant serendipitous sample search finding

Following up on sample unavailability, we examined mortality, which yields an expected rate: of white women aged 30, only 0.61 would be expected to die per 1000 (for age 32, 0.72, etc.). For black women, the risk is higher at 1.61 per 1000. For an ethnically mixed population, this would be, say, 1 in 1000. As an early and unexpected result, we note that, in testing the difference between proportions, HG patients proved significantly ($p = 0.001$) less accessible than migraine patients. What illness, mortality, mobility, time constraint, or cooperativeness factors may have contributed to this we do not know. In any event, the risk of mortality for women of average age 30 is exceedingly low. Any tracing methodology for death rates is seriously flawed when it relies on telephone contact; anyone not contacted could be dead. Taking the suspect records at face value: among the 57 HG women sought, none was reported dead. Among migraine sufferers in the sample of 50, at the hospital record number called, three were identified as dead. The death rate obtained here of 60 of 1000 is much higher than expected. Accidents, runs, and other odd things happen in sampling. There are no data supporting migraine or well-treated HG as a mortal risk. So this 60 times greater reported death rate may be treated as an error or blip. What if the deceased migraine sufferers were also HG women (because the migraine to HG link, and now conceivably the migraine–HG–death link, must be tested as 'causal' and not simply viewed as two conditions sharing commonalities of no known physiological and/or pathological consequence?) Unfunded, we had no way of pursuing verification/replication of this apparent high-risk mortality with its possible HG link. Were other workers to find it, it could be of importance. We leave this area with a troubled question mark.

Earlier migraine predicts to HG risk? $P<0.000001$

We used the binomial test to examine the relationship of earlier migraine to later HG; we found a rate of significance so great that it defied our statistician's computer, the zeroes running off the display, thus the predicted relationship of earlier migraine to later HG occurring at a probability of less than one in a million by chance.

In contrast, as a lesson on the importance of the choice of statistics for inference (the power weak on small samples), chi-squared yielded a p of only 0.001. However, there is no significant reverse relationship. The binomial test tells us that the risk of any HG woman having migraine, while presenting a trend, is with these small sample sizes not significant. Were this HG risk from migraine relationship (let alone the mortality) to be replicated, it would be an important demonstration of a heretofore unknown relationship.

The strength of the migraine to HG association, and the implied commonality, reciprocity, equivalence, or sequence of processes, is greater than any of which we are aware from the literature for prediction of HG risk. It is particularly important because it is a hypothesis based on reflecting the known commonalities between migraine and NV generally, their occurrence in relation to the reproductive cycle, and their preponderance in women. Obviously, more work beckons.

We close this discussion with an expression of our confidence that there is likely 'something really there' in the migraine–HG process. If our view of NV in general or PNV specifically is correct, a dynamic and interactive set of internal and environmental events will be found that are multi-leveled, from genetic and endocrinological, to psychological to situational.

PNV and olfaction: an adaptive immune connection?

Earlier we raised the question about whether immune activation occurs as part of any general mobilization, akin to Selye's stress response, when NV occur. Given a particular genetic/embryological link between olfactory cells/main olfactory bulb response and immune activation, one also asks whether, in those NV that are precipitated by odor, there should be future evidence of NV mobilization of T cells, as we expect, and whether the olfactory triggers lead to any greater than ordinary immune responsiveness. Our search of the literature has left us empty-handed except for one powerful set of findings linking the olfactory preferences of young women of reproductive age to the major histocompatibility complex (MHC) human leukocyte-associated antigen (HLA) status of similarly aged men whose HLA statuses are represented in the chemical signature of sweat secretions. The work of Wedekind et al. (1995), following that of Ferstl et al. (1992) cited in Doty and Muller-Schwarze (1992), found that, when presented with sweat-exposed undershirts of men, college women preferred the odors of those men whose MHC was characterized by HLAs that differed from theirs. Furthermore, the HLA-unlike self-odors (immune 'not me') preferred were recalled as being more similar to those of other men whom these women had actually selected as sex partners. In terms of an evolutionary selective advantage, the offspring from a more greatly diversified set of HLAs (as would occur from a mating of unlike HLA parents) would enjoy the advantage of this diversity as an expanded immune capability when confronted with infectious organisms. What has not been shown, because it has not been investigated, is that what we hypothesized as preference for an HLA grouping (found to be blocked when the woman is taking an oral contraceptive, and presumed to be blocked when endocrinologically equivalent as in pregnancy) has as its reciprocal not simply an aversion to a like-self HLA odor but that the description of this odor is 'nauseating,' particularly when intense or when the woman is in a fertile period of her cycle (and not wearing perfumes, etc.). The search for this critical link constitutes an early research priority.

As Ferstl et al. (1992) did find 'extremely adverse' odor responses in one pregnant woman to like-self HLA, they undertook to study perceived odor intensity as such. They found like-self HLAs to be characterized as intense more than expected. They did no work on preference or on NV. The clinical case was intuitively contrary to what one would expect from the findings of Wedekind et al. (1995). Although one may expect intensity as threshold sensitivity to be reached, and to be shown to be related to HLA mix, one must realize that odor sensitivity that is subliminal to awareness is common and can guide human preferential conduct. [For a macabre story of an overpowering but subliminal role for odor in human relationships, read Patrick Süskind's novel *Perfume*.]

New research should also test for a PNV immune mobilization response, and possibly a relationship to known cancer risk with spontaneous abortion, and possibly to severe PNV. The next studies should also test for neuropsychological traits such as Eysenck's introversion as an interaction to increase women's HLA sensitivity.

Threshold variables in odor sensitivity may be very important. All humans have individual chemical signatures detectable by others' noses (Schleidt, 1992). Schleidt finds that genetic factors contribute primarily to these. Microfauna contribute: bacterial products interact with proteins in cell secretions, with the outcome of a relatively consistent molecular complex as signature.

Basic work on mutant mice by Gold (1996) shows that whether any olfactory signal is transmitted from intact olfactory and vomeronasal organ system tissues in the mouse depends on the genetic integrity of the intracellular messenger cyclic adenosine monophosphate (cAMP). All odors appear to trigger olfactory neurons by increasing the production of cAMP. However, mice and humans as mammals may be presumed to require genetic cAMP central messenger presence. The question (ours, not Gold's) arises from the current all-or-nothing findings which show what fails to occur when genes are knocked out. Research designs cannot yet expand upon variations in what occurs in humans when intact, but there are diversely developed, genetically based protein elaborations resulting from interacting nature/nurture morphogenesis, although the aim is to learn whether cAMP signal efficiency measured as gradations in odor sensitivity may be found to be multi-gene dependent. One is reminded (Wasserstein, 1996) that life processes depend on multiple gene-to-gene interactions, including environmental interactions, with experience that is consequential for brain function development and work. Attention to the genetics of PNV might begin with cAMP and odor thresholds. It must not ignore earlier odor exposure, such as learning, and allow rhinencephalon development and limbic–cognitive 'definition' to be imposed on odor molecules.

Mate selection

The sensory preferential process of H-2-dissimilar mate selection in mice has been shown to be dominantly olfactory. Mice can distinguish the identities of mice according to odors of urine and other bodily secretions. Boyse et al. (1987) have shown that male and female mice can distinguish between MHC types through the scent of urine, even when the only genetic difference lies in the H-2K portion of the gene; in addition, they found at least three parts of the gene complex that could 'independently confer individuality of scent.' Yamazaki et al. (1983) support the theory of recognition as a result of MHC signals, with pheromones contributing additional information. Egid et al. (1989) found, in studies of mice, that H-2D and H-2K loci, both highly polymorphic (Boyse et al., 1987) with at least 50 alleles, are 'important in producing odor differences between MHC congenics,' and that MHC sensitivity depends on the state of estrous. Potts et al. (1993) believe that the ability to distinguish just a single polymorphic locus would be sufficient to avoid mating with those that are genetically similar, and they propose two mechanisms of recognition which describe the efficiency of inbreeding avoidance via recognition of a single polymorphic locus.

Although these studies support recognition of MHC type as the dominant factor in mate selection, the mechanism for this identification is not clear; several studies (Boyse et al., 1987; Zavazava et al., 1990; Roser et al., 1991) have shown that HLA exist intact and as metabolites in serum, urine, and sweat (though mice cannot distinguish MHC differences in the scent of serum), and that whichever molecule confers the MHC-related odor is volatile. Boyse et al. cite the appearance of soluble fragments of the H-2 gene complex (part of what they qualify as 'the only single gene so far tested and shown to participate in odor constitution,' the H-2K gene, expressed by all nucleated cells) in urine, and it may be that these fragments themselves are the odorants. Roser examined the possible role that bacteria may play in the distinguishing odor of urine, and found that the urine of germ-free rats could not be uniquely identified. However, Yamazaki has shown that germ-free mice can be trained to distinguish mice that differ only at the MHC (Yamazaki et al., 1990), so although it is certain that unique MHCs are the source of identifying odors, the mechanism by which they convey their message is still unclear.

Many studies have examined olfactory MHC recognition ability in mice; more interesting and relevant, however, are humans. Recall that Ferstl et al. (1992) conducted a preliminary investigation showing that rats can distinguish between specific human HLA class I phenotypes, and humans have shown an ability to distinguish by intensity the scents of mice differing only at the H-2 locus (Gilbert et al., 1986). There are a host of studies documenting the ability of mothers to identify the odors of their baby (and vice versa); in one study, mothers correctly identified the odor of their own child 17 out of 18 times; 16 out of 18 parents could distinguish between siblings, and 19 out of 24 children could identify the scent of their own siblings (Porter and Moore, 1981). Moreover, people reliably identify their own scent (Lord and Kasprzak, 1989).

Egid et al. (1989) and Doty et al. (1981) have shown separately that MHC sensitivity depends on the state of estrous, with a peak olfactory sensitivity occurring midcycle; this finding is logical because midcycle is the time during which olfactory skills should be most needed in determining an appropriate mate via MHC distinction. Other studies bear on MHC type functioning in human mate selection. Not surprisingly, given the problem of 'mechanism' seen as sole proprietors of process, they seem to draw different conclusions as to exactly how. The first of these, conducted by Ferstl et al. in 1992, examined 19 women (out of 400 interviewed) who identified at least two other men or women sensed as having 'intensive' odors during their pregnancies or over their menstrual cycles ('intensive' assumed, from the introduction, to indicate 'aversive'). A total of 51 subjects with aversive odors and 23 controls (people identified by the same women to have nonintense odors) were classified according to their HLA; significantly, 55% of the women studied shared one of two HLA alleles (class I A9 or B15) with 60% of the 'aversive' subjects, and only 23% of the controls. These results suggest that women tend to find men with similar MHC to be less attractive than other men, possibly, Ferstl suggests, as a result of the increased sweat production and therefore the increased number of odorants associated with subjects sharing the HLA-A9 and B-15 alleles. Problems existing in this study include the lack of definition of 'intensive' odors, and the unidentified state (pregnant or menstruating) of the women identifying those with the intensive odors. In addition, partners and relatives were excluded from the study, leaving questions as to mate choices made in relation to olfaction. However, this study provides some reliable evidence for the aversion via olfactory sensitivity of HLA-similar potential mates.

Also discussed earlier, Wedekind et al. (1995) showed that women not taking oral contraceptives find the odors of HLA-dissimilar men to be more pleasant than those of HLA-similar men, and that women taking oral contraceptives react in an opposite manner, rating the scents of men with similar HLA as more pleasant than those of HLA-dissimilar men, with sexiness ratings correlating with pleasantness for both groups; all women were tested in the second week after the start of menstruation. Also rated were the intensities of the men's odors, with more intensive odors tending to be more unpleasant in MHC-dissimilar men for women both on and off the pill, though no correlation for MHC-similar men was found. Finally, it was noted that odors of MHC-dissimilar men reminded women (most of whom were not on the pill) of a mate or ex-mate twice as often as did the odors of MHC-similar men.

One concludes that there is a compelling connection between the olfactory detection of MHC similarity/dissimilarity and mate choices, most strongly supported by the 'pleasantness/sexiness' ratings made by women not on the pill, as well as by the invoked memories of mates or ex-mates upon smelling the odors of MHC-dissimilar males by women mostly not using the pill. If Ferstl's study is to be interpreted as representative of pregnant women, however, a conflict arises concerning Wedekind's conclusion that the odor preferences of pregnant women or women on the pill change. Also difficult is the comparison of the 'intensity' rating used in both studies, because it is poorly defined and addresses MHC-similar men in Ferstl's study, although significantly it involves only MHC-dissimilar men (and correlates with increasing unpleasantness) in Wedekind's study. Wedekind believes that Ferstl's evidence concerning olfactory preferences of pregnant women is mostly anecdotal, though he concedes that variance does exist; he states that knowing MHC type and hormonal status of a given woman will only allow a 'good guess' as to her olfactory preferences, and that he and others continue to work for a better understanding of this topic (Wedekind et al., 1995).

Yet to be adequately addressed in the issue of identification via olfaction is the question of how these abilities and preferences develop. The dominant opinion appears to be that familial imprinting is responsible for recognition of family and preferences for mates, because mice raised with foster parents were found to prefer mates with MHC different from their foster parents, rather than similar to their own (Yamazaki et al., 1988), perhaps with environmental factors such as diet playing a part as well. But we bear in mind the general importance of other environmental features playing a role in differentiating postnatal brain development and thus, by implication, sensitivities and capabilities.

In sum regarding MHC, variability appears to play several key roles throughout the lifetime of mice as well as humans, with the advantages of MHC heterozygosity most clearly demonstrated in terms of spontaneous abortion. MHC heterozygosity may play a role in mate selection, with women preferring MHC-dissimilar men as mates, resulting in better chances of carrying a pregnancy to term.

Olfaction has been proposed and supported as the mechanism of these behaviors, with MHC-dissimilar men having generally more pleasant odors than MHC-similar men; the one exception appears in Wedekind's study, where women on the pill found MHC-similar men to have more pleasant odors than MHC-dissimilar men. The finding by Doty and Egid that women are more sensitive to smells at midcycle seems evolutionarily adaptive in light of the possibility that mate selection may be influenced by olfactory distinction of MHC similarity/dissimilarity.

If the hormonal state of women on the pill is considered to mimic pregnancy, it can be suggested that pregnant women, like pregnant mice in the first stages of pregnancy, prefer to be near males with MHC types similar to those of relatives. For mice, in fact, this preference is of utmost importance, because pregnancy block can occur upon the introduction of the scent of a new male. Higher olfactory sensitivity in women in the first trimester of pregnancy may indicate an evolutionarily adaptive role similar to that in mice, i.e., to incite pregnant women to seek the support of relatives rather than other males during this often difficult time of pregnancy. The hypothesized preference of pregnant women for the scents of men with MHC similar to their own can be applied to the phenomenon of PNV. As odors have been found frequently to trigger PNV, the aversive odors of MHC-dissimilar men (possibly, in some cases, including those of the father) may serve to reinforce the pregnant woman's preference to be around relatives, either by causing NV or by leading the pregnant woman to avoid further aversive odors when experiencing NV. Further investigation into the exact functions and consequences of MHC heterozygosity is required. And will assuredly be exciting.

Speculation as to further genetic contributions

Genetic contributions which we conceive not as rigid determinants for any complex behavior in the normal animal (thus ourselves) provides the building materials, limiting instructions, and opportunities for self-patterning developments. The field is a beckoning *terra incognita* for NV and PNV work. Environmental events, such as biological and ecological interactions with 'environments' recognized as internal and external, beginning embryonically, are the conceptual context.

There have been recurring proposals that PNV reflects a variation in prostaglandin (PG) levels in pregnancy. PG (it has several molecular structures) is almost universal in mammalian cells, and in fish PGs are emetics. Further, nonprostanoid metabolites which stimulate actual PG biosynthesis in the fish gastric mucosa are themselves emetic in fish; it appears thereby that precursors as well as PGs are emetic. Gerhart (1991) found that fish can discriminate between prey with emetic PGs and those without. A CTA is presumed, because, after exposure and V, experienced fish learn to avoid the emetic PG prey.

In women no such deep (sea) findings yet obtain. PG inhibits release of prolactin from the pituitary and of norepinephrine from sympathetic presynaptic nerve endings. Insofar as a prolactin hypothesis for PNV is favored, this must include the role of PG; similarly insofar as ANS activities, including end of the line muscular activity, PG production, delivery, utilization, and inhibition must be considered. PG actions are widely distributed including muscle contraction, inflammatory, immunological, and gastric responses. Kidney and cardiovascular functions are influenced. To date its primary recognized reproductive role is as one element in labor induction, derived from the late pregnancy regulatory role of estrogen. One process is increased cortisol secretion by the adrenals of the fetus itself (part of the 'I am ready to be born' or 'organ communication system' as it is called), then reduced placental secretion of progesterone and increased estrogen secretion, and then an increase in PG levels. It is accepted that fetal membranes play a profound role within the amnion in providing arachidonic acid and are related in PG biosynthesis. An inhibition of prostanoids lengthens labor; any premature increase yields a risk of abortion. PG measurement in cells is hardly a key to PNV, nor so far are measurements of its muscular function, although a demonstration of heightened presence in and activation of the gut during either first trimester PNV or third trimester HG would be dramatic.

PG is presumed to play an important early pregnancy regulatory role in placental hemodynamics (Speroff, 1975). Placental blood pressure is not known to differ between PNG and non-PNG women. But in a different vein (so to speak) PGs occur in human semen; were one to speculate on a proposal that semen absorption post-conception is not metabolized or secreted but incorporated as protein, some of which is non-self-immunological, one could imagine (reader indulgence is required) that an emetic role, in this instance circulating via the CTZ perhaps, might occur in humans. Or, alternatively, that PNV responsive to these semen-derived proteins might prove to be a PNV-inducing perturbation.

Far-fetched thinking receives some not so far-fetched support, although from the genetic world of fireflies, not humans. Rice (1966) reports chemical antagonism as part of the coevolution of the sexes. The consequences in fireflies are barriers to fertilization and species divergence. The seminal fluid of fireflies contains proteins toxic to the female. One functional effect, insuring an individual male's progenitorship, is that one peptide in semen encourages egg laying and dampens female sexual appetite, and therefore possible subsequent siring courtships. The female responds by suppressing chemicals that are hazardous to sperm survival in the oviduct. When Rice cloned males and eliminated female haplotypes (HLAs) that contributed to offspring characteristics, so that male-only genes were transmitted, a massive, genetic, evolutionary advantage appeared. One mechanism implicated seductive pheromones in the successful males. Females, on the other hand, died early, perhaps from the seminal toxin load. It is regrettable that the firefly, unlike the fish, cannot be an experimental model for V. Whether either provides ideas for work on the complex human remains to be seen.

To return to womankind and more limited PG speculation: an early test for PGs or more massive secretion by embryonic tissue, more so in women with PNV than in other parous women, would be instructive. A positive finding would confirm that PNV represents an adverse maternal reaction to the fetal stranger, here with PG endocrine compared with immune (the embryo as foreign tissue), physical (taking up space), blood transport (not enough to go around), or genetic survival itself: the mother and the embryo as competitors, their survival (however interdependent with the embryo far more so) by no means biosyntonic. One geneticist (Fernald, R., 1996, personal communication) characterizes this new school of thought as viewing the embryo as a 'parasite.' Implied in this is that the fetus, as an alien and parasitic 'not me,' leads after all to PNV as an immune activation expression. But this would not be an evolutionarily adaptive response were it to 'work' as an expulsive mechanism, for which there is no evidence. Nor would such PNV 'work' for the mother as immunologically competent riddance of alien tissue – except for the limited but pertinent evidence of HLA likeness and obstetric risk or reproductive hazard. What has priority is imaginative research on topics such as those identified in this section.

CHAPTER 13

Pregnancy nausea and vomiting: further explorations in theory

Pregnancy nausea and vomiting and odor sensitivity

The olfactory apparatus, and of course its anatomical situation and embryonic commonality with respect to the pituitary and hypothalamic, including limbic regions that constitute the triune brain (also termed the rhinencephalon), needs further investigation with respect to pregnancy nausea and vomiting (PNV), and indeed other NV. By way of an introductory literature there are fine works on olfaction. We recommend Engen (1982, 1983), Van Toller and Dodd (1988, 1992), Stoddart (1990), Doty and Muller-Schwarze (1992), Serby and Chobar (1992).

Understanding arising from this field will one day be incorporated into a comprehensive view of PNV–olfactory relationships, and those associated processes noted in the second section of this chapter. Recall that olfactory thresholds vary greatly during the menstrual cycle, as at the onset of PNV. This unequivocally demonstrates a hormonal base for sensitivity thresholds, and for the conditions for message processing – although not for their 'intelligent' selection [whether at glomeruli, the main olfactory bulb (MOB), or levels influenced by reticular or cortical vigilance] with respect to 'downstream' reactions such as hedonistic tone, emotional response, or NV triggering. Even after almost two decades of research, very little has emerged, although that little is critical.

Olfactory sensations, once synapsed in the cerebral cortex, become available for conscious awareness and learned associations. Direct and cerebrally routed information is presumed to connect with the area postrema (AP) and possibly other medullary NV trigger regions. One may allow for direct hormonal stimulation of the chemoreceptor trigger zone (CTZ) as noted. Le Magnen (1986) concludes that there is evidence to the effect that there is an olfactory–thalamic relay which could interact with the gate keeping of pain by the thalamus. In Le Magnen's view there is support for an interpretation of two systems. Extrathalamic projections prevailing in the olfactory system would be involved in emergency responses with internal or external environments; putative thalamic and thalamoneocortical projections would provide information for learning and thus for anticipation. Anticipation may include negative effects with stress-released hormones. Both might act as subassemblies of interregional patterning for a subset, i.e., one syndrome of PNV. A feedback loop to the hypothalamus and the olfactory bulb is proposed, thus providing a circuit for arousal, learning, and 'motivational' states, the last implying perturbations or stable state disruption in regulatory/homeostatic conditions. Le Magnen finds evidence that an odorant conditioned as an external insulin releaser will modify rat food intake via plasma insulin and blood glucose levels. A chemosensory neuroendocrine positive feedback loop suggests the involvement of olfaction in both feeding and sexual control systems – this possibly integrated reproductive system.

The work of Gibson et al. (1986) is provocative in showing the presence of the atrial natriuretic peptide (ANP) in both the olfactory apparatus and circumventricular areas, of which the AP and CTZ make up a portion. One may expect ANP in other nuclei regions to be capable of motor induction of NV. These investigators comment that ANP appears to function in the fluid and electrolytic regulation of homeostatic centers in the circumventricular region and, further, that its presence in the olfactory apparatus suggests additional complexity and function for and from these structures. There may be an ANP transmitter system which in itself is a messenger system linking olfactory and other NV trigger apparatus. Obviously it could not work alone. Hormonal and neural transmission, interdependent regulation, as well as interdependent dysfunctional critical instability are operative within the brain.

Uncommon pathways?

By the time the first international meeting on NV of any consequence took place in 1984 at Oxford University, a number of investigators had taken stock of the multilevel, multifactorial aspects of NV. Joss et al. (1981), Barnes (1984), Leathem (1986), and Harris and Cantwell (1986) had alerted the research community (a message still not heard by 1998 medical textbook writers) that the NV processes were very complex and interactive. Grahame-Smith, introducing the meeting, was clear: many sites of activity, many neurochemical messengers, widely diffused effects on muscle, other types of messengers, arousal, emotions, consciousness, other precipitating events were all acknowledged, as was the intrinsic uncertainty in the field. The notion of any NV, thus PNV, 'center' was discarded. With that conceptual ablation should have come an awareness that PNV (however much more specific and tied to pregnancy changes) is unlikely to have a 'one hormone' explanation. (It was also at this meeting that warnings were issued about surgical lesion-derived data.) As we note elsewhere, the studies show what can occur in a disrupted system, not what occurs in a functioning one. Andrews and Hawthorne (1988) propose that the work on the 'centers' could be viewed only as vagotomies done 'higher up.' If in 1984 there was awareness that a culture-borrowed, electrical circuit, or linear mechanism model was a poor schema, it becomes clear that the most focused and simultaneously broad-ranging research should have taken place in PNV work, with its now compelling information that potential biopsychological variables also interact, and conscious olfaction as a cognitive process – one of those capable of having learned components.

Stress and reproductive PNV links

We attend briefly now to the work, with its impetus in psychological stress research in the 1950s (Lacey's and Lazarus' work was dominant, but after Selye's) that became a great part of the field of psychophysiology. McGrath (1970) offered an excellent early review; for a more recent one, see Johnson and Anderson (1990). The cross-disciplinary relationship to the field of obstetrics has still to be made. A harbinger of this cross-disciplinary interest is provided by the International Society of Psychosomatic Obstetrics and Gynecology; a touch of wisdom which should remain in the mind of anyone working with women's NV or PNV was provided by Davis (1957):

> Our knowledge of somatic patterns is very meager indeed . . . early guesses of one, two, or three modes of variation are a long way short of the facts. Tangled as the relations are, there is an assuring hope for us in their very complexity. The peripheral patterns may (expose) the wealth of intermediate processes.

A stress–stress hormone–reproductive hormone PNV link?

Given the relationship between psychogenic features denoting maternal distress and a subset of PNV, one must employ a conceptual design for PNV which allows for these as etiological (at least interactively) and intermittently dominant descriptors of a PNV regulation hierarchy; alternatively, we can use interplay of critical patterning instabilities which intersect to provide the energy and amplitude that trigger NV. Anxiety and stress are estimated to be causally operative in 0–80% with the estimate depending on the investigator and his or her decade. One perspective conceives of anxiety/stress as separate psychological mechanisms (see Wruble et al., 1982); another is 'interactionist' (FitzGerald, 1984). Interactionism here is about the same psychosomatic position as that advocated by Morse and Van Hall (1987) for infertility. If the somatic aspects of psychosomatics are not to receive short shrift among those for whom 'psychogenic' translates only into ghosts as symbols, images haunting brain tissue, one must attend simultaneously to the reproductive hormone, neuroendocrine, gastric enzymes, and anatomical matters which (equally narrowly) have occupied non-psychosomatic (reductionist) NV workers.

One fruitful focus is on stress hormones in interaction with reproductive hormones, or gastrointestinal (GI) tract enzymes such as cholecystokinin (CCK) shown to be involved in NV. Jarnfelt-Samsioe et al. (1986, 1987) represent such an approach not simply in measuring pregnancy hormones, but in looking at individual organ sensitivities to these; they also measure those reproductive hormones released under arousal or maladaptively in stress. The concept is of a 'brain excitatory' role for estrogens (see Harlan et al., 1983), for which they cite Logothetis et al. (1959) and also Walker et al. (1985); when speculating on organ deficiency, they look at liver as an illustrative estrogen-responsive organ. Implicit in this is an organ system model which provides for lower threshold levels (i.e., greater excitability or less regulatory inhibition) for already distressed women who respond to normal reproductive hormones. Thereby NV pregnancy–neurotransmitter systems serve (or those constituting the medullar reticular formation – specifically implicated in Eysenck's 'neurotic' excitability) as a neurophysiological personality parameter, with the parvicellular reticular formation (PCRF) as a specific component operating in PNV activation. With an endocrine or BG protein-circulating messenger model in mind or a PI lipid system, and awareness of the operation of multiple neurotransmitter systems, an interactionist model suggests summating, potentiating, or inhibiting effects, or those critical instabilities that intersect as essentially a biochemical decision calculus that allows for messenger components from higher levels of the central nervous system (CNS).

This seems a tautological thesis for PNV unless one proceeds to demonstrate the theoretically predicted lower threshold levels (as Pennebaker has done for women's symptom awareness) at the level of PNV-activating synaptic or organ function. The model of a threshold level of individual single stimuli is related to predicting the dose–response and efficacy of particular medications; this efficacy is a somatic 'whole system' variable that is capable of being measured by taste. Joyce (1968, 1970) made the powerful demonstration (with a consequence that was not appreciated) that taste samples dosages necessary to produce a just-noticeable difference for gustation, when scaled interpersonally, differentially predicted for individuals a medication's dose-related efficacy.

Connotations of the word 'stress' may be misleading. There are constant perturbations in external environments leading, apart from to coma, to continuous multiple adaptive responses which invoke many bodily systems. 'Arousal' and 'activation' may be better terms within the NV context in which the definition of a 'stress' response is carefully restricted to a high arousal level that has nonadaptive continuation, and is psychophysiologically perpetuated. In that sense, 'stress' has common elements with the term 'neurosis' (now abandoned). It is well known that adrenal steroids are activated during arousal, releasing adrenocorticotrophic hormone (ACTH) and corticotropin-releasing factor (CRF). Andrews and Hawthorne (1988), reviewing the work of Stewart and that of Beleslin and Strbac, suggest that V caused by stress emesis is produced by increased epinephrine in the cerebrospinal fluid (CSF)-activating AP – what we would now refer to as interrelated medullary regions that are gates to the final V expressive pathway. Epinephrine levels would not be expected to be absolute predictors, but rather to vary with individual sensitivities. Once again, one has in mind the pioneering study of Hinkle and Wolff (1957a, 1957b) showing particular organ system sensitivity that varies among humans as the site, or sites, most vulnerable to the expression of stress-induced symptoms and pathology.

There have been proposals about how ACTH, CRF, and cognitive determinants might be involved further in the PNV chain of the first trimester or (insofar as those obstetricians who fervently believe that hyperemesis gravidarum (HG) is psychogenic) might represent a cumulative critical summating level. The psychogenic theory includes that subset of patients who can be treated by stress-reducing psychological interventions, including the use of hypnosis. Note here Henkin's (1974) work showing the adrenocortical insufficiency of Addison's disease, is associated with lower thresholds for sensory stimuli. The threshold for the accuracy of identifying responses is of interest, given the partially similar picture of menstrual cycle-related increase in acuity, e.g., smell in particular, and the same phenotypical sensitivity behavior in pregnancy.

Alternatively, one may propose that arousal stress hormones interact with any hormones with a level altered by pregnancy so as to produce either lower thresholds or specific or summating NV excitatory triggers that act on higher CNS-mediating centers to medullary AP and CPRH connections – not excluding the possibility of hyperthreshold, epileptic-like, explosive, medullary activity. One returns to the proposals of Harlan et al. (1983) that estrogen excites specific-ally for LHRH (luteinising hormone releasing hormoneand prolactin-like forebrain/hypothalamic effects which, in turn, influence circumventricular regulation. Jarnfelt-Samsioe (1986) also argues that estrogens are brain (and thus emetic reflex) excitatory. In 1986 they demonstrated that the common stress release hormone cortisol is lower, not higher, in PNV women, thus excluding that particular compound. There are, however, substances shown to be at higher levels in association with, but after, motion sickness. Stott (1986) found that an antidiuretic hormone was released; it is not yet evident whether this is vasopressin which is also increased during pregnancy. Vasopressin, along with CCK and ACTH, will continue to be compounds whose actions readily invite further PNV research.

Learning, hormones, and a stress PNV?

Recall that Verbalis et al. (1987) demonstrated that, in rats, noxious agents producing NV raise oxytocin levels, whereas in primates vasopressin plasma levels are raised. In primates CCK administration also stimulates vasopressin release and CCK will produce NV. These investigators propose that these oxytocin and vasopressin correlates of intestinal distress caused by irritants/toxins increase GI motility, leading to irritant/toxin expulsion, and also that vasopressin plays a role in satiety control in primates. Here again we introduce the theory of a dual function system employing common pathways for both NV as expulsion and nondistress satiety control – which may become a subjective discomfort only in overeating, if not a V response. Recall, also, the finding of Flood et al. (1987) that CCK enhances memory associated with aversive training in association with food ingestion. It is obvious that this learning has important adaptive, survival functions (i.e., caution) about previously ingested noxious materials (Garcia et al., 1974). But is there a possible function for PNV as satiety control? Even if atavistic and vestigial, this possibility once again demands interest in PNV. Do evolutionarily adaptive functions, perhaps again examined as obstetric risk consequences for eating patterns, control an overall weight gain or (more compatible with early populations at risk of danger) by selecting for foods that are optimally nutritive? The latter seems unlikely because humans have no innate tasting wisdom with regard to nutritive values (Taylor, K., 1990, personal communication).

Should PNV become functionally autonomous after a food (or food odor)-disliking experience as a possibly learned (i.e. anticipatory) conditioned taste aversion (CTA) response similar to anticipatory NV (ANV) in chemotherapy? Inferred CCK overload from its experimental administration does inhibit feeding. One sees this in rats where feeding 'memories' as CTAs, and 'satiety' attributable to inferred epigastric discomfort, can be induced by CCK overload; here CCK acts as an aversive memory enhancer that is retained as aversive, possibly as PNV in this case. It may be that CCK is active in a pathway: stress to hormone to enzyme to vagus and thence to efferent to medullary regions, and, in parallel, to nucleus tractus solitarius (NTS) to thalamus to PRVC to limbic awareness and memory, i.e., a conditioned response PNV chain. Even a set of long parallel sequences is probably too mechanistic a concept. It implies, however, that psychogenic stress, when expressed as one PNV syndrome, must be understood to have biochemical components that are not the same as those putative ones hypothesized for PNV caused by nonstress/nonanxiety at levels from the gastric to the plasma to memory storage.

Prolactin, ACTH, and growth hormone are released under stress, and the other catecholamines, norepinephrine (noradrenaline) and epinephrine. The latter make up Cannon's original arousal flight-or-fight substances (an early review was given in Sawin, 1969). Renaud et al. (1984) and Lambas-Schas et al. (1985) showed that the epinephrine transmitter system appears to play an active role in the NTS for NV production (see Chapter 9). Vasopressin may well play a double role; it has many functions with a raised level in pregnancy, including a measure of 'psychogenic stress.' Correlated levels both potentially inducing and generated by PNV seem to be possible with epigastric chemical irritants or CCK.

Edwards (1989) has proposed that vasopressin is such a reliable NV marker that it can be used as an efficacy marker in antiemetic drug trials. Here vasopressin becomes not simply a correlate of gastric motility distress, but is also associated with NV as part of an evolutionary, atavistic function. (Recall that its NV rise is also correlated with oxytocin level increases and hemostatic functions.) One is led to ask whether lactating dogs that feed their pups by predigestion/regurgitation show raised vasopressin–CCK levels, which are associated with hormone arousal that is not 'stress' released. We do not know whether an ethologist would say that the 'feed me' signals from pups are analogous conscious-activating signs such that dogs' 'minds' should be incorporated into a vasopressin–CCK model.

Olfactory projection

We learn from McLean and Shipley (1992) in Serby and Chobar (1992) that olfactory stimuli can activate visceral responses, including gastric secretions when these are part of autonomic nervous system (ANS) activity and, by implication, adaptive, escape, or homeostatic activities. There can be overlap, i.e., simultaneous or multiple functions in the same areas, between the structures handling visceral and olfactory information. For example, circuitry from the MOB to piriform and insular cortices in the mouse not only shows this multiplicity, but also these areas and the medial frontal cortex project to the ventral medulla and NTS. In other animals, we recognize that these last act in the final common pathway for V. Furthermore, integration of the limbic system, e.g., the amygdala with motor areas in the striatum where visceral and somatic effectors interact, may be via CCK. CCK is in turn involved as a neuropeptide active in some NV. McLean and Shipley (1992) also hold that MOB-projecting information may activate vasopressin. Although their emphasis is on water retention, we suspect that a vasopressin function, once it is released from the pituitary, will amplify the NV process. (As an aside one notes that carnosine may be a specific olfactory messenger compound.) In view of the fact that odor responsivity is fundamental to mammalian sexuality, although to a lesser extent in humans, in the mammalian brain the medial preoptic nucleus of the amygdala is active in this sexuality. Look for its role in PNV.

There are olfactory projections to the hippocampus and therefore probable higher-order perceptual coding including memory. As the thalamus is the arousal and awareness gatekeeper to the brain, and the medial thalamus is involved in pain processing, projections of the

MOB and piriform cortex to the dorsomedial thalamic nuclei and orbital prefrontal cortex indicate modulation or enhancement by failed inhibition or augmenting circuitry from reverberating limbic augmentation. The dorsomedial nuclei do in fact project, in turn, to the limbic system, including the amygdala which is connected to the olfactory apparatus in several ways, thus assuring olfaction a role in emotions and both conscious and vegetative 'preconscious' (our term) ANS arousal.

Kallman's Syndrome; are olfactory organs essential to PNV?

We hypothesized that given the proximity in the old brain of olfactory apparatus and function relating to the reproductive roles of the pituitary and hypothalamus, that PNV would not occur where there is an absent olfactory apparatus. (Since PNV is only a human function, no experimental ablations can be made.) We conceived of one clinical test involving Kallman's syndrome (sometimes termed Kallman/Swyre) patients. Kallman's syndrome is often a familial gonadotropin deficiency arising from under/absent development of the olfactory lobes, with subsequent reduced/absent odor detection capabilities. Most common in males, it is likely associated with renal and bone deficiency, facial deformity and color blindness. Associated gene deletions may produce correlated mental retardation.

In Kallman's syndrome, pregnancy cannot occur unless reproductive capability is induced by adminstering cyclical estrogen and progesterone to allow maturation, and then pulsatile gonadotrophin-releasing hormone (GnRH) over a prolonged period of ovulation. Such administered pregnancies are rare, and when they occur are obviously difficult to locate. We wrote to 12 physicians worldwide, identified by Medline query, 1975–1992 as having had pregnant patients with Kallman's or Swyre's syndrome or described (a limited evaluation) as having anosmia in pregnancy. For any test, attending doctors would have had to observe and record PNV. The accuracy of their replies to us depends on these observations. Three doctors replied, among whom were nine pregnancies. Seven of the nine were without PNV. Were that same proportion to be expanded in a larger sample, it would differ considerably from Western nation expected PNV rates, and demonstrate a genetic-anatomical-hypothalamic functional role for PNV (we would also suggest testing migraine risk in such expanded populations). But ours was an all-or-none hypothesis and as such failed to be supported. Our simple theory is dead.

Other researchers postulating alternative pathways to NV as triggers (cf. migraine processes) but testing for olfactory competence as a main contributor to PNV, (thus allowing the many-pathway probabilistic approach we have elsewhere seen as necessary) and able to generate larger Kallman/Swyre populations, may with attention to the validity of PNV observations, wish to try again. A further opportunity exists using Turner's syndrome women. They have chromosomal anomalies yielding phenotypical females but with sexual immaturity as gonadal dysgenesis. They are at risk of numerous severe anatomical abnormalities. Some Turner's syndrome women are anosmic with olfactory hypertrophy and sterility. They can become pregnant now by *in vitro* methods. Our hypothesis, untested, is that any pregnant anosmic Turner's syndrome woman will not have PNV – or if present, that patient group will have rates of PNV very much lower than expected in a normal population. Since odor does play such a role in PNV as a trigger, this expectation is not world shaking unless one shows that PNV cannot be induced by any stimuli, and that the anatomical dysgenesis is the critical element. In the meantime we confess to our disappointment over our Kallman test results; how fine it would have been to have a simple, linear, anatomically based demonstration of a kind of PNV causality after all.

Olfaction has the most powerful hedonistic tone of any sense. As noted elsewhere, it is the most negative in subsequent judgments about the biosphere. Put in folksier language, that old reptilian brain is an exceedingly sensitive, wary, suspicious, irritable, and easily displeased beast, prone to extreme reactions, including NV. Its currency, the odor molecule which activates patterns at levels where the sensing organs themselves have 'intelligence' (i.e., make decisions as to sensitivity, transmission, amplification) constitutes an unmediated direct chemical sense (no intervening nuclei, fewer energy transformations). It disallows much by way of objectification (abstraction–verbalization) and generates action without any requirement for cerebral cognitive participation, but after-the-fact awareness, even awareness of a vast number of subtle discriminations that are occurring, may be absent (as we see in mate selection with subliminal discriminations).

The range of odor discriminations, and hence their action which occurs at greatly varying rates, depends on sex and, among women, on their reproductive cyclical stage. In women, olfaction is a more important, sensitive apparatus than in men, and changes weekly, and also changes markedly when gravid. The woman's world, the important one of chemical signatures about potentially meaningful conditions, of events outside and within her, is comparatively unstable on a paradoxically regular basis. One may ask whether that inherent experience of more sensitive and fluctuating change, compared with men, generalizes either to PNV or to how life itself is experienced. Does constant exposure to a broader, moveable range of powerful, environmental, hedonistically toned events provide a broader and more tolerant field of aesthetics, even interpersonal relations? Or might it contrariwise be intrinsically destabilizing, contributing to lability of emotion and to cross-linked vulnerability to perturbation, including NV and PNV?

Regarding biomessengers, testosterone increases acetylcholine receptor numbers (in rats) whereas, as noted elsewhere in this text, serotonin receptor density in neurons is modulated by sex hormones. Furthermore, Dorries (1992) reports that, in the cholinesterase transmitter system, glomeruli in the olfactory bulb increase under conditions of mother–infant contact. Olfactory enhancement thresholds appear to be multiply influenced by second messenger systems, e.g., Anholt's work (1992) on adenylate cyclase. There is cross-talk between transmitter systems, and hormonal and CNS arousal state changes with particular emphasis on reproductive cycles. These changes include pregnancy, pheromone, or biosignificant odor presence that induces amplification; alternatively, from other studies, they include odor blocking, and the presence of 'biosignificant others,' such as an infant, potential mates, or (given clinical observations on pregnant women's sometimes severe olfactory aversion to the father) males present. This elementary summary provides some directional signposts to the anatomical map.

Among the most important studies demonstrating the power of olfaction in relation to reproduction are Bruce (1960) and Kaba et al. (1988). Be reminded that Bruce showed that a recently mated female mouse will abort if presented with the odors, or the presence, of a strange male mouse that is not the mate. But the abortion as a pregnancy block from a pheromonic effect is itself blocked if norepinephrine-mediated input to the accessory olfactory bulb is removed immediately after mating. Obviously, olfactory memory exists, and at the level of the bulb, i.e., within the sensory apparatus. Norepinephrine seems to be essential to establish, or to retrieve, this peripherally placed memory. Kaba et al. (1988), in turn, concluded that norepinephrine serves its memory role by inhibiting subsets of mitral cells after mating, by a localized augmenting or contrast effect which provides for particular odor patterning memory. These authors suggested that odor-responsive patterns of mitral cell activity at the time of mating, in the sense of being a memory of the mate, differ and are recognized as differing, at a later time when the strange male's smell is presented. We question whether conception itself induces 'centrifugal' (McLean's term) effects, for example, via circulating messengers from the pituitary, an immediate estrogen 'bounce' that reinforces peripheral sensory–memory discrimination. But it is certain that interpersonal ('intermouse') olfactory-based processes do profoundly affect post-conception reproductive system activities. Pheromones, memory, and neurotransmitters are players. By stretching this a bit, insofar as one allows spontaneous abortion to be categorized as rejecting behavior – its ultimate maternal psychosomatic language – then there is an analog to PNV.

Some of the foregoing 'hard science' material constitutes an overview of the olfactory map, the major activities, and an idea about messengers, but allows a folksy characterization of what can happen. It provides an incomplete set of locations and underlying processes for at least one demonstrable aspect of the PNV process. Importantly, the 'experience' of a woman's response may not involve conscious awareness of present and activating odors. There are a myriad of these in the biosphere – including reliably detected self-odor: signals and signatures (chemiotics as semeiochemicals, semeiotics as the broader science of the interpretation of signs and signals, including meanings). But these signatures, as messengers, are capable of being sensed chemically, so part of the woman's interaction with external and some internal environments will, whether or not consciously, nevertheless be detected and most often judged so as to interest, tease, tempt, please, arouse, compel, and, in the case of an adverse judgment, sensitize, warn, threaten, disgust, sicken, revolt, and/or repel. We presume seriously as well as in jest that the old reptilian brain is not simply where McLean says the 'unconscious' lurks and lives; it is a most responsive beast, and most likely useful when it is most expressive. An instance, probably olfactory, of its semeiochemical repulsion was reported to us while writing this chapter. A coed was forced into a car by three men intent upon gang rape. She vomited, spewing 'puke' on herself and them. They threw her unraped out of the car.

Maiworm and Langthaler (1992) report their work on axillary (armpit sweat) secretions working as pheromones. Axillary odor sensitivity is excellent in humans. Indeed, Albone and Natynczuk, discussed by Schleidt (1992), found that sex organs or secretory 'hot spots' are semeiochemical sources in which secreted pyrazine compounds have a 'universal alerting' capacity with low olfactory thresholds in mammals. Steroids also exist in plants; one wonders whether human response to plant odors may be linked to steroid chemistry (see Russell, 1996). Humans are much more scent responsive than they are aware. (And will surely respond aversively to disease smells such as vaginal infections, diabetic ketosis, etc., in a manner perhaps akin to revulsions from the sight of those who are maimed or deformed.) In humans, according to Stoddart (1990), axillary steroids can have a compelling influence on attractiveness. This impact is found possibly only when a man and woman have already made social contact and are physically close. We would add the expectation of considerable individual differences and population clustering into bimodal distributions as to acute sensitivity, following the work discussed by Labows and Preti and by Wysocki et al. (both cited in Van Toller and Dodd, 1992).

Maiworm and Langthaler (1992) have done an exciting piece of work, although not a refined design, on androsterone and androsterol axillary, urinary sexual steroids where the smell of the latter is akin to musk (itself a sexual attractant in the Himalayan deer described as having a 'warm, comforting smell' to humans) (Stoddart , 1990) and the former is said to be like sweat. (It is the latter to which truffle hunting pigs respond, because the truffle smell mimics a token of pig love.) They show that these affect women's assessments of male attractiveness, and do so in a way that varies with the menstrual cycle state. The attractiveness rating, under conditions of androsterol present or absent on the woman's lip, was made to photographs of men, an own-case control design, and required responding to a word checklist. During the estral phase, the men were more attractive, warm, masculine, and, a color preference rating, more 'black.' [On Osgood's Semantic Differential: warmer? heartier? deeper? Silver and Ferrante (1995) found that older women prefer 'black' and 'purple' compared with men.] For controls, no odors, only 'macho,' increased during the estral phase. Furthermore, 'androsterones' enhanced preexperimental evaluation: already handsome men got more so; less handsome ones got less so.

But now, the zinger! Women whose upper lip had been dabbed with androsterol, giving self-ratings of mood before and after the appraisal session, rated themselves as less tired, less 'sensitive' (we take that to mean vulnerable or unstable), and less depressed after looking at these good-looking chaps, courtesy of steroidal chemistry. But there was an unexpected (by us as readers) effect: when the very similar steroid androsterone was the odor, the rating was of a more negative effect. These findings of general mood effects are compatible with the work of Erlichman and Bastone (1992) in Van Toller and Dodd (1992), to the effect that pleasant odors affect performance, creativity, and other mental function. Schleidt (1992) discussed likeability as a function of existing relationships (with Maiworm and Langthaler these would be pending romances/dalliances) by citing work to the effect not only of specific odor recognition, e.g., infants of mothers (in humans odor senses mature earlier than others and are there to be put to use immediately prenatally, just as in other mammals), but also that the odors of friends, mates, and children are more pleasing. People generally like their own odors as well (Stoddart, 1990). The pleasing effect, compared with an aversive one with respect to other people, is dramatically a function of social situations; proximate strangers in a nonescape setting (the investigators used the subway) were judged as not being pleasant. It is also the case, consistent with the Swiss studies, that women given object choices for those scented or marked with androsterone will prefer these male scents to neutrally scented objects.

Male odors do affect whether a woman finds a man attractive. The effect can occur only during relatively close social (or physical) contact. The impact of steroids increases as a function of her own sexual receptivity/fertility, but there may be a 'realistic' visual esthetic which odors augment but do not override and which is affected by cultural or family standards, as to who is appealing, and real life factors such as compatibility, charm, power, wealth, etc. Delightfully for both parties in romance, odors, fertility, and a handsome face make the woman feel better physically and emotionally, even when only in an experiment over a short period of time. Furthermore, general mood and performance are affected by odor, and the nature of the relationship influences the hedonistic tone and sexual impact of a steroidal odor. We will be most surprised, and chastened, if PNV work fails to find that these factors do not contribute to PNV, especially that with proximate stranger males.

Stoddart (1990) concludes that science does not know much about human body odors in relationship to sexual behavior. But he reports that studies show women who spend more time with men and are more likely to ovulate than those women away from men (just as with mice) and that vaginal odors are more acceptable as smells during ovulation/fertility. There are, of course, major individual differences, not simply among rodents or between rodents and people, but among people. One suspects that readers will have their own experience of the attractiveness and stimulus values of whose odors when and where. The 'fragrance of Christ' and other allusions remind us of the power and meanings of smells. We do not learn everything about living, or about one another, from experimental data. The clinician and the reader are invited to move from their own experience to new ideas.

What the Maiworm and Langthaler work, however poorly designed but psychosexually sensible, has to do with PNV is not directly evident. But it suggests, as women are aversive to odors during PNV and likely to be in real pain from NV, that there may be some 'biosphere' signal that is either newly detected as sensitivity, newly self-produced, or 'interpreted,' i.e., inducing limbic/thalamic/cerebral reversals, compared with what happens during pre-pregnancy encounters with similar odors. Clinical reports from women we have seen tell us that powerful aversions occur in the pregnant woman's response to her own mate. Some women tell us that they cannot stand to sleep with their husbands, so offensive do they now find their odors. A workable theory must be able to account for these reactions.

The conscious interpretation and ensuing train of conduct, and consequently the action semeiotics, of odor molecules as input patterns change cyclically and during PNV. The sensitive stages have powerful esthetic, emotional, memory, and, as NV, sickening and expressively expulsive components. To what extent odors (male steroids or indeed female self-steroids) contribute to these reactions is unknown. That these reactions take place is taken seriously in the context of conscious psychosocial interactions, where sexual awareness or intent may or may not be present, and Maiworm and Langthaler's (1992) reassuring finding that the cultural–esthetic reality of how people appear to one another influences the magnitude and direction of olfactory influence. The olfactory mapping and messenger service, combined with maps, messengers, levels, and dynamics of NV, show the many levels of action involved, and comes closer to suggesting the routes, although still unsure about the functions of PNV.

PNV as a psychobiological esthetic

Chaucer would say that it is 'meet' to end this chapter about a mothering condition of women with a discussion of the elements of artistic judgment, because it is more than folkspeech that links women with beauty. Women are also the more sensitive judges of critical features of an olfactory, and therefore environmental, esthetic. Through the organ of unmediated chemical judgment, they are more alert and reactive to ugliness. PNV is revulsion pure and simple. To state that it is not is just semantic legerdemain.

We offer three premises: one is that PNV is an esthetic reaction. Revulsion names that which causes it as 'ugly.' At this holistic level of meanings, PNV is the esthetic sensitivity of the woman in her situation, a response reflecting innately determined triune brain judgments about what is ugly.

A second premise, based on consistency among studies done, holds that women consistently differ genetically, compared with men, in what they experience of the environment. Their perceptions, within defined spectral settings, may have lower thresholds and are accessible to a somewhat different range of stimuli. This does not exclude demonstrable superiority of men in many different perceptual motor tasks. When women are more sensitive to odor or audition, there is inherent risk because theirs is a heightened sensitivity towards perceived ugliness, when that is the brain's definition of the environmental patterns. The full parameters of this premise cannot be explored, because work in this field is just beginning. (See, for example, journals such as *Empirical Studies in the Arts, Perceptual and Motor Skills, Physiology and Behavior, Psychology of Music, Visual Arts Research, Hormones and Behavior, Perception and Psychophysics, Brain and Cognition, Neuropsychologica.*) A major problem is that researchers appear not to have much interest in esthetics as such, and rarely in ugliness and beauty and responses thereto. Instead, in perceptual work thcy try so hard to follow the psychophysics model which, generalizing to esthetics, must become our artfulness and point of view. The basic fact that cannot be denied by ephemeral political correctness is that women differ from men consistently and dramatically in their brain neurons, and therefore in those brain structures in which functions that are environmentally sensitive and interpretative occur (Kelly, 1991).

The third premise is a classic, non-relativistic one. There is a range of experience in which the psychobiology of the esthetic is fixed. Whatever may be learned, which is relative or individualistic, none is denied; deconstructivism, postmodernism as a general rule of relativity, and, ultimately, philosophical indifference are, in terms of perception of work of the brain, bunk. 'Recognition' could be an esthetic constant. Most of the work in support of this 'truth' (because it entertains absolutism) is by Arnheim, the experimental psychologist of art at Harvard until recently.

We begin with odor; as an awareness of reproductive cycle variance, women have lower thresholds, longer memories, can recall and recognize more odor names (see, for example, Lehner, 1993), and correspondingly are better at smell identification (Ship et al., 1993). Even dizygotic twin studies (Segal et al., 1995; Soussignan, 1996) have shown that girls, when observed in social situations, smiled in response to unpleasant odors, but when alone their facial expressions revealed whether they were smelling an unpleasant or a pleasant compound. Let us call this the 'Soussignan effect.' We infer from this not simply the social sensitivity of the female child (aged 5–12), i.e., her wish to appear pleasing, but also a conflict between her real expressive response (facial) to unpleasant odors and the imposed social demand that she does not display her real judgment. Obedience? Deceit? Shame? Harmonizing at the expense of self?

Maybe women who do not express PNV are more in learned control of an unpleasant response than others and maybe psychological conflict as such may exacerbate odor responses so that PNV risk is enhanced when conflict between what one experiences and what feminine norms dictates is oppressive and part of the meaning of PNV. An augmented ANS stress response to stimuli may be the expression of this conflict.

We have ranged over a variety of research findings from the limited sex/esthetics literature, from 1966 to 1996. Here we cite only those that are most interesting to us. We exclude most of the related and relevant literature on creativity. Amos (1978), comparing men and woman artists on personality tests, found that 'creative' females were more like creative males in personality than were their counterparts among less successful artists. We offer this in some sadness, because it suggests that, to be a 'success,' at least in 1978 (there are few women over the centuries or today who are considered to be top-notch creative artists), women had to become like men. Their perceptual esthetic differences are psychobiologically great, yet conformity, not expression, may be the requirement. In support of this, O'Kelly (1980), examining nearly 500 paintings and sculptures portrayed in Canadays' *Mainstreams of Modern Art*, and Janson's *History of Art* (covering 1750–1940) concludes that the presentation of men was as dominant, women as passive, regardless of the school of art, and that fine art is stereotyped by the social and historical dominance of men. 'Art is a record of male perceptions,' O'Kelly states. Both studies appear to support the earlier cited important 'Soussignan effect.' Generalized to PNV and conflict, the woman faced with her own perceptions of ugliness will be 'unauthenticated' or 'unempowered' to use the jargon, and thus in a conflict situation which will, one just proposes, enhance existing PNV risk perturbations.

Velle-Weiert (1987) in an overview concludes that, in olfactory differences, there are strong, consistent ones between men and women, with uncontradicted female superiority in sensitivity. Females are more sensitive to sound, whereas visual acuity is greater in males. If one assumes a more objectified, distance-mediated sensory skill among males, it is not unexpected that different visual processing in the retina and the CNS is proposed (Hoyenaga and Wallace, 1979). Consistent with this, Cobb and McCrossan (1978) show that female responses to colorimetric luminosity wavelengths show a narrower as well as a different range of responses compared with men.

How women's sensory perception differs from that of men: a range of findings

One seeks coherence among multiple studies of diverse esthetic-related performance. It is clear that multiple differences exist in visual elements which affect judgments. In women, not in men, these are affected by the emotional context of familiarity, affection, and pain. Performance failures and distortion arise more readily when, for women, pain and frustration are independently imposed. This 'stress'-induced distortion is greater for women in the absence of important others for whom there is otherwise more personal sensory acuteness – the 'Soussignan effect' again. Being with or being isolated, rapid responsivity occurs.

Women are more momentarily bound by the visual environment, but their responses are also biologically anchored, focused, and thus more constant and conservative when not disrupted by pain or frustration or altered by social requirements to please and conform, which introduce conflict. As conflict is a determining feature, we allow ourselves to infer that 'strcss' is a more dominant factor in women's actual perceptual response. As women, in a sensory processing task, are more affected by hemispheric lateralization, much that is exploratory or spatial specific within them is at risk of being altered or reduced.

By extrapolation, one may characterize these less lateralized response tendencies as leading to more holistic, integrating, and harmonizing response, and production tendencies. Klopfer (1978), making experimental prediction from Eysenck's neuropsychological scales and visual performance, concludes that women are better able to coordinate and harmonize external social stimuli in relation to (our interpretation) internal personality/neurosensory anchors and processes. Reduced exploratory willingness, greater (akin to field dependency) specific focus, and the apparent risk of magnifying error (at least in visual illusion and distortion studies) allow the proposal that, under conditions of stress and absent intimacy, personal involvement risks more freewheeling and unconstrained error.

As with odor, visuospatial and motor performance varies with menstrual phase. Being female is a challenge to felt personal and environmental stability. We propose that perceptual and organized conservative tendencies, which are built-in anchors in perception, serve as stabilizing social and neuroperceptive operations to counter reproductively and cyclical real instability.

Do these stabilizing, conservative, anchoring forces, faced with cyclical destabilization and greater social accommodation, suggest that a pregnant woman's vulnerability to perturbation triggers the extremely unconservative, destabilizing, anchorless, and messy response of PNV? Were one to allow that pregnancy is stressful, the answer would be 'yes.'

The greater pain of the unpleasant for women compared with men

The literature supports an internal sensory–emotional–tension reconciling 'program' as a functionally adaptive overview of a woman's world. That would be more painful to women than to men under the same perceptual, 'objectively' noxious conditions. Note that 'noxious' cannot be the same for women as for men and that 'objective' is only the viewer's standard. The research tends to be too simple; there is no observation of likely interacting variables such as absent intimacy, impersonal settings, topsy-turvy illusory events, forced projection of impending images, and the like. But Fredrikson et al. (1996) have examined phobias in a most welcoming and illuminating way. Presenting men and women with questions about situations/things/images such as darkness, spiders, snakes, injections, dentists, injuries, enclosed space, etc., they found, using a visual analog scale, that twice as many women as men (21%:11%) had one phobia and 5.4% of women, compared with 1.5% of men had multiple phobias. We conclude that living in a world in which (the same) things do hurt more, and in which the more important 'items' are people, not objects, women are more fearful even when the 'thing' feared is displaced, i.e., might not hurt and is not right there. The imagination in the real world of hurtful perceptions is generalized as 'phobia.'

The argument is circumstantial but the evidence for it consistent. There are sex differences in neuron and brain structures, region by region, and probably in the structure and processing of sensory organs: eyes, nose, perhaps ears, and touch. There are sex differences in how the world is literally experienced as sensation–perception–interpretation. For women, these experiences vary with reproductive phase and are by that definition unstable. Their external world is both more stably conserved and more cyclically unstable than men's. The experiments show that, in perceptual responses and follow-on tasks, women more than men opt for the stabilizing, focused environment. As a normative group, in studies of their perceptual behavior and brain organizing work, *Weltanschauung*, in looking for their world views, showed that women's response distributions have smaller standard deviations, sigma values, and are more sex coherent statistically than men's. Moderating synesthetic harmonies are imposed. There is female preference, and more acute sensitivities, for close and personal environments, rather than objects, spaces, or flights of fantasy. It appears that, to counteract the perceptually inevitable experience of an unstable physical environment, women, for all their cyclical liability, have inner and personal–social anchors of a psychobiological and esthetic sort. We argue that the esthetic anchor is bioecological. A woman knows by immediate direct experience what ugly is. NV state their presence and meaning.

This by no means rules out the imaginatively beautiful. There are differences in the environmental settings that work better or worse to influence judgments of what is going on in the world, i.e., realistically to avoid distortion, illusion, although not always phobic fears, probably confusion, perturbation, and therefore 'stress.' If stabilizing, personal and preferably hedonistically pleasing, supportive, cathected interactional settings are not there, the stability of experience itself, as mediated by the sensory–perceptual apparatus, is at risk. Distortions in what is actually seen, perhaps smelled, or heard occur, and a cascade of destabilizing, baseline awareness distortion becomes possible.

These are broad generalizations from a limited but consistent literature. They are readily assailable. They ignore individuality and exceptions. But our intent is to conceive of PNV in new ways. The *Anschauung* of the woman is made hormonally labile in her very experience of the world, her place, herself, her *Einstellung*. The esthetic of ugly is equivalent to pain sensitivity and threatens, obviously in PNV itself, systemic stability and psychological control, the integrity of intact being. Certainly NV can be and are precipitated by perceptions: motion, visual instability as in flickering film, tactile sensations of the gooey and squishy, the snaky and slimy, the scary, by dizziness and vertigo, by anxiety, pain, and, as our sample and the other data tell us, by fatigue and stress. One does not need a one-event or one-level theory of PNV. Instabilities of any sort, transformed in the judgment of sensations to repugnant and intolerable, may be at least contributory. In holistic language, which allows overall significance to be assigned, these are sufficient.

A sensory apparatus is in place, mostly for odor, which, if intensified, as happens in pregnancy and PNV, becomes undoubtedly painful (remember how our sample rated N and V as intensely painful) and an inner set of events take place that are destabilizing. Anchors are set adrift; they are only sea anchors and the process need not be conscious, because, as noted, many perceptions are subliminal. Remember the brain attends to the novel. Many studies show this and they also show how attitudes, feelings, and learning may induce 'repression' and cause sensitivity to associated arousal. Once again MacLean proposed, the 'unconscious' is the triune brain, at least for women and PNV. And if she doesn't like it intensely, whether or not it is a matter of the consciously ugly, PNV is no more remarkable a response than pupil dilation. PNV is, however, a total response, which is what happens when all of one's being is involved, whether ecstatic as in love or orgasm, mystical as in the union with the One, dedicated as in heroic deeds or passionate self-sacrifice, or with the whole body and mind speaking confusion, revulsion, telling her that the environment outside coming in is bad.

Some of what is normative female behavior is self-control in order to please others, that remarkable 'Soussignan effect'.

On other things

Arnheim (1986, 1991, 1995) and Eysenck's (1992) esthetics are as 'real' biologically as molecules, and should not be demeaned because they occur at the level of hedonistics as well as of protein messengers. Ugliness is real. It lies in the very nature of our response to a world that is with us interactively. Classically, the Devil exists autonomously. The boundary conditions between person and world are by no means as distinct as our practical minds conceive them. Ours are fluid and permeable boundaries; flora and fauna which are not quite us (and are sometimes hostile) inhabit us. We are a system of and with them. We breathe, ingest, at every moment take in the biosphere and exhale, perspire, void, speak, and move into it. Not quite the separation assumed conceptually as autonomous biological identity and environmental control, that 'I' versus 'otherness.' (Remember Walt Kelly's comic strip Pogo's remark to Albert Alligator, 'We have met the enemy and he is us'?) What is ugly outside that comes into us (as odors do but also sight and experiences) becomes ugliness inside ourselves and, when not either immunologically or biopsychologically excluded, is to be repelled. Ugliness is the 'not us.' When it is us, and cancer patients report the shock of the 'other self' horribly taking over and destroying the well self, we conceive of suicide, self-mutilation, religious conversion, heroic interventions, and psychological care. Or we may accept that we have made, with Faust, our pact with the Devil with whom we have accepted intertwined identities.

PNV is mostly about odor, although for Arnheim it is the visual that is the dominant instrument for dealing with the world and thereby for him the visual arts are the dominant esthetic. Our view must differ because we attend to PNV. The beauty of fragrance allows the poetry and literature of it, Catullus, the Song of Songs, Baudelaire, Zola, Proust, Herrick, or, as Stoddart tells us, the paintings of Bonnard or Ingres. Naturally the French are the perfumiers par excellence. Religious imagery ascribes the deepest experiences to odors, that 'fragrance of Christ' or the fetid sulfur of Satan. Mohammed's sweat produced roses. Socrates ascribed to the gods the best of odors. The Egyptians spoke of the sweet odors of sanctity. The contemporary mathematician Golitsin ascribes his Christian conversion to the moment of exposure to unguents emanating from the icon of the Montréal Mother of God. The direct experience of the 'One' is described by mystics as immediately sensory invoking the poetry of God as in Dionysios' *Mystical Theology* or in the poetry of William Blake.

We referred earlier to the observation, by Freud in his 'deferred action' of the Unconscious, by Triven and Stoddart of decreased sexual signal chemical sensitivity in humans, whether or not real. Giorgi et al. (1998) claims that most olfactory genes in primates are dysfunctional. Reduced human compulsory response to pheromones seems easy to demonstrate, but one does not rule out, in PNV women, that what is ugly is a sexual steroidal signal from a non-siring male (that pregnancy block analog?) or even from the siring male if her receptivity has plummeted. Research that should be considered here is a test of ratings of ugly among fertile estral, non-PNV, PNV yet receptive, and sexually nonreceptive PNV women. What is expected is the biological, genetic baseline for esthetics as set forth by Eysenck (1992) – one consistent with the work of the gestaltists, cognitive neuroscientists, and philosophers. These esthetics have in-built categorical judgments given contextual events, a concept that is in harmony with the philosophy of Kant and that derived from Plato. For Sartre, ostensibly a value-free existentialist, life itself is ugly; it is the tedium of G.B. Shaw's hell. Its 'statement' is nausea. Without 'Beauty,' there is Berdyev's Void, evil's equivalent: the emptiness of the absent God.

For NV, from PNV which is generally considered to be of no consequence, and by reflex disgusting even to study, we may have made some progress.

CHAPTER 14

Evolutionary biology: a radical view

This is a long chapter, but, consider, evolution has been going on a long time. For human nausea and vomiting (NV) it is 'work in progress.'

A new view of NV is necessary, one that includes reexamination and abandonment of one or more assumptions about its nature. For example, as evolutionary theory is itself in a state of considerable flux, with exciting discoveries and disagreement about principles describing processes, it is opportune to consider what appears to be evolutionarily the unique phenomenon of human NV. This is most particularly illustrated by pregnancy NV (PNV) but extends to other NV precipitants as well.

We ask the reader to evaluate the arguments – presented primarily in summary form by reference to outstanding advocates rather than by review of experiments – and decide for him- or herself what credence to give our 'hypotheses.' This term, implying exactness, probably gilds the lily, because ours are conceptions stated in a fashion denying null hypothesis experimentation. We are not presenting 'facts' about which there is little dispute, or a picture of the evolutionary, ecological, psychobiological world as if its nature and workings were a sure thing.

In this way the work of developing or at least of reflecting upon explanations for NV becomes the reader's task as well as our own, and that of workers who follow. Think of what follows in this chapter as material bearing on, pro or con, the theses that we advance. Consider whether or not the evidence allows the possibilities proposed, because they are radical compared with the content of current medical texts and conventional research approaches. One immediately sees that ideas about NV are only aspects of larger issues: levels and breadth of inquiry, which matter in understanding humans, their environment, and the features of evolution, are at stake.

Later in this chapter, there are further observations on NV themselves with respect to novel evolutionary considerations. There will be a respectful examination of some conventional theories of NV's evolutionary development but, in contradiction, there will also be a rejection of current doctrine about function. Challenge to doctrine requires that questions, some philosophical, be raised about a rigid Darwinian schema that has, to date, been applied to NV. One's familiarity with and openness to new schema is likely to persuade one to consider evolution, and therefore NV, in new ways.

An understanding of post-Darwinian theory is pertinent to examining NV. Some of this evolutionary thinking employs concepts as proposed new 'principles.' These are applicable to biopsychological phenomena such as clinical NV themselves as process and event. As a result of this theoretical correspondence, our species' developmental past can be connected conceptually to those 'principles' that describe NV workings as observed at any moment. This underlying partial equivalence of 'principles,' parsimony in theory, offers attractive simplicity even though the events past and present are complex. Indeed, it is an approach to that complexity which is, as in dynamic theory, uncertain in relating to the identification of morphological and energy constraints as the common ground. One finds that the same theoretical approach is applicable to both, even though in restricted ways.

For all the years of research in developmental embryology, genetics, and neuroscience, there is continuing controversy about evolutionary principles and processes. This excludes more dramatic advocacy on the part of religious 'creationists' and gives short shrift to cosmologist Fred Hoyle, and to Nobelist Crick who, in so far as he joins Hoyle, argues that the terrestrial geological record cannot offer explanations that sustain the observed complexity of life. They need not disagree with Darwinian principles as such, but rather claim that time has been too short. Biochemically conventional, but extraterrestrial evolutionary, origins that encompass 18 billion cosmic years, rather than 4 billion earthly ones, are invoked to account for our complexity. (Meteorite samples support the possibility of such organic molecule transport.)

Newer ideas about evolution as self-organizing intrinsic processes in living organisms may solve the problem of complexity in the evolutionary record. It is as though each cell can engage in an ongoing process of creation through interconnection of multiple cells. Given the immense complexity as multicellular organisms arise, it may be inner, rather than outer, space (i.e., the environment) that is invoked as the force for change. One must understand the stability of many structures and species, and conservation as such across important evolutionary levels. Random mutation is not the drive, yet still unresolved is a careful and testable definition of what constitutes the critical instabilities (such as NV) internal to an organism.

It may seem odd that one turns to evolution, and therefore to theoretical controversy about its nature and principles, for propositions that might lead one day to closure on a theory of NV. NV themselves seem so simple. We have, however, shown that they are not. To arrive at a better understanding of NV one turns to evolution. To set the stage for these considerations, we offer an exegesis on current evolutionary thought. Depew and Weber (1995) do that, and masterfully show its development as a chain of ideas. They do not address the particular and unique phenomena of NV. What is evident is that many scientists (Hartshorne, Dawkins, Gould, as exemplary progenitors) have moved beyond conventional Darwinism, and therefore beyond conventional reductionist mechanisms as the sole explanation for change over time. A 'paradigm shift' is under way.

The general propositions

- NV are evolutionarily expanded phenomena which, although possibly operating through conserved brain structures and biochemical messengers, represent in humans a primitive and transitional process in their expression. They are a self-organizing evolution in process (although possibly failing) defined as generating internal processes that become adaptive. They have little in common with an evolutionarily conserved 'escape' from physical danger because of its ordinarily explained origin in single-celled animals.
- On the whole NV in humans are not toxin ejection. One need not assume that V is simply a conserved function. With exceptions, in humans NV are expanded sensory emergency responses to a new class of experiences. We characterize these as psychobiologically experienced perturbations, conceptually here, 'threats.' Disequilibrating, at the cognitive level, the NV stimuli are transformed to take on a hedonistic sensory quality which, in turn, is elaborated as (our category for it) 'esthetic ugliness.' This negative hedonistic tone is a central functional feature. As for the perturbations generating NV, these are almost entirely 'synthetic' and made up of events arising from 10 000 cumulative years of urban invention, overpopulation, and ecological instability. Our

hunter–gatherer brain is sometimes unable to cope with these aspects of human invention.

- PNV is sometimes an exceptional case with immediately adaptive functions, although PNV itself is dysfunctional. A knowing, and thus competently evolved, mind need not induce complete disability through PNV which disability could conceivably increase risk to the pregnant woman and her offspring. Also, PNV's achievement of social support does not secure manipulative utility, for that is undermined by such an extreme form of pain. In so far as PNV represents an adaptive, selective social process, that PNV is quite new, although with respect to pheromone sensitivity NV are animally ancient and conserved.
- As a self-organizing process in humans, NV are biochemically mediated at DNA levels, which may be described as creative and 'intentional,' arising from the latent characteristics of biophysical structures. It is, in humans, a mostly failed reorganization of multiple environmental inputs into an emergency signalling experience that is dysfunctionally unpleasant. One predicts that this 'internal invitation' will, in short generational time, move toward a more reflective, representational, cognitive, individual, and also human social 'superorganism' as a socially organized warning system. Again human NV are posited as being evolution in process – an attribute relying on the greatly expanded flexible neo(iso)cortex. In so far as NV signals are primarily synthetic environmental perturbations impinging on the participating human, this awareness represents a new sensory = perceptual system: psychobiologically and potentially responsive to that class of ecological structures for which neither integrating perceptual nor adaptive capabilities immediately exist.
- The evolutionary operation in process is fully represented in the psychobiological formats: esthetic, olfactory, closely linked reproductive, biochemical, and brain space–time events of NV immediate processes. In NV, particularly PNV, evolution and current biological process are identities allowing similar, abstract, theoretical description. These 'intentions' arising out of structure and adaptation can be characterized at various levels of unfolding utilities (meanings or values; these help survival and define environments with opportunities for further self-organizing change). Note that not all NV can be so characterized. Those that come closest to the reflex (V only) mode in clinical presentation is not. One always keeps in mind the multiplicity of NV processes and is selective in identifying those embraced by these propositions.

Meanings and mind, for humans suffering NV from complex perturbations, are essential elements, and necessary for a 'super-organism' response. Indeed, meaning and mind may be correlates of biochemical changes affecting DNA, should what occurs in bacteria ever be demonstrated as an immediate source of change in higher animals. This cannot be argued here as a probability. However, for those whose philosophical positions are Hegelian or Aristotelian, it takes just one step to allow that 'intentions' imply that 'mind' has a more dominant executive position – as forecasting further, less painful, evolutionary adaptation, including definition of threatening events. NV are a marker for such events, although these are taken to be of much less mortal threat than synthetic carcinogens. (Whether one does something about known carcinogens – for example, cigarette risk – is another matter.)

Background views to consider

The multiple applications of dynamic theory imply a harmony of concepts that is not without philosophical foundation. Much of the new evolutionary view embraces schema familiar or attributable to philosophers. It may well be that this 'softer' thinking, which puts biology, psychology, and ecology in touch with synthesizing overviews, will be foreign to many readers. A particular problem for the scientist is the reemergence of a kind of mathematical or conceptual vitalism as intrinsic. The Jungian biologist Portman proposed quite early species-wide, self-realizing individuation, as, for example, in bird and fish speciation coloring. Species-wide intrinsic awareness toward organizing differentiation was seen as purposeful in evolution. One may compare Portman with modernists, such as the contemporary biologist Goodwin (1994) (attentive, for example, to leopard's spots), who quotes philosopher Alfred North Whitehead on evolution as a 'creative advance into novelty.'

Goodwin's work relies, as does much of post-Darwinism, on nonlinear dynamic system concepts such as Langton and Packard's 'life at the edge of chaos' or Kauffman's (1992) thesis that properties arise in systems, including evolutionary changes, that were not working as determinants in previous conditions. Instead, interaction of elements leads to new order, and to new structures of opportunity in relation to the biosphere. A summarizing view may be that derived from Fontana's calculus of algorithmic chemistry: polymers spontaneously transform into life-like systems; 'life doesn't need DNA to get started, it needs a rich network of facilitating relationships open to a flow of matter and energy across their boundaries.'

Some kind of awareness can be implied when chaos theory (Depew and Weber, 1995, citing Waldrop or Kauffman) proposes that living systems close to the edge of chaos transitions are pushed by natural selection to 'realizing opportunities.' One does not know if it is the observer stating this metaphorically or an intrinsic force imputed. When Salthe (1993) proposes differentiated patterns as specificities that are capacities for 'holding meanings,' the observer may consider that a restatement of information theory is to presume some kind of internally self-observing system – Pavlov's 'second system.' However, when concepts are introduced such as 'attentiveness to one's being in the world,' the 'self' as organizing agent in the context of encountering otherness, the posited observer seems internal and self-conscious. One could suspect that George Herbert Mead's seminal social–psychological view of the development of human self-concepts into formed intelligent awareness has been put into biodynamic contexts.

Information theory, whether cast as exchange, instruction, meanings, is by no means inconsequential for conceptions of the new evolution. Elitzur's (1995) explications of Schrödinger's thinking is superb, the latter viewing evolution as information processing, with Elitzur then discussing Lorenz' proposition, 'every organism constituting an hypothesis about the environment.' Implicit is that there must be close correspondence between structure and environmental conditions and that 'the most vital nutrient for life is order and information.' New information as novelty is, with Ornstein or Kosslyn and Koenig, who descend in the chain of ideas from Schrödinger, the only serious business of consciousness Consciousness as awareness of novelty, as instigator of plans for change, as assessor is in that metaphorical sense akin to a teleological view of evolution itself. Indeed, Elitzur says, 'the nervous system is the place where our species is still engaged in phylogenetic transformation.' We hold this to be so and will argue NV as the instance.

One can now turn to Shapiro who proposes, after work on bacteria, that an organism's molecules participate in adaptive mutations that are immediately selective. Biochemical complexes in cells reorganize DNA sequences and thus, at this level, the organism itself is an agent for genetic change. A similar analogy is the exchange of plasmid between bacteria, an immediate and well-known environmentally mediated genetic exchange. There is no blind, stochastic, passive domino chain here. Instead 'an ability to increase the frequency of useful mutations under selection can be evolutionarily quite significant' where 'biological requirements can feed back into genome structure.' Lamark, come home, all is forgiven!

That the genome is adaptive, particularly under stress, is becoming a more dominant idea among the new biologists. Consider the papers offered in the June (1998) New York Academy of Sciences Conference. Molecular strategies in biological evolution were summarized in *Science* (1998).

The new principles emerging suggest that, following the Nobelist McClintock's early insights 'the genome is a highly sensitive organ of the cell that in time of stress could initiate its own restructuring and renovation;' as Cairns' earlier controversial work demonstrated, when environmental pressure is greater mutation rates increase. We have, then, the concepts of adaptive or directed evolution. However, perfection is not inferred (implied) and a mutation that may provide advantage occurs with PNV; if we are correct for PNV and a lot of NV, we may have adverse affects as well.

With descriptive principles of self-maintenance, regeneration, and reproduction, the schema of open systems that is connotatively limited nevertheless relies on direction as an intrinsic force when defining life. 'Biology as a domain of emergent order in space and time,' with living creatures self-maximizing their strategies for survival, and therefore selection over time. This is more than natural selection arising from accident and momentary adjustments, however epochal. For species 'express a particular nature' rather than just 'moving about in a fitness landscape.' Evolution is by no means seen as passive or internally random.

Stephen J. Gould and Lewontin's work (1979) is central to the assertion that much evolves that is not 'adapted' – i.e., fitness selected. There is much life that is expressive but not adaptive. The tenure and structures of a species can be stable, and therefore ecologically a functioning interaction, but a species' characteristics need not be optimal for efficient observation. Emergence of a species is not explained by adaptation (see Gould, 1989, *Wonderful Life*) nor is there evidence that a Darwinian claim for only gradual emergence of novelty by the slow accumulation of minor adaptive modifications solely accounts for new creation. Ernst Mayr is an advocate of this view. Competitiveness as 'cause' for selection, yielding novel species or structures, becomes a minor consideration in describing evolution. There is room for being and becoming as well as for getting by.

This is seductively meaningful to the optimistic human observer, but where is the dividing line in time, among structural biological materials? Is there a line of demarcation between the anti-entropic inorganic, to organic, to 'self-intending' living hierarchy of complexity and intelligence?

For Goodwin and other new evolutionists, neither genes nor molecules are the basic materials 'causing' organizational novelty in living systems. Such reductionism is, instead, 'bad science.' Goodwin would replace such theories with those dynamic systems which, when expanded, become a 'science of qualities' and a 'holistic emerging order' where relational interactions as ordering patterns, not genetic determinism, are formative. Such theoretical ventures generate the responsive charge by traditionalists of 'romantic naturalism.' These folk – probably the majority – would reject intrinsic self-determining growth derived from here and now interrelationships, however many limits and directions are constrained by the surrounding available resources. 'Cells, DNA, evolution doesn't work that way,' they protest. 'Soft' may offer comforting explications but does not readily lead to null hypotheses for test in experimental work; Kelso is the exception here. The argument against Kauffman, Salthe, and the philosophical or mathematical biologists is that 'soft' may be comforting by way of explication but it is inexact. On the other hand, when 'exact' is neither exact nor predictive and does not become so, one looks for a new schema. Evolutionary biology and, if we are right, closely linked accountings for NV are in that transition.

That traditional position tends to emphasize genetic determinism. Interactions in such systems are recognized to be of consequence; certainly in any biochemistry, including neuropharmacology, they are central. It is apparent that neither approach is viable without the givens of energy, time, and space, and therein the laws of thermodynamics, physical forces, and chemistry. Yet in all approaches, except in those that might oxymoronically call for dead life, there are constructs vitally added, even at the viral or prion level, internally self-organizing, and reproducing the intentionality of function and outcomes.

There may be a greater affinity to inner directed vitalism for persons who are 'holistic,' 'molar,' or non-reductionist in their clinical and scientific work. It may also be that those workers who achieve in their education what C.P. Snow advocated (a bridge between the 'two cultures' of science and the humanities), and who are therefore able to employ philosophy in biology or psychology, will be more open to nonreductionist work. In so far as self-organization, intrinsic movements toward common mechanisms at any biological level go, then NV in action and in evolution may be approached in the same way.

It may be the case, as critics can claim, that vitalism is only disguised in its transformation, in psychobiological thinking, to the less easily observed and yet presumed regularities of chaos, or, more specific for psychobiology (e.g. the work of Kelso or Kauffman), in its dynamic theory, with its premises of synthesizing yet probabilistic patterns. These yield interpretation as integrating and therefore harmonizing the philosophical view. At issue is the psychology as well as the philosophy of positions in and about science. With Kuhn's work on earnest but wrong resistance to paradigm shifts in the mind (which seem to be occurring in evolution, neuroscience, and a psychology that is ecological and dynamic rather than one modeled on experimental physics), one must be mindful that new ideas in science are not necessarily wrong because they challenge established premises. But, as research workers, we acknowledge empirically that most new ideas require considerable shaping before they acquire practical utility.

Illustration of traditional evolutionary principles

'Principles' as such include genetic change by mutation which leads to natural selection as an environmentally adaptive process, optimizing conservation of mechanisms, materials, and function. One example in the brain is stability in neurogenesis, particularly in sensory systems. Lateral inhibition is locally opposed by stimuli in surrounding receptors to produce intensity differences where receptor fields evolve. This is where these patterning accentuations, as critical summations, produce cascade effects yielding perceptions and response. Another example (McLean and Shipley, 1992) is the organization of olfactory circuits in the cerebral cortex. This recently developed brain organization demonstrates the conservation of structures seen in less complex species with smaller isocortices. Examples in neurochemistry of continuity, including similarity in plant and animal kingdoms, are the building blocks of proteins and amino acids. The principle here is that nature keeps, and evolution expands upon, that which works – ergo, species survival.

This 'rule' must be qualified by noting that most species are wiped out by chance and without regard to immediate adaptability. This has been the fate of over 99.9% of all species in the geological record (see Leakey and Lewin, 1995). It is uncertainty and accident rather than evolutionary rules (slow increments of change) that play the much larger role. Presumably, then, this 'nature' in natural selection can be seen to conserve only the elements in those few species which accidental extinction misses. We see here two coexisting emphases: Darwinian order, rule and development, and that allowing alien events and probability in which a nonperfecting accident is dominant.

These two views are parallel and, although contradictory, are not exclusive. Philosophically or biologically they may 'pull' toward synthesis, but with respect to NV they work quite well when appropriately targeted toward (in one case) highly constrained, strongly canalized, or mechanically structured linear systems versus (the other case) highly complex, rapidly changing, and intrinsically probabilistic or extrinsically accidental phenomena that, at least for now, do not lead to ready predictions. Whether the latter, on examination, proves capable of some explication when exhibiting regularity is still in question. Leakey's accident and uncertainty, given a sufficient knowledge of variables accounting for meteorites, oxygen levels in the atmosphere, and cosmic events, become somewhat more regular in so far as eventual prediction is possible, unless we humans are not simply the cause of Leakey's great extinction of others, but will ourselves be the sixth extinction experienced. We shall ask whether NV are an inchoate and/or evolving measure of just that risk.

Continuing with principles of regularity we have the observation in the geological record of movement toward complexity. Complexity implies information, patterns, negative entropy, greater interconnectivity among subsystems, and observer systems that involve feedback and feed-forward methods. Casti expands upon the connotations of complexity as found in evolution: there will be multiple modes of operation, fast and slow time scales, and 'irreproducible surprises' observed. Indeed, with correlated views of independence for some as an example of complete systems existing independently of any observers, then any quality of an entity is independent. Dawkins (Dawkins et al., 1982; Dawkins, 1989) is widely cited for his work on evolving concepts of evolution, and in the case of complexity finds it contingent upon interaction with another system – a pragmatist's view. The demand for a 'new algebra of patterns' to assist in such formulation (Casti and Karlquist, 1986, citing Grenander) has been approached by Haaken and, in the behavioral neuroscience laboratory, by Kelso.

Growth toward complexity in the geological record, or as observed in living forms, can hardly imply the nonadaptability of less complex species and classes: compare insects, viruses, bacteria, fungi, and indeed the prions of BSE if their activity can be defined as 'life.' There is no lesser argument over the self-organizing characteristics of an amoeba than those of a human, except that magnified structures multiply, to *n*th powers, the opportunities for variation. But it is probably agreed, whether by Dawkins, Thom, Edelman, or Kauffman, that 'opportunities' are narrowly constrained. Quite a balanced position is to be found in Goodwin's experimental findings. He showed energy constraints forcing the embryo to develop, however self-organizing, along only one of a very small number of possible paths with 'archetypical' geometric forms, and tested by adaptation even with some degrees of freedom.

Unless . . . or until one is reminded that 'archetypical' is a Jungian term referring to powerful abstracted forms in the collective Unconscious and not to the emergence of new forms. These are instead repetitively emerging images for experiences that are ancient for the species. We cite this connotative matter because templates of some sort are implied in emerging patterns, and what are new or old are issues at the heart of Darwinian conservatism versus those of the biologist Goodwin. For example, on self-organization that occurs without reference to any genetic instruction: 'Systems produce something out of nothing . . . there is no plan, no blueprint . . . but the pattern that emerges.' Thom, by no means antithetical to Goodwin's constrained structures, moves from the geometry of event space to determinants, disallowing any mystery from noninteracting forces. As for ancient ones, these are mathematically, and physically, lawful. 'The principle of locality in biology is that all local processes inside living beings must be explicable of only local deterministic process, action . . . over a distance is prohibited.' This does not allow field forces as nonlocalized entities; they occupy the same space–time continuum either without interaction or, it seems, without simultaneous action with localized determinants.

The narrowing of processes and outcomes allowed by observers should be comforting to traditionalists hoping to grasp new principles of change and function: growth toward complexity, evident in the geological record allows 'yes, but' examples. Seely (1989), studying honey bee colonies as 'superorganisms,' describes the path of evolutionary sequence of subassemblies into nested hierarchies as certain. He agrees with Dawkins that complexity is selectively superior and cites him. If so, as more species are beetles than anything else, their subassemblies must satisfy nature as well as themselves. Leakey reminds us of the here pertinent story about J.B.S. Haldane who, upon being asked by clerics what his work in biology had revealed to him about God, said that it suggested that 'He had an inordinate fondness of beetles.' Complexity is indeed a matter of comparisons and the templates of the viewer.

The principle of genetic determination is obviously not agreed upon, except as providing a biochemical ground and a choice of templates for individual development-sharing species-wide characteristics. Nevertheless, the prediction that evolution directs toward a more intricately organized patterning is evident when more intricate subassemblies (in so far as prediction is made from knowledge of genetically available materials) ordinarily move towards new versions of known, classified forms and functions: e.g., wings, eyes, perhaps ants with new feeding adaptations. An instance of this principle is those endocrine organs in humans that evolved from earlier external and simpler structures. These have now become the more complex, internal, possibly multi-secretion, multi-neurochemically informed organ. Stoddart cites studies indicating that chemoreception was the original, i.e., earlier, evolutionary role for the pituitary. This suggests that endocrine organs originally had some other function. In higher vertebrates the pituitary and olfactory apparatus derive from the same patch of embryonic ectoderm. In evolution the nose became interposed – 'interposed itself' if one argues the extreme for self-organization – between the gonads and the external world, with the pituitary integrating information on internal status of the organism as it interacts with the environment. On the other hand, chemoreceptors, as found in the human nose, have showed no change throughout evolutionary history. Their response to steroids – quite important for human odor preferences and probably for PNV – is ancient [steroid bioregulators are widespread – recently found in plants – and in yeast there is a compound closely related to gonadotropin-releasing hormone (GnRH)].

Olfactory memory, so critical to pregnancy block and posited as active in PNV, has also been conservative; nonadrenergic, gamma-aminobutyric acid (GABA)-generating, and excitatory amino acid transmitters seem common in memory mechanisms, and occur economically at the first neural relay (Brennan et al., 1990). Adrenocorticotrophic hormone-like compounds are found in unicellular organisms, but in humans ACTH plays a much more expanded altered role. And conservation characterizes biochemical messengers as well as tissue structures.

Another principle relating to conservation and expansion is that brain structures in earlier forms are conserved yet also recruited and thus are more ordered to subserve new and other forms as well. This allows for multiple and simultaneous functions for subsets of brain tissue where functional, metabolic, and space efficiency are satisfied. Another example is cells moving toward greater differentiation from less differentiated forms. Constraints, their identification, and the principle of movement within those constraints will always be a descriptive, analytical aspect of developmental process viewed retrospectively, as evolution traditionally is.

Yet other principles are as follows: stability in well-adapted forms, passivity or accidentalism in the generation of mutation, and, for human evolutionary status, an implicit, frozen cross-section in the current moment of time of our species. This is opposed to the record of transitions of species observed as episodic: slow then fast; also known as punctuated evolution. Has the example disappeared or merged? What 'when' do we want as demarcating. Is it Neanderthal or the proto-human family emerging about 5 million years ago, the genus *Homo sapiens* about 2.5 million years ago, or biologically 'modern' environmentally refined hunter–gatherers perhaps 100 000 years ago, or urban humans simultaneous with the close of the Pleistocene Age, 10 000 or 12 000 years ago? In so far as experience generates enhancement of individual brain structure or morphological change, or introduces intrinsic self-generating change at cellular or sociobiological levels (including individual learning and cultural transmission), no human today is likely to be the same as any human in the Fertile Crescent's first village. But the brain, as Ornstein (1993) so coherently points out, and Leakey also appreciates, was at best an easier fit for the rugged environment of 100 000 years ago than the immensely more challenging environment of our own creation today. Individual development is not species evolution. However, selective and self-generating change processes cannot be assumed to be entirely independent, i.e., individual versus species. The change begins somewhere. Even flies of the *Drosophila* species are individuals.

In any event, all is not acceptable with traditional Darwinian principles, or indeed with scientists who would abide only by those principles. Being set beside them, and possibly soon in their place, are principles from other disciplines not derived from Darwin.

Current dynamic theory is in part an extension from earlier science as well as from philosophy. Most cited as origins are works by Boltzman, Maxwell, Bohr, Dobzhansky, or Schrödinger's (1944) 'negentropy' set forth in his *What is Life?* Derived chaos theory has been particularly attractive for its effort to deal with simultaneous complexities, emphasizing attention to instabilities and intrinsic probabilities operating in contexts where these contribute to latent or observable patterns. Granted there is overwhelming evidence of intrinsic self-organization within all matter, from atoms to neural networks; this is reasonably concluded as being operative in evolutionary change as well as current biological events. As Depew and Weber put it, 'change originates within itself.' But chaos theorists, however much they agree with traditionalists on non-specificity of genetic control, will face opposition from people such as the Nobelist Edelman (for a commentary, see Cohen, 1995). Edelman, while arguing against specific neural coding as a genetically determining specific function, nevertheless holds for a 'neural Darwinism' whereby populations of neurons develop individual networks via a Darwinian selection process.

Whatever view is taken, the very limited range of observed variability is apparent. These limits for Kauffman or Thom derive from the mathematics of interconnectiveness. Morphological structure, however self-organizing, is also self-limiting in variation (see Goodwin, 1994). Constraints generate orders of limited variability, whether in evolution or momentary event flows. Thus, even though a genome with 100 000 genes has a potential of 10 to the 30 000 for patterns of gene expression, in humans there are only 254 cell types. Among the newly proposed principles, there is still an argument; these principles are traceable to Aristotle and the era's cosmological inventor of hierarchy, Dionysios of Byzantium (about 600). One view proposes real hierarchies in which evolutionarily emerging capabilities such as the 'mind' dominate all subsystems.

For Salthe, hierarchies are distinguishable by the information they carry, whereas Sperry, Power, and others define them by the subunits that they command and organize. For Salthe, each scalar level contains information capable of being read as a kind of self-reflection, where hierarchies are to be measured by their components. This is defined as complexity, self-organization driven by anti-entropy, and an imposed system of interpretation which implicates the observer as part of the system. Nested systems of different scalar value are not in harmony, nor are they capable of single measurement or interpretation. Causes are within the system, even Aristotelian final causes, although one can allow purpose to be inferred from function. Survival is that kind of purpose as well as intricate self-reflection, or at least so some contend.

An implied larger context can be postulated where that 'boundless' complexity attracts events. Not inconsistent are principles set forth that emphasize individuality and individuation (see, for example, Wolf and Strohman, 1994, where whatever the uniformities in tissue structures, responses are individual and epigenetic).

Biological, and so evolutionary understanding moves from species and genes to individuals as self-organized and ecologically situated. They cite Claude Bernard, then Hughlings Jackson that 'Neural organization is dependent upon but distinct from anatomical structure.' The evolutionary situation of the individual is at best his beginning, but it is experience and meanings that shape, within defined parameters, all outcomes. As biopsychiatrist Danny Freedman (1992) wrote '. . . the brain, like DNA has blank spaces . . . a common human DNA produces any common human . . . all biomedicine might forego the rigid control of outcomes.' Or Rene Thom writing 'All modern biology has been trapped in the fallacious homonym associated with the phrase "genetic code". . . regulatory properties . . . rely on some geometric property . . . some abstract space of metabolic activities . . . [where] when [homeostatic] systems perform correctly . . . they assure canalization of metabolic states . . . around specific attractors.' Such thought is a far cry from bottom-up linearity.

We infer that the evolutionary moment is not to be divorced from the experiential one. It is happily coincidental that Wolf and Strohman make an example of sensory signals associated with N itself. As a final response to inner personal insult, these signals are described by their multiple organ involvement, using myriad neurons activated in an effector cascade involving somatic autonomic, immunological, and endocrine systems. The cell (citing Kauffman's work) sets its own order over its constituents. Individuals do so with respect to their inheritance, yet an organism's evolutionary status may be seen as experiencing events over time. Stein and Meredith's brilliant learning, interpreting, integrating, and instructing model of the superior colliculus is conceptually consequented as well as factual, that synesthetic structure having expanded and yet remaining conserved. When neuroscientist Harvey Karten affirmed that their fine work demonstrated that 'the consequences and principles of evolution are expressed in every feature of living brains,' it had not been decided how much the 'principles' are able to determine or allow.

Less debatably, and most importantly for NV, one allows qualifications as determining evolutionarily what sensory signals are to be enhanced. One moves into the biopsychology of affect, but thoughtfully. For example, in considering Humphrey, his observation is that evolution favored for sensation those that were affect laden (i.e., hedonistic or excitatory for events at the sensory boundaries of the organism). Humphrey holds that the nervous system is evolving toward a testing system of evaluation and response, in order to allow exploration of sites of stimuli. Evolution in vertebrates is therefore seen as providing for internal, necessarily complex representations, generated images than of what is 'out there' in the environment. The transmission of sensation results in perceptions where the brain can more safely and efficiently 'feel' the exterior world.

Just as thinking may be an exploratory substitute for doing, sensory perception short-circuits the work and exposure of immediate contact with the world. Consciousness is defined by the reverberating circuitry of the sum of evaluations. That attribution to the content of mind is consistent with a novel handling and appraising view of its functions. Emergency response is more readily admissible to this fairly mechanical view than creativity. Leahey (1994), reviewing Humphrey, is prompted to refer to William James. He argued that consciousness evolved so that survival would become an imperative 'decree,' accented with interests and adaptive striving. This of course is much more than 'survival,' because consciousness becomes an awareness aware of itself! (William James was a philosopher as well as a psychologist. He knew about elaborations, and as a previously depressed person may well have had doubts about the utility of consciousness as commanding only survival.)

When we look at mammalian brain evolution (see Allman, 1999), we rely particularly on Finlay and Darlington (1995) for an insight pertinent to NV. Their approach is intended to estimate the range of evolutionary change within the brain, and conservation of fundamental structures central to its isocortical size. It is reported that, where brain structures are measured and categorized as 12 non-overlapping anatomical divisions across 136 species studied, excluding the main olfactory bulb (MOB), there is essentially no correlation between the size of any one division and any other (the exception is the MOB with the high correlation, i.e., size predictability, accounting for about 35% of the variance, of about 0.70). A factor analysis showed that one factor, total brain size, accounts for 96% of the variance across the 131 species. In other words, the total size of the brain predicts mammalian neocortical and anatomical divisional size and, with it, MOB-correlated limbic components. A two-factor model encompasses these possibilities with 99% predictability. Patterns of brain enlargement across species, they emphasize, are conserved, as opposed to patterns of specificity.

Broad ranges across species size mean very great specific size differences across species; for example, the human brain is over 21 000 times greater than that of the smallest shrew, and the human neocortex is 142 000 times larger. The thrust of Finlay and Darlington's monumental work is that conservatism dominates over specificity as the main principle of brain enlargement. Also, there is an exponential leverage such that increases in brain size contribute to major expansion of the neocortex. They discuss as a basic variable the duration of neurogenesis allowed for cell division. It is the case that specific functions of brain tissue are not dependent only on brain size but on the proportion of differentiated cells available for a specific function. We draw on other work (Scheibel, for example, cited by Wolf and Strohman, 1994) showing that cortical localization for specific function is correlated with the richness of dendritic development as a function of daily activities. Be reminded here, however, that there is debate about whether brain growth in humans evolutionarily led to the capability of activity expansion, e.g., tool use, or whether activity led to brain dendritic cell development. There need not be exclusivity because exploration yields new activities that further yield new dendritic growth: cell preservation for new functions. In any event, paths in brain evolution may depend on which cell types are critical to a selected behavior, and whether neurogenetically their divisional duration in expansion is restricted or extended (see also Strohman, 1993).

This leads Finlay and Darlington to describe an easy and a difficult means for brain evolution. 'Easy' is the change in total duration of neurogenesis, i.e., over 250 million mammalian years and controlling for body size across mammalian species studied. Neocortical sizes now differ by a factor of 200. This can be attributable to minor variations in neurogenic duration. And, recalling measurement differences in divisional sizes supposed to be equal for this study, such as neurogenesis (even constant but certainly with any difference in duration), would allow for cumulatively great differences in division sizes. The 'difficult' way to evolve is via some co-ordinated enlargement of the independent components of a functional, or activity-directed, system across anatomical divisions. The authors opt for the former as the likely process (as would Allman, 1999), one where there is 'a conserved order but a nonlinear scaling of neuogenesis' across the whole brain. They propose that determination may be caused by pleiotropic effects (multiple changes induced by one gene) or two or more phenotypically unrelated effects by one gene.

This reference to gene dominance in trait origin will of course be debated, but Finlay and Darlington are skeptical about primary traits from which massive behavior categories are supposed to have arisen. Their point is that large primate brains will yield large isocortical size changes from relatively small total brain size change. The 'multiple facets and rapid rate of human evolution' are most easily attributed not to some controlling original trait that is conserved yet unrecognizable. Instead, if there is selection for one ability, i.e., expansion from motor/sensory activity (given the extremely high probability that all other brain areas will also expand) then nonselected multiple capabilities will also emerge. Their language is of 'greater processing capacity' and the 'isocortex as [becoming] a general purpose integrator that allows the organism to take advantage of the extra brain structure.'

The implications of this for any human function, or specificity of brain activity, are, in our view, profound. The brain, over its neocortically expanding time in primates, has been an available reservoir of capabilities whose interconnections may serve new adaptive activities. One should not assume that, because a structure is conserved and is put to use, it had selective advantage at an earlier time, or, in so far as there is ecological free space, there is no pain-enhanced sensory sharpening, or that it must be 'useful,' defined in Darwinian terms as reproduction for survival.

Freedom for the new brain to be put to new uses, such as availability for new problem-solving, would seem to be a critical principle. For the neocortex, the principle of its growing availability assures attention to new problems. If, during evolution, reflexive, individual, homeostatic, learned, habitual, or social group differentiated role assignments have not become routinized for adaptation (i.e., problem-solving is not 'routine'), then vigilance is required. An 'alerted mind' is implied. Other examples of routines or plans in place for problem detection/solving are autonomic nervous system (ANS) subsidiary vegetative routines (we may attend to breathing but do not ordinarily do so unless asthmatic, skiing, drowning, etc.) or responsive problem-solving ones at any level. Nor do brain regions recruited for response to problems escape that challenging function even if no coping apparatus exists such as one conserved from some earlier evolutionary stage.

The mind is condemned to wrestle with unsolved and unintegrated challenges, ones that appear to arouse the ANS only with or after NV (not as fight or flight), and are surely not homeostatic 'housekeeping' as an immediate response to the environmental perturbation. *This we propose is the NV phenomenon.* It is an obligatory one because the precipitants are recurrent and, when solutions are not learned (to seasickness by adaptation, to PNV by a cola drink), we are condemned to suffer it. Whether insolubility with the disadvantage of pain in turn generates a more competent biological adaptation remains a question for humans. An adaptively equivalent 'it' seems possible for bacteria, because during DNA plasmid transfer, rapid mutation is experimentally demonstrated.

In parallel, we propose that NV may provide enough biochemical impetus to DNA mutation to be searching for, if not selecting, either N or V as adaptive. This is demonstrable in evolutionarily new PNV, or pulled to generate sensory systems capable of handling perturbations without that disabling NV response.

'Cairnsian' mutation, its frequency in bacteria (e.g., *E. coli*, *Salmonella* species), and even its occurrence are subject to intense debate. Cairnsians most interestingly propose that it is during DNA damage repair (which occurs some trillion times a day in humans) that the mutation rates increase in undamaged DNA. Furthermore, repair not only enhances rates of change, but alters the nature of mutations. Workers in this field, where damage repair is termed 'SOS,' describe this rapid and altered direction of mutation as occurring during a 'stress' condition in bacteria. Nutritional stress has been proposed, but other challenges are allowed in this near Lamarckian process. Thaler calls it 'evolutionary bootstrapping of genetic intelligence.'

Were this to be the case for humans, one would expect NV themselves to be associated with experimentally observable DNA, or with chromosomal change, i.e., mutation. In particular, one would expect DNA damage and repair-related mutations (for example, those subsequent to increased oxidant exposure or to chemicals with DNA impacts measured by the Ames test) in the systems that are part of the NV process: cerebral cortex, amgydala, medullary paraventricular regions such as the locus ceruleus, gastrointestinal enterochromaffin cells, etc. These would be compared with DNA 'hits,' as Ames calls them, in other active cells in tissues not directly involved in NV but in the same organism.

There is another kind of evolution recently proposed: the human as a social animal, possibly associated with the NV and PNV that demonstrably yield social support in the form of assistance for the suffering person (Wilson et al., 1996). The initial thesis is that social interactions 'are . . . the most challenging aspects of the environment for higher primates . . . a major factor in the evolution of human intelligence.' Wilson cites Byrne and Whiten, and De Wall. One strategy for dealing with others is manipulation utilizing NV, often observed by pediatricians and psychiatrists (see Part V). Machiavellianism – psychologists Christei and Geis developed a test for it in 1968 – is such a strategy for self-interest. In a fascinating test of gender interrelationships, Barber and Raffield (1994) predicted and found that men manipulate both men and women, but women more so, whereas women are Machiavellian (Harold Bloom, 1998, would call them 'Machiavels') in conduct mostly with men, with women outmanipulating men. Wilson et al. propose that female Machiavellianism is via mimicry, but the very nature of PNV rules out this rather feminist favoring notion. There is a likelihood that NV, if considered a meaningful signal, may selectively evolve not simply as a signal but as a strategy for exploitation.

Such molecular selectivity would be expected to be responsive to environments even in those larger animals where the boundary between at least external environment and the DNA-repaired cell is quite removed. If nature continues to order priorities for DNA repair, which Ames' work finds is the case in rats (about one of the 10 needed per cell per day in rats, with repairs in humans at the rate of 10 000 repairs per cell per day), there will be priorities for the sometimes commanding, sometimes conflicted, but always problem addressing, neocortex.

This 'problem-solving' would seem less risky if achieved through representations, symbolic thinking, or fancies, i.e., as cognition, rather than the more chancy immediate physical immersion, which bacteria, for example, must abide by (although some genetic programs do very well as substitutes for deep thought: consider cockroaches or algae). Nevertheless, the 'physically immersed' animal faces the immediacy of trial and error, i.e., sink or swim, rather than the possibility of neocortical distancing, allowing the luxury of 'think then swim.' Grant that there is an exquisitely sensitive interdependence between organism and environment, even if the perception is of 'rugged landscapes' and improvised responses at the critical transition states, quite like DNA selectivity against a random mutation background. One turns here to Penrose (1994) who confronts the Nobelist Edelman's 'neural Darwinism' and says that consciousness – and thus the development of awareness and problem-solving – did not arise through the slow, neat, Darwinian accretion of complexities, but is a quite special characteristic.

Penrose argues in favor of 'entangled quantum states,' proposing 'gravitational self energy' to which one may then attribute the perceptual organization that occurs, for instance in the columnar visual cortex, as oscillation to rhythmicity. This is, for Penrose, the energy wave action of molecules over large distances (analogous to neuroscientific observations of conductance and volume transfer). Penrose, along with early psychologists concerned with gravity in infant development, credits gravity with the major operational role in the physics of consciousness. John Dewey, watching toddlers toddle with Myrtle McGraw, proposed that gravity was not simply acting upon, but was an internal property of, the central nervous system (CNS). One is reminded of Kelso and energy flow properties, although here gravitational not chaotic. The language of being 'well grounded' becomes profound.

This emphasis on gravity is evolutionarily of great consequence. If one views consciousness as an intertwined dual particle state that is indeterminate with respect to exact localization, but transient in the cortical tissue where gravity waves are a prime force in function, then NV (i.e., motion sickness) may well represent much more than a histamine messenger-mediated cognitive mismatch of vestigial and ocular input. It would be more than an externally generated sensory inconsistency. Assume greater consciousness in humans as a quantifiable measure, and therefore a greater role for gravity à la Penrose in their brains. Using gravity wavelength theory, one quotes Dalton, 'the nervous system [is enabled] to maintain a steady state of equilibrium' where cytoplasmic microtubules ('centrioles' with charged dimers) appear to offer gyroscopic stability, which is of considerable biological interest (Hameroff, 1989). These centrioles appear to generate a switching capacity allowing large behavioral and symbolic variability, including information exchange via frequency modulation. No particular biochemical would be of importance for consciousness per se, but, for canalized subsystems or substitutable brain 'soup', histamine transmission is a telling awareness (with an exclamation point in the gut) that gravity is not quite the steady-state wavelength required.

If this is so, is it not the case that gravitational complications experienced as motion sickness should interfere with imagery and other thought patterns to a greater extent than would other forms of intrusive NV? A testable hypothesis is the Penrose theory. That simple test is counterintuitive: all NV seems totally preoccupying. Hypothetically, there should also be a quantifiable increase in cognitive disability with destabilizing motion as neocortical size expands comparatively throughout the vertebrates. This is testable: shrews up through people, if one could develop a cognitive acuity test that is species specific, yet with species magnitudes previously scaled. Perhaps single photon emission computed tomography (SPECT) or other brain-imaging techniques of a conditioned signal before a learned choice for food would do it. Our point here is that it seems necessary to use theory, including evolutionary theory, to design NV experiments of quite a different, magnified range.

Returning now to Finlay and Darlington, the 'accidental' correlated growth of nondedicated neocortical areas obviously does not assure that the brain will be sensible about what its activities are. Randomness is not simply a principle of mutation (see again Lenski, 1994), environmental change, or intrinsic energy flows at points of critical repatterning instabilities. Randomness seems to be as involved in life as are plans, programming, and natural selection. Phenomenologically one reflects on brain awareness of itself – idle thoughts, the 'aha' phenomenon, the lucid creative dream, the Muse visiting, or the serial randomness of obsession, hallucinations (we all have them), or whom we meet on shipboard – as a kind of social Brownian movement. This is constrained of course, where the identification of constraints defines the parameters of randomness. It should not be ruled out that the evolution of so much undedicated isocortex allows for random activity via interconnections in so far as this is not immediately selected out (if everyone were absent minded enough to walk off cliffs or to engage in fugue state drift freeway driving, we would rule ourselves out of the game).

In another chapter we proposed epilepsy as an analog for NV or for motor pattern generators not conserved yet hyperactive, leading to explosive disinhibited nonhomeostatic action. (Also, see Chapter 8 for the great array of brain regions and neurochemical messengers sometimes involved in NV.) There need be no sense to its being an adaptive use, but there is some optimism with regard to unfolding genetic designs. A capability arising out of the evolution self-recruits to what is experienced, self and other, as revulsion. It is optimistic to describe this neuroactive recruitment as moving toward an ever-expanding signal system about difficult features of inner and outer environments. What brain regions beyond the isocortex and what biochemicals are involved in the activity may, however, be accidental. Implied is a latent value, intention, or 'attractant' having a response capability to otherwise nonspecified complexes of perturbations. If any of this is so, brain awareness and cognition are actively evolving us into what should be (given neuroscientific or evolutionary dynamic theory) a someday more efficient, dedicated and, therefore whether automated as ANS or consciously discriminating, organized perceptual sensory response system for now ill-defined 'perturbations' which will become more narrowly and 'sensibly' handled.

The failure of MOB growth to occur in correlation with (i.e., predictably with) other brain structure enlargement is reported in the Finlay and Darlington study. This observation is compatible with the work of Stoddart (1990). The thesis is of an evolutionary decline in humans in sensitivity to sexual pheromones, although for Freud it is one of active repression rather than rhinencephalon incapacity. Experimentally, it is demonstrated (Stoddart) that, compared with other mammals, humans are less responsive to compounds such as exaltolide (a synthetic musk to which women typically are twice as sensitive as men). Atrophy of olfactory capability is not indicated, given the potential great sensitivity humans have to training (see Moncrieff, 1944). However, human sexual preference is determined by much more than odors (although these play a subliminal or conscious role) as a function of that so greatly expanded neocortex and its socialized mass ownership, i.e., all of us as groups with norms, practicalities, etc. Nor can one rule out that the very comparative proportion in humans, MOB to brain mass, generates much by way of 'noise' to interfere with odor sensitivity.

Odor, increasing specificity, and disregarded evolutionary theses

The expanded human brain, for all its new capabilities and multiple functions for specific elements (tissues, messengers), is by no means necessarily 'perfected' or consistent. The very capability for adopting new functions in areas conserved for now abandoned or altered ones almost assures disparity as either earlier environments and functions appropriate for them, or the current activities of individuals whose work enriches private brains, are altered. It has disparate, conflicting functions, and its expansion has not been appropriate to solutions to modern life, as opposed to the dealings with the environment of early humans. This is Ornstein's (1993) thesis. His notion of neural evolution is of animal routines conserved but not necessarily integrated or known to us. Consciousness functions to warn and control, which is quite a job for a brain evolved for use in post-Pleistocene hominids.

Ornstein cites Haldane on brain size increase with the present iso(neo)cortex coming to its current state after perhaps 100 000 generations (at the primate level these are about 5 years per generation, totaling half a million years; at 15 years it would be 1500 000 million.) In any event the record suggests that this increase is the fastest known evolutionary transformation, using our own standards as a measure. There are a few problems with date setting, however, when Ornstein argues that differentiated hemispheres are among the most distinct hominid structures, dating such bifurcations to 4 million years ago. In any event the right hemisphere is credited with sensitivity to sensations, and becomes adverse to 'representations,' i.e., greater response specificity for hedonistic tone, most of which will be adverse. This will then involve the amygdala, limbic systems – parts of that reptilian, old, or triune brain – that are quickly responsive to unpleasantness and threat. This mostly negative hedonistic tone (a review of the olfactory studies compels that conclusion), given the direct chemical nature of olfaction, i.e., its unmediated intensity, is greater for olfaction than for any other external sensory function. When olfaction or other perturbations produce NV, its intensity matches direct pain itself, however briefly. Note that olfaction in response to pheromones plays a central role in reproduction for less complex species, and certainly plays some role in humans. (We have postulated a large role, such as esthetics, mating preference, possibly pregnancy safety, and mating immune strategy.)

It is not inconsequential as a Darwinian principle, then, that it is not individual survival, but species survival (the ability to reproduce successfully), that is the foundation for evolutionary success. Granting this, the activities associated with reproduction, those centered in the olfactory apparatus, pituitary, and hypothalamus, are central as are more specific mating and PNV-mediated ones. We have discussed elsewhere the obvious: NV of any kind are not a response that the brain can successfully mediate unless via culturally learned devices. Just as with the honeybee, we require the superorganism of social organization as intervention when V does not spontaneously terminate N. Whatever the centers involved (except perhaps the medullary connectivities that work to reduce N by inducing muscular efferents as a final common path for V, not N), the brain does not and cannot handle the experiences that produce NV. NV are in turn an undifferentiated report on the world as a momentarily very bad place indeed. The brain, and thus the aware mind, is simply not adapted to identify in advance, or to control, NV precipitants not 'forefended' by learning. Insofar as precipitants of NV are human-invented complexities, NV are the Frankenstein monster. As for PNV, the immunologically selectively adaptive response 'works,' but at a considerable subjective cost, because olfaction has no shortcut circuit 'revulsion' except to evolve away from it.

Much of the foregoing new evolutionary biology, involving new views of consciousness, reflects a sea change in biology itself, drawing from philosophy as well as from mathematics and physics. Critics will find this new view admitting what might be vitalism under the disguise of chaos. The scholarly Salthe, for example, enjoys philosophers Aristotle, Heidigger, Hegal, Uexkull; he praises highly Charles Sanders Pierce, draws from Kauffman (1992, 1995) and quantum mechanics, appreciates Henderson's 1917 *Fitness of the Environment*, cites Coleridge, Goethe, Herman Hesse, would not be uncomfortable with anthropic astronomers/cosmologists Barrow and Tipler, or with the geometries of Rene Thom, as he turns his erudition to the new biology of Maturana and Verela. Goodwin appreciates Kant and Cassirer, allows the esthetics of consciousness, moves on to Huizinga on play and to the psychoanalyst Winnicott from whom one may derive notions of its sociobiological creative and thus self-formative role. In evolutionary biology these days, C.P. Snow's hope for a bridge between 'the two worlds' of science and humanities is being realized. This allows broader definitions of 'evolution' as internal as well as social processes. The extreme question is: Are we 'inside' of evolution and thereby affecting it, rather than being non-interfering observers? Are we of those self-reflecting 'superorganism' levels that directly affect it? The next step is biotheological: Hartshorne's evolving humans as 'nerve cells of God.' By this time, the scientists (among whom are a disproportionate number of skeptics or atheists) will be heard to scream.

However, uniformities in species development appear less constant the more complex the structure, and thus offer the possibility for internally driven change. When it is recognized that experience itself is productive of permanent neural change (David Kresch was the first to show the much weightier brain in the problem-solving, and therefore learned, rat), serious questions arise as to the narrowness of the parameters of specificity for complex behavior derived from nonpathological genetic contributions. Differing cellular activity may derive not from different genes, but from networks of current intergenetic regulation, i.e., network states. For Kauffman, the quite narrow interneuronal constraints are described by Boolean mathematics. But one now faces the consequence of several genes governing one trait, as in Hammerstein's 1996 'streetcar' model, emphasizing phenotypic, not genotypic, interactions. One conceives a closely related reverse pleiomorphic effect of multiple genotypes converging to one cell structure or phenotypic trait. Also recognized is the possibility of observing naturally adaptive evolution as nature's work, like much of Cavafy's poetry, in 'progress', showing changes in island daisies over five generations. Change, as potentially current or inferable (beyond that 50% species extinction Leakey forecasts), is obviously possible. Is PNV, and thus other NV, also inferable?

Evolutionarily novel and expanding human NV

PNV is, quite remarkably, a new evolutionary development restricted to but widely present in women and (much less common) also in their partners. PNV itself appears to be the most dramatic instance of an expansion of NV in humans as a response to a range of quite diverse and often diffuse perturbations, including those that are 'psychosomatic' in the properly multilevel sense of the word. Thus NV occur dominantly in noniatrogenic settings as a response to stress, fatigue, ugliness, pain, learning, self-induction, odors, sight of food, and taste. The fact that NV are so readily precipitated becomes the signal and meaning of perturb-ation, and that they appear also as a behavioral, interpersonal, sometimes manipulative, almost always consciously meaningful action (see Sloan-Wilson et al., 1996), is consequential. Humans are responding with new PNV, more varied NV than other animals but with almost no utility. Even in strict Darwinian terms, it should be selecting itself out. That it is not, granting for a moment some importance even for the short timespan of our being *Homo sapiens*, justifies further examination.

Not useful, not toxin expulsive, and oddly conserved

We have found no text or traditional rendering of NV in reductionist accounting in which V, and by implication N as the prodrome, is not accounted for as being functional in humans for toxin expulsion and conserved from 'escape' activities back to our ancestral one-celled days. Conservation implies success and efficiency, yet allows altered functions and the multiplication of functioning tissues and messengers.

Toxin expulsion, except for the rare and diminishing use of antiemetics such as ipecacuanha C14H1807 in or through poison centers, is difficult to identify anywhere in human function. Ipecac emesis is also hardly a spontaneous expulsion, but is rather the social–organizational product of root gatherers, manufacturers, shippers, prudent mothers, carpenters building medicine cabinets, and poison center hotline personnel. One grants that one may ingest a bad tasting food and vomit. However, one does not know what proportion of these responses are to prevent bacterial illness. Small, no doubt. Even in mammals, where expulsion as in canids is pet owner evident, one sees V as the normal result of grass consumption by carnivores – its 'digestif' function no doubt known to veterinarians but not to us.

Andrews (1992), a fine traditional worker, reports that ejection of contaminated foods occurs throughout the animal kingdom: starfish, frogs, birds. However, he acknowledges (see below) that motor mechanisms for such an organized response differ in humans. He proposes that, for humans, there is a specialized system for each kind of 'dangerous' stimulus, but discussion of that system excludes the general states that our epidemiological sample of women reported as common. It is reasonable that NV precipitants are perceived via various sensory organs, and the mind, and will have some uncommon tissues, messengers, and perhaps medullary networks involved in processing. But there is no evidence for specificity of a linear route from ecological start to NV finish. Andrews does realistically observe that much observed V in animals is 'inappropriate.' In the same way he notes that most of what induces V appears to be circulating in the plasma where no expulsion is possible and where, we add, no evidence of 'toxicity' to vascular tissue or tissues is found.

Andrews and Hawthorne (1988) nevertheless characterize V as an 'appropriate protective reflex,' particularly for predators. And it may be. But food-bolting canids and birds (more moult than bolt?) also vomit in quite a different fashion from humans: a slow reverse peristalsis of regurgitation to feed the young. Whether this latter 'fourth trimester PNV' reflects any common predisposition, and thus any elements of circuitry in common among humans, canids, and some avians, is quite another matter. But, for work with severely handicapped humans whose post-feeding regurgitation seems a matter of an immature or defective CNS and other motor development, we are unfamiliar with the literature of adaptive regurgitative feeding. Whether any mechanisms are in common between this and expulsive V, except for directional flow, is unknown and seems doubtful. If there are elements in common, then one has an interest in the stimuli – think of minimal sensory pattern elements of the sort that trigger imprinting, as in the ethological work of the Nobelists Lorenz and Tinbergen, which may function as 'instinct' and initiation to trigger this maternal behavior with its unknown-to-us motor mechanisms. As questions of design, these are interesting. An understanding of PNV might benefit from cross-disciplinary studies of regurgitation studied from an ethological as well as a CNS enteric point of view.

Triesman (1977), writing on motion sickness, also attends to the obvious: NV are disadvantageous, as indeed the first Fertile Crescent Euphrates, marsh-dwelling coracle sailors, or ancient Britains, when first venturing to navigate (we invent this sea-going history), would have self-observed. Triesman cites Money's (1970) excellent review and that of Money and Miles which recognized that it was an 'evolutionary anomaly . . . without survival value.' True, unless Penrose is correct about gravity waves and centriole dimers as a fundamental force and structure for consciousness, and motion sickness is a serious warning about momentary brain dysfunction. Biederman and Davey (1993) are unusual in rejecting NV as adaptive in relationship to food. They report that NV are activated by bad taste and, as a conditioning process, are in fact an 'anti-sickness mechanism of evolution' (see discussion in Chapters 6 and 7). It is conditioned taste aversion which need not incorporate inefficiently evolved NV in humans, so that NV are, in these authors' view, an 'error' of brain process and (by inference) of evolution. Theirs is a rare and refreshing perspective, but gustatorily difficult to explain.

King (1988), on the other hand, finds a sensible efficiency. His proposal is that all homeostatic paraventricular nuclei 'have evolved from a prototypical behavior pattern of escape and subsequent avoidance of noxious stimuli.' King states that '. . . through this system of nuclei, blood pressure, respiration, GI motility and secretion of fluid and electrolytic balance and ingestion of food may all be influenced by noxious situations.' From our standpoint, one is hard pressed to see how at any evolutionary time the interruption of homeostatic function by noxious stimuli could itself serve the organism's survival. The exception seems to be only if no avoidance response could be induced by extant sensory systems so that direct interference with life-maintaining functions would be necessary to, in turn, trigger avoidance, or escape. This inference is not unlike the one that we have proposed for human NV: a correlated signal system within consciousness announcing the presence of serious perturbations otherwise incapable of being coped with. However, in humans this emergency awareness yields no avoidance or prophylactic behavior at all, only that physical immobilization, expulsive spasm, and mental preoccupation that accompanies severe N and almost any V. One does not see in this schema, either in lower animals or in humans, survival or adaptation served.

One might consider the environmental conditions to which a single-celled animal needs to respond adaptively. They are multiple, however simple the sensory and response capabilities. They include temperature, pressure, and density of the surroundings, and the milieu of moisture, including electrolytes, nutrients, available oxygen (for aerobic creatures), and absent cytotoxins or metabolic inhibitors.

Levels and duration of light, and habitat 'stability,' are potent as biosphere conditions. Destabilizing conditions are those of the sort that Leakey describes for extinction and predators, competitors, and species kin. For the early animal, response capabilities could be limited to ciliary, pseudopodic, drifting, etc., escape or approach, and cell permeability and ingestion/expulsion through the membrane. Much variation follows, such as syncytial cytoplasm, the variations of which are beyond our scope or knowledge. The point is that expulsion at this early level would by no means appear to be a dominant adaptation, and at the cellular level might well be handled by the same membrane permeability changes associated with expulsion of metabolic waste products. Is the rectum, as a toxin expulsion apparatus, equivalent to medullary nuclei? Why not?

The easy explanation (that what has been conserved evolutionarily in humans in NV is simply for toxin expulsion) is too narrow in any event – if it has merit at all. There is no evidence of the NV specialization in humans that King posits. When we look at the array of precipitating events (such as those just reviewed), sudden destabilizing or threatening conditions, or stimuli for single-celled or junior creatures, one finds that the most homeostatically disturbing conditions are capable of inducing human NV. Consider the range of categorical conditions: fluid pressure whether internal (baroreceptor response to brain trauma) or external (underwater hyperbaric pressure leading to divers' aspirating food – associated with direct pressure), temperature (heat exhaustion), air pressure (altitude sickness – also an oxygen phenomenon), life platform instabilities (under water for divers or on water, in air, or outer space, gravity changes on ground motion sickness but also 'virtual' presentations), moisture (excess humidity, dryness contributing to heat exhaustion), fluid molecular change (salt, other electrolyte depletion), milieu toxicity (internal bacterial, virus, external gases), nutrient intake (taste, texture, odor of foods), and other alien aspects of the milieu, etc. To what extent migraine photosensitivity can constitute an aspect of the migraine NV phenomena, and therefore NV as light 'sensitivity,' one does not know. We do know from a clinical case that PNV can be precipitated by color sensitivity, and therefore light wavelength (in this case, beige and brown).

The foregoing elucidation suggests that, in limited but consequential ways, the same survival conditions of the physical milieu of simple animals can trigger NV in humans. It is by no means clear that, at the single-cell animal or aggregated cell level, 'escape' is anything but a term encompassing whatever range of nonconfrontational survival devices an animal in a hostile environment may possess. Given the possibility that ejection may be aversion to and production of odoriferous contents, and thus a more interactional defense, 'escape' may not even be a retreat. In our view it is a poor term from which to derive 'conservation.' Expulsion is a much more specific activity, whether early on evolutionarily through cell membranes or later as in Andrew's spouting starfish. Yet here (with starfish we are out of our element for we can imagine but are not informed) we must ask whether the question of evacuation and/or defecation as toxin expulsion allows only a singular view of mammalian NV: only conserved escape or indeed expulsion?

Olfaction as ubiquitous evolved sensitivity?

At this point we introduce a remarkable finding, the full evolutionary and human functional implications of which will be of interest to workers in olfaction and NV for some time to come. It arises from the human genome project. Giorgi et al. (1998) report that two methods of gene analysis both demonstrate that olfactory genes are located on most, 19 or possibly 22 of 23, chromosomes in the human body. These olfactory genes constitute 1% of the human genome, although most (72%) of the 87 amino acid sequences that are taken to be olfactory receptor genes have been mutationally damaged and are deemed to be 'pseudogenes' and, in this light, not functional. To functioning genes the investigators attribute the many specific olfactory receptors in the nose, although here we must be reminded that incoming chemical signatures may be discriminated as patterns (by no means cognitively 'recognized' which does not prevent hedonistic tone assignments) by specific receptors acting in concert.

What are we to make of this massive array of genetic sequences, even if many are presumed to be, on the basis of current methodology and inference, now dysfunctional? The speculative dating of dysfunctionality by Giorgi et al. is common to primates, or at least to chimpanzees and macaques, as well as humans, with a proposed date before the emergence of the distinctive and initial human line as such, i.e., over 3 or 4 million years ago. Certainly distinctive among humans, and in contrast to this primate homogeneity, is PNV which has a large olfactory component.

Now for a burst of speculation: presume, for the moment, that the almost universal chromosomal genome design reflects or implicates primitive approach-avoidance sensitivities using cellular, and hence evolved reptilian brain, capabilities (see King, 1988; Andrews, 1992).

These are prototypical representations, preceding evolved 'olfaction' as we now know it. Presume further that the distribution of these initially cellular 'sensitivity' capabilities is widespread in human organ systems, perhaps even if they are judged to be mutationally damaged and thus not a classic olfactory amino acid sequence, but capable of perturbation. Assume further that perturbations experienced and transmitted by specific neuropeptides, or dynamic patterns thereof, are capable of arousing activation sequences in efferent-responsive structures of the human brain that are possibly diverse; these contain related and 'harmoniously' responsive, literally 'homogenous,' sensitivities that are sufficient, relying on a dynamic rather than a single pathway arousal model, to entrain N or V events.

Add to this concept a review by Williams (1997) (citing Denis Noble, Thomas Nagel, Jeffry Gray, Sydney Brenner, and Paul Nurse, presenting at a CIBA Foundation meeting) on the substitutability of gene-generated functions, the inability to predict function from genes, and Gray's proposal that as much as 50% of the genome codes for signalling, i.e., information-conveying functions. The same message (theoretically not quite the same) can be internally transmitted by multiple messengers, i.e., different genes generate chemical structures that perform the same message functions. Consider then the possibility that widespread 'olfactory' amino acid sequences may exist as part of the messengers themselves, whether neurotransmitters, neuropeptides, or hormones (these classifications themselves are somewhat interchangeable). If so, combining Gray and Giorgi with imagination, some of the signal enhancement from perturbations capable of initiating and carrying on a process that becomes N or motor-generated V may be from 'olfactory' gene-generated compounds within the messengers themselves. This does not disallow a preponderance of potentially NV activity within humans that can be characterized as involving olfactory and hypothalamic regions.

Does the Giorgi et al. (1998) finding suggest the possibility of a ubiquitous structural distribution of primitive sensitivity across multiple human organ systems identifiable by the 'olfactory' amino acid sequencing? We ask if these systems might, within the messenger compounds, play an active rather than a passive role in the dynamics of enhancing NV outcome potential. Might these provide a genetic structural basis for the multiple stimuli observed to induce NV as a nonspecific perturbation response? Could multiple brain regions and messenger systems be responsive to different messages from diffuse 'sensitivity' sites? Assume that it is established that NV activation sensitivity is conserved and concentrated in the olfactory–hypothalamic 'old brain' processing system which contains the final common pathway, the medullary oscillating motor networks of V, but also to an unknown extent GI motor and cognitive awareness networks for N.

An interactional self-state assessment

Human NV as a response range well beyond the instigating survival conditions of physical milieu leading to escape or ejection that confront lower animals. (Recall: among vertebrates fish vomit as a response to the noxious.) In humans the conversion or duplicated function metaphor is perhaps best argued when NV are symptomatic, and when the diagnosing physician or instructed sufferer bespeaks mortal threat, as in the milieu hazards discussed above (heat, altitude, pressure, etc.) or from morbid internal events such as radiation sickness, head trauma, cardiovascular, hepatic, renal, endocrinological and other organ system failures, febrile states, serious infection, and cancers. What is absent for comparative purposes is a count of V, or inferred N in lower animals or mammals of special interest, with similar conditions with respect to NV incidence as a behavioral marker. The field requires work with veterinary medical scientists. If the comparative incidence of NV in humans is greater than, say, the interactively expressive dog given the same morbidity, one may make further conclusions about NV elaboration in humans as a self-state assessment.

In humans, clearly interactional elements, rather than internal morbidity markers, are evolutionarily introduced as environmental responses, interpersonal communication, and strategic manipulation. In addition, assessments about the 'being' of a psychobiological esthetic, and about the ambiguous or disorganized perceptual process itself, are introduced. NV have evolved to become an expressive behavior about ecological situations and the self. For humans, and one does not rule out for pets as well, one can view NV as responsive to emotions, esthetics, symbols, thoughts, and intentions, and, strongly in PNV, preferences for mates, situations, and nourishment. One acknowledges that a strongly demonstrated evolutionary principle is conservation, and then elaboration of that which is conserved. The very massive expansion we posit for human NV over any lower animal function or apparatus suggests that its evolution is much less conservative than elaborative. In humans, NV are a general and (biosocially, evolutionarily temporary) dysfunctionally expanding response capability. Conserved tissues and messengers are inevitably involved, but emphasis on them risks the same simplification, or acceptance of unexamined premises, as does reliance on concepts such as reflex, toxin expulsion, and centers or one-locale motor pattern generators (see below). We propose that, for humans, acknowledging that the massive isocortex and mind do 'match,' NV as an evolved state must also be reflected on through a philosophy of psychobiology (about which Sartre was incisive) with respect to the quality of living, situation, self, and the invented environment bringing this about. It is to this point that we, and NV, have evolved, and may (now) be further evolving.

A careful and reasonable contradiction is seen in the evolutionary schema of Lawes which we present as part of the following.

Motor pattern generators, plus and minus . . .

'Motor pattern generator' is a term widely used by neuroanatomists doing work on the NV medullary and paraventricular (also termed 'circumventricular') areas specified as triggering V and its associated respiratory, ANS, and enteric nervous system (ENS) events. Beginning with the pioneer work of Borison and Wang, the search was on for a delineated, discrete cell group which would be 'the vomiting center.' The area postrema (AP) was soon identified. The term 'center' has tended to be replaced, although not yet in medical textbooks or other short shrift V accountings, by the term 'motor pattern generator.' It is our impression that the concept derives from the work of Brown in 1911 who showed that decerebrated animals ('spinal' animals) could still move rhythmically even with cut dorsal roots, i.e., independent of sensory or higher level input. This automatic capability for action of an organized reflexive nature when mechanically (whether electrically or chemically) stimulated in the spinal animal has been adapted for wider usage. So as 'vomiting motor pattern generator' is installed in the vocabulary, it also expands the concept to involuntary action and supra- and nonspinal mechanisms, i.e., to the CNS medulla and its connections – those 'downward' connections to the enteric organs.

There is most assuredly coordination of efferents in motor patterns for V, triggered from paraventricular regions. These were, beginning with Borison and Wang, shown to be capable of generation during surgical preparations by various emetics. But the notion of the AP as a single source for triggering action has been displaced, although the expanded motor pattern generator concept is widely used. Such locations and sources of activation remain the primary neuropharmacological research interest. In so far as antiemetics (AEs) can be shown experimentally to block triggering, one may hope thereby to develop AE compounds whose action directly or indirectly prevents NV. As we have seen in Chapter 4, there are clinical compounds that do this; new AEs are tested against emetics by this method. However, we have not been in a position to determine to what extent any existing AE compounds owe their discovery to 'rational' research relying on generator studies. We suspect, and will appreciate instruction otherwise, that most AEs in use have been trial-and-error clinical discoveries. At present there can be a kind of domain advocacy by competing investigators regarding the chemoreceptor trigger zone (CTZ), AP, the Bözinger complex, nucleus tractus solitarius (NTS), etc., which tells us that there is no agreement on centers or generator sites, or about the applicability of the otherwise more restricted 'generator' concept as defining a final common pathway. Finally, we apologize for being unable to be informative about the efficiency of generator research with respect to the rational, i.e., theory-based hypothesis-testing development of new pharmaceuticals. There is not perfect agreement as to which array of these restricted regions (Bözinger, NTS, locus ceruleus, general reticular medullary, or paraventricular) may ordinarily act as or on the final pathway.

Any typical CNS set of interconnected, reciprocal functions in which there is localized variation in neuronal involvement and/or multiple neuroactive messenger activity offers, in essence, a field of action for that 'plasticity' found at the medullary–enteric level. One has distributed capabilities, conductance, and network self-patterning organization, and all information resides in and is generated, or modulated, in such groupings across CNS levels. At each level one may narrowly but not inaccurately speak of 'intelligence' as information processing, and pattern recognition and generation.

Too many authors of texts that give in passing short shrift to explanations of NV have failed to appreciate the work of Lawes, and have continued to offer the mechanistic medullary–vagal structure as 'explaining' both N and V. It is therefore useful to distinguish between the special usage of the term 'motor pattern generator' in the case of NV, as opposed to a more common homeostatic or motor application where such nuclei/regions are found to drive or contribute to continuing rhythmic behavior such as walking or breathing. The AP, for example, is open to much circulating material, including cerebrospinal fluid (CSF) and neuroactive transmitter information (it is not insulated by the blood–brain barrier). It is, as Rowland et al. say, in Kandel et al. (1991), 'leaky' with respect to that barrier. The AP in turn projects to most areas of the brain. It appears regularly involved in sodium and water balance, may be responsive to circulating lithium chloride, and is believed to contribute to taste aversion as well (Adachi et al., 1991). Broadly speaking, it participates in appetite and electrolytic function.

The AP's functions are consonant with the larger paraventricular system where its regular operations are involved in blood pressure, respiration, gastrointestinal (GI) motility secretion, fluid and electrolyte balance, temperature and osmoregulation, cardiovascular control, and, in Lawes's view, some ingestion control (not satiety). The common premise is that the GI 'sensorium' communicates to the paraventricular with respect to the chemical 'appropriateness' of intestinal contents, and therefore nutrients, and to food and pathogen-generated toxicity. Evolutionarily, what might have been a sensory system for potential food touching the cell wall of a paramecium, or being passed through that wall, and thus capable of immediate rejection or expulsion, is conserved, modified, elaborated in vertebrates. As far as toxins are concerned, particularly those excreted by bacteria, NV could be the consequence of bacterial secretions detected too late. Such 'poisoning' is a done deal and, in so far as the paraventricular system is viewed as still attempting expulsion, it is not only V which has come likely too late but, as we see from the range of precipitants for NV (see Chapter 3), it has become a misguided, overextended, disruptive stimulus–response (S–R) system indeed. It will thus, for humans, require another and less optimistic functional description. For Lawes, the behavioral–functional description includes arousal, aversion, emotion, defense, pain reception, and analgesia. We take it as implied that such nonhomeostatic activities must be only participatory or subsidiarily invoked roles, because other brain regions (some emergingly dominant as the conscious whole for any threatening or person-involving ecological interaction) as well as a range of neuroactive compounds are demonstrably involved in these functions. Indeed, for NV themselves there will be disagreement among workers with respect to structures, modulators, functions, network complexity and reach, levels, and dominance with respect to nested patterns, or microdetermination.

In any event, the original paraventricular sensors have evolved, in a deeply internalized and wonderfully interconnected way, to become a reticular medullary system and are by no means independent of their CNS, ANS, ENS, and 'neuroendocrine commonalities.' Given an almost unlimited interconnectivity, where the to and from of most of the brain is within reach, learning exists and evolved as well. (Learning is present in all of the simplest animals, with planaria and aplysia as favorite laboratory examples.) This experience of negative or positive reinforcement would appear to be facilitated (we follow Lawes' exposition or implications) for ingestion associated with paraventricular 'responsibilities' when hedonistic intensity can facilitate learning. Thus, as one finds the amygdala with pathways to the AP, Lawes proposes, this constitutes circuitry that could provide for conditioned taste aversion (CTA). Our dissenting commentary is that one must remember that NV and CTA are but remotely and unpredictably associated.

An illustrative study among many is that of Rain and Hunt (1992). Aversive learning, particularly associated with stress and corticosteroid concentrations, and also alert to environmental novelty, occurs. For Lawes, CTA is a paraventricular–amygdala behavioral expression, in the production of which vasopressin and oxytocin release plays a particularly important role. We know that vasopressin is implicated elsewhere not only in NV, but in learning facilitation as well (as is serotonin). For Lawes, vasopressin 'is the indisputable marker of paraventricular system activation.'

Before working out a straightforward evolutionary view for paraventricular functions that incorporates V as an example of an elaborated and adaptive noxious escape system, one must be reminded that the paraventricular functions are subsumed under those of the hypothalamus (the paraventricular region is ordinarily considered only a 'nucleus' of the hypothalamus) and in close association with the limbic system. It is also to be kept in mind that the hypothalamic–limbic region is the homeostatic regulatory/maintenance system, which produces and regulates emotion and reproduction, directly controls the endocrine system via direct and indirect secretion, and is heavily peptidergic (contains vasopressin, oxytocin, but also cholecystokinin, substance P, and many others). The interest in NV study of the paraventricular arises from the discoveries of Borison, Brizzie, and Wang about the roles played by the AP and CTZ in NV. What may be said about the paraventricular will be in the context of its hypothalamic–limbic setting.

For Lawes, it is assumed that, before homeostatic self-contained (and thus more protected) organismic systems evolved, each of the separate regulatory functions of the paraventricular was, at the level of the single-celled animal, achievable only by living in sustaining external environments. This required great response immediacy and thus a range of externally oriented sensors linked to a 'see-and-avoid' motor apparatus. Escape was dictated from those environments hostile in terms of their temperature, chemistry, pressure, and nutrients. It is proposed that these senses were internalized in a region well served with endocrine and neuroactive messengers. These would (and here we continue to elaborate upon Lawes's elegant work) report from what are now both external and internal sensory systems to a region mediating what are now internal environmental changes – behaviors such as food aversion, altered intake, V. In Lawes's schema, those once external sensors remain, but at a distance, removed from external surfaces. They continue to innervate behavior, although they no longer power some tiny creature to scurry away or toward, or die for the lack of ability to do so. Today, instead, the system monitors and rhythmically intercedes, and initiates complex, mostly ANS-mediated, neuroactive messenger and organ-acting endocrine activities.

This schema of the paraventricular system's elements which sense and respond to environments in terms of their survival qualities is a cogent one, including as it does the evolved amygdala complex which facilitates learning. Indeed, the idea of enhanced non-NV behavioral and cognitive response remains intriguing, even if we dispute its validity as being unreliable for CTA; for NV in humans, it is too historically grounded in Darwin.

Nevertheless, as a neural 'sampler' the foregoing is useful. Aversive behaviors have a reciprocal (but a disruptive) effect on homeostatic functions. Lawes implies that regulatory functions (specifically osmotic) and stress responses may be seen as interchangeable, or at least co-localized neuroactively. This is because both corticotropin-releasing factor and vasopressin occupy the same cells of paraventricular nuclei, and become analogous in functionality where defense/stress leading to regulatory adaptation are sides of the same systemic coin. From this it was easy to conclude, as Lawes did, that all of the functions of the paraventricular, however now subsumed as hypothalamic homeostatic server states, including NV, derive from and continue to act essentially as escape and avoidance mechanisms. In humans, more complex physiological states have replaced the single-cell elementary behaviors. But the functions seen, Lawes explains, are visceral and endocrine concomitants that have evolutionarily expanded. This view is entirely consonant with the accepted function of the quite large telencephalon (embryologically generating cerebral hemisphere, hippocampus, etc.) of which the hypothalamus (and thus the paraventricular) is a part. The function is to be in touch with the outer world, and includes some control of motor responses for approach thereto and avoidance thereof. But we keep in mind that sensory systems – probing and selective as they are – may also be seen as a structure in an ecological context. It may also be characterized biologically as 'irritable' or 'knowing' as a more philosophical definition of sentience.

Pioneering work has identified the AP as 'the vomiting center' (along with the CTZ), although the following earlier views must all be revised: the 'center' as identifiable neurons consistently firing as a trigger, the AP being the only source of such efferents, and equating the unusual and behaviorally explosive motor activity of V with other motor pattern generation. Note that in some animals the AP is never involved in V (Matsuki et al., 1993). Miller and Ruggiero (1994) using c-fos gene-expressed immunoreactivity as their methodology concluded that, although a number of anatomically identifiable locales (the AP, nodose ganglia, NTS, reticular zone of lateral tegmental field, nucleus retroambiguus, inspiratory propriospinal cell region, dorsal vagal and phrenic motor nerve nuclei, raphe magnus, subretrofacial nucleus, and spinal dorsal horn; see Chapter 8 for mapping) were responsive in cats given a variety of putative emetics, 'No unique well defined group of labeled neurons that might function as a vomiting center could be identified.' That study, being currently definitive, helps show that the AP is one of several small V-related networks, a sometimes active area depending on what emetics are present, what pathways to the enteric plexus are intact, and what other unknown processes are occurring to constitute 'plasticity.' This reminds us of multiple functions in the CNS providing for substituted efferent origins – and for NV uncertainty.

Consonant with the work of Miller's group, and that of Lawes, the AP, like adjacent locales, is an abstract geometric concept. This does not deny the pragmatic utility of places where neurons, messengers, and energy fields are at work. This work for the mid-stations of the medullary centers invoking V will ordinarily be engaged in other business. The AP will be routinely and (for the NV student) undramatically engaged in biochemical network activities attentive to sodium, water balance, and other synchronizing, adjusting, and homeostatically 'advising' functions: distributive, interactive, and momentarily localized conductance. If the AP is like other points in this distribution, and thus a typical motor pattern 'generator,' it will oscillate between two stable states; its individual neurons should be inherently rhythmical and should generate reciprocally responsive/controlling networks (see Kleinfeld and Chiles, 1990). Thus, it alternates with one or the other active partner cell. Should three cells become active, then one would expect rhythms based on self-patterning to emerge. What produces instability in these tiny reciprocally stabilizing cell assemblies, varying as networks, is not clear from our reading of Kleinfeld and Chiles.

The proposition differs from Lawes's in that it suggests that V may be an 'accident' of cascading sensory integrative failure, and thus local medullary sensitivity to destabilization beyond efficiently organized homeostatic function. This proposition allows a cumulative effect beginning with sensory input that cannot normally be accommodated (neither statistically nor in terms of adaptation). Matches with memory also occur (one presumes hippocampal) and would also trigger or enhance, as in anticipatory nausea and vomiting (ANV). One would then have a statistically abnormal, nonconsonant process leading to accidental consequences, with a presumed extreme destabilization as an outcome of NV. Epilepsy is an analog, but one without any potentially adaptive emergency signal or environmentally evaluative use. Once again, processes are proposed that are not useful either with respect to adjustment, survival, or ingestion, or as the normal function of the regions that induce motor patterning.

Instead, one would allow that the disrupted 'self-disorganizing' patterning has become the proximal cause of V, and of the N that involves prodromal muscle spasms. Remaining focused on the medulla, one would then look for the biochemistry, the neuroactive information exchange, the regional patterning conductance, and the sensory precipitants that disturb the balance of any medullary center capable of initiating critical instabilities in the region which, in turn, produce the extreme activity that is V. By no means does this rule out that it is N that constitutes the proximal event for probable V and that it is V that, though a feedback system, inhibits further N, becoming its 'cure.' The foregoing is only speculation about new approaches and is intended to be provocative.

Yet, in so far as the AP is shown to participate in one of those partnerships that induces those extravagant oscillating efferents constituting V motor activity, this activity may itself represent an unstable mode, rather than 'normal' activity typical of the homeostatic balancing work of this region. Also, if what occurs constitutes a destabilized mode of noncanalized energy flows diffusing to the morphological limits of tissue capability, it would be this hyperactivity that could lead to V. If this should be the case, one may conceive of quite a different view of V and its distributed 'origins' – whichever location may be involved in the final pathway action. Perhaps seen only in humans where there can be greater cerebrocortical activity to generate more NV threshold activity, this radical view would propose that it is oscillatory destabilization in which network neurons lose their network balance that in turn triggers the unusual V muscle activity. Thus, normal rhythms are supplanted by intensive, extreme ones with emotion-arousing, memory-instilling activities that produce the motor phenomenon of human V.

Some take a more specific view of motor pattern generation. The generator triggers genetically available produce patterns ordinarily associated with appetitive, consummatory behavior, and preceded by behavior in which input is modified so that sensory stimuli are internally transformed. Quite importantly, fixed action patterns – species inherent – may occur in the absence of any eliciting stimulus as 'vacuum activity,' most likely in animal experiments occurring when an animal is in a conflict situation. According to Kupferman, these instances are 'displacement' activities. One may take issue with the characterization of cognitive conflict as not constituting a 'stimulus,' although it is better characterized as a complex situational challenge. A 'vacuum' activity may well fit the definition of an 'unprogrammed response' to unexpected, and thus perturbing, events outside the loop of ordinary experimental afferents where experimenter and animal constitute the 'loop.' Yet the motor response occurring maladaptively, i.e., not in relationship to the appetitive behavior to which this definition is attentive, would be entirely compatible with our earlier proposal for oscillatory disruption as energy inputs incompatible with paraventricular neurons triggering patterned events. Epilepsy, which can produce V, is perhaps an analogy, if not a source of research notions. It is by no means adaptively evolved.

'Motor pattern generator' is a concept central to the anatomical work (all on animal preparations) carried out to date on NV. It is a concept central to evolutionary accountings, seen in humans as a conserved, internalized nucleus or nuclei directly derived from lower animal 'escape' designs.

Quite a different view of V and its distributed origins arises when the pathway is seen as a final common pathway action for at least V, although not necessarily N. This view allows that it may well be an oscillatory destabilization which leads to medullary triggering discharge of V, where this is a loss of interregulatory network balance. The inhibitory control of the network, which requires only two cells to be interlinked, is lost. The concept is one of overexcitation and loss of normal homeostatic function (whether water balance or other). Normal rhythms are supplanted by extreme ones which become motor spastic for GI and respiratory apparatus, with associated emergency ANS activity and alerting of the consciousness. Unquestionably, some NV rely predominantly on neocortical, mental events, but others (for example, brain injury and spinal cervical manipulation are reflex-like forms of V) appear after the fact. In any event, the extreme nature becomes preoccupying and in many instances memorialized either for later ANV or, more happily, for preventive or adaptive learning. In this view, compatible with the concepts of Ornstein, and Finlay and Darlington, human NV are the accident of CNS evolutionary development.

This proposition differs from that of Lawes in suggesting that V is an accident, a cascading sensory integrative failure that leads to destabilization as abnormal function, not a parallel homeostatic one. The proposition allows a cumulative effect beginning with sensory input that is not accommodated either initially or at limbic or cerebrocortical levels. Memory matches, presumably hippocampal, would augment disinhibition, or instabilities, or centriole dimer destabilization, whatever conceptual scheme is used descriptively. To consider medullary networks as receiving inputs beyond the thresholds for controlled pattern output puts into question the essence of the conserved elaborated 'escape,' yet still homeostatic, evolutionary schema. There is no escape, nor are medullary networks involved. A feedback design is still allowed if N is shown to be the critical response feature. In this case V is as functional as the 'cure', and future research, other than focusing on N itself as it must, would look for the difference between N signals that lead to V and those that do not, and, within those V patterns, those that interrupt or terminate N or NV occurring together. Learned self-stimulation – Roman feathers or the drunken finger – which effectively terminates N via V is not excluded from interest, here, either.

Lawes, in working out an evolutionary view for paraventricular functions that incorporate V as a conserved system, the optimism of evolution, conservation, and human adaptation, may be summarized as defining V as a homeostatic, self-contained, sensory-signalling apparatus that evolved very early. Each of the observed regulatory functions of the human paraventricular was, at the level of single-celled animals, only achievable by living in sustaining external environments where manipulations of the ecosystem by the immersed animal are considered minimal. This situation required great response immediacy across a range of milieu characteristics, and thus a range of externally oriented sensors linked to a seek-or-avoid motor apparatus. Escape was dictated when environments were entered, or changed, so that their temperature, chemistry, pressure, nutrient capability, etc. were adverse. These sensors over evolutionary time came to be internalized in higher mammals into regions well served with endocrine and neuroactive messengers. They were capable of reporting on assessments made by a newly evolved class of sensors testing external and internal environments for essentially the same features that the now internalized apparatus would respond to, but no longer assess, at a distance from a body boundary. The nuclei and networks in the responding region (in humans now hypothalamic) mediated what are now proximally internal environmental changes or messages. They induce behavior such as food aversion and altered ingestion patterns, and such adjustments that can be made to adverse physical–chemical, milieu features, and V. N as internal sensation is ignored, or perhaps again assumed to be prodromal, in a unified linear event sequence.

Beautifully and sensibly set forth, but not a sufficient account or description of either human NV, or PNV.

Once again asked, an evolving response to modernity?

Hesiod, the Greek poet of about 800 BC in his *Works and Days* harkened to the Golden Age:

> Since before this time the races of men
> had been living on earth
> free from all evils, free from laborious work
> and free from all wearing sicknesses that bring/their fates down on men
> . . . there are other troubles by thousands
> that hover about men/for the earth is full of evil things . . .
> (Hesiod, translation by Richard Lattimore, Ann Arbor, University of Michigan Press, 1991)

It may be a siren song to harken to simpler times, but even Leakey, with Lewin and Ornstein, would suggest that for all its uncontrolled terrors, our brain coped better with early *Homo sapiens* Africa, however 'rugged' the landscape. He cites a study of landscape preferences by unprompted modern adults; they preferred grassland and hills much like the Africa of Leakey's emerging human. Jungian, to be sure, in its implications, but, as a perception, a good story about what is pleasing.

On the other hand, the *American Journal of Public Health* editor Mervyn Susser quotes himself and associates Watson and Hopper in a 1996 editorial to the effect that 'Societies in part create the disease they experience and . . . materially shape the ways in which diseases are to be experienced . . . the varieties of human affliction owe as much to the inventiveness of culture as they do the vagaries of nature . . . [disease] status as a culturally constituted reality becomes apparent' (see also Link and Phelan, 1996).

Our proposal that NV are primarily a response to our own inventions partakes of both views: Hesiod and the Golden Age, and recognition that, in building a technologically advanced nest, we not only 'foul' it, but line it with troublesome stickers. Consider once again some precipitants for NV: stress, fatigue, iatrogenic procedures, vehicular motion, medications, ipecac for ingested manufactured toxins or house planted phylodendron, bulimia, cancers of which most are believed to be triggered by man-made sources, radiation itself, urban centers, and the infections from heterogeneous populations transferable by water- and food-handling systems. As for foods, compare the limited known varieties shot or picked by hunter–gatherers 'safe' in traditions. The folk wisdom of safety and narrow choice against our own range: fish from a sea thousands of miles away, vegetables from a dozen lands some still fertilized with feces or canned with botulism, meats packed even today in facilities Upton Sinclair (recall *The Jungle*) would have exposed (think salmonella chicken and warning labels or hard boiled egg sandwiches at summer company picnics).

Antonovsky (1980) demonstrates that predictable environments, or those with primarily intentional sensory variation, are less productive of anxiety and morbidity. The present high-tech world surely is more controlled, and therefore less terrorizing, yet the multiplicity and literal inhumanity of the multiple presentations of hidden or implicit threat are perturbing. We live longer, suffer less pain, and by no means dare protest that we were not born to slavery, leprous sores or blood sacrifice in Ur of the Chaldees or Catal Hulyuk (but perhaps those times and places better those than modern S. Sudan or Ruanda). But we do not live in perfect compatibility, no matter that Darwin believed, himself a product of the Enlightenment, Empire and Christianity, that evolution was working '. . . by and for the good of each being (where) all corporeal and mental endowments will tend to progress towards perfection' (*Origin of the Species*).

Consider Catal Hulyuk 7000 BC (Mellaart, 1967) as the progenitor of urbanization, of later Babylon and myriad inventions.

Consider the great urban leap come the eleventh century invention of the steel plow and the shod horse to pull it, with its food abundance, and more people, commerce, invention, and sufficient abundance of food and drink for more overindulgence per capita than Roman feasting, in spite of the bread baskets of Roman Syria. Mark vehicular progress, camel to coracle to chariot to sailing ships to space ships – all a challenge to coordination if not to Penrose's basic gravity of consciousness. With urbanization come role specialization, bureaucracy, and the relevance of power hierarchies. Panetic studies show that governments and 'respectable' institutions inflict far more suffering than do individuals. The great rush of it all began with urbanization about 10 000 years ago. It is not only the newborn who is confronted with that 'bloomin' buzzin' confusion' which William James described empathetically; it is anyone living with change and invention, and thus more risk of NV. It may be the same set of risks to the biosphere that Gea theory encompasses, here at the level of individual perceiving worlds. Long is the list of poets, artists, and ecologists who have expressed, without being Luddites, their concern with rapid change and technological impact. Be reminded of Charlie Chaplin's film *Modern Times*.

Pursuing this speculative thesis of human NV as an expanding marker of 'too much to cope with' but also 'on the evolutionary road to utility,' one returns to discussion of the empirical findings in Chapter 11 re PNV. The range in lifetime incidence of PNV across cultures is remarkable, although better estimates await methodological refinement. About the data available, it may be that at least a few isolated cultures are without PNV. In so far as they continue to lack the major categories of perturbations for modern NV, any such isolated culture should show less incidence of NV. In contrast, most of the PNV studies among modern women approximate a rate of 75%. One way to account for this is to consider that allopathic speciation, which allows for quite differentiated and rapidly occurring rates of genetic change, does give rise to new traits, of which PNV is the one of interest to us.

Given the range of brain structures, messengers, and sensory systems involved, by no means dare one assume that it is only a one-gene affair, although population genetic formulae might require that assumption. Most importantly, one keeps in mind from Chapter 11 that PNV does show obstetric risk advantage as measured by observable lower rates of spontaneous abortion. If these were to confer consistent reproductive advantage as a PNV-inheritable trait, they then imply that women with that trait (for whatever reason, but resulting from some immune system advantage derived from the mother's HLA-diverse odor preference for the father), would constitute a group whose offspring's numbers would survive at a rate higher than those of non-PNV women. Surely, such a phenotypic trait as PNV cannot occur via a single gene; and one keeps in mind that 'offspring advantage' would not be consistent, because PNV can occur in one pregnancy but not in another (its occurrence cannot yet be predicted) among primiparae. Keep in mind as well that, in the modern world, there is very considerable protection for the newborn, as well as for adult lives during reproductive periods. Thus traits occurring in groups not able to provide health care, nutrition, and safety may even so not be disadvantageous in humans.

This all leads to a fascinating possibility for the evolutionary 'dating' of PNV as a function of differing values entered for selective advantage, dates of origin, and complexity of assumptions about alleles involved. Those competent in population genetics, and better equipped with such PNV research knowledge yet to be developed, may enjoy continued refinements of this approach. One gives credit to Profet (1991), who has been the only one to ask the question how PNV came to evolve in humans. (See Chapter 12 for discussion of Profet's theory and our basis for concluding that it is not tenable.)

Consider the following possibilities: the expansion of PNV as a marker for other NV, but with the quality of uniqueness in humans and the only form with evidence of recent adaptive advantage, began coincidentally with the development of urban society and thus massive inventiveness. That would place it roughly 10 000–12 000 years ago. We make the simple assumption that there is only one allele, and therefore no more than paired genes coding for DNA with PNV potential. 'Potential' is a critical notion, compatible with development on an 'as challenged' or 'opportunizing' rather than a genetically compelled basis. Further, as a selective advantage occurring much less than the differential of some spontaneous abortion rates shown in studies, i.e., 3%, only a minuscule selective advantage is conferred by data on obstetric risk protection, but not necessarily consisting only of that. Accept the evidence that cultural groups exist with no PNV, and that these represent isolation from otherwise massive population diffusion. Accept also that (given this recent PNV 'origins' thesis) the ancient evolution of *Homo erectus* and emigration out of Africa (say 1.5 million years ago) is irrelevant, for any advantage at all now would be to find only PNV women in any population – so great is the exponential growth when selective advantage (and no extinction!) occurs. Even the relatively recent diffusions (as, for example, roughly 30 000 years for *Homo sapiens* into Europe or New Guinea) seems 'before the beginning' (see Powledge and Rose, 1996). This does not rule out a trait randomly present as potential. Assume further that the 75% observed PNV statistic may be generalized to apply to modern populations. And assume a generation is 20 years. (Ornstein, working from the early Pleistocene, sets a primate one of 5 years.) One presumes that, with 40-year and shorter lifespans as measured in Roman cemeteries, and with a normal age for a woman giving birth for the first time being 15 years (assume also the higher risks associated with childbirth at that age), that 20 years is a safe definition for a generation.

What then would be the advantage ratio of 3% more live births per reproductive life of 100 women – a high average from current work on obstetric risk, our Stanford sample, for example, at 85%. That would yield, say, a 75% advantage over, say, 12 000 recent years? That was a hunter–gatherer milieu but also including some settled almost agrarian, tamed livestock, altered grains, probably village but pre-urban folk, as, for example, in the Fertile Crescent, perhaps the still wet Sahara, certainly the caves of France and Spain. The formula employed by Hartl (1988) requires the assumption of a 1% prevalence of a trait at year one of the trait's presence. This is not difficult to assume. At generation 1 the selective advantage would be 1:9895, PNV vs non-PNV for every 10 000 women. The next generation, G + 1, would see non-PNV women's offspring number 9895 to PNV offspring at 1000. In the second generation, there would be 10 more PNV than non-PNV mothers' offspring per about 20 000 people.

Not much of an advantage? Assume, in generation 2, that before the great early civilizations – Indus, Babylon, Egypt, China – there were 1 million nonisolated, mating-available PNV trait-accessible humans (not true, of course). Each generation of the PNV advantageous trait in reproduction would add 5000 more PNV per 1000 000 where the calculation is only arithmetic, not exponential. Assuming a generation of 15 years, or six generations per 100 years, there are 30 000 more, at 1000 years, 300 000 more PNV trait carriers in the presumably stable 1 million. In 2000 years 'everything equal' (of course not so), more than half of the population would be PNV trait positive. This assumes dozens of constants none of which are conditions that are met. But roughly, for 1000 000 people in a mating-accessible mix, with our artful calculation based on constants instead of granting random periodic famine, pestilence, war, celibacy, gonorrhea, and discounting the possibility that our own work suggests of severe PNV being disadvantageous, 3000 years would yield 75% in those populations where PNV would somehow, some way continue to be a selective advantage.

It is all almost nonsense, but not quite. If we assume less than the 3% advantage, acknowledge diversity in populations from 0 to 85 PNV trait positive, allow for 1000 000 mating-accessible folk, and discount the additional major histocompatibility complex (MHC) advantage for immune diversity, we allow that 4000 years ago is as good a date as any, given the introduction of war horses, chariots, barcques, and inevitable motion sickness, for a 1% trait advantage of a spontaneously mutating set of interacting genes capable of a systemic PNV response-centered history.

Each reader may well generate a different conclusion depending on what theoretical premises, particular assumptions, and formulae are accepted, and numerical values substituted. For ourselves, and emphasizing the rather more substantial obstetric risk advantage apparently served through PNV, one possibility is not that the conferred advantage data may be spurious, but that PNV would be of more recent origins than agriculture and/or urbanization. If Fairweather (1968) is correct, PNV was described in ancient Egypt about 2000 BC and in Greece by Hippocrates about the time of Christ. If the Egyptian reference is accurate (one wishes to verify it), we have a fixed point for the appearance of PNV historically. Thus any calculation of selective advantage must begin at least 4000 years ago. One does not have to assume a straight line projection; such advantage could be greater or lesser during a particular time period (introducing one more variable as a value in the formula). It is a good search for a scholar to make. It is also possible that this conferred advantage differs much more markedly than is currently known from group to group, i.e., the illustrative 0–75% (Minturn and Weiher, 1984) range which is in only one point of a diverse geoethnic demographic distribution. If so, ahead of us is much more intensive ecological and genetic study of groups not accidentally selected, but representative of genetic lines and environmental situations.

As with much else about NV, we close this chapter with proposals set as questions, and with ideas in need of researchers to generate and pursue them.

PART V

THE PRACTICAL CLINICIAN: A SUMMARY OF HANDS-ON ADVICE FOR CLINICAL CARE

The clinical topics and content of the chapters in this part have been written by practitioners at Stanford Health Services and at the University of California at San Francisco, with (except for the section on space medicine in Chapter 32) primary emphasis on how they think about and respond to patients with nausea and vomiting (NV). The content is practical and is neither exhaustive nor always substantiated by evidence, or references, from controlled clinical trials.

Thus, the experience of physicians and surgeons and nurses is richly in evidence and may vary from other regions of the country and world. Diffusion of knowledge is slow and much of the new emphasis on therapy has been promulgated by pharmaceutical companies offering new, and always better, remedies. The continued use of therapeutic 'cocktails' for correction of chemotherapy-induced NV indicates the paucity of real advances in clinical practice. The new attention to smoking marijuana for relief of N, and as an antiemetic, suggests the depth of our darkness about logical prophylactic and therapeutic agents. So read and enjoy these chapters with the feeling of 'front-line' medicine, and grow with us!

We, the editors, were surprised to learn from students upon their return from preliminary discussions with the authors of these clinical chapters that almost all of the co-authors believed that the topic of NV was well covered in the standard textbooks of their discipline. However, on inspection, most found their belief to be inaccurate, often commenting that the terms 'nausea' and 'vomiting' were not even referenced in the index. Rather, they were mentioned in the context of the descriptions of the clinical conditions. From this seminal understanding stemmed the enthusiastic co-operation of the authors of these clinical chapters. Only one potential collaborator declined! We are in the debt of our colleagues for learning along with us, and organizing the information so thoughtfully and carefully.

Readers, particularly those in primary care to whom this book is importantly addressed, will see that there is no chapter within Part V entitled 'Primary Care and Family Practice.' The primary care doctor, nurse, physician's assistant, paramedic and other such caretaker are, necessarily, multispecialists. No single organ system confines their work. In organizing the material on NV and its differential diagnostic significance and treatment we elected to do so by specialty, but with full awareness of, and respect for, addressing the needs of primary caretakers. All chapters in Part V (and Parts I and II as well) are relevant to their work, but perhaps most commonly encountered are the areas treated in Chapters 17, 23, 24, 25, 26, and 30.

Beyond recognizing that particularly outside North America, (and increasingly within North America), it is mostly primary care personnel who will be called upon to treat NV (albeit, were the research available, one would surely learn that the giant's share of ordinary NV is self- and family-treated) we wish to affirm that the sufferer becoming the patient by no means needs to feel a compulsion to run to a specialist. Primary care personnel, *providing they inform themselves*, will do quite well. Specialists have the same obligation.

As a final point, introducing Part V, all caretakers, however specialized, provide their best service to the patient, do their best for the doctor–patient relationship, when they give NV, and the information herein about its importance, their full and compassionate attention.

CHAPTER 15

Allergy and immunology

Allergic disorders are among the most common diseases afflicting humans, with a prevalence of 10–20% of the population. Two-thirds of the patients with asthma and allergic rhinitis are managed by either family physicians or allergists, making communication between these physician groups essential in understanding these diseases. As immunology is the basic science of allergy, these two fields are combined

How allergy and immunology are related to nausea and vomiting (NV)

NV are subjective or observational findings of several allergic and immunological reactions. There are two cat-egories of reactions associated with allergic and immunological disorders that involve NV. The first is those reactions stimulated by inhalants or ingested material such as monosodium glutamate (MSG), food, environmental excitants, or drugs used to treat allergic or immunological diseases: intravenous immunoglobulin, methotrexate, azathioprine, cyclophosphamide, interleukin-2 (IL-2), and sulfa drugs. The other category involves reactions caused by immunological diseases such as mastocytosis, graft versus host transplant disease, serum sickness, diffuse cutaneous systemic sclerosis, anaphylaxis, and immune hemolysis.

Differential diagnosis

For those reactions that are a result of ingested or inhaled substances, the NV reaction is generally accompanied by other gastrointestinal (GI) tract malaise, such as diarrhea and cramps. Another major symptom that nearly always accompanies NV is mild-to-severe abdominal pain. The other symptoms resemble those of a prototypical allergic reaction: wheezing, burning sensations, chest pain, inflammatory reactions, and headache.

NV caused by immunological diseases are usually in conjunction with diarrhea, abdominal pain, and fever, but are not as likely to be accompanied by the 'allergy' symptoms mentioned previously.

NV produced without treatment

Ingested material

MSG

MSG contains glutamic acid, which is a nonessential amino acid that makes up 20% of dietary protein. It occurs naturally in some foods (cheese), but the highest exposure to glutamic acid is when it is used as a flavor enhancer. It is heavily used in Chinese food, and is one of Kentucky Fried Chicken's 'secret spices.' Generally recognized as 'safe' by the Food and Drug Administration, glutamic acid causes adverse reactions when large amounts are ingested, which are rapidly absorbed in solution or on an empty stomach.

'Chinese restaurant syndrome'
About 15–20 minutes after ingestion, symptoms appear that are characterized by headache, chest tightness, nausea, and sweating. This reaction is related to dosage of MSG, and varies from person to person (prevalence in the Chinese restaurant eating population is about 30%). More recent tests suggest that the three major categories of symptoms are burning sensations, facial pressure, and chest pain, rather than headache and chest tightness.

Food

Immune-mediated adverse reactions to food are often mediated by immunoglobulin E (IgE) and follow passage of food through the mouth and oropharynx. Nausea, cramps, abdominal distention, vomiting, flatulence, and diarrhea may be observed as food comes into contact with the gastrointestinal mucosa – this is sometimes referred to as gastrointestinal anaphylaxis.

Inhaled material

Environmental illness

This is characterized by adverse reactions to environmental

excitants, as they are modified by individual susceptibility in terms of specific adaptations. The excitants are present in air, water, drugs, and our habitats – most people have multiple symptoms which are referable to multiple organ systems.

The most common complaints are fatigue, headache, nausea, malaise, and pain (all nonspecific). Specific causes are often formaldehyde, phenol, ethanol, ammonia, hydrocarbons, and petrochemicals (e.g. cleaners, paints, perfumes, pesticides, smoke, gasoline)

The theory behind environmental illness suggests that the human body cannot always adapt to industrial synthetic chemicals, and failure to adapt will produce a hypersensitivity to these chemicals.

Immunological diseases

Anaphylaxis

The visceral manifestations of this disease are N, V, abdominal colic, diarrhea, and fecal incontinence. Cramping, abdominal pain, and hyperperistalsis can also result from visceral smooth muscle contraction. Almost 95% of anaphylactic reactions to intravenous drugs occur within 5 minutes of injection, and severity is directly proportional to the rapidity of onset of reaction. There is the possibility of recurrence for 8–12 hours afterwards, and people with asthma are at greater risk.

Mastocytosis

Gastrointestinal involvement is more common than was recognized in the past for this disease. Abdominal pain is the most common symptom, but NV either separately or together may be severe and are usually related to pulmonary disease.

Graft versus host disease

Bone marrow

After bone marrow transplantation, donor T cells can reject the recipient. The HLA identity between recipients is required for successful unfractionated bone marrow transplantation. When recipient class II HLA antigens do not match, the graft antigens stimulate genetically different donor T cells to proliferate and become cytotoxic, causing graft versus host reactions. The symptoms are: a high unrelenting fever, a morbilliform, maculopapular, erythematous rash, and severe diarrhea (can be bloody). NV and severe abdominal cramps occur as a result of GI involvement.

Liver
The symptoms are mediated by T-cell release of cytokines, including: tumor necrosis factor, IL-2, and interferon. The main symptoms are: fever in 70–100% of patients, rigors in 30%, NV and diarrhea in 15–20%, hypotension, chest pain, dyspnea, and/or wheezing.

Many factors, including drug toxicity and viral infection, have been implicated in the cause of post-transplantation liver disease. Viral infections, GI infections (enteritis), and hepatic infections are common after liver transplantation. The principal source of these diseases is the transplanted organ.

Enteritis

This involves the duodenum and stomach, and produces NV, early satiety, mucosal erythema or aphthous ulcers seen during endoscopy.

Serum sickness

Early observations indicated that NV and abdominal pain, mild and abated, occurred in 6% of patients, but later studies showed that 20 of 30 patients experienced abdominal bloating, abdominal cramping, NV, or diarrhea in decreasing order of frequency.

Diffuse cutaneous systemic sclerosis

Gut involvement is almost universal in patients with systemic sclerosis. Pseudo-obstruction is a main result of sphincter dysfunction and dysmotility from smooth muscle fibrosis or atrophy, which presents an acute abdominal process with anorexia, NV, constipation, and abdominal pain.

Immune hemolysis

This disease may occur intravascularly or extravascularly. Intravascular disease involves antibody-mediated complement activation which releases free hemoglobin after the red blood cell membrane is lysed. The most common symptoms are fever, chest pain, N, flushing, and dyspnea.

NV produced with treatment

Pharmaceutical agents: the following drugs are used to treat allergies or immunological diseases and have side effects that involve N and/or V. It is not implied that the following drugs invoke allergic or immunological reactions themselves; they are merely used in treating such disorders.

Intravenous immunoglobulin administration

Used primarily for people with immune deficiencies, intravenous immunoglobulin (IVIG) consists of IgG antibodies. The adverse reactions to this treatment are: vasodilatory and inflammatory reactions including flushing, headache, NV, chest tightening, and abdominal and lower back pain. These symptoms occur about 10% of the time. These effects have been attributed to immune complexes formed between passively administered IgG antibodies and antigens from infectious agents present in the host.

Methotrexate

This is a pharmaceutical agent that mediates enhanced adenosine release by fibroblasts and endothelial cells which inhibit adherence to these cells. Over 90% of patients who take it will experience an adverse reaction, which includes gastrointestinal reactions ranging from anorexia and mild N to severe NV. This reaction usually occurs within 24 hours of administration

Azathioprine

An inactive prodrug that differs from 6-mercaptopurine by virtue of addition of an imidazole group to the sulfur moiety of 6-mercaptopurine. Gastrointestinal complaints are common upon administration and vary from mild N to severe abdominal pain and V.

Cyclophosphamide

Treatment with this is given intravenously and in pulses for the treatment of lupus nephritis. Patients frequently have severe NV and require pre-treatment with antiemetics.

Sulfonamide antibiotics (sulfa drugs)

This set of drugs is associated with high rates of minor and severe skin rashes. NV and abdominal pain are the most common causes for discontinuing sulfasalazine.

Interleukin-2

A 133 amino acid protein which can render lymphocytes cytotoxic to a broad range of tumor cell targets, centered on the treatment of cancers. The GI side effects include NV and diarrhea in many patients.

Case study

A 3-year-old girl vomited every time she ate shellfish. Her parents thought that the cause was psychological because she just didn't like the texture of the 'slimy fish.' In actuality, their daughter was allergic to a chemical component of the shellfish. Vomiting is an important manifestation of allergy in infants and small children, but not usually in older children and adults. It indicates a severe sensitivity to the food which older patients recognize and avoid, and may indicate a real food allergy.

CHAPTER 16

Anesthesiology

This chapter differs from the other clinical chapters in Part V because it does not offer practical guidance for those working in primary health care because we believe that anesthesiology is a specialty that only exceptionally comes within the domain of primary care. Given that assumption, we have chosen instead to alert the practitioner who is interested in the control of pre- and post-operative nausea and vomiting (NV) to the complexity, delicacy, and uncertainty of that aspect of anesthesiology itself. We seek to achieve this by providing references to recent reviews, clinical trial conclusions about anti-emetics, or analyses of trial implications. These are intended to be signposts to guide interested readers.

We remind the reader that the pharmacological control of perisurgical NV is often incomplete and uncertain. The research which would allow more accurate outcome prediction has not been done, nor do the literature references cited below consider many of the variables which have been shown or suggested to influence perisurgical control of NV.

The risk of perisurgical NV or the outcome of efforts to control them with drugs may vary with and depend upon a great many factors. These include the nature of the hospital, day surgery center or other setting in which surgery takes place; the characteristics and approaches of the medical personnel present during surgery; the nature of the surgery itself, including the site; type (abdominal, bone marrow, orchiopexy, spinal above T4 or strabismus are reported as carrying the highest risk); the extent and duration of the procedure. It will also depend on which drugs are used presurgically, for example the use of nitrous oxide does alter NV risk outcomes; the manner of administration, (IV, inhalation, local etc.), and what, if any, compounds are administered postsurgically to control pain, (e.g.

morphine or its analogs). Other factors to consider are the sex of the patient, (females being the greater risk), age, obesity of the patient, the quality of care received by the patient postsurgically. It also seems that postoperative side effects, including delayed effects of anesthesia such as dizziness or blurred vision, may themselves precipitate NV. In addition there are likely to be a variety of interactions between all these factors and medications, which at this point are not clear.

One must also acknowledge the anesthesiologist's deep concern for the risk which V itself can pose postoperatively. Pressure caused by V can lead to esophageal tears or ruptures, blood vessel damage near the operative site creating a hazard to wound closure, or internal bleeding around sites of hoemostatic sutures or clips. Visceral anastomases can be damaged, and electrolyte disorders from chronic V may also occur with the risk of metabolic alkalosis and thence hypokalemia or hyponatremia. Aspiration pneumonitis can also occur and the patient's pain and disability from anesthetically induced NV is a major concern.

The following abstracts highlight recent literature on the treatment and PONV. As can be seen the results can be bewildering, confusing, and at times contradictory, often as a result of pooled data. The many different surgical operations cause endless biases like age, sex, disease, duration of surgery, hydration etc., thereby making comparisons difficult. The successful treatment and/or prevention of PONV is a real puzzle, as some patients respond satisfactorily and others do not. The abstracts indicate the many ways people have attempted to 'skin the cat.' They also illustrate the frustration and difficulty in treating and or preventing PONV. Furthermore, they show clearly that despite all our efforts some unfortunate patients suffer from N and/or V. Large prospective clinical trials are necessary before we can hope to claim victory. These trials must be conducted according to laid down standards. Without them, interpretation of comparisons will continue to be difficult, if not impossible.

We suggest that the reader who wishes to learn more should look first at the broad systematic review by McQuay and Moore (1998). The reader interested in the outcome of randomized controlled clinical trials or their meta analysis of antiemetics used to control postoperative NV (PONV) should read those that follow.

Reviews on postoperative nausea and vomiting: annotated abstracts

(Abbreviations used in abstracts: postoperative nausea and vomiting, PONV; ondansetron, OND, droperidol, DROP; metoclropramide, METO; dolasetron, DOL)

PONV especially after day-case surgery

An extensive review of the use of analgesics and antiemetics in day-care surgery practice: only the authors' recommendations for future research appear here. This report highlights what is known, and what is widely believed about this topic, but is not really understood. This review emphasizes the complexity of N, V, and pain symptoms, the halting success made toward their amelioration, and recommends research for achieving advances.

McQuay HJ, Moore RA
Pain Research & Nuffield Department of Anaesthetics, University of Oxford, Churchill Hospital, Oxford, UK
Postoperative analgesia and vomiting, with special reference to day-case surgery: a systematic review. Health Technol Assess 1998;2(12): 1–236

Paraphrased Abstract
Research recommendations:
(1) Extend the number of systematic reviews to include other analgesics, including the newer non-steroidal anti-imflammatory drugs (NSAIDs), to provide a more comprehensive ladder of relative efficacy.
(2) Establish pilot audits of the implementation of the information included in this report; both 'before' and 'after' audits are needed to put the existing evidence into clinical practice to good effect.
(3) Investigate the effect of chance in clinical trials. Because of the many analgesic trials, usually performed using standard methods and including patients with similar entry criteria (moderate or severe pain), the effects of chance in clinical trials may be usefully studied with them. Variability between trials is large and investigators need to be able to understand the effects of chance in the accurate assessment of any new drugs(s).

(4) Investigate how to minimize PONV. Efficacy varies considerably between trials. This may be the result of chance, or due to components of the overall package of care other than anesthesia or antiemetics.

Authors' Conclusion:
There is an obvious and important research agenda here in understanding how best to minimize PONV. However, this is a complex area which will not easily be understood.

How effectively does ondansetron prevent PONV?

An analysis of 53 randomized, controlled trials using OND: the largest meta-analysis currently available on this topic.

Tramer MR, Reynolds DJ, Moore RA, McQuay HJ. Oxford, UK
Efficacy, dose–response, and safety of ondansetron in prevention of postoperative nausea and vomiting: a quantitative systematic review of randomized placebo-controlled trials. Anesthesiology 1997 Dec;87:1277–89

Paraphrased Abstract:
Fifty-three clinical trials for efficacy and safety data for OND for preventing PONV included 7177 patients receiving 24 different OND regimens and from 5712 controls receiving placebo or no treatment. Average early and late PONV incidences without OND were 40% and 60%, respectively. With an IV dose of 8 mg and an oral dose of 16 mg the estimated number-needed-to-treat to prevent PONV with the best-documented regimens was between 5 and 6. Anti-vomiting efficacy was consistently better than anti-nausea efficacy. Efficacy in children was poorly documented. OND significantly increased the risk for elevated liver enzymes (number-needed-to-harm was 31) and headache (number-needed-to-harm was 36).

Authors' Conclusion:
If the risk of PONV is very high, for every 100 patients receiving an adequate dose of ondansetron 20 patients will not vomit who would have vomited had they received placebo. The anti-nausea effect is less pronounced. Of these 100, three will have elevated liver enzymes

and three will have a headache that they would not have had as an adverse effect without the drug.
See also: Comment in: *Anesthesiology* 1997 Dec;87(6):1271–3

How well does ondansetron relieve established PONV?

A critical review of seven trials with 1043 patients describing OND's efficacy for PONV.

Tramer MR, Moore RA, Reynolds DJ, McQuay HJ. Oxford, UK
A quantitative systematic review of ondansetron in treatment of established postoperative nausea and vomiting. BMJ 1997 Apr 12;314(7087):1088–92

Paraphrased Abstract:
Evidence for a dose–response was sought with OND for treatment of PONV in seven, published, randomized, controlled trials from 1991 to January 1996. Among four placebo-controlled trials with 1043 patients studied IV OND 1 mg, 4 mg, or 8 mg, all doses were more efficacious than placebo in preventing further episodes of PONV. For combined data, the point estimates for the number-needed-to-treat were between 3.1 (8 mg) and 3.8 (1 mg) for early efficacy (within 6 hours) and between 4.1 (8 mg) and 4.8 (1 mg) for late (within 24 hours) efficacy, without significant differences between doses. No difference was found between OND and DROP in two trials with 129 patients or between OND and METO in one trial with 80 patients.

Authors' Conclusion:
Further nausea and vomiting could be prevented in 25% of patients who had N or V with ondansetron compared with placebo (number-needed-to-treat, about 4). There was no evidence of a clinically relevant dose–response between 1 mg and 8 mg or a difference between ondansetron and either droperidol or metoclopramide in a limited dataset. A false impression of ondansetron's efficacy may arise because one-quarter of all relevant published reports are duplicates, and reporting of study results is uncritical.

Individual trials

Ondansetron compared with dolasetron in prevention of PONV

Comparison in 514 patients of OND and DOL for prevention of PONV.

Korttila K, Clergue F, Leeser J, Feiss P, Olthoff D, Payeur-Michel C, Wessel P, Nave S, Hahne W, Brown R
Department of Obstetrics and Gynaecology, University of Helsinki, Finland
Intravenous dolasetron and ondansetron in prevention of postoperative nausea and vomiting: a multicenter, double-blind, placebo-controlled study. Acta Anaesthesiol Scand 1997 Aug;41(7):914–22

Paraphrased Abstract:
In a double-blind, placebo-controlled, randomized, multicenter trial, 514 patients at 24 sites received one of four single IV treatments placebo, 25 or 50 mg DOL, or 4 mg OND. PONV efficacy was measured by complete response (0 emetic episodes and no rescue medication), nausea severity, and patient satisfaction as measured on a visual analog scale (VAS), investigator's rating, of nausea severity, and total response [complete response with no nausea (< or = 5 mm VAS)]. Fifty mg DOL and 4 mg OND doses were statistically equivalent, and superior to placebo, for all efficacy measures. Complete response rates were 49%, 51%, 71 %, and 64% for placebo, 25 and 50 mg DOL, and OND, respectively. DOL, 50 mg was statistically superior to 25 mg, for complete response, total response, VAS maximum nausea, time to first emetic episode, and patient satisfaction. The majority of adverse events were of mild-to-moderate intensity. Headache was the most frequently reported treatment-related adverse event with a 3%–5% incidence across treatments.

Authors' Conclusion:
When given at induction of anesthesia, 50 mg IV dolasetron is equivalent to 4 mg ondansetron and superior to 25 mg dolasetron and placebo for the prevention of PONV. All treatments were safely administered and well tolerated.

Anesthesia with propofol causes less PONV than the use of other anesthetics

Occurrence of PONV among 6069 patients after propofol anesthesia.

Tramer M, Moore A, McQuay H. Oxford, UK
Propofol anaesthesia and postoperative nausea and vomiting: quantitative systematic review of randomized controlled studies. Br J Anaesth 1997 Mar;78(3):247–55

Paraphrased Abstract:
Among 84 studies with 6069 patients randomized in controlled trials of propofol anesthesia compared with other anesthetics (control), PONV depended mainly on the method of administration, time of measurement and range of control event rates. Cumulative data of early (0–6 h) and late (0–48 hour) PONV were recorded as occurrence or non-occurrence of N or V. Combined odds ratio and number-needed-to-treat were calculated for propofol as an induction or maintenance regimen, early or late outcomes, and different emetic events. This was performed for all control event rates and within a range of 20-60% control event rates. The number-needed-to-treat to prevent PONV with propofol was more than 9 when used for induction of anaesthesia and at best 6 when used for maintenance. Within the 20–60% control event rate range, best results were achieved with propofol maintenance to prevent early PONV: the number-needed-to-treat to prevent early nausea was 4.7 (95% confidence interval 3.8–6.3), vomiting 4.9 (4–61) and any emetic event 4.9 (3.7–71). Within the 20–60% control event rate, of five patients treated, one will not vomit or be nauseated who would otherwise have vomited or been nauseated, perhaps clinically relevant. In all other situations the difference may have reached statistical significance but was of doubtful clinical relevance.

Authors' Conclusion:
Treatment efficacy should be established within a defined range of control event rates for meaningful estimates of efficacy and for comparisons.

Ondansetron v. metoclopramide in preventing PONV in orthopedic surgery

An analysis of the efficacy of antiemetics in preventing PONV in 124 orthopedic patients.

Alexander R, Fennelly M

Department of Anaesthetics, Royal National Orthopaedic Hospital, Stanmore, UK

Comparison of ondansetron, metoclopramide and placebo as premedicants to reduce nausea and vomiting after major surgery.
Anaesthesia 1997 Jul;52(7):695–8

Paraphrased Abstract:
In a randomized, double-blind study, PONV in 124 patients undergoing major lower limb orthopedic surgery following oral premedication was compared with temazapam and OND 8 mg, METO 10 mg or placebo. Patients received a standardized epidural and general anesthetic. An epidural mixture containing bupivacaine 0.1% and fentanyl 10 mg/ml was infused postoperatively. Assessment every 4 hours for 24 hours demonstrated that V significantly decreased from 55% and 43% in the placebo and METO groups, respectively, compared to 26% in the OND group ($p = 0.03$). The incidence of PONV in patients who had previously suffered was also significantly reduced from 67% and 68% in the placebo and METO groups, respectively, compared to 29% in the OND group ($p = 0.035$).

Authors' Conclusion:
Oral premedication with ondansetron 8 mg was superior to metoclopramide 10 mg and placebo in preventing PONV following major orthopedic surgery in patients given epidural opioid analgesia.

Ondansetron v. placebo in outpatient surgery

A clinical trial of the efficacy of OND for preventing PONV in 468 men.

Kovac AL, Pearman MH, Khalil SN, Scuderi PE, Joslyn AF, Prillaman BA, Cox F
Department of Anesthesiology, University of Kansas Medical Center, Kansas City, KS, USA

Ondansetron prevents postoperative emesis in male outpatients. S3A-379 Study Group. J Clin Anesth 1996 Dec;8(8):644–51

Paraphrased Abstract:
A prospective, randomized, stratified, double-blind study in 24 medical centers with 468 ASA physical status I and II males at least 12 years of age, the efficacy and safety of 4 mg (IV) OND or placebo in the prevention of (PONV) in male outpatients, prognostic factors for PONV in males, and their perceptions of the debilitating effects of PONV was determined in the ambulatory surgery setting after undergoing general balanced (opioid) anesthesia. Emetic episodes, vital signs, adverse events, and nausea assessments were recorded by a blinded observer, and after discharge, patients completed a diary that collected emetic episodes, adverse events, nausea, and pharmaco-economic data. The number of patients with no emesis and no nausea during the 24-hour study period was significantly greater ($p < 0.05$) with OND 4 mg compared with placebo. Finally, 38% of patients experiencing PONV perceived PONV to be as, or more debilitating than, the after effects of surgery itself.

Authors' Conclusion:
Ondansetron 4 mg was more effective than placebo in preventing PONV in male outpatients. Males at potential risk for developing PONV include: (1) those with a history of motion sickness and/or PONV; (2) patients undergoing nonorthopedic procedures; and (3) procedures lasting longer than 1 hour. Such patients may benefit from receipt of a prophylactic antiemetic. PONV has a debilitating effect that can be differentiated by patients from the effects of surgery itself.

Ondansetron to prevent PONV in women: a dose–response study

A clinical trial for the efficacy of OND for the prevention of PONV in 175 women.

Dershwitz M, Conant JA, Chang Y, Rosow CE, Connors PM
Department of Anesthesia and Critical Care, Massachusetts General Hospital and Harvard Medical School, Boston, MA, USA
A randomized, double-blind, dose–response study of ondansetron in the prevention of postoperative nausea and vomiting. J Clin Anesth 1998; 10: 314-20.

Paraphrased Abstract:
In a prospective, randomized, double-blind study, 175 women aged 18 to 80 years received one of six doses of OND (0.5 mg, 1 mg, 2 mg, 4 mg, 8 mg, 16 mg) or placebo prior to the induction of general anesthesia with propofol to determine the dose–response relationship of OND in preventing PONV in women undergoing elective surgery. Maintenance was with nitrous oxide, isoflurane, opioid, and muscle relaxant. Data collected were nausea scores, a 0 to 10 scale taken at multiple time points during the 24-hour study period, patient satisfaction by a visual analog scale at 1 and 24 hours after awakening, and use of rescue medication for severe nausea (three emetic episodes within 15 minutes), or if requested by the patient. The primary efficacy variable was the need for rescue antiemetic therapy. The dose–response curve (by logistic regression) of the percentage of patients not rescued v. dose indicated an ED_{50} of 0.54 mg (95% confidence interval 0.03–1.05 mg). Survival analysis of the need for rescue, and nausea score v. time curves, also both suggested the superiority of the 4 mg dose compared with lower doses. In addition, a highly significant correlation existed between the lack of need for rescue and satisfaction with anesthesia at 24 hours after emergence.

Authors' Conclusion:
The recommended dose of ondansetron for PONV prophylaxis in women remains 4 mg.

Ondansetron v. metoclopramide for preventing PONV in minor gynecological surgery

Comparison of OND and METO in minor gynecological surgery for preventing PONV.

Monagle J, Barnes R, Goodchild C, Hewitt M
Department of Anaesthesia, Monash Medical Centre, Clayton, Victoria, Australia
Ondansetron is not superior to moderate dose metoclopramide in the prevention of post-operative nausea and vomiting after minor gynaecological surgery. Eur J Anaesthesiol 1997 Nov; 14(6):604–9

Paraphrased Abstract:
A randomized study of 96 patients undergoing minor gynecological surgery investigated the relative benefits of OND compared with METO used at a dose higher than used in previous studies for the

prevention of PONV. After OND 4 mg or METO 0.4 mg/kg, patients were assessed in the recovery room, in the day ward prior to discharge and the following day for the occurrence of PONV. Emetic symptoms were similar between both groups, and nausea scores, similar between the groups in the recovery ward and 24-hour follow-ups. Patients had higher postoperative nausea scores in the OND group in the day ward (p = 0.001), and no significant side effects were recorded.

Authors' Conclusion:
Moderate dose metoclopramide is an effective alternative to ondansetron in the control of PONV

Ondansetron v. droperidol in women having laparoscopic surgery

Comparison of OND and DROP in women having laparoscopic surgery.

Koivuranta M, Laara E, Ranta P, Ravaska P, Alahuhta S
Department of Anaesthesiology, Oulu University Hospital and Lappi Central Hospital, Finland
Comparison of ondansetron and droperidol in the prevention of postoperative nausea and vomiting after laparoscopic surgery in women. A randomised, double-blind, placebo-controlled trial. Acta Anaesthesiol Scand 1997 Nov;41(10):1273–9

Paraphrased Abstract:
This study among 439 women having laparoscopies was designed to ascertain primarily the relative difference in efficacy of OND and DROP and secondarily between these drugs and placebo in the prevention of PONV. The proportion of patients with nausea was 48%, 50%, and 67% in the OND, DROP, and placebo groups, respectively; with a significant difference when both OND (p = 0.02) and DROP (p = 0.04) were compared with placebo. Vomiting occurred in 18%, 26%, and 37% of the patients in the three groups, respectively (p = 0.05 between OND and DROP, p = 0.004 between OND and placebo, p = 0.16 between DROP and placebo). The proportion of patients given rescue medication was 34%, 28% and 49%, respectively (p = 0.23 for OND and DROP, p = 0.07 for OND and placebo, p = 0.007 for DROP and placebo). During early

recovery the patients treated with OND were significantly more alert than after OND. Headache was significantly more common after OND than after DROP treatment, and no serious side effects were observed.

Authors' Conclusion:
The efficacy of prophylactic ondansetron and droperidol in reducing postoperative nausea associated with laparoscopic surgery in female inpatients was similar, but ondansetron appeared to be slightly more efficient than droperidol in preventing vomiting. Ondansetron and droperidol were both significantly better than placebo in the prophylaxis of PONV.

Dolansetron v. placebo in major gynecologic surgery

A clinical trial for the efficacy of DOL for the prevention of PONV in 789 women having major gynecologic surgery.

Diemunsch P, Korttila K, Leeser J, Helmers JH, Wilkey B, Nave S, Radke AJ, Hahne WF, Brown RA
Department of Anesthesiology, Les Hôpitaux Universitaires de Strasbourg, France
Oral dolasetron mesylate for prevention of postoperative nausea and vomiting: a multicenter, double-blind, placebo-controlled study. The Oral Dolasetron PONV Prevention Study Group. J Clin Anesth 1998 Mar; 10(2):145–52

Paraphrased Abstract:
A randomized, double-blind, placebo-controlled trial in 32 hospitals included 789 ASA physical status I, II, and III female patients, ages 18 to 60 years, weighing between 45 and 100 kg, having major gynecologic surgery (abdominal hysterectomy, laparotomy, or vaginal hysterectomy). The efficacy and safety of four single oral doses of DOL mesylate (25, 50, 100, or 200 mg, or placebo), administered 1 to 2 hours before general anesthesia, was evaluated for the prevention of PONV. Efficacy was assessed for 24 hours post-recovery by measuring complete response (no emetic episodes, no rescue medication), total response (complete response with no nausea), time to first emetic episode or rescue, and patient visual analog scale evaluations of nausea severity and satisfaction with antiemetic therapy. Complete and total response rates were statistically greater in the

three largest dose groups than in the placebo group ($p = 0.012$). The percentage of patients with no nausea and patient satisfaction scores were significantly higher for each DOL dose group than placebo ($p <$ or $= 0.047$ and $p <$ or $= 0.004$, respectively). Efficacy peaked at the 50 mg dose. The incidence of adverse events, about 30% was similar in both groups; 2% to 5% of patients had headaches from either drug.

Authors' Conclusion:
Dolasetron administered 1 to 2 hours before induction of anesthesia, is safe and effective for PONV. Maximal antiemetic response was seen with the 50 mg oral dolasetron dose.

Ondansetron in children having ENT or eye surgery

A randomized, double-blind study of the efficacy of OND for the prevention of PONV in 320 children having ophthalmologic or otolaryngologic surgery.

Lawhorn CD, Kymer PJ, Stewart FC, Stoner JM, Shirey R, Volpe P
Division of Pediatric Anesthesia, Arkansas Children's Hospital, Little Rock, AR, USA
Ondansetron dose–response curve in high-risk pediatric patients.
J Clin Anesth 1997 Dec;9(8):637–42

Paraphrased Abstract:
In a prospective, randomized, double-blind study of 320 ASA physical status I and II patients between the ages of 2 and 12 years undergoing tonsillectomy and adenoidectomy or strabismus surgery, individuals were randomized into eight groups before anesthesia was administered to establish a dose–response relationship for OND, and to evaluate any effects of oral premedication with METO. Groups 1, 2, 3, and 4 received IV saline or IV OND at doses of 0.05 mg/kg, 0.1 mg/kg, and 0.15 mg/kg, respectively. Groups 5, 6, 7, and 8 received oral METO 0.15 mg/kg as well as IV saline, and OND 0.05 mg/kg, 0.1 mg/kg, or 0.15 mg/kg. OND 0.05 mg/kg, 0.1 mg/kg, and 0.15 mg/kg were significantly more effective than placebo in reducing the incidence of emesis prior to, following discharge, and during the first 24 postoperative hours ($p < 0.001$). No significant differences in the occurrence of emesis between the

groups receiving OND 0.05 mg/kg, 0.1 mg/kg, and 0.15 mg/kg were noted, and addition of oral METO 0.15 mg/kg had no effect on any group.

Authors' Conclusion:
Ondansetron is an effective medication for the treatment and prevention of PONV, and a dose of ondansetron 0.05 mg/kg is as effective as 0.1 mg/kg and 0.15 mg/kg. Metoclopramide 0.15 mg/kg has no effect on the incidence of PONV.

Ondansetron v. droperidol v. placebo in middle ear surgery

A randomized, double-blind study of the efficacy of OND for the prevention of PONV in 120 patients undergoing middle ear surgery.

Jellish WS, Thalji Z, Fluter E, Leonetti JP
Department of Anesthesiology, Loyola University Medical Center, Maywood, IL, USA
Ondansetron versus droperidol or placebo when given prophylactically for the prevention of postoperative nausea and vomiting in patients undergoing middle ear procedures. J Clin Anesth 1997 Sep;9(6):451–6

Paraphrased Abstract:
In a prospective, randomized, double-blind study, 120 ASA physical status I and II patients presenting for elective middle ear surgical procedures were randomly assigned to receive either placebo (Group 1), OND 4 mg IV (Group 2), or DROP 25 µg/kg IV (Group 3) 10 minutes before induction of general anesthesia using thiopental 5 mg/kg IV with fentanyl 2 µg/kg IV and maintenance anesthesia with isoflurane 1% to 2% end-tidal in a 50% air/oxygen mixture. The intergroup incidence and severity of N, V, and pain along with rescue antiemetic administration were similar except that the male to female ratio was higher in the OND group. Stewart scores, reflecting emergence from anesthesia, were higher with OND compared with DROP. The incidence of nausea was similar between the groups but the severity was less after OND therapy. Vomiting was more frequent after placebo than when given with either DROP or OND, and at 24 hours, more patients who received the placebo persisted with N or V.

Authors' Conclusion:
Ondansetron 4 mg IV is as effective as droperidol and better than placebo in preventing N and V in patients undergoing middle ear surgery. No cost advantage as determined by lower use of rescue antiemetics or shorter times in the postanesthesia care unit (PACO) was noted after the prophylactic administration of ondansetron.

CHAPTER 17
Comforting

Providing comfort is the all-encompassing goal of the nursing profession. It is the pervasive theme of all nursing programs and students in the profession are taught that this ability is what will make them 'a good nurse.' Nurses are taught to elicit histories from patients, to assess the patients, to make a nursing diagnosis, to implement a plan, and to evaluate those measures employed. Yet, despite this very logical methodology, the pressures of high technology, time, and short staffing may prevent the nurse from the very thing she or he does best: listening and comforting.

Nursing theory

Nursing is a profession that is both an art and a science. Documentation by early theorists, such as Florence Nightingale in *On the Art of Comforting*, is based on a theoretical framework supporting its validity as a true intervention that makes a difference in patient outcomes. Nurses use theory in the form of concepts, principles, and processes to guide their observations and to understand the phenomena that are a focus of their interventions (ANA, 1980). The profession is defined by the Social Policy statement of the American Nurses Association (ANA) 'as the diagnosis and treatment of human responses to actual or potential health problems.' This covers a wide range of health responses in people who are well or sick. The response is what nursing focuses its diagnosis and treatment on, while medicine deals with the actual health problem. The response is based on the client's biopsychosocial adaptation to stress from any time frame in their life. The nurse interacts by contracting with the clients in a partnership and by helping them to find solutions to their dilemma. The nurse helps them to assess their lifestyle, their interactions with others, and their responses to stress and crises, in order to help them cope using appropriate responses. This is achieved by employing their strengths and any alternative methods, other than medicine, to maintain their integrity. The nurse uses nursing functions, independent from physicians' orders, to help alleviate stress, pain, suffering, or any other discomfort, such as nausea (N), that her or his client may be experiencing. The nursing profession uses an interactive, problem-solving process in a systematic and individualized way to fulfill the goal of nursing care and to maximize the clients' positive interactions with the environment, their level of wellness, and their degree of self-actualization. It also differs in that the problem-solving process can be done in isolation and the nursing process involves a partnership with the client in the helping relationship (Sundeen et al., 1994).

All individuals face circumstances and interactions that daily produce stimuli and reactions. These arise from within and from environmental encounters. The person then reacts and responds appropriately or inappropriately, strongly or not so strongly, based on the cognitive appraisal of the perceived threat. The evoked responses may vary from one individual to the next. The responses are both emotional, such as fear and anger, and physiological, such as rapid heart rate, elevated blood pressure, tense muscles, N, or flushing. This exposure to life's stressors enhances one's dynamic nature and adaptability to life and promotes growth and development from childhood on.

Nursing process

The dance of human life, as it is so often referred to (Dossey et al., 1988), polarizes attributes of strength and weakness, illness and wellness, peaks and valleys, and stress and tranquility. Clients seek help in dealing with these polarities. A nurse healer is a guide who helps clients with the art of cognitively choosing new health behaviors, appropriate therapies and solutions, and proper tools for self-care and self-healing. This guidance helps clients to be in control of their destiny, thus producing a harmony in their existence.

Earlier, the nursing process and the use of standards of care was discussed. The standard that we will look at is specific to comfort, in relationship to the phenomena of nausea and vomiting (NV). The standard, nursing process and desired outcome are as shown in Table 17.1.

Table 17.1: Comfort

A: standard	The patient's symptoms are managed to the patient's and family's satisfaction
B: outcome criteria	The patient and family: (1) feel that the reports of alterations in comfort level are accepted without value judgment (2) feel that their suggestions for modifying physical and emotional comfort are sought and considered (3) feel satisfied with the management of the symptoms
C: process criteria	The nurse: (1) assesses symptoms, e.g., pain, anxiety, sleeplessness, loneliness, N, etc. (2) considers patient/family input in planning and evaluating symptom management (3) uses creative problem-solving techniques to relieve symptoms (4) evaluates the efficiency of interventions (Dossey et al., 1988)

When it is the result of emotional origins, N can be controlled throughout life, from childhood to adulthood. It can surface as a reaction or control mechanism in any situation or conflict. It is subjective in nature, not totally measurable, and, therefore, its degree of affliction is totally in the hands of the victim.

Nursing interventions

Gastric distention from fluid/food ingestion can trigger the vagal visceral afferent pathways that stimulate the medulla oblongata (Rhodes, 1990b). N precedes V in most instances and frequently exists by itself. N may be a prodromal signal of disease, injury, or purely a normal physiological adjustment to pregnancy. In any of these situations, nurses are often the ones to provide interventions that make a difference. Medicines can alleviate V, but persistent N, which is often not alleviated by medicine, subsides or decreases most often because of nursing interventions. Nurses are present around the clock in inpatient settings, and are the ones to respond to the patient's complaint of N. Nursing assessment looks at duration, frequency, associated symptoms such as V in relationship to: meals, position, medications, activity, time of day, pain, and specific foods, as well as documenting the measures that offer relief of N (Carpenito, 1995).

Comfort measures that help the patient with N are:

- assessment for risk of V and aspiration
- assessment for cleanliness of client and environment
- oral care, with or without V
- cool cloths to neck, forehead, and wrists
- reducing stimuli from pain – such as planning procedures away from mealtimes
- preparing the client's psyche by letting them know what will take place and how long it will last
- medicating the client before meals and before painful procedures
- providing a pleasant, clean, quiet, relaxed atmosphere (do not rush activity)
- serving small, appealing servings
- having the client rest before meals
- if client is at home, having them prepare large quantities for future meals or arranging for help to prepare meals
- avoiding odiferous foods (fried food, coffee brewing)
- trying cold foods
- walking before meals
- using foods that avoid preparation if N is triggered by cooking.

Carpenito (1995) also suggests diversional activities, a quiet environment, and restricting activities and the number of visitors. She advises clients to breathe deeply, to swallow frequently, to avoid sudden changes in position, and to keep the head of the bed elevated.

These interventions are measures that demand consideration in addition to those alternative measures discussed in Chapter 18, such as massage, music, meditation, yoga, herbal remedies, and biofeedback.

Nursing research

N has existed forever, but its management has been ignored, except for the traditional medical standby of a few pills and suppositories. As it is not life threatening, and is self-limiting, subjective, and has a degree of psychological overlay, clinical research has been minimal. The nursing profession has probably been the leader in research in this arena. This is because nurses most often are the people dealing with the clients suffering from the symptoms of N. The few studies available have shown that the frequency, duration, and distress of N differ from patient to patient. It is believed to have a strong psychogenic component. Antiemetic drugs and behavioral interventions are most often effective because they produce changes in neurotransmitters in the area of the brain responsible for controlling N and V (Cotanch, 1988). Currently, antiemetic drugs are used because they all have a common effect of sedation, which is the goal in alleviating the N and then distracting the client. However, the major, most successful interventions are still the behavioral ones, such as relaxation and self-hypnosis.

There are scales to measure N and V (Lundberg and Frankhauser, 1980), but N alone is most difficult to measure and therefore its nature has been much less studied. More work and research need to be done on measurement scales, self-care models, and the use of behavioral interventions and their usefulness in clients suffering from N. Issues of functioning and quality of life are most important and N is still one of the most elusive symptoms that affects both of these. From the terminally ill patient to the healthy pregnant woman, N can greatly impact on the patient's day-to-day comfort and well-being.

Orem's self-care theory (1985) is usually the guide that nurses use in assessing the client's capacity to respond appropriately to the demands of self-care. The self-care act is based on the client's knowledge of what to do for their symptoms, the skills required to do it, and the ability to perform the acts of self-care. Nursing interventions are effective inasmuch as they influence the coping responses. Nurses can increase their list of interventions by asking patients what they have done that has made them feel better. Self-care journals can facilitate this helpful knowledge for both the patient and the nurse. As for the use of medication as an intervention, it is well known that a pre-load before precipitating therapies or experiences can help; the use of regular dosing to avoid a crescendo of symptoms is also beneficial.

As members of a caring profession, nurses are always concerned with how their clients feel, more from the aspects of the signs and symptoms than from the response to these symptoms. The major contribution of nursing is in helping the ill patient to cope with distress. The interventions used should be the basis of future research to assess their reliability and applicability to the symptoms of N. The UCSF Symptoms Management Facility Group (Facione et al., 1994) has designed a conceptual model of symptom management.

Some of the most significant work on N and its relief measures has been with pregnant women (Voda and Randall, 1982; Abney, 1985; DiLorio, 1985). Studies rated the N on a three-point scale: mild, moderate, and severe. Most of the symptoms fell in the mild range, and most experienced the symptoms for 12 hours a day with no interference to their daily functions. The major contributing factor to the N was fatigue. Other factors were eating, hunger, and odors. Less commonly reported factors were driving, stress, thoughts of food, and vitamins. Eating produced the most severe symptoms.

Lying down and resting were frequently reported as a relief measure by the women. Crackers, toast, and small, more frequent meals were also cited by the women as offering relief from their N. Some used carbonated beverages, milk, tea, or medicines. Other measures cited were vitamin B, low fat intake, high carbohydrate intake, high protein intake, hypnosis, and acupressure for relief of N. These were all rated on a 1–5 scale and eating was rated more effective than lying down, even though fatigue was listed as a major factor contributing to N. Lifestyle changes were necessary in seeking relief for symptoms of N. Nurses can give clients permission to do whatever it takes to obtain relief from the symptoms of N, thus making it acceptable to interrupt their busy schedules and to take time to do this. Emotional support, at any time, is cross-transferable and a commodity that nurses can easily dispense to all clients. Nurses' most valuable contribution may be that of identifying those clients at risk for developing N and helping them, through anticipatory guidance, to plan effective coping measures for their symptoms. This not only can help to decrease and possibly avoid the symptoms, but it can also alleviate anxiety and other forms of distress, because anxiety has been identified as a factor linked to N.

Conclusion

Contemporary nurses are broadening their experience of themselves as healers. By paying attention to their philosophy, values, and beliefs about their profession, nurses empower themselves to recognize their own unique qualities; as this recognition evolves, caring grows, and the true philosophy and art and science of caring emerge in their nursing practice (Dossey et al., 1988). This caring can benefit only those clients who are experiencing the discomfort of N, and offer hope in the future that ongoing research by nurses will discover new interventions that will be successful in managing symptoms and offering better quality of life.

CHAPTER 18

Complementary therapies

In the USA, the UK, and Europe, there appears to be an expanding use of nonprescribed, medically unconventional therapies for healing and alleviation of discomfort. Some physicians embracing 'holistic' medicine participate. Herbal, medical, psychological, environmental, and mechanical means are employed, as are religious ones. For herbalists, the first known published materia medica, plant pharmacognosy, the Ebers Papyrus of about 600 BC, Egypt (followed by Dioscorides in the first century AD and Soranus in the second century, who focused on midwifery and herbals useful for women's and children's disorders) shows the systemization of knowledge likely accumulating over thousands of earlier years. There has been a continuing interchange among healers of various schools and cultures. No one today, for example, would be surprised by Soranus' pregnancy nausea and vomiting (PNV), obstetric–gynecological recommendations for rest, fasting, massage, easily digested food, weak wines, passive exercise, and pleasant odors.

But self-care, when based on skepticism among educated persons about the profession of medicine, may, in one particular, be an American tradition, because it includes surprising anti-intellectual components and what may be a peculiar ability to market 'snake oil' (see Starr, 1982; Fuchs, 1993). It may also be a response to the strenuous efforts in the last century on the part of American physicians toward a social distance and expensive exclusivity. On the other hand, in Europe and Asia folk medicines are part of the enduring cultural histories where mothers, 'wise women,' *brujos*, as healers, have been taught for generations about the tools and methods of caring, just as nurses have been. What we see today in alternative or 'complementary' therapies, when used along with medical ones, is that they are part of these thrusts ancient and modern, and that they certainly constitute a cultural phenomenon.

There is an understandable comfort in dealing with familiar plants or with tender care, in using a vocabulary that one can understand as opposed to that 'mystification' of which medicine stands accused – sometimes rightly so. Complementary care has gained popularity because of its focus on giving individuals the responsibility and control of their own health care and state of well-being. Nowhere is a feeling of loss of control more predominant than among patients suffering from nausea and/or vomiting (NV). We know that people suffer from NV for a myriad reasons. For women, stress, fatigue, and entirely uncomprehended biological events contribute to their NV vulnerability and their comparatively lesser responsitivity to NV drugs given for serious emesis.

Persons might wish to avoid taking prescribed pharmaceutical antiemetics (AEs) to manage NV symptoms because they are already taking multiple drugs for the primary illness, or the side effects of the AE or the drug–drug interactions are undesirable, because the pharmaceutical doesn't work, or simply because they, or those caring for them, have an antipathy to medical care as such. And it may be that, for NV, people know that pharmaceuticals have the risk of not working, or are seen as possibly harmful. For example, a pregnant woman will want to avoid any drugs that could be harmful to the fetus. Even when demonstrated risk is very slight, the woman in this age of exaggerated warnings may worry. Alternative interventions because they are 'folk' or 'herbal' may be used instead.

Using methods other than going to the doctor for 'normal' ailments is, probably for most, the first choice. There is, after all, a great market for over-the-counter (OTC) compounds, and surely people visit their 'drug stores' or 'chemists' far more often than they visit a doctor. Nowadays 'pharmacies' as a kind of supermarket make a great business of selling herbal remedies and aromatherapies. Western pharmacists, these days, may emphasize homeopathic 'natural' remedies more than prescription ones, especially if they are independent retailers, because the advent of major discount pharmaceutical suppliers has meant that the 'old-fashioned' independent 'chemist' will be undersold for any prescription drug and must find another stock in trade.

Keep in mind, however, that any herbal can be as powerful as and, if unstudied, more unpredictable than a pharmaceutically manufactured compound. 'Natural' includes the world of plant, mineral, and insect products, some of which are clearly powerful, and some of which are poisons. Complementary care offers a wide spectrum of therapies, including human interventions, that are not the ordinary medical model, such as hypnosis, relaxation, aromatherapy, herbalism, prayer, imaging, and diet. Undoubtedly some of these can be helpful in the management of one or another pattern of NV. We have seen this (in Chapter 3) in the report of our sample of women recounting what they find makes them experience less NV, and how their own remedies are felt to be superior to, and no doubt cheaper and easier than, ones that doctors prescribe. Or, as in the case of PNV, doctors dare not prescribe for greater fear of lawsuits than fear of the rare outcome of infant defects (teratogenicity).

One keeps in mind that, in the alternative therapies as much as in medical or formally professional cultural ones, and Chinese herbal remedies or acupuncture or East Indian Aruvedic ones come into the latter, expectations play an important role. We have discussed placebo effects elsewhere. There is nothing at all wrong with these, because they can be of major value, including having strong biochemical components. But with all folk remedies, and perhaps particularly those that are sold today with much commercial trumpeting, shout, and drumbeat, one is reminded of the rule of caution. One does not believe whatever one is told. Herbals can be dangerous. Compounds not tested with randomized controlled trials are not capable of description of outcomes on large samples. And Barnum was right, there is a 'sucker born every minute.' For a healthy introduction to skepticism about healing claims of any sort (and be assured, conventional medicine when not experimentally based deserves the same caution) read Mark Twain's caustic, funny, self and other critical book, *Christian Science*. (Not that one need believe Twain either, but his is a witty, although sometimes bitter, reminder of our foibles of faith, belief, self, and tomfoolery.)

The economics of complementary care are probably underplayed, whether as an industry itself producing herbs, oils, and potions, or as a rational response not simply of consumers to increased health care costs, at least in the USA. These have risen about 14% a year over the last few decades, and with no measurable improvement in US morbidity, quality of life, or mortality – at a national cost twice that of other industrialized nations, most of which enjoy better health by conventional measures. After all, the biggest variable associated with being healthy in any technologically advanced nation is being educated, and economists such as Fuchs

(1993) challenge whether or not modern medicine, beyond alleviating pain and demonstrating some powerful technology, has done much at all to improve health above and beyond the gains that education and affluence, along with their public health correlates in foods, sanitation, etc., bring.

A new force for alternative medicine is the new profession of the health maintenance organization (HMO) executive or stockholder. Some HMOs encourage alternative healing, advertised as greater 'choice' but in fact much cheaper for the HMO. When asked about a cancer patient who might die because she had elected a cheaper alternative therapy under the HMO plan, one HMO executive went so far as to be quoted publicly saying that it was to the patient's advantage because she did what she wanted, and to the HMO stockholders' advantage because she cost them less to die. But profitability without health gain has also driven conventional medicine. Among the few studies extant, it can be shown that the recent reduction in 25% of referrals for consultation or tests, and reduced time with patients by HMO expensive procedures, has made no difference in the morbidity/mortality of the population studied. HMO patients may dislike it, but so far their health has not suffered en masse. At the very least, one must conclude that there is a large 'cushion' of unnecessary profit-making, otherwise useless care within the practice of modern medicine. This is one of the arguments for evidence-based medicine, for alternative healing, and also for evidence-based alternative care itself. One dare not, however, discount the 'clinical' evidence that thousands of years of safe use in the hands of family or cultural healers constitutes. Table 18.1 lists various complementary therapies for NV.

Self-care therapy

One of complementary care's goals is to promote self-care and empowerment of the patient. Not only are hypnosis, guided imagery, visualization, massage, and relaxation inexpensive and pleasant, but there are many claims about their effectiveness. Perhaps at this stage in the nonscience of alternative healing, the person will be his or her own best clinical judge. Almost all of these interventions can be directed either by a facilitator, such as a nurse or loved one, or by the person as patient. The most important factor for self-care interventions is that the patient wants to take control and be a participant in the process. And if something is clearly not working or going wrong, the patient should stop and look again.

Table 18.1: Complementary therapies for NV

Food therapy	Environmental therapy
Avoid a high-fat diet Eat foods high in fiber (vegetables and whole grains) Keep dry toast or soda crackers by the bed and eat some before rising Glass of fruit juice in the morning Drink Coca-Cola syrup or any warm nonfizzy liquid (Note Coca-Cola was often prescribed by pediatricians; one wonders if that began in the pre-FDA days when it contained coca leaf, now prohibited – compare derivative cocaine. But used by Andean Indians for analgesia, NV control) PNV women like crackers and take small, not large meals	New age/classical music Positive visual stimuli Avoid any stimuli associated with adverse experiences Social support including TLC (tender loving care) Hot water bottle or low-temperature heating pad
Herbal and aromatherapy	**Self-care and other relaxing, diverting, interventions**
See Table 18.2	Hypnosis Guided imagery Visualization Relaxation Massage Brisk walks Short naps Acupuncture Acupressure

Hypnosis

Hypnosis is a method in which a patient is placed into an induced trance and a therapist/facilitator attempts to reach the patient through suggestion. Even though facilitators are usually necessary, they are just what the name implies, facilitators. The patient is still in control. Guided imagery can be used to relax the patient and induce a sedated 'trance-like' state. The patient is asked to imagine a time when or a place where they feel happy, comfortable, and relaxed. An example could be a walk along the beach or sitting in a field of wild flowers. Once the patient becomes relaxed, the therapist can begin to discuss the patient's concerns and help the patient gain more control over how he or she is feeling. Hypnosis has been widely practiced as a relaxation technique and with patients who are suffering N during drug treatment or pregnancy, and after surgery. Its results, measured experimentally, are uneven.

Visualization and relaxation

A similar technique to hypnosis, but one that can be learned and practiced by an individual, is a technique that combines visualization and relaxation. The goal of this therapy is to achieve a positive state of mind and a healthy balance between the mind and body. This positive state of mind and balance can be practiced so that, when achieved, it can induce physiological changes, such as the reduction of N. The first step in this method is for the patient to lie down in a comfortable and relaxed position with no crossing of legs or arms. The individual begins by breathing deeply and visualizing an experience in which he or she felt relaxed and peaceful. He or she eventually achieves muscle relaxation by moving down the entire body, contracting a muscle and slowly releasing it. While the patient is breathing and relaxing the muscles, he or she can visualize breathing in the 'good' air and exhaling the 'bad' or 'nauseous' air. This method is highly effective in that it gives an individual a sense of well-being and control over the mind and body. This method does, however, require practice in order to elicit the physiological changes.

Massage therapy

There are other simple forms of self-care that use the body to achieve a physiological change instead of a change in one's state of mind. Massage therapy is a popular technique used to induce relaxation and to create a therapeutic environment. All that is needed for a massage is a quiet place where the patient is comfortable and the session will not be disturbed.

It has been widely documented that simply taking several deep breaths before one gets out of bed in the morning can significantly reduce morning N, especially in pregnant women. Exercise has also been highly recommended as a mechanism to reduce NV. Although strenuous exercise may not be favorable, taking a brisk walk every day can help tremendously. On the other hand, taking a brief nap, or lying down for 20 minutes, can also relieve a bout of N. Generally speaking, an individual suffering from NV should do whatever activity offers relief, but therapies as basic as breathing, walking, and resting do work.

Environmental therapy

The environment can play a significant role in both the onset and relief of NV. Although the exact mechanisms of NV are still unknown, it is widely recognized that certain sounds, smells, sights, etc., can trigger acute and severe bouts of NV. At the same time, these same senses can be used to help manage these symptoms. Environmental factors play the greatest role in anticipatory NV. For example, if one knows that chemotherapy causes N, the individual can try to create an environment to curb the extent to which he or she feels ill. Music, especially soft classical or new age, has a very calming effect on most people. The medical specialties of oncology, pediatrics, obstetrics, and dentistry are beginning to use music therapy as an adjunct in their practice. Even visual stimuli, such as a favorite picture, can induce a calming effect. Obviously, the rule for environmental factors is for the patient to avoid those stimuli that are associated with negative and aversive experiences such as previous NV and surround him- or herself with stimuli that create a peaceful and relaxed environment.

Food as therapy

Food therapy has also been a widely used tool for NV management and includes the general diet, vitamin and mineral supplements, and herbal therapy. In regard to one's general diet, any individual suffering from N and/or V should avoid high-fat foods and eat a wide variety of vegetables and whole grains. This type of high-fiber diet will help to maintain a clean and motile digestive tract. N is often most common in the morning because the patient has an empty stomach. To relieve early morning N, it is recommended that one keep some dry toast or the proverbial soda cracker by the bed, and to eat a little before rising. The bread will absorb some of the excess acid in the stomach, reducing any feeling of N. A small glass of fruit juice is also suggested for the morning. Coca-Cola syrup, sugar syrup, any warm nonfizzy liquid, and gelatin desserts seem to work. Emetrol, a popular OTC remedy for NV, basically contains sugar syrup: glucose, fructose, and phosphoric acid. Ice chips are recommended for women experiencing morning sickness for any time during the day in an attempt to calm a spastic stomach.

Herbal and aromatherapy

Most people are generally familiar with the ideas of herbal medicine, i.e., using herbs for medicinal purposes by ingesting or applying the herb to their body. Although there are many warnings that herbal medicine should not take the place of our regular medical care, for many users it has proven to be a remarkably effective complement. And where there is experimental literature, as, for example, in European studies on ginger for use in PNV (one cannot recommend it in the USA for fear of lawsuits because one component is a mutagen), a herb may show itself to be efficacious as well as pleasant and inexpensive. In more recent years, aromatherapy has been introduced as an extension of herbal medicine. In actuality, the two are very different, despite the fact that they both use natural extracts and plants for the same purposes.

Aromatherapy suggests something that works exclusively through our sense of smell, but this need not be the case. Apart from their scents, each essential oil has an individual combination of constituents which interact with the body's chemistry in a direct manner. They are absorbed into the skin and affect certain organs or systems as a whole. It is not only the aroma that is important psychologically, but also the chemical interaction between the oils and the body, which takes about 20–120 minutes to have an effect. There are few aromatherapy studies with strict controls.

Most of the essential oils are taken from plants also used in herbal medicine, i.e., the two treatments are complementary. The differences between herbal medicine and aromatherapy are that, taken as a whole, the overall effect of the herb is the action of all its pharmacologically active constituents, but the oil used in aromatherapy is more concentrated, extracted from specific parts of the plant, and thus less suited for internal use. The oil is primarily used as an inhalant and is thus very well suited to respiratory ailments, and also affects an individual's mood or feelings. Some herbalists view essential oils in the same way that they regard synthetic drugs, as being only a 'part' of the whole, rather than the entire herb; they do, however, play an active role in the modern pharmaceutical industry.

Aromatherapy and herbal medicine will be considered together, because many of the essential oils used come from the whole plants used in herbal medicine. For some plants we note whether this plant or extract is used as an herbal remedy, essential oil, or both. There are many books on herbal and other alternative treatments.

Let us begin with Soranus of the early second century. He recommended aloe, alum, barley meal, mastic, myrtle, pomegranate, roses, and saffron for PNV. In the 1960s, a Yacqui Indian medicine man gave, approvingly, to one of the authors the list of carminatives of Dr Alvarez-Gonzales, a Mexican medical school professor. This list included caraway, angelica, anise, cardamom, costicpatli, costomate, cilantro, fennel, laurel, manzanilla, mint, and poleo. There was also a tincture on hand which, on analysis, was found to be coca root and another unidentified local plant in alcohol. The point is that historical and cross-cultural interchange, and folk, tribal, peasant, and urban professional exchange do occur. Some hoped-for remedies are widely known; others are known only locally. Some clearly act via olfaction, others through absorption, some as sedatives, some psychedelically, and in the same context of expectations and physical change that characterize compounds now known as pharmaceuticals, but whose 'roots' may be in herbal medicine. Table 18.2 is a list compiled from herbal texts or local practitioners.

Acupuncture and acupressure

Acupuncture

Acupuncture is the ancient Chinese technique of stimulating points on the body to control pain or relieve systems. Maps of these points have been around for hundreds of years. Needles are inserted into these specific points, and then the needle is rotated or heated for further stimulation.

Acupressure

Acupressure is noninvasive and involves applying pressure to the acupuncture point. The relevant acupressure point for emesis is the Nei-kuan point, which is on the inside of the wrist, and can be supplemented by the Tsu-san-li and Chung-kuan points, on the lower kneecap and above the stomach on the ventral side, respectively. Some home remedy books also suggest firmly massaging between your first and second toes, between the thumb and index finger, or directly on the thumbnail. Acupressure is more commonly used as a real medical treatment because it is much less expensive, and can be used continuously by patients themselves. Special wrist bands have been created especially for chemotherapy and postoperative patients, which contain a plastic stud over the Nei-kuan point. The patient or outpatient presses on the stud at regular time intervals, thus stimulating the acupressure point.

Table 18.2: List of plants used as herbals and for aromatherapy

Alexandrian senna: A laxative that can cause N.

Allspice: In the herbal tradition, allspice has been used in solution for flatulent indigestion and externally for rheumatic pain. The essential oil extracted from the shell of the fruit can be used for cramps, flatulence, indigestion, and N. Used mostly in aromatherapy for treating N.

Angelica (or anselica): Used for N relief. Claimed to have special usefulness for motion sickness.

Aniseed: Can quell N. Laboratory studies suggest action in the liver.

Artichoke, globe: Used for N relief.

Balm, lemon: This sweet-scented herb was one of the earliest known medicinal plants. It is used particularly for digestive and respiratory complaints. The oil from the leaves and flowering tops is used in aromatherapy for colic, indigestion, and N. Aromatherapy and herbal.

Basil, French: A tender, dark-green herb with a strong fragrance, it is used to improve blood circulation and the digestive system. and in China for stomach and kidney ailments. The oil from the flowering herb is used for dyspepsia, flatulence, and N. Aromatherapy and herbal.

Bergamot: Used against N.

California Bay: Strongly scented, used as many herbals are to spice foods; can cause N but shows the same paradoxical effects as observed in AE pharmaceuticals by dose, preparation, timing. It is used as a tea to relieve N.

Cardamom: Reed-like herb native to Asia, used especially in India and Europe for pulmonary disease, fever, and digestive and urinary complaints. The oil from the dried fruit is used for anorexia, colic, cramp, indigestion, and V. Aromatherapy and herbal.

Cascarilla bark: Large shrub often made into tea leaves which treats diarrhea, dysentery, N, V, and bronchitis. The oil from the dried bark is used for dyspepsia, flatulence, and N. Aromatherapy and herbal.

***Cannabis indica* (marijuana)**: In folk use against NV, but now, under facilitating laws in California, used medically. States are in combat with the US Federal Government with advocates in the latter, including many physicians, offering evidence of demonstrated medical utility in NV control. In some jurisdictions it (or the active ingredient of tetrahydrocannabinol) may be prescribed.

Chamomile: A small stocky herb which is widely employed in the treatment of N, anorexia, pregnancy NV, and flatulent dyspepsia. It appears in the *British Herbal Pharmacopoeia* for treatment of these ailments. The oil from the flower heads is used for treatment of N; specifically, German chamomile is used most often. Aromatherapy and herbal.

Cinnamon: Used to treat N.

Clary sage: A digestif with possible anti-N qualities, especially if claims for its stress-reducing effect were to be proven.

Cloves: Have been used as a powder or as a tea for gas, N, and V. Well known as a domestic remedy for toothache, they are said to allay NV, and to relieve flatulent colic and other gastrointestinal disorders. The part of the plant employed is the unexpanded flower buds, which are either boiled (tea) or ground (powder). The oil from most parts of the plant can be used to treat colic, dyspepsia, and N. Aromatherapy and herbal medicine.

(contd)

Table 18.2: (contd)

Cola nut: A West African native, a bitter seed used as a condiment and to improve digestion. May relieve food-induced NV risk.

Cola syrup: Cola drinks widely used for stomach distress, sometimes recommended by physicians for N may have, as with Coca-Cola, secret proprietary contents. However, sugar compounds typically compounded by apothecaries may contain as sugars levulose, dextrose, sucrose, fructose, etc. which we recognize as contained in home or OTC remedies. Likewise, apothecaries may compound phosphoric acid, caffeine, caramel for color, flavorings. Proprietary labeling denies our knowing whether a given beverage may contain cola nut extract (distillate, etc.) or what other non-FDA submitted 'natural' ingredients there may be. One would not be surprised if vitamins B6 and 12, as once in the prescribed (and effective) anti-PNV medicine, Bendectin, would be added when nausea control is claimed for a beverage.

Coriander: Strongly aromatic, this herb has been used since ancient Egyptian times to treat diarrhea, digestive upsets, and N. The oil from the seeds is used for the same maladies. Aromatherapy and herbal medicine.

Dill: Claimed to ease a variety of digestive pains.

Fennel, sweet: Native to Europe, this herb has been used for digestive complaints such as colic, indigestion, and N. The sweet fennel oil is obtained from the crushed seeds, and treats anorexia, colic, constipation, and N. Herbalists warn against its use by epileptics or during pregnancy. Aromatherapy and herbal medicine.

Garlic: Has been used for centuries in all parts of the world, but only used a lot in the USA for 25 years. It kills round and thread worms, so it can be classed as an anthelmintic. Twelve case histories show that garlic cured NV over administration from a week to a month. It is a drug of 'noteworthy usage' and an excellent medicament for a diversity of conditions, not just NV. Used in herbal medicine.

Ginger: Commonly used and recommended as a digestive aid, and recommended by the *British Herbal Pharmacopoeia*. European clinical trials show it to be useful in PNV. NASA sends it with astronauts to control NV because it has no sedating effects. It is often used in tea and as a sweet. Essential oil comes from the root, and is used for diarrhea, colic, cramps, indigestion, and N. Aromatherapy and herbal medicine.

Goldenrod: Held to be useful for some NV. (Given its allergenic properties, the researcher will once again think of relationships between olfaction, allergy, and immune response, and N.)

Grapes: Claimed as useful against N. One is reminded of research showing that wine aids appetite, as well as having other healthful effects. But, as with alcohol in large doses, it can be teratogenic

Lavandin: This plant is a hybrid between lavender and spike lavender. It is larger, grows in France, and its oil and herbal properties are very similar to those of lavender. It does not have a long history of herbal use, only about 60–70 years. Mostly used in aromatherapy.

Lavender: A woody shrub that is cultivated all over the world, this scent is familiar to almost everyone and has been used for thousands of years to 'comfort the stomach.' The essential oil from the flowers is used for cramps, colic, and N. Aromatherapy and herbal medicine.

Lilac: Can cause N when inhaled; mechanisms are of scientific interest.

(contd)

Table 18.2: (contd)

Lobelia, giant: As with lilac, V may be precipitated by inhalation.

Mace: Claimed to be useful for NV in small doses; higher doses may be hallucinogenic and become toxic. As toxicity is established and AE efficacy is not, caution is the better part of home experimentation.

Marjoram: Said to have benign effects on the GI tract.

Megsulia: Claimed to be useful against V.

Mint, peppermint: Remedy for indigestion, N, and gas pains. Regarded as an excellent carminative and gastric stimulant, and widely used. Sometimes incorporated into olive oil for local application for inflammation. The oil from the flowers is used for dyspepsia, flatulence, and, directly or by inhalation, for N. Aromatherapy and herbal medicine.

Mint, spearmint: The actions are essentially the same as peppermint, but less powerful; thus some feel it is better for upsets in children. It is often used in combination with peppermint. Aromatherapy and herbal medicine.

Nigella: Said to enhance sense of smell, thus by implication may affect odor-induced NV, particularly PNV. Of research interest.

Nutmeg: A spice and a remedy for digestive and kidney problems used for centuries. The oil comes from the shell and is used for flatulence, indigestion, and N. Possibly hallucinogenic in larger doses, with asserted toxicity risks. Aromatherapy and herbal medicine. Caution.

Opium: Used at least since 2000 BC and still employed in peasant cultures to alleviate pain, including GI tract disorder. Availability depends on local farming, but worldwide it is now outlawed because of high addictive potential. As with its derivative prescribed compound morphine, it is heavily analgesic and, although it may control NV temporarily, and for some produce euphoria, for many people it induces GI distress including N and sometimes V. For the heroin user this may be called 'the good sick' because of its association with euphoria. Once again there are paradoxical effects and widespread individual differences in response.

Patchouli: A strong smelling 'incense' from a Malay plant best known in California to conceal marijuana smoking odors. Nevertheless claimed to be useful in the control of V.

Pepper, black: Comes from a vine native to the tropics, and used for stomach ache, digestive problems, and to 'fortify the stomach.' Extraction of the oil from the peppercorns can treat colic, constipation, and N. Aromatherapy and herbal medicine.

Persimmon: Used by some Californian herbalists as juice or when dried as tincture.

Plum, Chinese salted/dried. Part of Oriental medicine as well as a condiment and an aperitif. Claimed to be useful for NV.

Rose (cabbage and damask): The rose usually used for oil is a hybrid between *Rosa centifolia*, a pink rose, and *R. gallica*, a dark red rose. It is not often used in herbal medicine anymore, but used to be taken for menstrual and digestive disorders. It is effective as an oil, and is used for liver congestion, cholecystitis, and N. Used in aromatherapy.

Rosewood: The oil is distilled from its wood chips. Claims are made for its relief of stress-related conditions which can produce N. Used in aromatherapy.

(contd)

Table 18.2: (contd)

Sandalwood: Comes from a small evergreen tree native to tropical Asia, it is one of the oldest known perfumes, and in China is it used to treat stomach ache and V. The oil from the roots and heartwood is used for diarrhea, N, and other stress-related complaints. Aromatherapy and herbal medicine.
Sickle hare's ear: As a decoction used to combat V.
Thistle, holly: Induces V; in small doses said to be useful for digestive disturbance. If so, it is another example of the paradoxical effect of compounds both eliciting and serving to reduce NV.
Thistle, milk: Said to counteract motion sickness. The seeds are said to be toxic, although, as they are a naturally occurring food enjoyed by ruminants, one should, as with much that is said about herbals, ask about the evidence.

Although there is definitely a psychological component to this treatment, it has also been proven that acupuncture and acupressure produce benefit in the majority of patients. A study of 105 patients after chemotherapy shows that 99 of them benefited from acupuncture; most were completely relieved of symptoms. Four randomized trials in PNV are cited in Chapter 6 (page 127). Providing people with a 'dummy' acupressure point somewhere else on their body also has positive effects, but is not as effective as using the true acupressure point. Acupressure not only has a real physiological component, but also gives the patients an active role in their own treatment.

Homeopathic therapies for N

Homeopathic therapies generally use exceedingly small doses, sometimes of ordinary medications, based on a theory of bodily competence in self-healing which can be assisted by giving minute amounts of medicines that produce the symptoms of the disease. Immunization is a successful example when applied to preventive immune system enhancement. The homeopathic approach to NV appears to rely entirely on the paradoxical effects commented on earlier with respect to emetics and AEs. Neither conventional medicine nor homeopathy has attended sufficiently to this important phenomenon by way of theory and research.

Compounds used by homeopaths, now often sold in drug stores, at chemists, etc., for the treatment of N include promethazine ZPLO gel administered transdermally for PNV, antimonium tartaricum,* calcarea phosphorica, cocculus indicus, echinacea angustifolia, ipecacuanha* (as a primary emetic used in animal studies but only rarely now in poison centers to induce V), nux vomica,* podophyllum peltatum,* phosphorus.*

For the treatment of V those starred are recommended as well as kali bichromicum and veratrum album. All are available at chemists carrying homeopathic remedies. As the dosage is so small, safety is not usually a concern. The scientific evidence for efficacy, using research models used in biology, is almost entirely absent.

CHAPTER 19

Emergency medicine/trauma/ poisoning

In emergency rooms, the staff are unable to anticipate the next patient's problem. Therefore, the staff must have a good understanding of the commonly occurring conditions associated with the various symptoms that patients are likely to present with. Acute nausea and vomiting (NV) is a very common complaint, most commonly caused in adults by gastroenteritis, febrile illnesses, or drug misuse. Chronic NV may present patients with an intestinal obstruction, with chronic analgesic therapy, or with emotional illnesses. Serious illnesses such as myocardial infarction, cerebral hemorrhage, volvulus of the bowel, and Reye's syndrome are less frequently the etiology of repeated V.

The conditions that commonly precipitate NV attacks are listed below under the topics of pediatric conditions, cancer, pregnancy, food poisoning, migraine headache, insect bites and mushroom ingestion, common poisons and drug overdose, and trauma. Metoclopramide is described as a therapeutic remedy. Many of these conditions are addressed in specific chapters on those topics (see Chapters 20–27). Rather, those unexpected emergency situations that are not addressed elsewhere are emphasized in this chapter.

Children

NV in children occur commonly from:

- Formula intolerance
- Improper feeding techniques
- Gastroenteritis
- Appendicitis
- Necrotizing enterocolitis
- Duodenal hematoma from trauma

- Pyloric stenosis: this rare, but dramatic condition typically affects 3- to 6-week-old boys (4:1 male preponderance), causing forceful V after feeding. V in pyloric stenosis produces a more extreme hypochloremic/hypoalkemic metabolic alkalosis than in other V conditions (Aghababian and Fleisher, 1992).

Less frequently occurring pediatric conditions with V as a primary symptom include:

- Sepsis
- Elevated intracranial pressure
- Cystic fibrosis
- Whooping cough
- Adrenogenital deficiency
- Congenital metabolic disorders.

(See Chapter 30 for descriptions of these conditions.)

Vomiting by patients with cancer

Vomiting by cancer patients may be a result of increased intracranial pressure from cranial metastasis, or from bowel obstruction. Metabolic disorders such as uremia, hypercalcemia, and hyponatremia may result from renal failure, ureteral obstruction, and dehydration. Administration of chemotherapeutic drugs usually causes NV soon thereafter, and opiate analgesics advisable for the relief of pain may also be the source of chronic N (see Chapter 27).

Hyperemesis gravidarum

This condition occurs when pregnancy NV (PNV) is severe, causing weight loss, dehydration, and starvation. The etiology of severe PNV remains unknown; however, preliminary data suggest an association with the risk for experiencing migraine headache (see Chapter 26).

Staphylococcal food poisoning

Food poisoning often results in severe NV (see Chapters 21 and 24).

Migraine headaches

Some patients may experience NV associated with migraine headaches. Such NV are probably a result of intravascular pressure in the cranium (see Chapter 25).

Spider bites and mushroom poisoning

Neurotoxic black widow spider bites

The black widow spider's venom contains proteins that bind to the calcium ion channels in the synaptic endplates, resulting in a massive release of acetylcholine and norepinephrine. Within 1–2 hours, clinical features include pain in the lymph nodes and muscle spasms in abdominal and upper truncal muscles, anxiety, NV, dizziness, and headaches. Recovery usually occurs at this point; however, in more severe cases, the patient experiences further pain, anxiety, dyspnea, dysphagia, ptosis, and edema of the eyelids, a low-grade fever, skin rash, sweating, lacrimation, salivation, bronchorrhea, and elevation of arterial and cerebrospinal fluid pressures. Death is rare (Schwartz et al., 1992).

Amatoxin mushroom poisoning

Amatoxin is a cyclic octapeptine found in species of mushrooms: *Amanita* (*A. phalloides*), *Galerina*, and *Lepiota*. It inhibits the following RNA polymerase II, blocking protein synthesis. Amatoxin produces toxic effects within 6–24 hours and can lead to death.

Coprine mushroom poisoning

Coprine, a protoxin found in the genus *Coprinus*, is an aldehyde dehydrogenase inhibitor and blocks ethanol metabolism at the acetaldehyde stage. The autonomic nervous system is rapidly affected, and symptoms include NV, flushing, dyspnea, diaphoresis, and chest pain.

Cyclopeptide mushroom poisoning

Early symptoms of cyclopeptide poisoning include colicky abdominal pain, watery diarrhea, and NV. Late symptoms are pain in the right upper quadrant, hepatomegaly, asterixis, jaundice, and encephalopathy. This compound found in mushrooms destroys cells and its effects are delayed from the time of ingestion.

Gyromitrin mushroom poisoning

Early signs and symptoms include dizziness, bloating, NV, and headaches followed later by hepatic failure, seizures, and coma.

Gyromitrin has a delayed action and causes cellular destruction (Bongard and Sue, 1994).

NV in drug poisoning

Digoxin poisoning

After overdosing, diagnosis of digoxin poisoning relies on symptoms of weakness, N, anorexia, fatigue, and visual complaints. Other symptoms that may present include V, headaches, diarrhea, and dizziness. Digitalis preparations first increase the vagal tone which leads to a conduction blockade at the atrioventricular node, thus causing a decrease in chronotropy, and, second, they inhibit the myocardial Na^+/K^+ ATPase pump. This causes an increase in intracellular calcium and thus an increased contractile force of the heart. In toxic concentrations, the results are excessive extracellular potassium and an increase in intracellular sodium and calcium causing cardiac, gastrointestinal, neurological, and electrolyte abnormalities.

Acetaminophen (paracetamol) poisoning

NV, jaundice, right upper quadrant pain, asterixis, lethargy, coma, bleeding, and hypoglycemia are essential for diagnosing acetaminophen poisoning. Toxic amounts of acetaminophen lead to liver failure as a result of a depletion of hepatic glutathione which metabolizes acetaminophen in the cytochrome P450 oxidase system. This leads to an accumulation of toxic intermediates and metabolites of acetaminophen. In 24 hours, NV present as well as lethargy. During the 24- to 48-hour interval, the patient may feel well, but, 3–4 days after ingestion, there is an increase in liver damage, NV, and presentation of the symptoms listed above.

Salicylate (aspirin, etc.) poisoning

Salicylate's effects are dose dependent. Therapeutic levels are 20–30 mg/dl. Blood levels of 30–50 mg/dl often produce tinnitus, N, and abdominal pain, and 50–70 mg/dl includes lethargy, disorientation, and confusion. Levels over 70 mg/dl may precipitate convulsions, seizures, coma, and cardiovascular failure. After an overdose, hepatic enzymes become saturated, leading to a change in the metabolism of salicylates by the body. The half-life increases from a few hours to 18–36 hours. Respiratory alkalosis may occur because of the stimulation of the central nervous system (CNS) response center and the increased sensitivity to changes in carbon dioxide and oxygen concentrations in the blood. Overdoses also result in an uncoupling of oxidative phosphorylation, leading to an increased metabolic rate, increased glucose and oxygen consumption, and increased heat production. Hypoglycemia and fever may be the result. The drug also inhibits the citrate cycle enzymes forcing a build-up of pyruvate and lactate, and thus a high anion gap metabolic acidosis.

Theophylline poisoning

Theophylline overdose is characterized by NV, tachycardia with atrial or ventricular arrhythmias, hypotension, agitation, hyperreflexia, seizures, and hypoalkalemia. Theophylline is a phosphodiesterase inhibitor and increases intracellular cyclic AMP. In overdoses, the drug stimulates catecholamine release from the adrenal medulla which causes excessive beta stimulation. The CNS is also affected (by unknown mechanisms). NV in patients are from local gastric irritation and central effects, but NV are not universal.

Methanol or ethylene glycol poisoning

Visual disturbances, NV, abdominal pain, lethargy, confusion, seizures, coma, and abdominal tenderness occur 12–24 hours after ingestion of methanol or ethylene glycol. (Effects are similar to intoxication by alcohol.) These substances are CNS depressants found in antifreeze and de-icing products. The toxic intermediate of methanol (14–18 hours) is formic acid, a product of metabolism by the hepatic enzyme, alcohol dehydrogenase. Methanol in small doses (30–60 ml) can be toxic and lethal. Ethylene glycol (half-life 3–8 hours) is broken down into oxalic acid which is toxic in high doses. Patients progress in three stages (for ethylene glycol): the first stage consists of CNS effects – basically, intoxication, slurred speech, hallucinations, perhaps NV, mild hypertension, stupor, seizures, and coma; the second stage is cardiopulmonary in nature – hypertension and tachycardia; and the third stage is renal based.

Isopropyl alcohol poisoning

Patients who suffer isopropyl alcohol poisoning complain of headaches, dizziness, confusion, intoxication, poor coordination, abdominal pain, NV, tachycardia, miosis, and nystagmus. This compound is found in rubbing alcohol, skin and hair products, and antifreeze. Most people can manage isopropyl alcohol in large amounts (of the order of 1 liter). The effects of excessive isopropyl alcohol include gastrointestinal and CNS effects and, as it is a gastric irritant, it may cause gastritis. Isopropyl alcohol is also a CNS depressant, and half of the quantity consumed is excreted while the other half is metabolized into acetone.

Lithium poisoning

Therapeutic serum concentrations of lithium are typically 0.6–1.2 mmol/l. When the concentrations rise to 1.5–2.0 mmol/l, symptoms include NV and diarrhea. From 2.0 to 2.5 mmol/l, drowsiness, dizziness, vertigo, nystagmus, confusion, slurred speech, scotomata, blurred vision, weakness, syncope, and hyperreflexia are often witnessed. Concentrations of 2.5–3.0 mmol/l produce myoclonic twitches, choreoathetoid movements, urinary and fecal incontinence, and increasing stupor leading to coma. Higher levels, 3.0–4.0 mmol/l, often result in seizures and cardiac arrhythmias, and over 4.0 mmol/l evidences hypotension and peripheral vascular collapse.

Management of acute alcoholic intoxication

One way to treat acute intoxication from alcohol is to administer fructose, but this treatment is often accompanied by such adverse affects as 'abdominal and retrosternal pain, apprehension, itching and burning of the skin, nausea and vomiting, ketoacidosis, and osmotic diuresis' (Aghababian and Fleisher, 1992). Hydration with balanced intravenous fluids may be dramatically helpful in severe cases.

Trauma

Hypovolemic shock

Symptoms include cool and pale skin, decreased capillary flow, thirst (as a result of elevated levels of antidiuretic hormone), low peripheral venous pressure, NV, and a decreased core body temperature.

Airway management

A main cause of pulmonary and airway complications after trauma is the V of stomach contents. Approximately 10–20% of all patients undergoing general anesthesia vomit small amounts. Anesthetics have the effect of decreasing the tone of the lower esophageal sphincter.

General factors predisposing to regurgitation, aspiration, and subsequent pulmonary pathology

Pain, fear, anxiety, alcohol intoxication, narcotics/opiates, sedatives, shock, impaired consciousness, trauma, as well as elevated intra-abdominal pressure produced by intestinal distention, intraperitoneal blood, and/or increased muscular activity, can all result in elevated intragastric pressure and a predisposition to vomit. When the normal difference in pressures between the esophagus and the stomach is reversed, developing a lower pressure in the esophageal section than in the intragastric portion of the gastrointestinal (GI) tract, V is likely to occur. Further, when the lower esophageal tension is lowered, usually as a result of trauma specifically of the brain, upper abdominal organs, or the diaphragm, V may occur. Anesthetic drugs may also decrease the sphincter's tone [except succinylcholine (suxamethonium), pancuronium, and neostigmine].

NV treatment: metoclopramide

Metoclopramide has powerful effects on the lower esophageal sphincter, GI motility, and the 'vomiting center' of the brain stem. It increases anterograde gastric motility, synchronizes gastric and duodenal movements, and increases lower esophageal barrier pressure. At intravenous doses of 10 or 20 mg it reduces the gastric volume within, in about 20–30 minutes. It does not have an effect on gastric acidity and its effects are antagonized by simultaneously administered anticholinergics, opiates, and diazepam. Side effects may include irritability, flushing, dizziness, extrapyramidal symptoms, and hypotension. This drug is particularly useful in relieving NV.

Case history

A 23-year-old woman, driver of an automobile that was hit broadside on the driver's side by another speeding vehicle, was transported to the emergency room by an aid vehicle. She had not been wearing a seatbelt, and the window was shattered in the crumpled driver's door. The attendants had administered oxygen by facemask after the patient, still conscious, had 'air hunger.' She had also vomited undigested food that apparently contained a small quantity of blood. On arrival, her BP was 110/68, pulse 90, respiratory rate 30, temperature 37.2°C. She complained of headache, and pain in the left chest wall and the epigastric region. A history obtained partially from the patient and her husband, who was summoned by the police, indicated that she had been healthy, and that she was 5 months' pregnant. She had been having daily episodes of V, but was using no medication for it.

Physical examination indicated a left-sided bruise of the temporal area of the head, with normal neurological evaluation, and point tenderness over the eighth rib laterally, but with normal breath sounds. The abdomen was negative for rebound tenderness, and no masses (except for the pregnant uterus at the umbilicus) were palpable. The fetal heart sounds were present. A CT scan of the chest demonstrated a fractured rib, but the skull film was negative. An ultrasonographic study of the uterus indicated no evidence of retroplacental bleeding, and the upper abdomen was negative for masses or gall stones. Laboratory tests indicated a hematocrit of 34%, with hypochromic indices, and a white blood cell count of 9800/mm^3. Serum amylase was 20 units, and the urine analysis was normal.

The conclusion was that the injuries were mild, and that the V was the result of the anxiety from the accident, having a full stomach, and rather protracted N of pregnancy. The apparent blood was not accounted for, but may have been pigmented food items. The chest was taped, and she was discharged after 2 hours' observation with fetal monitoring that was normal. Her obstetrician visited her during the emergency room admission, and scheduled seeing her in 48 hours. Soft foods were advised for 12 hours, and the hypochromic anemia was noted for future iron therapy.

The case report is typical for the complexity of intercurrent problems involving several organ systems that must be resolved in a short time. The chronicity of the V reduced concern about it in this setting. The case also emphasizes that pregnant women are more likely to be injured in accidents if seat belts and shoulder straps are not worn.

CHAPTER 20

Endocrinology

Although many endocrine disorders and conditions have been found to be associated with nausea and vomiting (NV), there is a tremendous lack of information regarding these subjective and observational findings in the field of endocrinology. Even the major endocrinology texts make no index reference of any kind to NV. However, endocrine factors should not be underestimated. One must presume that, somewhere in the complexity of the endocrine system, its interactions with other systems and compounds may be partly, in one way or another, responsible for inducing NV. Thus, it is essential for us to examine the endocrine disorders that are commonly associated with NV. Although many studies have indicated a correlation between vasopressin levels and NV, there remain many unanswered questions and contradictory findings.

In this chapter, we consider conditions in endocrinology that often accompany emesis and then suggest possible mechanisms about how NV are produced. We also explore treatments and measures, both pharmacological and nonpharmacological, that may help prevent or reduce the occurrence of NV.

Conditions/disorders commonly associated with NV

Adrenal insufficiency

Both acute and chronic adrenal insufficiency are often associated with gastrointestinal (GI) symptoms. Anorexia and weight loss are early manifestations in most cases and may progress to N and intractable V (Becker, 1990).

The clinical features of the syndrome may vary depending upon whether the patient has primary adrenal failure (deficiency of both glucocorticoid and mineralocorticoid hormones) or pituitary adrenocorticotropic hormone (ACTH) deficiency with secondary adrenal insufficiency (deficiency only of glucocorticoids).

In chronic primary adrenal insufficiency, the entire adrenal is usually destroyed by the underlying process. The most prominent clinical feature in these patients is weakness and easy fatiguability. The patient may feel well upon awakening in the morning, but tires rapidly after only minimal exertion. A loss of appetite, occasionally with V, is also a prominent feature, and most patients have noted some degree of weight loss as a result of the anorexia. Symptoms of volume depletion, such as low blood pressure, postural dizziness, and hypotension, as well as hyponatremia, hyperkalemia, and hyperpigmentation, are also common in the presentation of patients with primary adrenal insufficiency (Hare, 1986).

The clinical presentation in secondary adrenal insufficiency is slightly different. As they lack ACTH, these patients are not hyperpigmented and, as they produce mineralocorticoid normally, they also lack the prominent symptoms of volume depletion. However, the symptoms of weakness, anorexia, weight loss, and easy fatiguability (symptoms of cortisol deficiency) closely resemble those seen in primary adrenal insufficiency.

Acute adrenal insufficiency is characterized by a 1- to 2-day course with NV, hypotension, and often fever. In the absence of steroid therapy, patients may deteriorate rapidly and the outcome is almost universally fatal.

The exact mechanism of these manifestations is unknown, but usually symptoms are relieved with correction of the hormone deficiencies.

Differential diagnosis of adrenal insufficiency

Many of the symptoms listed above help to differentiate the patient with adrenal insufficiency from those with depression. Although depressed patients may share many of these symptoms, they do not get hyperpigmentation, hypercalcemia, or hypotension (Camargo, C., unpublished observations).

When the clinical presentation suggests the possibility of adrenal insufficiency, routine laboratory tests may provide some supportive evidence. In acute adrenal insufficiency, particularly when primary, hyponatremia and hyperkalemia are often noted. Hypoglycemia and eosinophilia are also seen. The definitive diagnosis must rely on the measurement of actual hormone levels in the blood and urine.

Syndrome of inappropriate antidiuretic hormone secretion (SIADH)

Excessive antidiuretic hormone (ADH) secretion causes SIADH and reflects an impaired capacity to dilute the urine and thus excrete solute-free water, which leads to hyponatremia and hypo-osmolality. SIADH is characterized by volume expansion, a low serum sodium level, decreased serum osmolality, an inappropriately high urine osmolality, and continued renal excretion of sodium. It is often associated with tumors, and central nervous system (CNS) and pulmonary diseases (Becker, 1990). Early symptoms consist of anorexia, NV, as well as lethargy; later, irritability and personality changes occur, which can be followed by confusion, stupor, and coma. Other endocrine disorders, such as adrenal insufficiency, myxedema, and anterior pituitary insufficiency, may be associated with SIADH secondary to hypovolemia and impaired renal excretion of free water (Hare, 1986; Greenspan and Baxter, 1994).

N is the most potent stimulus of bioactive arginine vasopressin secretion. However, chronic N is usually not a causal factor for hypo-osmolality. Often, NV are overlooked in hypo-osmolar patients as signs of dysfunction of the CNS. The NV associated with hypo-osmolality should be assumed to be of CNS origin and, hence, as significant as other neurological symptoms, particularly because hypo-osmolality does not have a known direct effect on the GI tract (Becker, 1990).

Differential diagnosis of SIADH

The diagnosis of SIADH is established by the presence of hyponatremia and hypo-osmolality in the presence of concentrated urine and increased sodium in urine excretion, with normal renal and adrenal function. Over 100 clinical entities may be associated with this syndrome, including ectopic secretion of ADH by tumors, many neurological conditions, intoxication of certain drugs, and metabolic disorders such as porphyria (see Chapter 23).

Diabetes mellitus

The severity and frequency of NV in people with diabetes vary greatly. Some may have NV several times a week or even daily, whereas others may have NV attacks accompanied by persistent abdominal pain lasting for days to weeks. In diabetes, the NV most likely has many causes, ranging from GI factors to psychiatric disorders.

Diabetic gastroparesis

Some people with diabetes will have 'attacks' of N, V, and abdominal pain lasting days to weeks. During these periods, plasma glucose may be difficult to control and weight loss may occur. Besides gastrointestinal causes (e.g., infection, inflammation, obstruction, or motility disturbance), there are many other causes to consider. These include: metabolic disturbances (e.g., diabetic ketoacidosis, uremia); side effects from medications; disorders of the biliary tract, pancreas, heart, and CNS; and psychiatric disorders. Acute-onset NV are usually explained after an appropriate history, physical examination, and standard laboratory evaluation. However, chronic, unexplained NV are more challenging. It is customary to label those people with diabetes as having a gastric motor disturbance, or diabetic gastroparesis (Becker, 1990).

The incidence of NV in diabetic gastroparesis has been described in Feldman and Schiller (1983). In a survey of 136 patients attending a diabetic clinic, 26% complained of intermittent or chronic NV. Fasting and postprandial contractile activity in the pylorus region of the stomach was increased in people with diabetes who had recurrent NV, but the exact interrelationships of pylorospasm, gastric emptying, and NV remain unclear (Kucharczyk et al., 1991).

Differential diagnosis of gastroparesis

In some diabetics with chronic, unexplained NV, psychogenic V may be suspected. Even if symptoms of anxiety, depression, or hypochondriasis are present, the diagnosis of psychogenic V can never be made with certainty. V in diabetic gastroparesis typically occurs hours after eating, and the vomitus contains old food; psychogenic V tends to occur immediately after eating. However, there are many exceptions to these typical patterns. It may be necessary to refer some patients for psychological or psychiatric evaluation (Schiller and Feldman, 1990). It is of course necessary always to rule out metabolic disorders such as acidosis and electrolyte disturbance (Camargo, C., unpublished observations).

Diabetic ketoacidosis

When the insulin lack is severe (type 1 diabetes), ketoacidosis results. Not only are polyuria and polydipsia present, but also general malaise, fatigue, NV, and abdominal pain are all common. If profound, acidosis results in Kussmaul's respirations and, if it is sufficiently severe and accompanied by marked dehydration, hypotension may ensue. Ketoacidosis may be precipitated by several causes, and it may be the first manifestation of diabetes mellitus type 1 (Camargo, C., personal observation). In a patient with established diabetes, omission of an insulin dose may also be the cause. Most patients will not leave out their insulin dose because they are aware of its necessity. Infections of a variety of types, both viral and bacterial, may also precipitate ketoacidosis. Another cause, myocardial infarction, is not uncommon as either a precipitant or a consequence of ketoacidosis (Hare, 1986).

Differential diagnosis of diabetic ketoacidosis

The differential diagnosis includes all types of metabolic acidosis and coma. An accumulation of ketone bodies sufficient to cause metabolic acidosis may be seen in the absence of diabetes in poorly nourished, alcoholic patients with repeated bouts of V. This dysfunction is called alcoholic ketoacidosis (Felig et al., 1995; Weatherall et al., 1996).

To diagnose diabetic ketoacidosis, ketone bodies and glucose should be measured (Hershman, 1980). Lactic acidosis, resulting from accumulation of lactic acid, may occur in older people with diabetes who have vascular insufficiency and tissue ischemia. Phenformin and its derivatives are also associated with lactic acidosis (Camargo, C., personal observation).

Hyperthyroidism and hyperemesis gravidarum

NV may occasionally be the predominant presenting symptoms in patients with hyperthyroidism, or hyperactivity of the thyroid gland. Graves' disease is the most common result of hyperthyroidism. When this occurs during pregnancy, it may present as hyperemesis gravidarum (HG). In one series of patients with HG, two of 39 patients were found to be thyrotoxic. However, elevated levels of free thyroxine (T_4) and triiodothyronine (T_3) may be found transiently in up to a third of subjects presenting with HG. These increased thyroid hormone levels probably result from stimulation by human chorionic gonadotropin (hCG) because serum hCG levels were increased by about 50% in those subjects with elevated free T_4 levels and correlated with the free T_4 levels. On the other hand, there is considerable overlap of hCG levels with those of normal individuals, so that some authors have postulated that, in those cases associated with transient hyperthyroidism, the hCG may have some structural variation resulting in increased biological activity. In most patients, the free T_4 levels fall to normal over 6–133 days (mean 35.1 days) while still pregnant. Therefore, patients with hyperemesis and elevated free T_4 and T_3 levels present a considerable diagnostic dilemma (DeGroot et al., 1985).

Differential diagnosis of hyperthyroidism

The most efficient screening test for hyperthyroidism is the free T_4 and thyroid-stimulating hormone (TSH) determination. Also, thyroid uptake of radiolabeled iodine is elevated in most hyperthyroid patients. A low thyroid uptake of radiolabeled iodine (< 5% at 24 hours) is found in thyroiditis because the damaged gland does not trap and bind it. As painless chronic lymphocytic hyperthyroidism may account for 10% of hyperthyroid patients in some areas, the thyroid uptake of radiolabeled iodine should be measured in all patients who do not have the eye or skin manifestations of Graves' disease (Hershman, 1980).

Hyperparathyroidism

Symptomatic primary hyperparathyroidism most commonly presents with renal or skeletal disease, but GI manifestations may be seen in up to 35% of the patients. The reported frequency of abdominal symptoms varies according to the patient population and selection bias, the degree of hypercalcemia, and the duration of illness. With the advent of multichannel serum auto-analyzers, up to 50% of patients with hyperparathyroidism are now being diagnosed on the basis of asymptomatic hypercalcemia.

The most dramatic presentation of gastroenterological manifestations occurs in the syndrome of so-called acute hyperparathyroidism. Such patients often present with severe abdominal pain, NV, lethargy, dehydration, and altered mental status, which may progress to coma and seizures. In many of these cases, digestive tract symptoms predominate and peptic ulceration or pancreatitis is common.

Severe primary hyperparathyroidism is also associated with frequent GI symptoms which include anorexia, weight loss, NV, abdominal pain, and constipation. Although several reports describe an increased incidence of peptic ulceration in hyperparathyroidism, others have disputed this (Becker, 1990).

It has been postulated that the V in hyperparathyroidism is one manifestation of generalized CNS hyperexcitability that may lower the threshold of excitation of the chemoreceptor trigger zone (CTZ) or the medullary V center (Kurcharczyk et al., 1991).

Differential diagnosis of hyperparathyroidism

Hypercalcemia is the hallmark of hyperparathyroidism, but many other conditions can be associated with hypercalcemia, such as neoplasias, vitamin D intoxication, milk–alkaloid syndrome, and the familial disorder of the calcium sensor. The association of hypercalcemia with elevated serum levels of parathyroid hormones (with intact molecule radioimmunology assays) establishes the diagnosis of primary hyperparathyroidism (Camargo, C., unpublished observations).

Hypercalcemia

Hypercalcemia, a common complication of malignancy, occurs in 5–10% of patients with solid tumors, and usually occurs in later stages of disease. Hypercalcemia is most commonly seen in the setting of an increase in bone resorption over bone formation, increased renal calcium reabsorption, and impaired glomerular filtration. Symptoms of hypercalcemia include anorexia, N and/or V, polyuria, confusion, coma, and progressive muscular weakness. Symptoms are evident when serum calcium levels are greater than 11.5 mg/dl (Becker, 1990).

Hypoglycemia and uremia

Acute hypoglycemia often occurs as a result of insulin excess and from a rapid fall in plasma glucose, either exogenous or endogenous, and it often accompanies conditions associated with arterial hyperinsulinism. Uremic patients occasionally have troublesome hypoglycemia, possibly caused by impaired gluconeogenesis.

Acute hypoglycemia is a relatively weak stimulus for vasopressin release. The receptor and pathway that mediate this effect are separate from those of other recognized stimuli, because hypoglycemia stimulates vasopressin secretion in patients who have lost the capacity to respond selectively to osmotic, hemodynamic, or emetic stimuli. However, the vasopressin response to hypoglycemia is accentuated by dehydration and is abolished by water loading. Thus, glucopenic stimuli probably act in concert with osmotic influences, even though the osmoreceptors are unnecessary for the response.

Vasopressin release may be triggered by an intracellular deficiency of glucose or one of its metabolites, because 2-deoxyglucose is also an effective stimulus.

Differential diagnosis of hypoglycemia

It is important to separate fasting hypoglycemia (which is always clearly the result of organic causes such as insulin-producing tumors of the pancreas, insufficiency of hormones inducing gluconeogenesis, or enzymatic defects in glycogenolysis or gluconeogenesis). Also, reactive, postprandial hypoglycemia is often 'functional' in nature and usually not life threatening (Camargo, C., unpublished observations).

Stress and N

The secretion of arginine vasopressin (AVP) is affected by inputs from various parts of the 'visceral brain' and the reticular activating system, regions that are involved in maintenance of consciousness and in emotional expression. N is accompanied by intense AVP release, presumably by reflex stimulation from the medullary V center (area postrema).

When Verney began his studies of water regulation in dogs, he was struck by the marked effect of emotional stress on antidiuretic activity (Schrier and Goldberg, 1980). It has been generally believed that humans and rats also release AVP in response to emotional stress, but Robertson (1989) showed that pain or other stresses that are incidental to human physiological experiments rarely influence plasma AVP concentrations. The same is true for deliberately applied severe stress in rats. Nevertheless, the influence of 'higher' neural centers on AVP secretion can be demonstrated by experimental induction of diuresis or antidiuresis, through hypnotic suggestion in humans or neurogenic disturbance in regulation of AVP secretion, to be the disturbed control of water excretion in patients with anorexia nervosa and in some schizophrenics who have succeeded in overhydrating themselves to the point of water intoxication.

Other endocrine-related diseases and disorders

Anorexia and bulimia

Anorexia nervosa in its classic form is a serious but uncommon disorder characterized by extreme malnutrition and hypogonadotropism. It is considered to be a severe behavioral disorder, with endocrine changes secondary to both psychological and nutritional disturbances. Amenorrhea may precede weight loss. Malnutrition may result from refusal to eat, induced V (bulimia), and excessive use of laxatives (Greenspan and Forsham, 1986). Self-induced V is usually activated by a gag reflex with fingers or a toothbrush. Some people with bulimia actually learn to vomit spontaneously (Foster, 1992).

Pheochromocytoma

Pheochromocytomas are common tumors arising from chromaffin cells in the sympathetic nervous system. They release epinephrine or norepinephrine (or both) – and in some cases dopamine – into the circulation, causing hypertension and other signs and symptoms, such as headache, sweating, anxiety, fatigue, abdominal or chest pain, and NV. About 50% of those affected with a pheochromocytoma exhibit NV (Becker, 1990).

Hypothyroidism

Hypothyroidism is a clinical syndrome resulting from a deficiency of thyroid hormones, which in turn results in a generalized slowing down of metabolic processes. Hypothyroidism in infants and children results in a marked slowing of growth and development. In adults, there is a generalized slowing down of the organism, resulting in fatigability, coldness, weight gain, constipation, and N (Greenspan and Forsham, 1986).

Treatments/drugs for endocrine disorders that cause NV

Angiotensin and other peptides

Numerous studies have shown that N is a powerful stimulus for vasopressin secretion in humans. It can be activated by a variety of drugs and conditions, including apomorphine, morphine, nicotine, alcohol, and motion sickness.

Emetic stimuli probably mediate many pharmacological and pathological effects on vasopressin secretion. Furthermore, emetic stimulation may be at least partially responsible for the increase in vasopressin secretion observed with IV administration of cyclophosphamide and with vasovagal reactions, ketoacidosis, acute hypoxia, and motion sickness.

The renin–angiotensin system has been implicated in the control of vasopressin secretion. The precise site and mechanism of action have not been defined, but central receptors seem likely to be involved, because angiotensin is most effective when injected directly into brain ventricles or cranial arteries. The levels of plasma renin or angiotensin required to stimulate vasopressin release have not been determined, but are probably quite high. When administered intravenously, pressor doses of angiotensin increase plasma vasopressin two- to fourfold. The magnitude of the vasopressin response may depend upon the concurrent osmotic stimulus, because angiotensin increases the sensitivity of the osmoregulatory system. This dependency on osmotic influences resembles that seen with glucopenic stimuli, and may account for the inconsistency of the vasopressin response to exogenous angiotensin.

Several other peptides have also been shown to affect the CNS and to induce emesis. These peptides are neurotensin, oxytocin, and somatostatin (Becker, 1990).

Bromocriptine

Bromocriptine (2-bromo-α-ergocryptine mesylate), a semisynthetic ergot alkaloid, is often used for the treatment of prolactinomas. If the goal is to achieve lasting normalization of prolactin after discontinuing therapy, then surgery or radiotherapy might be more effective; however, bromocriptine will control prolactin levels in more patients than either surgery or radiotherapy. This alkaloid specifically binds to and stimulates dopamine receptors.

Side effects are usually dose related, with a rapid development of tolerance. Many side effects are potentiated by alcohol, use of which should be avoided in sensitive patients. N is the most common side effect, occurring in up to 25% of treated patients. The N is usually mild, may be minimized by administration of the drug with food and by the initial use of low doses, and generally improves with time.

Calcitonin

Treatment for hypercalcemia is to correct the primary disease, if possible. General measures include saline and diuresis to increase urinary calcium excretion. In longer-term treatment, phosphates, calcitonin, mithramycin, bisphosphonates, corticosteroids, and gallium nitrate can be administered. Calcitonin is also used to treat osteoporosis and hypercalcemia (Camargo, C., unpublished observations). However, a major side of effect of calcitonin is N and tachyphylaxis is also common (Becker, 1990).

Possible mechanisms

Vasopressin

Many stimuli and factors other than osmotic and baroregulatory have been implicated in the control of vasopressin secretion, but careful studies by Schrier and his group have indicated that the effect of many is mediated by baroregulatory mechanisms (DeGroot et al., 1985). Independent of those two main controlling influences are N and emesis, which in humans are remarkably potent stimuli of vasopressin. The pathway that mediates this effect has not been defined but probably involves the CTZ in the area postrema of the medulla, which can be activated by a variety of drugs and conditions. Its effect on vasopressin is instantaneous and extremely potent. Increases of 100–1000 times basal levels are not unusual even when the N is transient and unaccompanied by V or changes in blood pressure. Pretreatment with fluphenazine, haloperidol, or promethazine in doses sufficient to prevent N completely abolishes the vasopressin response. The inhibitory effect of these dopamine antagonists is specific for emetic stimuli, because they do not alter the vasopressin response to osmotic and hemodynamic stimuli. Water loading blunts but does not abolish the effect of N on vasopressin release, suggesting that osmotic and emetic influences interact in a manner similar to the interaction of osmotic and hemodynamic pathways. Emesis is the only vasopressin stimulus known to exhibit significant species differences. In rats, apomorphine has little or no effect on vasopressin but produces marked increases in oxytocin (Felig et al., 1995).

Intracellular pH changes

It is possible that the NV associated with deficiency states, such as hypothyroidism and hypoadrenalism, and electrolyte imbalance, ketoacidosis, and uremia, are the result of an effect on the CTZ in the medulla or on other synaptically connected hypothalamic or medullary centers in the brain. A recent preliminary study explored the role of pH in the induction of emesis in experimental dogs. The results indicate that changes in intracellular hydrogen ion concentration may be the final step leading to activation of chemoreceptors mediating emesis. The data also suggest that ammonia entry into chemoreceptor neurons may precipitate the critical intracellular pH changes (Kucharczyk et al., 1991).

Hormonal changes

Changes in the levels of a number of hormones have been observed during motion sickness. These include increased serum levels of vasopressin, epinephrine, norepinephrine, prolactin, growth hormone, vasoactive intestinal peptide (VIP), ACTH, and the adrenal hormones aldosterone, corticosterone, 11-deoxycorticosterone, 17-hydroxyprogesterone, 11-deoxycortisol, cortisol, and androstendione. Increases have also been noted in the urinary output of the thyroid hormones T_3 and T_4, with an accompanying decrease in serum levels of TSH. Most of these changes have been related to the increased stress associated with motion sickness. With the exception of VIP, epinephrine, and norepinephrine, these hormones are either secreted by the pituitary or dependent upon pituitary hormones for their release. In addition, the synthesis of epinephrine and, to a lesser extent, of norepinephrine by the adrenal medulla is regulated by glucocorticoids from the adrenal cortex. In general, the plasma level of epinephrine is a measure of adrenal medulla secretion, whereas that of norepinephrine reflects sympathetic nerve activity.

Therefore, most of these hormonal changes are probably not essential for the appearance of many aspects of motion sickness because the latency to motion-induced V is unchanged after removal of the pituitary, and as V and related prodromal activity can be produced by natural or electrical vestibular stimulation after decerebration. However, the increased levels of VIP may be at least partly responsible for the decreased gastric tone and motility observed during motion sickness. Some of these hormones have also been related to susceptibility to motion sickness (Kucharczyk et al., 1991).

Control efforts for NV

In endocrinology, the treatment for NV, in general, should first consist of specific therapy for the underlining disorder (i.e., hypercalcemia, hyperparathyroidism, etc.) (Camargo, C., personal communication). If these specific therapies do not alleviate NV, then the antiemetics and methods listed below can be used.

Dopamine antagonists

Dopamine-blocking agents, such as the phenothiazines or butyrophenones, and drugs such as metoclopramide and domperidone, are very effective in blocking apomorphine-induced V (Davis et al., 1986).

For patients with gastroparesis, NV may respond to treatment with oral metoclopramide (5–20 mg, half an hour before meals and, perhaps, at bedtime). Initially, the drug can be given parenterally. As this drug also acts centrally as an antiemetic, it may be effective in NV as a result of various causes other than gastroparesis. Dopamine antagonists, particularly metoclopramide, occasionally have serious CNS side effects, including extrapyramidal motor disorders (e.g., dyskinesis). These can be permanent. Domperidone penetrates the blood–brain barrier less well than metoclopramide and has fewer CNS side effects. Both drugs can also cause hyperprolactinemia and galactorrhea. Thus, these drugs should not be used indiscriminately and, when effective, they should be used at the lowest effective dose for as short a time as possible. An investigational, prokinetic drug, cisapride, may offer symptomatic relief in people with diabetes who have delayed gastric emptying without the risk of neurological side effects.

Rarely does gastroparesis become life threatening. When it occurs, it may cause patients to go into hypovolemic shock, necessitating hospital admission. Check the patient's vital signs immediately. Signs of shock include: a fast, thready pulse; rapid breathing, cyanosis, or pallor; extreme lethargy; and neurological impairment, including altered mentation in older children and adults. Once the patient's stability has been established, his or her hydration status should be checked. Signs of dehydration may include sunken eyes, cold and clammy skin, and, in young and middle-aged patients, poor skin turgor. Patients with severe NV often require temporary nasogastric intubation for gastric decompression, as well as parenteral nutrition and metoclopramide. A few patients with refractory chronic NV have been treated with antrectomy, gastrojejunostomy, or pyloroplasty in order to improve gastric emptying. These operations have had limited success and should be considered only as a last resort.

As N has been shown to induce vasopressin secretion, pre-treatment with fluphenazine, haloperidol, or promethazine usually prevents N. These pre-treatments completely abolish the vasopressin response. The inhibitory effect of these dopamine antagonists is specific for emetic stimuli, because they do not alter the vasopressin response to hyperosmolality, hypovolemia, or hypotension (Becker, 1990).

For N induced by oral contraceptives, phenergan, an oral antiemetic, is also routinely prescribed 1 hour before breakfast and the evening meal. Rectal suppositories may also be used. The high-dose estrogen is then taken after the meal. This administration method will decrease NV (Cunningham, 1993).

Caution is warranted when prescribing an antiemetic to a patient who is also taking other medications. An over-the-counter antiemetic, for ex-ample, may mask an ototoxic response to certain prescription drugs which results in permanent loss of hearing. Thus, it is important to obtain a record of the medications that the patient is currently taking and to get a pharmacist's advice before prescribing an antiemetic (Chase, 1993).

Non-drug remedies

Although dopamine antagonists have been found to be quite effective in treating NV, conservative, non-drug methods should be tried first before drug treatments or operations. The majority of patients can be reassured of the benign nature of this disorder and can be managed with simple maneuvers. For the patient with slight-to-moderate NV, clinicians and family members should provide reassurancc and relieve any fears, ensure rest, and reduce the patient's workload.

As noted above, gastroparesis is hardly ever life threatening. Thus, conservative therapy, which includes control of plasma glucose with insulin and frequent, small meals, is often recommended first because it usually leads to recovery (Becker, 1990).

Once the patient is recovering after a bout of severe V, one should warn the patient not to go right back to his or her regular diet. What seems to work best at first are bland, easily digested foods such as: bananas, rice, apple sauce, toast, boiled eggs, baked or mashed potatoes, plain pasta, crackers, oatmeal, and boiled chicken or turkey. Milk and milk products and carbonated, caffeinated, alcoholic, or sugary beverages should be avoided for the first day or two (Cohen and Moss, 1994).

For those with anorexia and bulimia, psychiatric treatment is required, and hospitalization may be necessary to prevent death from starvation, suicide, or intercurrent illnesses (Greenspan and Forsham, 1986).

Case study

A 27-year-old patient came to Stanford Hospital with severe NV and weight loss that lasted for 3 months. He was initially diagnosed with a malignancy; however, his attending physician overlooked the enlargement of his thyroid gland. A consulting physician noticed the enlargement of the patient's thyroid gland and measured a very high calcium level of 14 mg/dl (the normal level is 8.5–10.2 mg/dl). The patient was thus successfully diagnosed with hyperthyroidism. This case study demonstrates that hyperthyroidism can lead to severe NV and drastic weight loss.

CHAPTER 21

Gastroenterology

Prevalence

The gastrointestinal tract is the organ system of the body directly associated with nausea and vomiting (NV). These symptoms can be considered as an 'early warning system' for the body's internal homeostasis. Therefore, although the symptoms of N, with or without V, may seem trivial, they may be symptomatic of serious medical conditions. Examples of such conditions are: peritonitis, cholecystitis, pancreatitis, intracranial lesions, hepatitis, pregnancy, gastrointestinal obstruction, addisonian crisis, and others.

In some cases, the presence of NV indicates a life-threatening situation such as occurs when appendicitis is unrecognized, or its treatment is delayed. In other circumstances characterized by post-anesthesia, stroke-related paralysis, or coma, or with other restricted movements, controlling the NV is important because V may lead to aspiration pneumonia or, less frequently, the Mallory–Weiss syndrome, and esophageal rupture may occur. Plasma volume and electrolyte depletion, acid–base imbalance, and malnutrition are the predictable result of protracted V of gastric contents.

Primary caregivers must be able to establish effectively the appropriate diagnosis producing the NV, and initiate treatment. Complex situations require referral of the patient to a medical or surgical specialist.

Differential diagnosis

When a patient presents experiencing NV to a medical facility, a careful personal history, the circumstances surrounding the onset, the duration, associated events such as pain, headache, photophobia, diarrhea, abdominal distention, characteristics of vomitus, etc. must be learned. Often, from that history alone, an accurate clinical diagnosis can be made. In children, observations of parents or caregivers are the only, often-uncertain guide. Further, the timing of V in relation to meals, the relief of pain by V, the content of the vomitus, the odor, and other considerations taken during a patient's history may indicate the appropriate diagnosis.

Relation to meals

The timing of V in relation to meals is broken into three relevant periods: immediate, delayed (> 1 hour), and early morning. V that occurs immediately after meals indicates psychogenic V or a peptic ulcer near the pyloric channel. Delayed V is a sign that there may be some gastric outlet obstruction. V rarely occurs 12 hours after a meal. Finally, V that presents itself in the early morning is common with morning sickness in pregnancy, in postgastrectomy patients, as well as in those with uremia, alcoholism, postnasal drip, and increased intracranial pressure, perhaps as the result of a brain tumor.

Pain

Pain may be relieved or caused by V. V relieves pain in those with gastritis or peptic ulcer disease, but pain caused by pancreatitis, biliary tract disease, peritonitis, or pyelonephritis is not relieved by V. In addition, projectile V followed by 'dry heaves' with increased respiratory activity helps to eliminate the diagnosis of increased intracranial pressure.

Appearance/odor of vomitus

The content and odor of the vomitus can aid in the differential diagnosis of the patient's condition. Undigested food present in the vomitus indicates gastric outlet obstruction or upper, small bowel obstruction. Bilious V usually occurs after gastric surgery, and the presence of bile hints at a connection between the proximal duodenum and the stomach, ruling out obstruction in that segment. If feculent odors accompany the vomitus, intestinal obstruction is the normal culprit. However, there may also be peritonitis with ileus, gastrocolic fistula, ischemic injury to the gut, or a long-standing obstruction to the gut with bacterial overgrowth. Other considerations when diagnosing the patient involve: age, weight loss, chronic or acute, and history of alcohol consumption.

Gastroenteritis

The most common ailment producing the symptoms of NV is gastroenteritis. The origin can be either bacterial or viral, depending on the exposure history of the patient. Often the best way to diagnose the condition is by taking a careful history. Food poisoning causes similar acute V of epidemic proportions among others, and a careful history will frequently document the source of contamination. Normally, in bacterial food poisoning cases, there is a 6–12 hour incubation period before the onset of V. Some of the common offending agents are: *Staphylococcus* species, *Clostridium perfringens*, and *Salmonella* species. Patients who travel internationally will frequently be contaminated with a distant region's 'turista,' representing new species of common organisms, and have severe NV.

Cyclic/repetitive occurrence

Cyclical V is V that occurs over regular time intervals. In some rare cases, patients may vomit regularly every 60 days. There are usually three causes for such V: first, *psychogenic V* normally occurs in young women (15–25) who are under the stress of parents, a new marriage, etc. In more cases than not, psychogenic V is the direct result of some sort of emotional disturbance. The second cause of cyclical NV is *increased intracranial pressure* from brain tumors or hydrocephalus. Finally, *pregnancy* NV (PNV) is frequently accompanied by 'morning sickness.' In addition, hyperemesis gravidarum (HG) is a rare condition in which a woman must be treated for severe PNV. It occurs in about 1% of all pregnancies. New data suggest an association with the risk for migraine headache.

Peptic ulcer disease

Another common cause of NV is peptic ulcer disease. The diagnosis of peptic ulcer disease is not possible through physical examination. V is rare in duodenal ulcers and the pain is often marked by rhythmicity, periodicity, and chronicity. Relief can occur when a patient drinks a glass of water to dilute the acidity of the area. It is difficult to separate gastric and duodenal ulcers – the actual identity may never be known. Gastric ulcer patients tend to be older and their relative population frequency is 5 of 10 000 per year. A good diagnostic tool is a barium radiograph which will appear on the film as a clump of barium lodged within an ulcer hole. Also, endoscopy can detect about 85–95% of all lesions. The normal diagnosis procedure is to complete the barium X-ray before the endoscopy. Still, the endoscopy is a powerful tool in determining whether the ulcer is malignant. Other methods employed are measurement of gastrin level tests and a search for the bacterium *Helicobacter pylori.*

Gastric ulcers are accompanied by the traditional 'ulcer pain' and are associated with dyspepsia and heartburn. Milk or antacid alleviates the pain associated with gastric ulcer. About 20% of patients with duodenal ulcer signs end up having gastric ulcer upon endoscopic examination. V, fullness, and distention may signify gastric ulcer on the lesser curvature which is sometimes associated with reflex gastric retention. Gastric emptying is often delayed in gastric ulcer and pain may radiate through the back. Bleeding recurs in roughly 50% of gastric ulcer cases. Weight loss and delayed healing are also further signs. As with a dudodenal ulcer, a barium X-ray is the most common method of determining the presence of a gastric ulcer. However, it is first important to rule out gastric cancer as a possibility. This is done by further endoscopy and a biopsy if the ulcer changes in form. Biopsy with endoscopy has roughly an 80% accuracy rate.

Appendicitis

Acute appendicitis is another gastrointestinal inflammatory condition that is accompanied by NV. The patient will present with NV in about 95% of cases, pain in the lower right quadrant of the abdomen, a slight fever (on average over 37.8°C), and possibly diarrhea. For men, the frequency of acute appendicitis is 8.6% in a lifetime. For women, that frequency drops to 6.7%. The differential diagnosis of acute appendicitis can be made with a careful history, a thorough physical examination, and the appropriate tests. Acute appendicitis is often very difficult to determine in young and old people because its presence in young patients is accompanied by a significant amount of V whereas older patients tend to endure the pain more easily.

In the physical examination, the most likely finding is tenderness at McBurney's point, midway between the anterior superior iliac crest and the umbilicus. Also, the abdominal wall is sensitive to pressure inward, followed by sudden release, producing 'rebound tenderness,' and muscle spasms. Next, the obturator sign should be sought by passive extension of the right lower extremity with the patient lying on the left lateral side, and the knee flexed. If these signs are positive, a white blood cell count (WBC) may be useful. The common range for acute appendicitis is 10 000–16 000 cells/mm^3. Abdominal films and ultrasonography may also be carried out if the diagnosis is still uncertain. Abdominal films occasionally show a fecalith close to the midpoint of the right iliac crest. Ultrasonography shows the lumen surrounded by an edematous, distended, and inflamed wall shaped like a doughnut. Diagnoses that mimic acute appendicitis include: inflammation of the small intestine, mesenteric lymph nodes, gynecological diseases, urinary tract diseases, and Meckel's diverticulum. Intravenous urography can be used to differentiate acute appendicitis from diseases of the urinary tract.

Cholecystitis

Diseases of the gallbladder frequently result in NV. These symptoms are often precipitated by eating a meal with high fat content that causes the gallbladder to contract and release its enzyme/bile salts load. Inflammation or gallstones may become evident from the pain that accompanies fatty food ingestion. One of the cardinal signs of a gallbladder problem is the appearance of jaundice. There are many types of gallbladder disease that cause NV: carcinoma of the gallbladder, carcinoma of the bile ducts, and dysfunction of the sphincter of Oddi. Diagnostic techniques include computed tomography (CT), magnetic resonance imaging, oral cholecystography, and ultrasonography.

Foreign bodies

Frequently, physicians may examine patients, often very young or elderly people, who have ingested a foreign object. In these cases, the challenge is to select the right application of endoscopy, surgery, and expectant management. Perforation may also occur and one in 12 patients will die after perforation from hemorrhage or peritonitis. The signs that an object is lodged in the esophagus include choking while eating, stimulating the gag reflex, and the regurgitation of the bolus. Proper diagnosis can be made with X-rays and the soft tissue technique. Barium radiographs are not useful in these cases because they add an additional foreign body to the esophagus.

A foreign object in the stomach will cause few, if any, symptoms.

Phytobezoars, accumulations of hulls, hair, and other objects ingested by some people, may persist for months and years. Pain, fever, bleeding, or V suggests either a pyloric obstruction or mucosal disruption, or penetration by the object. Plain films should be used to diagnose a foreign body in the stomach and an abdominal X-ray should be used to see if the object remains in the stomach before endoscopy.

Foreign objects in the duodenum and the small bowel are common because of the curvature of the organ. Long, thin objects are likely to get caught in this area and repeated X-rays may be necessary for observation of movement. However, the size and shape of foreign objects in the gut are of critical importance. Normally, objects pass through the gut without a problem. Some patients, for instance small children, require prompt diagnostic effort and treatment because of the small size of their luminal cavities and uncertainty about the exact features of the ingested object. One always hopes that the history will provide the answer.

Hepatitis

Hepatitis is the final diagnosis we consider within the gastroenterology specialty. Each year, about 100 000 cases are reported in the USA. Hepatitis comes in five forms: A, B, C, D, and E. The virus is transmitted orally, through serum and semen, and from fecal contamination. A personal history might determine the possible source of infection and be helpful in the diagnosis. In the preicteric stage, hepatitis is indicated by fever, fatigue, NV, anorexia, and abdominal pain in the right upper quadrant. The icteric stage of the infection is marked by dark urine, jaundice, fever, headache, and arthritis. A physical examination will yield large lymph nodes in the posterior cervical chain, and a swollen throat in the preicteric phase. In the icteric phase, the liver enlarges and can usually be detected by direct physical examination.

The diagnosis for hepatitis involves taking a blood sample. A patient with hepatitis will have a normal WBC and an atypical number of lymphocytes resembling those from mononucleosis. Antigen testing in blood should also be able to determine the exact strain of hepatitis (see Chapter 24).

Procedures and treatment priorities

For patients diagnosed with gastroenteritis or food poisoning, the main priority is to remove the source of the infection. The patient is requested to drink at least 1 quart (about 1 liter) of fluid daily to help the body combat the infection. Patients with pyelonephritis, endometritis or salpingitis, and bacterial enteritis are subjects for antibiotic treatment; NV usually cease several hours after initiation of effective therapy. Patients who are diagnosed with peptic ulcer disease are treated in a variety of ways depending on whether their ulcer was duodenal or gastric. For duodenal ulcer patients, therapy may be divided into three categories: antacid measures, anti-*H. pylori* agents, and promotion of 'cytoprotective' restitution. It is important to remember that, without acid, a duodenal ulcer will not cause the patient pain. Some physicians recommend a variety of diet changes, H_2-receptor blockers, and antacids. Also, it has been shown that the elimination of *H. pylori* can delay the recurrence of the ulcers for some time. Surgery necessary for patients with duodenal ulcers has been halved since the introduction of the H_2-receptor blockers. However, some patients still need to have portions of the duodenum removed in extreme cases.

The treatment for gastric ulcers is quite similar to that for duodenal ulcer patients. Patients with gastric ulcers diagnosed should also be examined for gastric cancer. Like duodenal ulcer treatment, the removal of *H. pylori* can substantially reduce the number of occurrences of gastric ulcers. If surgery is inevitable, part of the stomach may have to be removed.

Foreign bodies present in the gastrointestinal tract normally pass through the system. However, for long, thin objects, observation of the stool and frequent X-rays may be useful to see if the object has passed. If the object lodges in one of the angulations of the esophagus or small intestine, the endoscopic or surgical removal of the object is urgent. Without removal, the obstructed area may become infected and more serious conditions such as peritonitis may result.

Treatment for hepatitis emphasizes personal responsibility of the patient and less of doctor intervention. Patients with hepatitis should be educated about the proper hygiene necessary to avoid its spread after it has been acquired. Also, patients should be encouraged to get bed rest and urged to eat small portions of food, at increased intervals. Supplementary B vitamins are prescribed. Steroids have no place in the treatment of hepatitis and surgery is never considered. Patients with severe NV as well as an uncertain diagnosis should be hospitalized and a liver biopsy should be performed.

Several different medical therapies are possible for those patients experiencing NV that result from morning sickness or drug toxicity. Antihistamines are widely used in the amelioration or prevention of PNV. Phenothiazines are employed to combat V related to drug toxicity. Also, dopaminergic antagonists are popular antiemetics. Patients who suffer from psychogenic V may also require counseling.

Case study

A 29-year-old woman came to an emergency room with NV and abdominal pain. Her temperature at the time of admission was 38.0°C. The pain was localized in the right lower quadrant. Initially, the pain was centered in the periumbilical area. She had mild tenderness and guarding in the right lower quadrant of her abdomen. Upon pelvic examination, there was right adnexal tenderness. Her WBC is 12 200/mm^3.

The attending physician, uncertain as to whether the patient had acute appendicitis from her personal history or physical examination (clinical manifestations), ordered supine and upright plain X-rays of the abdomen. These showed a relative paucity of bowel gas on the right side of the abdomen. Also, irregularities in the folds of the loop of bowel in the right lower quadrant were observed. There was no sign of an appendicolith or intraperitoneal air. However, several gas–fluid levels were witnessed. All of these signs indicated an inflammatory process in the right lower quadrant resulting from small bowel ileus.

The attending physician also requested an ultrasonogram of the lower right quadrant of the abdomen. The monitor showed a thick, tubular structure that measured approximately 2.2 cm in its outer anteroposterior diameter. The presence of periappendiceal fluid may have represented a perforation. However, the size and location of the tubular structure were consistent with an inflamed appendix.

The patient was scheduled for emergency appendectomy with the diagnosis of appendicitis. The operative findings were consistent with the clinical picture and the pathological diagnosis: acute suppurative appendicitis.

Comment

Up to 70% of the patients with lower right quadrant pain do not have appendicitis. Similar afflictions with similar clinical manifestations are salpingitis, Crohn's disease, bowel obstruction, ureteral calculi, or degenerating uterine leiomyomas. In addition, most cases of acute appendicitis are diagnosed clinically. However, if necessary, ultrasonography or graded compression sonography may be used. The sonographic criteria for acute appendicitis may include: outer anteroposterior diameter of at least 7 mm, mural thickness of 3 mm or more, and the presence of an appendicolith. Periappendiceal abscesses may be drained, under either CT or ultrasonic guidance. Appendectomy and excision of the abscess may be necessary if the response to antibiotic therapy fails.

CHAPTER 22

General surgery

How nausea and vomiting appear in general surgery

In general, nausea and vomiting (NV) reflect altered homeostasis within the circulation (electrolyte imbalance or severe, acute anemia), within the gastrointestinal tract (as with a viral gastroenteritis or diverticulitis), within the peritoneal cavity (as with pelvic inflammatory disease or other peritonitis), or, finally, efferent stimuli from anatomical structures adjacent to the peritoneum or viscus, e.g., the kidney (pyelonephritis) and the ureters (ureteral stones or the bladder). In many cases, NV may be the only findings that indicate a life-threatening situation.

General surgeons are often consulted to assist in establishing the diagnosis of a large variety of conditions signaled by NV. Most of the patients who require the expertise of general surgeons have no prior history of surgically related NV; however, such symptoms may also occur as a result of prior intra-abdominal surgical procedures. Most conditions seen by general surgeons relate to the upper and lower gastrointestinal tracts, and their appendages, the hepatobiliary–pancreatic duct system, and the appendix.

Innervation of the abdomen

To understand NV, one must grasp the innervation of the abdominal organs. The efferent innervation of the abdomen is composed of the sympathetic nervous system (SNS) and the parasysmpathetic nervous system (PNS). These systems provide innervation for the same organs, but have generally opposing activities, e.g., the SNS decreases motility and visceral blood flow and increases sphincter action; the PNS opposes these actions. The parasympathetic fibers originate from the vagus nerves and the pelvic splanchnic nerves.

The SNS arises only from the thoracic spinal cord. The afferent flow from the abdominal viscera is distinct from the above systems.

Clinical scenarios

Surgical conditions associated with NV may reasonably be considered in two groups: those occurring with a 'virginal' abdomen, indicating no prior surgical experience, and those that occur with the 'postsurgical abdomen' (Table 22.1). NV-related conditions may occur independently as new illnesses, or may overlap with prior surgical experiences. For example, an individual with acute pancreatitis may have had a previous laparotomy unrelated to this new condition. The age of the patient, whether infant, child, adult, or older individual, also delineates the types of conditions heralded by NV. Sex is yet another factor that may influence the occurrence, severity, and differential diagnosis of NV. The general surgeon is often called upon to assist with the diagnosis of conditions ultimately attributable to the urinary and the reproductive tracts, particularly in women.

Table 22.1: Surgical conditions associated with NV

'Virgin' abdomen	'Postsurgical' abdomen
Gastritis	Any of the 'virgin' abdomen in column 1
Gallbladder disease	Adynamic ileus
Peritonitis (diverticulitis, etc.)	Anastomotic leak
Congenital defects	Small bowel obstruction; adhesions
Volvulus, intussusception	Large bowel obstruction; adhesions
Traumatic viscus rupture	Abscess
Incarcerated hernias	
Hemorrhagic shock	

An important consideration about NV, associated with the gastroesophageal and upper bowel organs, including the hepatobiliary–pancreatic tracts, is that the lower in the gastrointestinal tract the offending lesion is, the less the likelihood of N. V is not such a reliable indicator as N.

Vomitus: bilious or nonbilious?

With a patient of any age, the nature of vomitus is important for establishing a diagnosis; nonbilious vomitus indicates obstructive lesions proximal to the sphincter of Oddi, whereas bilious vomitus indicates a distal obstruction. This observational finding is particularly important in newborn babies and children who may not be able to describe other clinical components, e.g., N and pain. The corollary finding of abdominal distention assists the clinician in localizing lesions. Malaise and anorexia are the inferred observational equivalents of N in neonates and young children.

Neonates and children

Lesions with nonbilious vomitus

Atresia or narrowing of the esophagus, producing gastroesophageal reflux, possibly in association with a tracheal fistula, is the most commonly occurring surgical lesion of newborn babies who fail to retain feeds. Indeed, the concern for an undiagnosed tracheoesophageal fistula is diminished by the resuscitative efforts of gastric aspiration of newborn babies, and the first feeds of clear fluid to establish normal, nonfenestrated tracts. These lesions result in nonbilious regurgitation, and often, hypersalivation. Another rare lesion producing this observational finding is hypertropic pyloric stenosis, a lesion that develops by weeks 4–6 of life.

Lesions with bilious vomitus

Examples of lesions associated with bilious vomitus are midgut malrotations often with volvulus, meconium ileus, or, occasionally, Meckel's diverticulum. Necrotizing enterocolitis is another condition of the neonatal period, particularly for those born pre-term. Lesions associated with respiratory difficulties always suggest a pulmonary component, as with a diaphragmatic hernia. The greatest and most feared complication of gastroesophageal regurgitation is pulmonary contamination and aspiration pneumonitis.

Older children and adults

Appendicitis is a common, acute, surgical condition of youth, with a peak incidence (6–7%) between the ages of puberty and 25. It remains a thoughtful reminder that the 25% incidence of appendiceal rupture in this age group increases as the age decreases (35–60% below age 10) or increases (50–70% over 50 years), and surgical mortality risk is directly proportional to rupture (Davis et al., 1991). The risk in pregnant women is also elevated because the typical anatomical site of the pain associated with appendicitis rises higher and higher in the abdomen as the pregnancy proceeds, and confuses the diagnosis.

Acute and chronic cholecystitis

Acute cholecystitis is usually characterized by right upper quadrant abdominal pain, V, and fever. Gallstones are found in 95% of these patients. Chronic cholecystitis is usually aggravated by ingestion of fatty foods or alcohol, and is characterized by NV, belching, bloating, and flatulence; pain and fever may also accompany it.

Peptic ulcer disease

The classic symptoms of epigastric distress and dyspepsia relieved by ingestion of food, especially fatty foods, or temporarily by fluids, are not usually accompanied by NV, especially early in the development of the disease process. Only as the ulcerogenic, chronic phase of the condition persists do NV result. This may be the result of the inflammatory nature of progressive disease, and some obstructive consequences. Mostly in modern general surgical practice, the need for surgical duodenal diversions (Bilroth I and II procedures) has become infrequent. Peptic ulcer disease has become the responsibility of generalists, because the condition often responds to medical therapy, including antibiotics.

It is important to distinguish between edema and obstruction caused by a reactivated acute ulcer because scarring from an acute ulcer may require surgical intervention. The two cases can be separated by the use of a nasogastric tube and H_2-receptor blockers. After 5–7 days of this type of therapy, gastric flow rates are reassessed and an operation is the recommended procedure. Finally, intractability of the ulcer suggests the presence of a malignant gastric tumor. Endoscopy with biopsy is a useful tool for reducing the possibility of cancer.

Acute pancreatitis

Back pain is the foremost, early, subjective finding in acute pancreatitis, often aggravated by respiratory actions of coughing or deep breathing. NV, either spontaneous or induced by food, are a consequence of the paralytic ileus that often accompanies pancreatitis. Recurrent acute pancreatitis may indicate the presence of a gallstone in the common biliary duct, a history of alcoholism, or may be caused by a variety of anatomical, metabolic, drug-induced, infectious, or vascular causes.

Gynecological conditions

Advanced ectopic pregnancy is a surgical condition, particularly if the patient has ruptured the fallopian tube and a hemoperitoneum has developed. Such individuals commonly experience NV, in relation to hemorrhagic shock, but also caused by peritoneal 'irritation.' Unruptured ectopic pregnancies may be treated effectively (85–95%) with methotrexate, a folic acid inhibitor used for the treatment of hydatidiform mole, thereby avoiding surgery.

Any cause of hemoperitoneum may provoke NV. Other commonly occurring examples are ruptured ovarian cyst or a bleeding corpus luteum. Patients taking large doses of anti-inflammatory medications, or aspirin, often for chronic pelvic pain, are at risk. The diagnosis of pelvic inflammatory disease occupies a central role in the assessment of pelvic pain with fever, leukorrhea, and often NV. This condition is effectively treated with antibiotic therapy, even in the presence of pelvic abscesses. These are often best approached surgically with laparoscopy, if the diagnosis is uncertain or if intervention becomes necessary because of the failure of antibiotic therapy.

Urological conditions

Ureteral stones typically are characterized by severe flank pain which radiates to the groin, possibly with hematuria. Visceral afferent nerve stimuli effectively provoke NV in most patients. This propensity may be aggravated by the analgesic therapy prescribed. If stones do not pass with smooth muscle-relaxing analgesics, surgical extraction may be required. Acute testicular torsion or other testicular trauma usually causes NV.

Older people

With advancing age, an additional, new set of surgical conditions appears. These include the increasing incidence of intra-abdominal neoplasms and inflammatory lesions. Upper gastrointestinal neoplastic lesions are slow to produce NV as early findings, unless obstructive lesions develop. These may include pancreatic or common biliary duct obstruction, or gastric tumors. Rather, the increasing incidence of ovarian cancer, and the development of diverticulitis and colon cancer, may include N among their rather nonspecific, subjective findings. NV usually appear only late in these diseases, or with complications of bowel perforation or rupture of abscesses or cystic lesions, all producing peritonitis. Ascites is another stimulant of NV.

Postsurgical patients

NV in the postsurgical patient (excluding the immediate postoperative NV attributable to anesthesia) may occur in the short term, as with adynamic ileus, or months or years later. For instance, adhesions may develop after an intra-abdominal procedure, producing a small or large bowel obstruction, with NV as a consequence. Such adhesions, which occur to some degree in 40–60% of all postoperative patients, may 'strangle' the gut and eventually lead to tissue necrosis, rupture of a viscus, and death from sepsis. Thus, immediate medical attention is needed to establish the diagnosis, and relieve the obstruction to allow for normal bowel function.

Differential diagnosis

When the bowels cease peristaltic movement and any forward propulsion of the intestinal contents, the condition is called adynamic or paralytic ileus. The diagnosis of paralytic ileus is often confused with small bowel obstruction because the flow of the contents of the intestine is interrupted. Postoperative ileus may also occur after thoracic operations, indicating a neurogenic cause. Other causes include: extensive body trauma, long bone fracture, potassium deficiency, and thrombosis of the mesenteric vessels. Ileus is thought to be related to the use of anesthetics, the extent and the manner in which the bowel is manipulated during surgery, metabolic disturbances, and sympathetic overactivity. It is accompanied by the gaseous distention of the bowel produced by swallowed air. A dynamic ileus without circulatory impairment or peritonitis is accompanied by decreased bowel sounds, distended abdomen, V, and indications of extracellular fluid loss from fluid secretion into the bowel.

One of the clinical features of ileus is V. This occurs as long as the ileus persists. During pelvic surgery, resection of the colon, retroperitoneal vascular surgery, and genitourinary surgery, injury to the ureter or bladder may occur. Urine leakage from unrecognized injuries (urinoma) or partial or complete ureteral ligation often leads to paralytic ileus and V.

The diagnosis of paralytic ileus can be confirmed with a supine and upright or lateral decubitis X-ray examination. Such analysis will normally indicate the presence of air and fluid levels within the small intestine and colon. Ileus is most common after operative manipulation of the small intestine. However, thoracic and retroperitoneal operations as well as infections of the spine and pelvis carry with them high incidence of ileus.

A general surgeon may be presented with a patient with small bowel obstruction which is almost always accompanied by V. Small bowel obstruction can often be attributed to three main causes: peptic ulcer disease, postoperative adhesions, and malignancy.

Obstruction that occurs as a result of a gastric ulcer normally suggests malignancy. Duodenal ulcers are, however, the normal cause of peptic ulcer obstruction. The clinical signs of obstruction of the small intestine resulting from gastric outlet obstruction that complicates a duodenal ulcer are distention and frequent episodes of V. In addition, obstruction may occur as a result of scarring which results from frequent bouts of the peptic ulcer disease.

The most common source of small bowel obstruction in the USA is intestinal adhesions from previous surgical procedures. In addition, either intrinsic or extrinsic malignancies may be the source of small bowel obstruction. The clinical sign of small bowel obstruction includes feculent vomit, failure to pass gas or feces, and active, high-pitched bowel sounds. Abdominal tenderness is not always present and any rebound tenderness may call for immediate surgery as a result of interference with intestinal blood flow.

The diagnosis of any type of small bowl obstruction is confirmed with X-ray examinations of the abdomen. Air levels may also be observed but are more common in patients who have suffered gastroenteritis and V. However, a barium X-ray may be used if the diagnosis is still unclear. If the barium is seen to pass beyond the cecum, then small bowel obstruction is ruled out. It must be noted, however, that barium by mouth is dangerous in these cases because it may convert a partial large intestinal obstruction into a complete one. Therefore, a barium enema is much safer in diagnosing small bowel obstruction if the flat and upright films, the patient's history, and the physical examination do not delineate the situation. If all results are still inconclusive, computed tomography is likely to yield the final, although expensive, diagnosis.

Peritonitis, another condition that produces V, may be caused by exogenous bacteria including *Pneumococcus* species, β-hemolytic streptococci, or gonococci. Further, secondary peritonitis may result from release of enteric pathogens, *Escherichia coli, Klebsiella* species, or *Proteus* species. Peritonitis can be aseptic as well. Glove powders containing talc or starch, or blood, bile, gastric juice, and pancreatic juices entering the peritoneal cavity, may also cause peritonitis. Secondary peritonitis can result from four contributing factors: postoperative anastomosis failure, diverticulitis, inadvertent bowel perforation during surgical procedures, and abdominal trauma. Postoperative peritonitis is commonly found in resections of the stomach, large and small gut, and pancreas. Resections of the larger intestine are the most common source of postoperative peritonitis as a result of anastomotic leakage from the suture areas. Postoperative peritonitis accounts for about 34% of all cases. Colonic diverticulitis involves the formation of a pseudofistulous tract through the muscle of the sigmoid colon, creating an external pouch. There are two types of diverticulitis: true and false. True diverticulitis involves the pouching of all three layers of the intestine. Meanwhile, false diverticulitis consists of the pouching of only the mucosal and serosal layers. False diverticulitis has a tendency to perforate. In the Western World, because of the lack of fiber in the diet, diverticulitis of the descending colon and rectum is the most common.

The most effective tool for diagnosing diverticulitis is a barium enema. In addition, the perforation of the gut by foreign bodies may also be observed in this fashion (see Chapter 21).

Another possible source of V, although rare, is large bowel obstruction. The large bowel can become obstructed either by a malignancy or volvulus of the colon. In both cases, a barium enema should reveal the appropriate diagnosis. X-rays may also be used and the presence of volvulus may produce a kidney bean-shaped pocket of air in the upper left quadrant of cecal volvulus and a coffee bean-shaped air collection in the right upper quadrant in the case of sigmoid volvulus. One must also be careful not to confuse ovarian cancer with volvulus because many of the same clinical symptoms appear.

Priorities and procedures

Nasogastric decompression is the primary treatment of ileus after surgery. Intravenous fluids are used to reverse the metabolic and electrolyte abnormalities, and provide for intrinsic losses. Narcotic substances or opiates should be discontinued as such agents are likely to contribute to the ileus. The removal of the large pocket of air from the colon can be achieved with a rectal tube. Finally, the compound metoclopramide can, in some cases, stimulate the neuromuscular coordination in the mesenteric and submucosal plexus with resultant peristalsis.

Peptic ulcer obstruction of the small bowel is traditionally observed for 5–7 days under nasogastric tube and treatment with

H_2-receptor blockers. If the barium radiograph indicates that the obstruction has remained, surgery is immediate. The types of surgery applicable to this illness include vagectomy, gastro-enterostomy, pyloroplasty, gastrectomy, and partial cell vagotomy. All of these procedures involve manipulation of the stomach and intestine in order to remove the portion of the stomach or duodenum responsible for the recurring ulcer and blockage of the small intestine.

Foregut obstruction usually requires operative intervention. Midgut obstruction can often be improved with intestinal intubation which removes air and accumulated fluid, providing relief of the distention. Acute inflammatory adhesions are frequently treated with this method. Patients with chronic adhesive obstruction may also be converted to a partial obstruction so the intestinal tract seems to function properly. However, it is important to remember that other types of intestinal obstruction are not as easily reduced by intubation and suction. In these cases, as with nonstrangulated mechanical obstruction, surgery becomes unavoidable.

Treatment for peritonitis depends on the exact cause of the illness. If postoperative peritonitis is the cause and internal leakage is found, steps must be taken to stop it. These include:

1. Excision of the anastomosis site and primary repair
2. Colostomy
3. Suction drainage of the anatomical region.

Nonsurgical treatment for peritonitis is less complicated. In the case of a perforated diverticulitis, if the septic process is localized, the patient should receive nothing by mouth. In addition, nasogastric suction is used to prevent the distention of the bowel by swallowed air. Intravenous fluids are used to maintain appropriate hydration levels. Antibiotics such as gentamicin and clindamycin may be used and white blood cell count, temperature, and abdominal findings are monitored. In the case of any free peritoneal air developing from abdomen or chest X-rays, early operation is strongly advised.

Volvulus of the colon is treated with a laparotomy and a right hemicolectomy. Malignancies identified must be excised with a partial colectomy and node dissection.

Case study

A 67-year-old man came to the emergency room with rectal bleeding and NV. A single-contrast barium enema showed a solitary, smoothly marginated filling defect of the ileocecal valve region. There was no apparent mucosal irregularity and the barium showed a normal looking appendix and distal ileum. The mass was probably a neoplasm of the ileocecal valve, a rare cause of small intestine obstruction. The smooth margins as well as the absence of mucosal irregularity hinted at a submucosal tumor. Lipomatous hyperplasia of the ileocecal valve is an incidental finding of a barium enema. It is more common in women and in patients less than 40 years old. An abdominal CT scan may be helpful for diagnosis.

CHAPTER 23

Hematology

Nausea and vomiting (NV) occur occasionally as a sign or symptom of a hematological disease. Hematological conditions that are associated with NV may be congenital or acquired, life threatening or transient. However, NV themselves are rarely a serious danger for the hematology patient, aside from problems encountered as a result of dehydration, alkalosis, etc. The following is an examination of the most common conditions within hematology that precipitate an NV response.

Acute intermittent porphyria and variegate porphyria

Porphyrias are caused by inherited defects in enzymes of the heme synthetic pathways. There are seven causes of porphyrias – all of which involve deficient enzymes that are transmitted genetically. The porphyric causes that have neurovisceral manifestations include acute intermittent porphyria (AIP), which is the most common variety, variegate porphyria, which is most common in South Africans of Dutch ancestry, 5δ-aminolevulinate (ALA) dehydratase deficiency which has been found in only four patients to date and manifested only in homozygotes, and coproporphyria, which is uncommon. In this text, we consider only the two most common acute porphyrias with neurovisceral symptoms: AIP and variegate porphyria.

Clinical manifestations of acute porphyrias include neurovisceral and psychiatric deficits. An acute attack, usually characterized by an autonomic neuropathy, causes abdominal pain, V, constipation, and segmental intestinal spasm. Other common symptoms include tachycardia, labile hypertension, and urinary retention. The link between these symptoms and their biological mechanisms remains unclear, although three biosynthetic mechanisms have been outlined (see the third point):

- block in heme synthesis leads to
- critical heme deficiency which leads to
- increase in tryptophan from liver, or increase in ALA synthase which increases ALA, or increase in neuronal adenosine triphosphate (ATP) production, which leads to
- neuronal dysfunction, and to
- neurovisceral symptoms.

The clinical expression of porphyria is variable, and genetic, metabolic, and environmental factors may contribute to its expression. Clinical attacks of acute porphyria occur rarely, if ever, before puberty and are more common in women.

Hormonal, nutritional, and pharmacological agents may precipitate acute porphyric attacks. Gonadal hormones, especially the 5β-steroids (e.g., etiocholanolone), and androgenic or progestational ovarian hormones and their metabolites, can induce hepatic ALA synthase activity, worsening the metabolic abnormality. Some women are prone to attacks during the luteal phase of the menstrual cycle (high progesterone). Oral contraceptives with their large doses of progestational hormones, some androgenic, may worsen porphyric symptoms in some women, or may be used as preventive therapy for others. Likewise, pregnancy may aggravate the porphyria, have no effect, or temporarily remedy its symptoms.

Barbiturates, phenytoin, estrogen preparations, ethanol excess, griseofulvin, mephenytoin, meprobamate, sulfonamides, and valproic acid are among the drugs considered unsafe for patients with AIP or variegate porphyria. Barbiturates and sulfonamides can precipitate porphyric attacks because they increase the need for hepatocellular heme to metabolize the drug.

Treatment of acute attacks remained limited until recently. In the past, AIP and variegate patients with neurological abnormalities had a 30% mortality rate, but now, with supportive care and intravenous hematin (ferric heme), the mortality rate in patients with neurological symptoms is reduced to 10%.

Most often, hospital treatment of patients suffering an acute attack consists of morphine analgesia, and NV symptom control during the first 24 hours with phenothiazines and chlorpromazine 325 mg, four times a day. Carbohydrates are given orally or IV (300–500 g glucose/day; high carbohydrates can prevent experimental porphyria in rats). If no improvement is apparent in the patient's condition within 24 hours, IV hematin, which suppresses ALA synthase activity, is administered in a dose of 4 mg/kg body weight every 12 hours.

Prevention of attacks consists mainly of avoiding drugs known to be unsafe. Fasting should also be avoided. In women whose attacks are menstrually regulated, oral contraceptives may be used to suppress ovulation. However, as previously mentioned, oral contraceptives can worsen symptoms in some women. Another preventive measure is use of a long-acting gonadotropin-releasing hormone (GnRH) agonist to suppress ovulation, and the production of progesterone and its 5β metabolites, using low-dose, add-back therapy with estrogen.

Acute intermittent porphyria

Also known as AIP, pyrroloporphyria, and Swedish porphyria, this porphyria is a dominantly inherited trait located on chromosome 11 which results in half-normal activity of pyrrole porphobilinogen (PBG) deaminase. Both PBG deaminase and ALA synthase are important regulatory enzymes in the heme biosynthetic pathway. Thus, the deficient function of PBG deaminase results in accumulation of its substrate, PBG, which leads to a deficit of cellular heme. The lack of sufficient heme supply induces ALA synthase which only serves to increase the accumulation of porphyrin precursors. The substrates, ALA and PBG, are excreted into the plasma and bile, and ultimately in the urine.

This genetic defect is distributed equally between the sexes, but 60–75% of those with the clinically active type of AIP are women. First symptoms usually occur in the third or fourth decade of life, but symptoms may present immediately after puberty or even late in life. From 1.5 to 10 per 100 000 people are affected by AIP, and the condition is most common in Scandinavia, Britain, and Ireland.

Most individuals with AIP do not develop symptoms. Some experience acute attacks of mental, abdominal, and neurological symptoms, which may last several days to several months (with latent periods), and which are probably related to the disease's effect on the nervous system. Acute attacks consist of an acute painful crisis associated with autonomic dysfunction. These attacks usually begin with abdominal pain, which is described as moderate to severe in degree, crampy and colicky, either generalized, periumbilical, or localized in the lower abdominal quadrants, and often accompanied by constipation and V. Mild-to-moderate weakness in the upper extremities and proximal musculature may also be noted. Respiratory problems and sinus tachycardia are common. All cranial nerves may be involved; blindness has resulted from both optic nerve and occipital lobe involvement, but sensory abnormalities are less common. Autonomic neuropathic manifestations include hypertension, postural hypotension, inappropriate sweating, and bladder distention. Mental symptoms resemble toxic delirium; symptoms include hallucination, confusion, and acute anxiety attacks. Tonic–clonic seizures appear in about 20% patients with a severe attack. Depression and suicidal tendencies may follow the attack. Severe attacks are associated with peripheral motor neuropathy and can progress to truncal and cranial nerve involvement, delirium, seizures, coma, and death (usually by respiratory paralysis).

Chronic lymphocytic leukemia (CLL)

Leukemia, in general, is a group of diseases characterized by neoplastic proliferation of one or more of the blood-forming cellular elements. CLL most commonly affects elderly and middle-aged people. It is a disease characterized by the accumulation, rather than overproduction, of long-lived, mainly B-cell lymphocytes in the blood, lymphoid organs, and bone marrow. Mild-to-severe immunological dysfunction, usually in the form of hypogammaglobulinemia, results, sometimes accompanied by autoimmune hemolytic anemia and increasingly delayed hypersensitivity reactions (i.e., to insect bites). On average, patients do not experience initial symptoms until 4 years after the onset of disease processes.

Malaise is the most common symptom experienced. This symptom may commonly be accompanied by fatiguability, loss of appetite and weight, low fever, and night sweats.

Hypercalcemia in multiple myeloma

Multiple myeloma typically involves the bone marrow and is a malignancy of the plasma cells in which several lines proliferate to produce a specific protein as if they are constantly stimulated. The cause of multiple myeloma is unknown.

Hypercalcemia can accompany multiple myeloma and cause the following symptoms: N, V, apathy, weakness, polydipsia, polyuria, anorexia, confusion, constipation, stupor, and coma. Hypercalcemia is also often accompanied by renal insufficiency and dehydration.

Treatment of hypercalcemia can include rehydration therapy, calcitonin, gallium nitrate, aminohydroxypropylidene bisphosphonate, and hemodialysis using a low-calcium dialysate.

NV triggered by hypercalcemia as a result of hyperparathyroidism may be found in Chapter 20.

Acute lymphocytic leukemia (ALL)

ALL is the most common malignant disease affecting children: it makes up 30% of all childhood cancers. The highest incidence of ALL is among children aged 1–5, although it can affect any age group. This form of leukemia is more common among white children, and among boys (57%).

The most common symptoms of ALL are fatiguability, lethargy (both caused by anemia), fever (probably a result of the leukemic process itself because there is no infectious agent), and bone and joint pain (from erosion of bones and leukemic processes in periosteum, or by bone marrow necrosis). A small number of patients complain of headaches and V (about 1%) resulting from the leukemia affecting the central nervous system (CNS). Reduced numbers of leukocytes and increased numbers of white blood cells are characteristic.

Infiltration of organs as a complication of hemopoietic neoplasm

The leukemias, lymphomas, myelomas, and related diseases cause morbidity and mortality through three general mechanisms:

(1) deficit in normal cell number or function
(2) invasion of vital organs with impairment of organ function, and
(3) systemic disturbances as manifested by weight loss, pruritus, or metabolic alteration, such as hypercalcemia.

The CNS, spinal cord, and cranial and peripheral nerves can be affected by infiltrating or compressing tumors. For example, patients with acute lymphocytic anemia (ALA) often suffer from infiltration of the cerebral leptomeninges by lymphoblasts. Other areas that can also be infiltrated include the spinal meninges and cranial nerve sheaths. Manifestations appear as perivascular infiltration of the meningeal vessels, or perivascular infiltration of the intracerebral vessels (less common).

Signs and symptoms of this infiltration include headaches, lethargy, and NV. The symptoms are mainly those resulting from increased intracranial pressure.

Infectious mononucleosis

Infectious mononucleosis is caused by the Epstein–Barr virus (EBV), a DNA family virus. EBV is also associated with lymphoproliferative diseases, nasopharyngeal carcinoma, African Burkitt's lymphoma, and other non-Hodgkin's lymphomas.

The incubation period of the virus is not known precisely, but can range from 33 to 49 days. Symptom onset is abrupt and includes excessive fatigue, general malaise, and perhaps even feverishness, sweating, and chills. Anorexia is also an early, common symptom accompanied by a sore throat and dysphagia. N is as common as anorexia (50–70%); however, V is rare. Smoking may precipitate attacks of N, and smokers often develop an aversion to cigarettes when infected with EBV. Some patients have vague abdominal distress, including discomfort in the upper left quadrant when active. Diarrhea is uncommon, but a small minority complain of soft stools. Headaches also occur early and may be retro-orbital. Most patients recover fully by 2 months, though there is the potential for fatal complications (about 1 in 3000).

No specific therapy is recommended for infectious mononucleosis. Adrenocorticosteroids may have a dramatic effect in the reduction of fever and lymphatic hyperplasia. Steroid therapy can also be used for patients with complications such as hemolytic anemia, immune thrombocytopenia, progressive neurological complications, and incipient airway obstructions. Aspirin makes recovery slower. The primary goal for recovery is to preserve immune system function.

Acute iron intoxication

Symptoms of acute iron intoxication occur in four stages:

- Gastrointestinal symptoms such as V, diarrhea, and melena followed by shock as well as dyspnea, lethargy, and coma; all occur within the first 6 hours.
- Six to 24 hours after ingestion, transient improvement occurs.
- Metabolic acidosis and death may occur within 12–48 hours of ingestion.

- Intestinal obstruction occurs as a complication of intestinal scarring.

These stages are caused by the local irritative action of iron which causes mucosal bleeding and ulceration. Other signs of acute iron intoxication include capillary dilation and diapedesis of red blood cells. Shock may have one of several causes, including the absorption of iron in amounts exceeding the plasma's binding capacity. The cause of metabolic acidosis is uncertain. Coma is caused by hypoxia, metabolic disturbances, and hepatic damage.

Therapy of iron intoxication utilizes deferoxamine, which binds the excess iron.

Acute mountain sickness

The incidence of acute mountain sickness is higher among younger people as well as among those who fly to high altitudes (7500–10 000 feet), spend little time acclimatizing, and ultimately reach higher altitudes. Symptoms include fatigue, dizziness, pulsating headache, NV, insomnia, anorexia, and irritability. These symptoms usually first appear 4–6 hours after rapid ascent to high altitudes; however, symptoms may appear as much as 96 hours later. Progression of the symptoms to confusion, coma, and death related to pulmonary edema may ensue but can be prevented by returning to low altitude. Acute mountain sickness may involve hypoxia, but is not caused solely by hypoxia. Excessive secretion of antidiuretic hormone (ADH) and adrenal steroids, with increased fluid retention, increased blood volume, and cerebral edema and/or pulmonary congestion, may also by noted. Symptoms can be mitigated by the use of diuretics such as acetazolamide or furosemide. Dexamethasone is also effective.

Prevention of acute mountain sickness includes spending several days acclimatizing to higher and higher altitudes. The physiological processes of acclimatization are not fully understood but probably include the following:

- an increase in erythrocyte 2,3-diphosphoglycerate (2,3-DPG) levels, with a shift to the right in the oxygen–hemoglobin dissociation curve
- an increase in plasma and urinary erythropoietin levels, in plasma iron turnover, reticulocytosis, and in red cell mass and blood volume
- a subsidence of original excessive ADH and adrenal steroid

secretion followed by a return to the normal diurnal variation of plasma steroid levels

These three mechanisms would thereby increase alveolar ventilation, respiratory frequency, and red cell mass.

Autoerythrocyte sensitization and related disorders

Autoerythrocyte sensitization is one of various forms of purpuras. Although the condition itself is uncommon, NV are a common symptom of autoerythrocyte sensitization. The disease is characterized by spontaneous painful ecchymoses, lesions surrounded by erythema and edema, and associated symptoms of headache and NV. Occasionally intracranial, genitourinary, and gastrointestinal bleeding occur. With an enigmatic etiology, one hypothesis purports that the purpura is the result of autosensitization to some component of the red cell membrane. In many clinical patients, this autosensitization is related to a history of severe injury with bruising; in others, it is related to severe emotional trauma.

Autoerythrocyte sensitization almost exclusively affects middle-aged women. Some hypothesize emotional factors in its pathogenesis. Findings supporting this conjecture include data that these patients have a propensity to express emotional problems in a physical form through both hysterical mechanisms and psychophysiological reactions. Other patients manifested a prominent element of masochism in their character. Purpuric bouts were found to occur at times of emotional stress. Psychological testing revealed a remarkably uniform personality pattern characterized by difficulty in handling aggressive feeling as and by other features that favor the view that this condition may be psychosomatic in nature. In some patients, purpura apparently was induced by hypnotic suggestion.

In the related disorder of DNA autosensitivity, the ecchymoses are found only on the extremities and can by produced by intradermal injections of a suspension of the patient's leukocytes or a solution of DNA. This condition, localized to the extremities, reflects hypersensitivity to DNA specifically.

Unfortunately, no treatment for either disorder exists. Corticosteroids and antihistamines have no effect, and psychotherapy seldom has a permanent effect. Patients with DNA autosensitivity can be treated with chloroquine and primaquine (250 mg four times daily, followed by 250–500 mg daily), or hydroxychloroquine with a good response. Relapse, however, follows with cessation of drug therapy.

Antibiotic prophylaxis

Antibiotics are sometimes used in treating patients with neutropenia. With the goal of selectively decontaminating the gastrointestinal tract of patients, health care practitioners administered oral non-absorbable antibiotics, such as colistin, kanamycin, or gentamicin. The antibiotics are only partially effective in reducing the host bacterial load and result in significant NV and diarrhea.

CHAPTER 24
Infectious diseases

'Infectious diseases' are caused by microbial agents or constituents of microorganisms and encompass a diverse spectrum of diseases. The main paths by which an infectious agent or microbial factors can enter the body include: inhalation, a common vehicle (e.g., water, food, needles), contact (e.g., sexual), and if vector borne (e.g., arthropod). Regardless of the acquisition, once the microorganism or microbial factors are present, there are two general methods of pathogenesis of disease. In one process, the microorganism colonizes the host's tissue. Thereafter, it begins to multiply and can eventually cause tissue damage if sufficient noxious factors or microbial agents directly affect the host's structure and function. There are myriad numbers of microbial pathogens that can affect all organ systems (e.g., the gastrointestinal tract, the respiratory system, the reproductive system). The other method does not require live microbial agents to cause disease. The basis for infection with diseases by non-activated microbial agents requires host exposure to microbial toxins. In this case, it is the toxin that causes the tissue damage rather than the organism itself. The manifestations or the host response to an infectious agent depends on numerous factors including quantitative factors (e.g., amount of toxin or the number of organisms), the site of infection, and the immunological status of the host. As the range of infection can be very broad (e.g., viral gastroenteritis, bacterial meningitis, scarlet fever), it is not surprising that infections can be manifested as an asymptomatic state to moribund status. Overt clinical manifestations are present only when there has been sufficient tissue damage response.

Nausea and vomiting (NV) are two of the most visible and common consequences of infectious diseases. There is, however, no typical form of NV to differentiate one infectious disease from another. This is because there is a common mechanism for stimulating them, irrespective of whether the cause is an infectious disease or not. NV are merely the result of the stimulation of the emetic center in the central nervous system (CNS). Stimulation of emesis can occur by a variety of noxious insults, including exposure to toxins in the blood, neural signals from the gut via the enteric nervous system, or increased cranial pressure as a consequence of mass effects (e.g., neoplastic process).

Establishing a differential diagnosis

NV are, in themselves, nonspecific symptoms of infectious disease. Therefore, they offer no definitive diagnostic clues for a physician to make a diagnosis of the cause of illness. In most cases of infectious disease, it is impossible to make a specific diagnosis on clinical evidence alone. To obtain an accurate diagnosis, biochemical, microbiological, and histological testing of both host tissues and body fluids is essential. The prerequisite for a rational process to make a diagnosis requires a thorough patient history. This must include details about all symptoms (e.g., onset, duration, frequency, and severity), as well as recent activities (e.g., hobbies such as having animals), dietary habits, occupation, and possible exposure to other ill individuals. Obtaining a thorough background can provide helpful clues as to what infectious agent a patient may have been exposed to and acquired. Although NV are nonspecific manifestations of many diseases, there are several classic examples that help to describe certain types of infectious disease illnesses.

Food-borne disease

Food-borne diseases make up an estimated 9,000,000 illnesses a year in the USA. They are caused by the ingestion of foods contaminated with microbial toxins, chemicals, or pathogenic microorganisms. In the case of a food-borne disease, knowledge about what food the patient ingested in the last 72 hours is extremely helpful, especially if two or more people shared the same meal and are both presenting themselves with gastrointestinal and/or neurological manifestations.

If a patient suffers from NV within 1–6 hours of a meal, the disease has probably been caused by preformed enterotoxins. Enterotoxins produced by *Staphylococcus aureus* and *Bacillus cereus* are the most common causes of toxin-induced NV. Close to 80% of individuals intoxicated by the enterotoxin *S. aureus* suffer from V and diarrhea after recent ingestion of contaminated ham, poultry, potato, or egg salads, or cream-filled pastries. Patients intoxicated with *B. cereus* enterotoxin suffer from NV after recent ingestion of fried rice, meats, or vegetables.

Table 24.1: Common diseases that cause NV

Organism	Disease
Bacteria	Cholera Bacterial meningitis Botulism Helicobacteriosis Nontyphoidal salmonelloses Scarlet fever Typhus fevers Relapsing fever Yersiniosis Diarrheagenic *Escherichia coli* Staphylococcal enterotoxin *Bacillus cereus* enterotoxin
Rickettsia	Colorado tick fever Ehrlichiosis Rat bite fever Rocky Mountain spotted fever Rickettsiosis spotted fever
Virus	Viral meningoencephalitis Viral gastroenteritis Common 'flu AIDS Influenza Ebola Lassa fever Hepatitis A Dengue fever
Fungus	Blastomycosis Candidiasis
Parasitic	Intestinal nematodiasis Amebiasis Giardiasis Visceral larva migrans Larval cestodiasis Fascioliasis Intestinal cestodes

If a patient is suffering from fever, abdominal cramps, diarrhea, and V within 16–48 hours of ingestion of food, the disease is more likely to result from eating food contaminated by live salmonellae, shigellae, *Campylobacter jejuni*, *Vibrio parahaemolyticus*, and enteropathogenic *Escherichia coli* strains. In such cases, the microorganism survives transit through the stomach. Thereafter, they attach to enterocytes in the small intestine, colonize the mucosal surface, multiply, and affect enterocytes directly by invasion or indirectly by the *de novo* elaboration of enterotoxins. Salmonella poisoning often results after the ingestion of contaminated beef, poultry, eggs, or dairy products, whereas shigellae are more often associated with the ingestion of contaminated potato or egg salads and other cool, moist foods. In general, foods likely to be contaminated by bacteria that cause diarrhea and NV include: poorly cooked beef and poultry, all unpasteurized dairy products, and raw shellfish and other sea food.

If a patient is suffering from NV, diarrhea, and paralysis within 18–36 hours of the ingestion of food, the patient is most likely suffering from food-borne botulism. The NV usually occur at the onset of illness and are followed by a relentless pattern of descending weakness or paralysis. Food-borne botulism is caused by the ingestion of preformed neurotoxins produced by the spores of clostridium botulism.

A patient suffering from abdominal cramps, severe watery diarrhea, and V within 16–72 hours of the ingestion of food or drink is most probably suffering from cholera. This disease is caused by enterotoxins produced in vivo by *Vibrio cholerae* 01 strains. The V may last for up to 5 days and is characterized by abrupt projectile vomiting in the absence of any N. Cholera may last for up to 12 days, although it will usually resolve itself within 72–96 hours.

A patient suffering from abdominal cramps, mild fever, V, and some watery diarrhea within 16–72 hours of food ingestion may be suffering from viral gastroenteritis. There are several strains of viral agents that cause gastroenteritis: including common agents such as the Norwalk viruses, calicivirus, astrovirus, enterovirus, and enteric adenovirus. Viral gastroenteritis is commonly referred to as the 'intestinal 'flu' and usually resolves within 24–48 hours after the onset of symptoms.

Water-borne disease

Although food is often the carrier of pathogenic microorganisms, water can serve as an equally efficient vehicle for transmission. *Giardia lamblia* is one of the most common pathogens transmitted by contaminated water in the USA. It is especially prevalent among the campers and backpackers of the mountainous western USA. The disease can have an incubation period of up to 4 weeks. Giardiasis is characterized by abdominal cramps, bloating, diarrhea, and less so by NV. Also, many food-borne diseases can be transmitted through contaminated water. These include: shigellae, hepatitis A, non-typhoidal salmonellae, and cholera.

Miscellaneous and vector-borne disease

The diseases mentioned previously are classic prototype infectious diseases transmitted via contaminated food or water. However, most other food-borne diseases have less well-defined symptoms. Many parasitic infestations are asymptomatic, even among heavily infected individuals. When symptoms are present, they are usually vague and can consist of abdominal pain, N, a feeling of weakness, and intermittent diarrhea. Common examples of poorly defined parasitic illnesses associated with N include: intestinal cestodiases (tapeworms), intestinal nematodiasis (whipworm), and amebiasis (*Entamoeba histolytica*). In these cases, a microscopic examination of a stool sample is necessary for a diagnosis because the clinical manifest-ations are not pathognomonic for a specific microbial agent.

Vector-borne diseases frequently arise after a host has been bitten by a carrier (e.g., tick, mite, or rat). The most prominent symptom in many of these cases is fever, and not NV. A few examples of vector-borne illness in which NV do constitute a common feature of the illness include: Colorado tick fever, rat-bite fever, ehrlichiosis, relapsing fever, Boutonneuse fever, Rocky Mountain spotted fever, Dengue fever, and typhus fevers.

There are thousands of infectious diseases and the number and variety are continually growing as new pathogens are recognized. NV are two very common consequences of many different types of disease. Table 24.1 gives a list of infectious diseases that can cause NV and the antimicrobial agents that can also produce NV.

Management of NV

Even though NV are the symptoms for a very broad spectrum of infectious diseases, the treatment is similar for all of them. The first step in treatment should be to treat the underlying agent and, subsequently, the NV will be treated as well. Almost all food-borne diseases, with the exception of botulism, are self-limiting and it is necessary to allow the NV to run their course. This is also true with viruses, such as viral gastroenteritis, which cannot be treated with antibiotics and have no specific therapy. Regardless of the situation, hydration and maintenance of electrolyte balance are imperative. The optimal way to treat any associated NV is to keep the patient comfortable while administering oral fluids and glucose solutions. In extreme cases (e.g., botulism), enemas or cathartics may be administered to remove any unabsorbed toxins from the intestines. If V is unremitting, an antiemetic can be prescribed in conjunction with the disease therapy. If a patient has incessant V and cannot retain any liquids in the stomach, intravenous therapy, and even hospitalization, may be necessary. Ideally, the best care to give a patient is supportive care, making them as comfortable as possible while maintaining hydration and treating the underlying disease.

It is also common that the treatments for many diseases have the adverse side effects of NV. The management of this type of NV is also the same as mentioned above, namely, supportive care. If the clinician has the option of discontinuing the drug causing the adverse effects and trying a different one, then that measure should be taken. Table 24.2 lists all the antimicrobial agents that have N and/or V associated with their administration.

Case study

The patient was a 20-year-old Stanford coed with no chronic medical problems. She attended a picnic party celebrating the end of the school year on a hot Saturday afternoon. She ate a hamburger grilled on the barbecue, as well as green salad and potato salad. Shc complained of abdominal cramps and severe NV about 2 hours after attending the party. She had no bowel movements and did not feel feverish. She is unable to keep any fluids down over a 3-hour period and then proceeded to have a friend take her to the emergency room where she saw six other party members with similar complaints. On physical examination, she appeared to be in distress and was frequently observed about to vomit into a bowl. Her vital measurements were:

- BP: 110/80
- Chest: normal
- Neurology: normal
- Respiratory rate: 18
- Head, eyes, ears, nose, and throat: normal

Table 24.2: Commonly used antimicrobials likely to cause NV

Antimicrobal	Agent	NV	Comments
Antibiotics	Erythromycin	NV N	Frequently the result of oral administration
	Tetracyclines	N NV	Intravenous administration does not cause NV
	Sulfonamides	NV N	Most common with oxytetracycline dose
	β-Lactams:		Both oral and parenteral route
	penicillins	N	Associated with fast infusion
	cephalosporins	NV	Most common if renal failure present
	monobactams, imipenem	NV NV	Most common if orally administered
	Quinolines:		Only parenteral administration
	norfloxacin		Only parenteral administration
	ciprofloxacin, enoxacin		Only with oral administration on an empty stomach
Antifungals	Amphotericin B	NV	Associated with intravenous infusion
	Ketoconazole	NV	Especially with underlying gastric motility problems
	Flucytosine	V	Associated with oral administration
	Griseofulvin	NV	Associated with oral administration
Antivirals	Acyclovir	NV	Worse with renal failure
	Vidarabine	NV	Oral administration
	Zidovudine	NV	Oral administration

- Heart rate: 100 bpm
- Heart: normal
- Abdomen: hyperactive, bowel sounds, mildly tender, but soft and no rebound.
- Laboratory:
  - Na^+: 135 mmol/l
  - creatinine: 2.0 mmol/l
  - K^+: 3.0 mmol/l
  - blood urea nitrogen: 80
  - Cl^-: 100 mmol/l
  - WBC: 8000/mm^3 (no shift)
  - HbB: 14.5 g.

Impression

In the setting of NV within 2–8 hours of food ingestion, especially of salad foods with mayonnaise, and of other party members having similar symptoms, the physician assumed that the likely diagnosis was staphylococcal enterotoxin intoxication. Treatment was intravenous fluids for moderate dehydration because the patient was unable to take fluids by mouth. In addition, a mild antiemetic (promethazine) was administered to control V, after leaving the emergency room, once rehydrated.

CHAPTER 25

Neurology

In the field of neurology, nausea and vomiting (NV) are prominent symptoms in a variety of disorders. However, even with its rather common occurrence, neurology textbooks yield surprisingly little information on NV. From the limited information available, Table 25.1 presents a list of neurological disorders associated with emesis.

How is neurology associated with NV?

Severe pain

Acutely occurring, severe pain is often associated with emesis. As indicated in Table 25.1, events such as myocardial infarction and other painful episodes are frequently described as inducing NV. This is also true in cases of extreme headaches which may result from intracranial bleeding or from classic migraine headaches.

Table 25.1: Neurological disorders commonly accompanied by emesis

Intense pain	Central disorders
Neuropathic pain	Intracranial hypertension
Tabes dorsalis	Meningitis, tumor, hydrocephalus
Thalamic pain	Fourth ventricle lesions
Headache	Tumor, cyst
Migraine	Brain stem ischemia, hemorrhage, tumors
Closed head injury	
Spontaneous intracranial hemorrhage	Cerebellopontine angle tumor
Cluster headache	Miscellaneous
Muscle tension headache	Periodic cyclic V

Neoplasms

Tumor formation often leads to elevated intracranial pressure because the growing tumor is too large for the brain tissue and the skull to accommodate. Tumors provoke edema, leading to increased volume and hence increased pressure. The increased pressure may then lead to direct stimulation of the medullary centers, obstruction of the cerebrospinal fluid (CSF) circulation, or deformation of the brain stem, all of which can result in V. However, in cases of severely increased intracranial pressure, there may be inhibition of V. For tumors occurring at the floor of the fourth ventricle and surrounding structures, i.e., the area postrema, V is especially prevalent, because the structures around those areas are believed to be important for V. Accordingly, surgical damage to the floor of the fourth ventricle may result in protracted emesis, or may also inhibit intractable V.

Intracranial bleeding

Along with brain tumors, intracranial bleeding can lead to elevated intracranial pressures and trigger NV. For patients with brain tumors, such as those resulting from the von Hippel–Lindau disease, V is usually preceded by headaches. N is more often prevalent than V, which only occurs in about a third of the tumor patients. However, for patients with tumors of the posterior fossa, NV are particularly more frequent.

NV also occur during the onset of subarachnoid hemorrhage, when the leakage is considerable and the chance of the patient losing consciousness high. Coma patients have also been commonly observed to experience V. For NV not resulting from obvious peripheral stimuli, such as pain, ingestion of emetics, gastrointestinal disorders, or vestibular dysfunction, the term 'central V' has been coined. Those occurrences of NV often result from abnormal intracranial pressure, fourth ventricle lesions, and other causes.

Migraine headaches

Migraine headaches are a common cause of NV. Emesis often occurs about an hour after the onset, especially during the painful phase of the migraine, with N prominent throughout the whole migraine attack. It appears that V somewhat relieves the migraine – in classic migraine the headache usually disappears after emesis. N is also more prevalent than V; in a 1995 study (Silberstein, 1995) of 500 patients, over 90% developed N whereas only 70% vomited. Migraines in childhood may be associated with cyclical V.

Emotional causes

Other occurrences of NV in neurological disorders include hysterical V. Hysterical V refers to V in hysteria or other abnormal illness behavior. The patient often vomits after a meal and is left hungry, resulting in weight loss and pain in the lower abdomen, which often leads to unnecessary appendectomies and pelvic organ removal in young women. Not much is known about the cause, but hysterical V may be induced by unpleasant circumstances and may last for weeks. It is not known whether the patient has voluntary control over the V, nor is there any mention of concurrent N. Perhaps a link can be drawn to induced V for bulimic patients.

Intoxication

In a more familiar guise, NV can result from intoxication; severe intake of alcohol will sometimes result in NV for patients. NV are also initial symptoms of chloral hydrate intoxication. The inhalation, ingestion, or injection of arsenic also produces NV.

Vertigo/vestibular dysfunction or neoplasia

In vertigo/vestibular dizziness and associated neurological diseases, NV are associated. From studies in this area, the dorsolateral reticular formation is believed to be important for NV. Vertigo, a particular type of dizziness, is the only kind that has a common NV association. Neurological V is usually accompanied by vertigo but lesions close to the floor of the fourth ventricle are sometimes likely to give rise to positional V without vertigo. Another disease with N associated is vestibular neuronitis, vertigo of abrupt onset. As vertigo is often related to the functioning of the inner ear, dysfunction of the labyrinthine (inner ear), vestibulocochlear nerve, or vestibular nucleus also causes vertigo with N and nystagmus. Ménière's disease, a recurrent vertigo syndrome in which there are recurrent attacks of severe giddiness, usually leads to V and the development of severe N. It is found that the NV last as long as the patient remains very giddy. Another kind of V, 'effortless V,' may be seen in those with severe diabetic autonomic neuropathy.

Establishing the diagnosis

For the diagnosis of tumors, repetitive V in the early hours should raise suspicion of an intracranial mass. V of this nature is not usually related to liquid or food ingestion, often occurring before breakfast. Also, V generally correlates with the severity of headache and the presence of raised intracranial pressure. Some patients suffer from both NV, whereas others (usually children) vomit forcibly without preceding N (known as projectile V). Some patients say that V sometimes helps relieve some of the headache, whereas others claim that V increases intracranial pressure and worsens the headache. Specifically in children, V is associated with headache, which is indicative of elevated intracranial pressure. It is unusual for V to occur in children without other signs of raised intracranial pressure.

For hydrocephalus, the following indications apply. V may occur in a very young baby or child, but it is difficult to evaluate because it is rarely explosive or projectile. In children less than 6 years old, V associated with a headache is a reliable indicator of elevated intracranial pressure.

Table 25.2: Drugs and treatment for common causes of NV

Example	Possible mechanism	Treatment used
Digitalis	Stimulation of chemoreceptor mechanisms	Dopamine antagonists
Levodopa		
Apomorphine		
Ménière's disease	Stimulation of labyrinthine mechanisms	Anticholinergic drugs
Anxiety, high emotion	Cortical stimulation	Benzodiazepines
Cerebral hemorrhage, tumor	Increased intracranial pressure	Prednisolone
	Stimulation of abdominal afferents	Pyridoxine
Migraine	Central and gastric effects	Gastrokinetic antagonist, e.g., domperidone, metoclopramide

Most dopamine-like drugs used in the treatment of Parkinson's disease cause V whereas dopamine antagonists are mostly antiemetic. There is evidence showing that the effects of dopamine-like drugs affect the gastric system in addition to stimulating brain regions. In patients with vagotomy for pyloric stenosis given levodopa for treatment of parkinsonism, the drug produced no V.

However, the relative importance of a gastric and central mechanism is unknown. Other drugs used in the treatment of other diseases also facilitate NV. Digitalis is a treatment for congestive heart failure that may lead to neurological complications characterized by NV.

CHAPTER 26

Obstetrics and gynecology

Many epidemiological studies and self-reports indicate that women are at a much higher risk for nausea and vomiting (NV) than men; thus, it is critically important for us to look at NV in the field of reproductive medicine. NV are symptoms associated with a diverse array of clinical disorders and conditions in obstetrics and gynecology, ranging from pregnancy to intra-abdominal diseases. These symptoms can be very distressing to the patient and can have important physiological consequences and, thus, greatly affect the patient's quality of life. This chapter outlines the different disorders and conditions in obstetrics and gynecology that are often accompanied by emesis. Possible pathophysiological mechanisms that provoke such emesis and treatments that appear to be successful will also be considered, but pregnancy NV is discussed in more detail in Chapters 11–13.

Conditions/disorders in obstetrics and gynecology commonly associated with NV

Pregnancy-related conditions

Morning sickness

Many myths and few facts describe sickness in early pregnancy. Textbooks often perpetuate the former and the latter have not been available. NV in the early morning, which have been given the name 'morning sickness,' are so common that it is accepted as a symptom of normal pregnancy. Despite its name, morning sickness can occur almost any time of the day, although many women report greater severity in the morning. N is often precipitated by heavy cooking odors or pungent smells such as cigarette or cigar smoke, or petroleum or wax fumes (Benson, 1984). For some women, morning sickness may be mild and sporadic and may last only up to week 14. In a much smaller proportion of cases, probably not more than 2% of pregnant women, the V becomes more serious and persistent, occurring throughout the day and even during the night. To this serious form of V, the term 'hyperemesis gravidarum' (HG) is given.

N occurs in 50–90% and V in 25–55% of all pregnancies (Kucharczyk et al., 1991). According to the American College of Obstetricians and Gynecologists, nearly half of pregnant women experience some N or V during the early months of pregnancy, with varying degrees of severity. The specific percentage varies from study to study, but they all indicate that a majority of pregnant women experience morning sickness. In general, the NV of pregnancy begin about 2 weeks after the first missed menstrual period and ordinarily abate spontaneously by the end of the first trimester. It may persist to 14 weeks in as many as 40% of pregnant women, to 16 weeks in less than 20% of pregnancies, and to 20 weeks in less than 10% of pregnancies. Its prevalence has been reported to be greater in multiple than in single gestations. NV also occur occasionally before and frequently after rupture of an ectopic pregnancy. Morning sickness is typically felt in the first trimester upon waking up, often before any food has been ingested, and its occurrence does not seriously affect the nutritional state or the fluid–electrolyte balance (Davis et al., 1984).

In a survey of 1000 women, 85% experienced N and 52% V. Of these, 70% and 40% reported daily N and V, respectively. An analysis of the time of day at which women felt nauseous or vomited clearly shows that the term 'morning sickness' is a misnomer. Only 17% of women who had N reported that their symptoms occurred exclusively in the morning. Of all the women who reported N, 57% said the symptom occurred both in the morning and at other times during the day. In contrast, only 10% of women reported that they never suffered from pregnancy sickness in the morning, only at other times of the day. In a third of the women, the onset of pregnancy sickness occurred within 4 weeks of the last period and, in three-quarters, within 6 weeks. Furthermore, the earlier the onset of symptoms, the more likely women were to suffer from frequent bouts of NV. Positive correlations were found with the occurrence of pregnancy sickness and age, parity, and the development of food cravings (Whitehead et al., 1992).

In 1985, Klebanoff and colleagues reported observations from more than 9000 women enrolled during the first trimester into the Collaborative Perinatal Project. They found that slightly over half of these women had V in early pregnancy. They also found that V was more likely during the first pregnancy in younger women, and that it usually recurred in subsequent gestations. Intriguingly, women with early pregnancy V had better outcomes than women without V (Cunningham, 1993).

Differential diagnosis

Pregnancy results in widely varied alterations in multiple organ systems, particularly in the reproductive system. As marked subjective and objective variations among individuals occur and can result from physiological and pathological processes other than pregnancy, diagnostic criteria for pregnancy are classified as: (1) presumptive, (2) probable, and (3) positive. NV are considered presumptive manifestations of pregnancy. Any symptom compatible with presumptive or probable symptoms of pregnancy may lead to an incorrect diagnosis of pregnancy. The most common causes of diagnostic error are abdominal, adrenal, and uterine masses. Amenorrhea as a result of emotional, endocrine, or systemic causes may also be mistaken for amenorrhea caused by pregnancy. Pseudocyesis is the emotionally induced condition in which the symptoms of pregnancy appear, but without a prior conception.

All the presumptive and probable symptoms and signs of pregnancy can be caused by other physiological conditions as well. These include, but are not limited to, the following: endocrine dysfunction; malnutrition; peptic ulcer disease; infectious process; urinary tract disease; galactorrhea; pelvic congestion syndrome; uterine myoma, sarcoma, hematometra, or pyometra; ovarian or tubal tumor; uterine sacculation; and an intrauterine fetal demise. As there are so many possible differential diagnoses, one must be sure that the symptom does not represent the development of other disorders, although usually there are distinguishing features that assist in differential diagnosing (Benson, 1984; Creasy and Resnick, 1994).

HG

Morning sickness can be distinguished from the severe V of HG, a condition that often requires hospitalization. The term HG is reserved for those few patients developing intractable V and disturbed nutrition, with dehydration, acidosis from starvation, a weight loss of 5% or greater, and disturbances in electrolyte balance and protein metabolism, which may persist well after the first trimester. Although hyperemesis now has a low incidence in Western industrialized countries, in severe untreated cases, ketosis, metabolic alkalosis, neurological disturbances, and death can occur. Intractable uncompensated V can be fatal, but induced abortion is justified only in extreme cases.

Hydatidiform mole

Hydatidiform mole is an abnormal pregnancy characterized grossly by multiple grape-like vesicles filling and distending the uterus, usually in the absence of an intact fetus. Most hydatidiform moles are recognizable on gross examination, but some are small and may seem to be ordinary abortuses. Abnormal uterine bleeding, usually during the first trimester, is the most common symptom, occurring in over 90% of patients with molar pregnancies. NV, frequently excessive but at times difficult to distinguish from similar complaints normally occurring in pregnancy, have been reported to occur in 14–32% of patients with hydatidiform moles. Ten percent of patients with molar pregnancies have NV severe enough to require hospitalization (Decherney et al., 1994).

Differential diagnosis

In women with this disorder, it is important to consider other causes of NV and to maintain hydration and provide nutrition. The differential diagnosis of severe NV in early pregnancy includes gastritis, hepatitis, appendicitis, partial intestinal obstruction, diabetic ketoacidosis, molar pregnancy, and hyperthyroidism. These disorders may be excluded on the basis of history and selected laboratory tests. Patients who have no other causes for severe NV have HG.

Ptyalism

One problem that may worsen NV during pregnancy is ptyalism, or the hypersalivation that some women experience with pregnancy. Occasionally, these patients may be identified by the cups or piles of tissues that they carry to accommodate their saliva. Not only are NV an inconvenience, this condition may lead to loss of fluid and electrolytes. Although anticholinergic drugs are frequently effective, they should be used with caution during a pregnancy.

Labor

NV of undigested food eaten after the onset of labor are not uncommon in normal labor. This may be because gastrointestinal motility and absorption and stomach emptying time are delayed during labor. It may be secondary to analgesic treatment or may indicate full dilatation of the cervix. It may also be the result of a serious undiagnosed medical or surgical disorder. The V carries the risk of aspiration of acid gastric contents and associated Mendelson's syndrome with severe bronchospasm, cyanosis, tachycardia, and collapse. This is most likely to occur if the pH of the aspirate is below 3. The risk is small while the patient retains her cough reflex, but is significant should a general anesthetic be required (Ledward et al., 1991).

Infections and cancers of the urinary tract

NV are frequently seen in patients with urinary tract infections, especially when these are associated with gastroparesis, as well as in patients with uremic encephalopathy. Urinary tract infections are one of the most common types of infections in women. Pregnant women are especially vulnerable to urinary tract infections because the altered secretions of steroid sex hormones and the pressure exerted by the gravid uterus upon the ureters and bladder cause hypotonia and congestion and predispose to ureterovesical reflux and urinary stasis. Asymptomatic bacteriuria occurs in about 5% of all pregnant women, and up to 20% of all women will suffer from a urinary tract infection during their lifespan. Urinary tract infections are manifested as infections involving the bladder, referred to as cystitis, the kidney, as pyelonephritis, or the urethra, as urethritis. Pyelonephritis, infection of the renal parenchyma, is sometimes characterized by high fever, chills, flank pain, and NV (Benson, 1984).

Ovarian cancer

Ovarian cancer is the second most common cancer of the female genital tract. However, it is the most lethal, accounting for more than 50% of all deaths from gynecological cancer. Early ovarian cancer is usually asymptomatic, or symptoms are so vague that they are not recognized by either the patient or her physician. Symptoms occur with progressive enlargement of the tumor and invasion of the surrounding structures. The presenting complaints are often of short duration and most commonly consist of abdominal distention and pain. Less frequently, abnormal vaginal bleeding may occur. Vague abdominal symptoms, including dyspepsia, mild anorexia or N, and indigestion may precede other symptoms by many months.

Acute intra-abdominal diseases

Appendicitis

Appendicitis is a common acute surgical disease usually seen in patients under 30 years of age. Anorexia and NV are frequent symptoms of appendicitis. Diagnosis is more difficult in the female than in the male because of the proximity of the diseased appendix to the internal reproductive organs. This is particularly true if appendicitis is associated with disorders such as acute salpingitis, ovulatory bleeding, or ectopic pregnancy.

Appendicitis occurs no more often during pregnancy than at other times. However, it may be more difficult to diagnose because the symptoms of appendicitis are the same as the more common gastrointestinal upsets that occur during pregnancy, such as NV. Also, the enlarging uterus may obscure the diagnosis. The location of the appendix changes as the pregnancy progresses. As the uterus enlarges the appendix is pushed upward, so that by the middle of the second trimester it is at the level of the umbilicus; by the end of pregnancy it may be in the right upper quadrant. The frequency of abortion and premature labor is increased by the disease (Benson, 1984).

Acute pancreatitis

Pregnancy may be a predisposing factor to pancreatitis, and acute pancreatitis occurs in 1:1000 to 1:10 000 pregnancies. Ninety percent of cases in pregnancy are caused by cholelithiases. Other causes include excess alcohol, abdominal surgery, trauma, drugs, peptic ulcer perforation, hyperparathyroidism, pre-eclampsia, hyperlipidemia (often after contraceptive use), and viral infection. The chief symptoms of pancreatitis are midepigastric pain, N, V, and low-grade fever, and jaundice (Milheiro et al., 1995).

Differential diagnosis

The differential diagnosis must consider common duct stone or the rare perforated peptic ulcer with elevated serum amylase. Other problems with similar symptoms include mesenteric thrombosis, renal colic, acute cholecystitis, pre-eclampsia, appendicitis, myocardial infarction, aortic dissection, and intestinal obstruction (Benson, 1984).

Acute cholecystitis

Acute cholecystitis occurs in about 1 in 4000 pregnancies. It is more common in older women, during late pregnancy, and in those who have had previous attacks. Patients often complain of upper right quadrant pain, anorexia, N, and V. Displacement or compression of the extrahepatic biliary system by the enlarged pregnant uterus may interfere with circulation and drainage of the gallbladder. This often predisposes to acute cholecystitis (Benson, 1984).

Differential diagnosis

The differential diagnosis includes pancreatitis, appendicitis, pyelonephritis, peptic ulcer disease, and hepatitis.

Acute fatty liver

Acute liver failure occurs in the third trimester of pregnancy and may be caused by fulminant viral hepatitis, drug-induced hepatic toxicity, or acute fatty liver According to the reviews by Schorr-Lesnick and colleagues (1991) and Watson and Seeds (1990), its incidence is about 1:10 000 to 1:15 000 pregnancies. Mortality may be as high as 85%, but with improved recognition and immediate delivery, the mortality range is 20–30%. The disorder is usually seen after week 35 of gestation and is more common in primigravidas and those with twins. Typically, there is onset over several days to weeks of malaise, anorexia, NV, epigastric pain, and progressive jaundice. In many women with acute fatty liver, V is the major symptom. In perhaps half of these women, there is hypertension, proteinuria, and edema – signs suggestive of pre-eclampsia (Cunningham, 1993).

Differential diagnosis

The differential diagnosis is that of fulminant hepatitis. However, liver function test results for fulminant hepatitis are higher (greater than 1000 IU/ml) than those for acute fatty liver of pregnancy (usually less than 500 IU/ml). It is also important to review the appropriate history and perform the appropriate tests for toxins that may cause liver failure. Pre-eclampsia may involve the liver but typic-ally does not cause jaundice. The elevations in liver function tests in patients with pre-eclampsia usually do not reach the levels seen in patients with acute fatty liver of pregnancy (Cunningham, 1993).

Drugs/treatments in obstetrics and gynecology that cause NV

Pregnancy-related drugs

Drugs for uterine contraction

Many drugs used to stimulate uterine activity cause NV. Such drugs include: gemeprost, which is used to soften and dilate the cervix before transcervical operative procedures; dinoprostone, which is used in the form of gels or vaginal pessaries for softening the cervix before legal abortion or the induction of labor; and ergometrine, a uterotonic drug used in the management of spontaneous and legal abortion, for the management of the third stage of labor, and in post-partum hemorrhage caused by uterine atony (Ledward et al., 1991). Indomethacin, in sufficient doses, can inhibit uterine contractions and prevent pre-term labor. This agent may be effective for pharmacological control of pre-term labor but it may also cause NV.

Bromocriptine

Bromocriptine mesylate is a stimulant of dopamine receptors in the brain that inhibits release of prolactin by the pituitary gland. It is found to be quite effective in suppressing lactation; however, it has disturbing side effects, such as N, V, constipation, headache, dizziness, postural hypotension, and drowsiness.

Analgesics

Many methods are available for analgesia for labor, and they include good antenatal preparation, nursing care, psychological care, as well as physiotherapy. Methods available for the relief of pain in labor include parenteral drugs as well.

The most commonly used obstetric analgesics are diamorphine (a derivative of heroin) and pethidine hydrochloride (a synthetic opiate), a powerful analgesic and atropin-like antispasmodic with actions on both the brain and spinal cord. Both drugs can slow labor down and are supposed to provide pain relief, but women who have had these drugs often report side effects of NV. Other analgesics that cause NV include: meptazinol hydrochloride, which has antagonist activity against opiate analgesics and is used for short-term treatment of moderate pain; and morphine sulfate, which is more effective than pethidine and has a longer duration. Morphine, a short-term rapidly acting sedative for acute situations, has a complex emetic effect, stimulating the chemoreceptor trigger zone (CTZ) but depressing the V center, stimulating the inner ear but decreasing gastric motility. This is probably how it causes NV (Kucharczyk et al., 1991; Ledward et al., 1991).

Sedatives

Many sedatives used during pregnancy can induce NV. For more routine indications, phenobarbitones are often used as sedatives in pregnancy. Given in late pregnancy, phenobarbitone has been shown to decrease neonatal serum bilirubin by enhancing hepatic enzyme activity in the fetus and newborn infant. The side effects of phenobarbitone include hypersensitivity, which may cause skin rashes. In daily doses, phenobarbitone is cumulative and drowsiness, vertigo, headache, and N may occur. Another sedative often used for hypertension and eclampsia is chlormethiazole edisylate, which is a sedative hypnotic derived from the thiazole part of the vitamin B_1 molecule. It is also an anticonvulsant. A patient treated with chlormethiazole edisylate may have temporary hypotension, local thrombophlebitis, a tingling sensation in the nose or sneezing, conjunctival irritation, dyspepsia, and NV. In the USA, magnesium sulfate is also often used for pre-eclampsia; it is quite effective for seizures (Witlin and Sibai, 1998). Other sedatives commonly used to treat hypertension during pregnancy that may lead to NV include: hydralazine hydrochloride, a drug that lowers blood pressure and exerts a moderate but significant antihypertensive effect and tends to improve renal, uterine, and cerebral blood flow; and propranolol hydrochloride, used to control mild or moderate hypertension (Ledward et al., 1995).

Oral contraceptives

Estrogens and progestins

An estrogen administered after intercourse to prevent unwanted pregnancy has come to be known as the morning-after pill. Kucharczyk et al. (1991) reported no pregnancies in 1000 women who had inadequate contraceptive protection at the time of intercourse but within 3 days began to take stilbestrol, 25 mg twice daily for the next few days. The morning-after pill has proved to be quite effective, but it can cause disturbing side effects. The chief side effects appear to be NV, and these symptoms may be quite severe, especially with stilbestrol, which is no longer used for contraception, and ethinyl estradiol (Cunningham, 1993; Boodman, 1995).

N caused by the pill is likely the result of its estrogenic component. A shift to a combined pill with less estrogen or a progestin-only pill may alleviate N (Greenspan and Forsham, 1986; Cunningham, 1993). Also,

N often decreases after the first few cycles or else occurs on just the first day of the cycle once a woman begins the pill regimen (Rosenwaks et al., 1987). Promethazine, an oral antiemetic, may be prescribed 1 hour before breakfast and the evening meal, but it is strongly sedative. Rectal suppositories may also be used. The high-dose estrogen is then taken after the meal. This administration method will decrease NV.

Hematinics

To provide sufficient iron for the conceptus, the normal woman's daily iron need of about 1.5 mg is increased to 3.5–4.0 mg. Oral iron is usually the first line of treatment, and folic acid is also preferably given. The possible side effects of almost all iron tablets, including folic acid, are N, dysphagia, epigastric pain, diarrhea, and constipation (Ledward et al., 1991).

Antimicrobials

NV are also typical side effects of antimicrobial agents. Examples are: sodium fusidate, an alternative preparation for penicillin-resistant staphylococcal infection in patients who are penicillin sensitive; metronidazole, which is recommended both prophylactically and therapeutically for infections caused by *Bacteroides* spp. and also *Clostridium* spp. and other anaerobes; nitrofurantoin, bactericidal in renal tissue and throughout the urinary tract; and spectinomycin, an antimicrobial substance produced by the growth of *Streptomyces spectabilis*.

Treatment of NV in obstetrics and gynecology

Non-drug remedies

In the past, the suggested therapy for pregnancy NV has been antiemetic drugs, but, because of the possibility of teratogenic effects, there has been an understandable reluctance to use drugs of any kind during early pregnancy. The majority of patients can be reassured of the transient and benign nature of this disorder and can be managed with simple maneuvers. For the patient with slight to moderate NV of pregnancy, clinicians and family members should provide reassurance and relieve any fears, ensure rest, and reduce the patient's workload. Clinicians generally recommend the following for NV of pregnancy:

- Eat frequent small meals with a high carbohydrate content (that is, crackers, toast, potatoes) to avoid being too hungry or too full, and avoid strong-tasting or smelling foods. A woman's sense of smell is much keener during pregnancy, making odors and tastes more intense (DiLorio et al., 1994).

- Avoid N-triggering smells, such as onions, perfumes, trash cans, diaper pails, vehicle exhaust, and cigarette smoke.
- Wear wristbands (aka Morning Garde, Sea Band, or AcuBand): the Nei-kuan point is the anti-N point on the inside of the wrist used in acupuncture and acupressure, located about three finger-widths up from the wristfold in the midline between two tendons. Originally developed to prevent motion sickness and seasickness, these bands have been found to reduce NV in 60% of pregnant women who used them (Aikins Murphy and Cruikshank, 1995).
- Take ginger capsules or drink a cup of ginger root tea in the morning. Several studies have demonstrated that ginger reduces the frequency of NV bouts in pregnant women. A report (Fischer-Rasmussen, 1991) showed ordinary ginger powder in capsules to be effective even against the most severe form of pregnancy-related NV, HG. Another study found it to be useful in preventing postoperative N after major gynecological surgery.
- Acupuncture: several studies have shown that acupuncture will relieve the symptoms of NV during pregnancy.

Medication

If the simple, nonpharmacological maneuvers do not work, antiemetic drugs may be prescribed. Antiemetic agents are available for the symptomatic control of V of early pregnancy (Table 26.1), during labor, and also for postoperative V. In general, pharmacological management is more effective in prevention than in treatment of the condition (Benson, 1984; Scott et al., 1994).

When morning sickness is of the severity that hospitalization admission is required, the patient should be hospitalized in a quiet, cheerful, well-ventilated, single room. Immediate management may involve correction of electrolyte problems and sedation, while investigations to exclude an organic basis for the V proceed (Gleicher, 1992). The patient should be confined to bed in the initial phase and have routine observations performed. If ketonemia occurs, administration of intravenous fluids may provide relief. Measurements of weight, urine testing (particularly bacteriology of the urine to exclude urinary infection), maintenance of fluid balance charts, and recording of hemoglobin and electrolytes is essential. It is also reasonable to employ parenteral sedatives which have antiemetic properties on a short-term basis in cases where the V does not

Table 26.1: Antiemetic agents for pregnancy-related NV (see Chapter 6, p.126)

Vitamin B6	Vitamin B6 (pyridoxine) has no major side effects and no contraindications for N and V in early pregnancy but its effectiveness remains uncertain. It may be tried first.
Doxylamine	Is an antihistamine that is available over the counter as Unisome. A combination similar to Bendectin can be made. Vitamin B6 and Unisome at bedtime, one half of each in the morning, and one half of each in the afternoon, can be used, but whether B6 contributes usefully is doubtful. (See Ledward et al., 1991; Decherney, 1994; Scott et al., 1994; Vutyavanich et al., 1995.)
Promethazine	This is a long-acting antihistamine with antiemetic and sedative effects. Promethazine is often used for morning sickness or V of late pregnancy. Promethazine is also used in patients suffering from HG and in labor to enhance the effect of pethidine (meperidine). (See Ledward et al., 1991.)
Metoclopramide	This drug has been widely employed for symptomatic relief of NV in early pregnancy and is often useful. It promotes esophageal and gastric peristalsis, increases tone of the cardiac sphincter, and tends to speed gastric emptying. It also has a central (hindbrain) antiemetic effect and is a dopamine receptor antagonist. (See Ledward et al., 1991; Walder et al., 1994.)
Meclozine	A small, randomized, placebo-controlled study suggested that meclozine might be teratogenic in humans. In 1014 patients in thc Collaborative Perinatal Project and an additional 613 patients from the Kaiser Health Plan, no teratogenic effect was found. (See Ledward et al., 1991; Scott et al., 1994.)
Dimenhydrinate	No teratogenicity has been demonstrated for fetuses exposed to dimenhydrinate (Dramamine), but a 29% failure rate and significant incidence of side effects, especially drowsiness, have been reported for mothers. (See Scott et al., 1994.)
Diphenhydramine	The infants of 595 patients treated with diphenhydramine (Benadryl) in the Collaborative Perinatal Project showed no signs of teratogenicity. (See Scott et al., 1994.)
Emetrol	Emetrol is a phosphorylated carbohydrate solution that acts locally on the wall of the gastrointestinal tract. It reduces smooth muscle contractions in direct proportion to the amount used. (See Scott et al., 1994.)

resolve with hospital rest and correction of plasma electrolytes, and where an organic disease such as infective hepatitis is not suspected. Some antiemetics should be given intramuscularly; an injection of amobarbital sodium (Amytal) will reinforce the antiemetic sedative action if the antiemetic itself cannot control the V. Subsequent care of intractable and recurrent cases may include psychiatric consultation. Godsey and Newman (1991) studied 140 women with HG and demonstrated that, in many instances, social and psychological factors contribute to the illness. Steroids are also occasionally useful in controlling recurrence (Ledward et al., 1991).

Parenteral antiemetic drugs with sedative properties, suitable for use in pregnancy for 1–3 days at a time, include:

- Promethazine: this long-acting antihistamine is used for morning sickness as well as HG, as mentioned earlier.
- Phenothiazines and related drugs (chlorpromazine, promazine, and trifluoperazine): phenothiazines are antiemetic drugs with sedative properties effective in treating HG, and the most common side effect is drowsiness. Teratogenicity does not appear to be a problem with the phenothiazines as a group.

Drugs available for treating V in labor include antacids such as magnesium trisilicate and parenteral antiemetics such as promethazine. Magnesium trisilicate forms a gel in the stomach, which may protect the mucosa. If given, this should be the only oral medication given to the pregnant patient while she is in labor. Other antiemetics used for V in labor include cimetidine, ranitidine, promazine, and sodium citrate. This sodium citrate solution mixes well with gastric contents and acts rapidly in raising gastric pH, but its duration of action is short, 45 minutes or less. It is therefore best used shortly before general anesthesia.

As mentioned earlier, however, drugs are only used as a last resort and non-drug treatment should be attempted first, especially if the patient is pregnant. This is a particularly important factor to consider in sexually active women of reproductive age.

The treatment of postoperative NV and of NV related to cancer chemotherapy is discussed in Chapters 16 and 27 respectively.

Case study

Splenic avulsion in pregnancy is a rare condition that carries a high risk of death to both the mother and the fetus. A 30-year-old woman with HG had spontaneous avulsion of the spleen at 30 weeks' gestation. She underwent a splenectomy and cesarean section, resulting in a stillborn fetus. It was most likely that violent V resulted in splenic avulsion. Prompt surgical intervention by a general surgeon and obstetrician is required in such cases. This case study illustrates how severe V can lead to tragic results.

CHAPTER 27
Oncology

Nausea and vomiting (NV) are common concerns for oncological patients. Although several types of cancer can induce NV, most occurrences of NV result from the treatment of cancer attributable to radiotherapy, chemotherapy, and/or surgical procedures. These subjective and observational findings can be very distressing to the patient and can have important physiological consequences that reduce the quality of living for patients suffering from cancer. Among the dangers of prolonged or recurrent NV are dehydration, electrolyte abnormalities (for example, potassium), nutritional depletion, esophageal tears, fractures, wound dehiscence, and negative nitrogen balance already present in some cancer patients. These could also lead to the degeneration of self-care and functional ability.

Although many cancer patients develop NV as a result of their treatment, there are also many factors related to the malignancy itself that can cause NV. Examples are gastrointestinal (GI) metastases, hepatic metastases, brain metastases, uremia, infections, bowl obstruction, ascites, fluid and electrolyte abnormalities, and psychological stress.

Differential diagnosis of conditions associated with N

About one-third of the patients in hospice care as a result of terminal cancers suffer from NV. Various types of cancers are known to induce NV; the primary cancers include those of the GI tract. The formation of a tumor impinging extrinsically on the GI tract may cause NV as a result of nerve impulses sent from the upper GI tract to the V centers or network by the way of vagal and parasympathetic nerves. Physicians can use the incidence and likelihood of NV as part of the diagnosis of the cancer.

Gallbladder cancer

Gallbladder cancer is frequently diagnosed during the late stages of the disease when curative surgery is no longer possible. Seventy-six percent of patients with gallbladder cancer experience abdominal pain, 38% with jaundice, 39% with weight loss, and 32% with NV. In addition, these symptoms may be present for diagnosis: acute cholecystitis, chronic cholecystitis, biliary tract tumors, and gastrointestinal hemorrhage. Advancement of gallbladder cancer can lead to extreme N, V, anorexia, and weight loss.

Gastrointestinal cancers

NV are affiliated with upper GI malignancies, particularly gastric cancer. Of the patients with tumors located in the upper GI tract, 75% experience V accompanied with ulcer-type pain, and pain unrelieved by alkaline food or V. Symptoms related to GI cancers may vary with the extent of disease. Ulcerated lesions (types IIc and III) are more likely to have epigastric pain and V as a major symptom as opposed to (type I) lesions in which bleeding is more common. Furthermore, weight loss becomes less prevalent in the advanced stages of the disease.

Esophageal cancer

Very small tumors in the esophagus usually do not cause symptoms; however, as the tumor grows, swallowing becomes difficult. Patients may have a feeling of fullness and pressure in addition to the dysphagia. As the tumor grows larger, the pathway to the stomach becomes narrower. Cancer of the esophagus can also cause indigestion, heartburn, V, and frequent choking on food. As a result of these problems, weight loss is common.

Small bowel cancer

NV are also associated with small bowel obstruction from advanced or recurrent cancers. NV occur frequently in small bowel cancers along with recurrent cramps in the mid- to upper abdomen. A neoplasm may act as the lead point for an intussusception, with the attending obstructing symptoms. NV are more prominent symptoms in duodenal and proximal jejunal neoplasms. If there is a suspected blockage in the ileum, the patient tends to have moderate cramps with little or no V. Large bowel cancer patients also tend to develop

NV. Unlike patients with small bowel cancers, patients who have large bowel obstructions usually experience cramps in the mid- to lower abdomen but V may not be present until the later stages.

Colon cancer

NV also arise frequently in colon cancer. Obstruction of the GI tract by tumor may result from intraluminal growth of primary colorectal carcinomas. Twenty-five percent of those diagnosed with colon cancer experience N and 23% experience V. Those with right colon cancer, on the other hand, tend to experience only N (25%) without V.

Hepatic cancers

In some patients without cirrhosis and with good hepatic function, hepatic carcinomas may grow to huge proportions before becoming symptomatic. The common presenting symptoms include: right upper quadrant abdominal pain, weight loss, abdominal distention, weakness, fatigue, anorexia, and NV. NV occur in 19–40% of patients with liver metastases.

Gynecological cancers

Other cancers also induce NV. In gynecology and obstetrics, clinicians may confront gestational trophoblastic disease and choriocarcinoma, an epithelial tumor composed of syncytiotrophoblastic and cytotrophoblastic cells. These tumors tend to follow pregnancy and can be diagnosed histopathologically. NV are frequent and excessive; however, at times, it is difficult to distinguish from similar complaints normally occurring in pregnancy. Of patients with hydatidiform moles, 14–32% tend to vomit and 10% of patients with molar pregnancies have such severe NV that hospitalization is required. NV are also prevalent in epithelial ovarian cancer through its effect on the GI track. Accumulation of ascites leads to electrolyte imbalance and increased abdominal pressure.

Pancreatic tumors

Pancreatic endocrine tumors may cause NV; 45% of patients with pancreatic cancer experience NV. Insulinomas, β-cell tumors, can cause many symptoms, including NV. Other diagnostic symptoms include hypoglycemia, flushing, and sweating which may be related to the sympathetic nervous system. Carcinoid syndrome is also affiliated with NV. When these tumors metastasize to the liver they can cause flushing, diarrhea, and asthma-like attacks with NV.

Brain tumors

Brain tumors can also cause NV. The 'classic' brain tumor headache is severe in the morning and associated with NV at times. In general, 24% of the patients diagnosed with brain tumors experience NV. Those patients who have increased cranial pressure will experience N 67% of the time as opposed to those having a supratentorial tumor without increased cranial pressure. Clinicians should monitor patients who have a history for headaches. If any new symptoms, especially N or V, should occur, additional evaluation perhaps leading to computed tomography (CT) or magnetic resonance imaging (MRI) is necessary.

Increased cranial pressure is believed to be associated with a decrease in arterial oxygen concentration, increased arterial carbon dioxide concentration, and decreased blood–brain flow. The baroreceptor hypothesis thus invoked provides an alternative mechanism for NV. There is an apparent pattern with the incidence of NV and an increase of internal body pressure. NV also occur in intracranial hyper- as well as hypotension. The primary integrating center for the baroreceptor reflexes is a diffuse network of highly interconnected neurons in the medulla oblongata of the brain stem called the medullary cardiovascular center. The neurons in the receptor receive input from various baroreceptors. As part of the baroreceptor reflexes, angiotensin II generation and vasopressin secretion are altered so as to help restore the blood pressure. Sometimes the input from these receptors can bypass the medulla center. Certain neurons in the cerebral cortex and hypothalamus synapse directly on the sympathetic neurons in the spinal cord.

Oncological therapies that induce NV

Chemotherapy

The most prevalent occurrences of NV in the practice of oncology, however, result from the side effects of many chemotherapy drugs. NV from chemotherapy are both drug and dose dependent. More than 75% of the patients receiving cisplatin are affected by NV. Although NV itself is not life threatening, it can pose detrimental effects on nutritional status and the quality of life of these patients. Severe NV may lead to serious psychosocial consequences that produce depression, anxiety, and helplessness. On the third day after cisplatin chemotherapy, 23% were unable to go to work and 12% were so ill that they could not care for themselves. There are also a number of other medical complications such as the Mallory–Weiss tears of the esophagus, pathological bone fractures, severe dehydration, electrolyte imbalance, metabolic alkalosis, malnutrition, vitamin deficiencies, and GI hemorrhage. These serious complications occur in a small minority of patients. The dosage of chemotherapy agents used is the most important determinant factor in relation to the amount of NV that follows. The severity for NV induced by the various chemotherapeutic agents differs for each of the various reagents as shown in Table 27.1.

Table 27.1: Potential of chemotherapeutic agents for producing NV. Some drugs appear twice because the incidence of NV depends on doses used

High potential (>80% incidence)	Moderate potential (50–80% incidence)	Lower potential (25–50% incidence)	Lowest potential (0–25% incidence)
Cisplatin	Actinomycin D	Asparaginase	Bleomycin
Cyclophosphamide	Carmustine (BiCNU)	Carboplatin	Busulfan
Cytarabine	Cyclophosphamide	Mitomycin	Etoposide
Dacarbazine	Cytarabine	Paclitaxel	5-Fluorouracil
Nitrogen mustard	Methotrexate		Melphalan
Streptozocin	Daunorubicin bolus		Methotrexate
Mechlorethamine	Doxorubicin bolus		6-Thioguanine
Ifosfamide	Ifosfamide		Vinblastine
	Indarubicin		Vincristine
	Picamycin		
	Paclitaxel		
	Hexamethylenamine		
	Procarbazine		
	Lomustine		

Cisplatin is one of the most commonly used agents that induce NV. It increases the plasma and urinary levels of 5-hydroxyindoleacetic acid (5HIAA) but does not affect the platelet and free plasma serotonin. The changes in 5HIAA are believed to be associated with the onset of V. V begins 1–2 hours after administration, reaches maximal intensity after 5–6 hours, and thereafter NV appear sporadically. Patients who do not vomit after the first 8 hours rarely vomit during the following 16 hours. Delayed emesis begins 24 hours after the chemotherapy and is present in 20–85% of the patients. The reason why some chemotherapy agents induce NV more severely than others is not known.

Hypothesis of the mechanisms of NV in chemotherapy

There are many proposed hypotheses as to how chemotherapy may cause NV. One hypothesis suggests that there is a chemoreceptor trigger zone (CTZ) located in the area postrema in the dorsal portion of the lateral reticular formation of the brain. The area postrema is high vascularized with fenestrated blood vessels with tight junctions between capillary and endothelial cells. Chemotherapy drugs are believed to act on such receptors located in the CTZ which is specialized to sample chemicals present in the circulating blood readily. Chemotherapy initiates the release of neurotransmitters from the CTZ which activate the V center. The CTZ is more permeable to substances carried in the blood and cerebrospinal fluid than in the rest of the brain and is only activated by chemicals. There are believed to be over 17 putative neurotransmitters near the CTZ such as serotonin, dopamine, histamine, norepinephrine, apomorphine, angiotension II, neurotension, leucine-enkephalin, vasoactive intestinal polypeptide, thyrotropin-releasing hormone, gastrin, vasopressin, and substance P (see Chapter 9). Of these neurotransmitters, the one that appears to the most specifically linked to chemotherapy-induced NV is dopamine. Many effective antiemetic drugs are dopamine antagonists that specifically bind to the D_2 receptor. From the effects of these antiemetic drugs, it shows that neurotransmitters may be important in mediation of NV at some sites in the overall reflex pathways.

Problems, however, exist, within this hypothesis. It is unlikely that the CTZ has a large enough number of receptors sensitive to each of the chemotherapeutic drugs. Second, the long latency time for the onset is not consistent with a direct action of the emetic drugs on the CTZ. Last, there is a vagotomy- and sympathectomy-abolished, cisplatin-induced emesis in a ferret, indicating an indirect action of chemotherapy.

Another hypothesis, the humoral model, suggests that endogenous factors formed after chemotherapy are released in the circulation and stimulate NV. The delayed time of onset is in agreement with this possible mechanism. Vasopressin is believed to induce NV. When cisplatin is given to a dog, the vasopressin increases 30-fold. Serotonin is also believed to be increased. 5HIAA may be a marker of the released serotonin that circulates on the $5HT_3$ receptors to trigger NV. Damage of the gastrointestinal mucosa caused by cytotoxic agents induces the release of serotonin. Chemotherapeutic drugs may also stimulate neural fibers increasing the release of acetylcholine, which then acts on receptors located in the enterochromaffin cells to induce the release of serotonin. The actual mechanism of chemotherapy-induced NV could entail the combination of both of the above hypotheses. As with the CTZ hypothesis, there are pitfalls to the later hypothesis. When the blood from a dog with NV was injected into another asymptomatic dog, NV were not induced. This indicates that endogenous factors may not directly stimulate NV.

Radiotherapy

In general, patients receiving radiotherapy to the GI tract or brain have the greatest potential for NV as a side effect. As GI cells divide quickly, they are sensitive to radiotherapy. Radiation to the brain is believed to stimulate the brains' CTZ V center. Radiotherapy causes NV in addition to anorexia, fatigue, and weight loss. Experiencing NV is not an indication of whether the drug is or is not destroying cancer cells. The V is usually less severe than for those patients receiving aggressive chemotherapy. Typically the latent period is about 1 hour and NV occurs at intervals for a period of 2–3 hours. No changes in pulse rate, blood pressure, body temperature, or respiration rate are usually observed associated with the act of V. Factors that must be taken into account are the site of irradiation, the field size, dose per fraction, the age of the patient, and the anxiety of the patient.

The site of irradiation is a major determinant of NV. The incidence of V tends to be higher after irradiation of the abdomen than when irradiation is confined to the upper part of the trunk. NV tend to occur more frequently also when the upper half of the body is irradiated as opposed to the lower half. Irradiation of the extremities seldom produces NV. The radiation size also affects NV. The V response may be influenced by the volume of the tissue irradiated. Total body irradiation has been shown to induce NV more frequently and to a greater intensity than partial body irradiation. The dose is also directly related to NV. The higher the daily dose of irradiation, the greater amount of V. Raised intracranial pressure resulting from irradiation of the head and neck may also create direct pressure from the brain stem and stimulate the CTZ. Adults tend to experience more NV than children, and those patients who are apprehensive tend to develop more NV than those who are less anxious. More frequent administration of radiation may increase side effects if high doses per fracture are used. Recently, the development of CHART (**c**ontinuous **h**yperfractionated **a**ccelerated **r**adiotherapy **t**reatment) has been shown to produce a better tumor response than the conventional radiotherapy in advanced lung cancer. This new therapy, however, increases the risk of NV.

Hormone therapy

Hormonal agents are generally tolerated much better than chemotherapy and radiotherapy. The efficacy of the drug treatment depends upon the apparent sensitivity of a tumor to the drug and upon whether or not the tumors have hormone receptors. Hormonal drugs do not have a curative potential themselves, although they might increase the cure rate of some tumors when used with additional local treatment. Hormonal drugs can be used in prostate, breast, endometrial, thyroid, ovarian, and renal cancers. Various types of hormonal drugs such as fosfestrol, progesterone, and estrogen used for prostate cancer have been shown to induce NV. Used for breast and prostate cancer, diethylstilbestrol's main side effects also include NV, along with fluid retention, thromboembolism, gynecomastia, and impotence. Tamoxifen used in breast cancer has been shown to cause N, fluid retention, hypercalcemia, and warfarin toxicity.

Surgery

NV may also result from anesthesia and surgery, can occur in the immediate postoperative period and are usually anesthesia related. NV later in the postoperative period may demand diagnostic attention because the symptoms may be the result of either adynamic ileus or partial bowel obstruction.

Ileus is characterized by abdominal distention, absence of bowel sounds, and generalized abdominal tympany on percussion. This complication is noted 48–72 hours after surgery. A diagnostic abdominal radiograph can indicate generalized dilatation and gaseous distention of both the large and small bowel. Obstipation or urological trauma with extravasation of urine may also be a cause of ileus. If NV become severe, insertion of a nasogastric tube into the stomach may be necessary to rest the bowel and to supply nutrients.

Intestinal obstruction can develop 5–6 days after surgery. Fibrous adhesions can develop and entrap the bowel. Protracted V results and is accompanied by cramping abdominal pain, large fluid shifts, and vigorous hydration.

Priorities and procedures

Not all cancer patients experience NV. The most common causes are emetogenic chemotherapy drugs and radiotherapy to the GI tract, liver, or brain. Other possible causes include electrolyte imbalance, tumor growth, infection or septicemia, uremia, and constipation. Clinicians treating NV must be aware of all the potential causes and factors especially in cancer patients who may be receiving combination treatments and medications. Past medical histories and use of antiemetics should be taken into consideration when establishing a diagnosis.

Chemotherapy-induced NV can be divided into three discrete clinical syndromes, which have specific therapeutic implications: acute NV, delayed NV, and anticipatory NV.

Acute NV occur within 24 hours of the chemotherapy administration. The NV in this phase are the most severe. With most chemotherapeutic agents, such as cisplatin, NV occur 1–2 hours after intravenous administration. With other drugs, such as cyclophosphamide, the onset of NV may not occur until 9–18 hours later. This suggests that various mechanisms of inducing NV may exist.

Delayed NV usually occur 24 hours or more after chemotherapy administration. They are less severe than acute NV and the course can be more protracted, leading to difficulties in dehydration, nutrition, and performance status. Cisplatin frequently causes delayed emesis usually 24–72 hours after chemotherapy. In some patients, emesis may not occur or may last 4–5 days after treatment. Delayed NV have a great impact on the quality of the patient's life.

Anticipatory NV occur in patients who have experienced poor control of emesis with previous chemotherapy treatments. The onset can occur before or during chemotherapy administration. This type of NV is a conditioned response and may be induced by a stimulus which reminds the patient of chemotherapy treatment such as the hospital environment or the oncologist's office. Factors that may increase the risk of developing anticipatory NV include: emetogenicity of chemotherapy received, sweating after last chemotherapy, feeling warm or hot after last chemotherapy, post-treatment dizziness and lightheadedness, number of chemotherapy cycles received, age under 50 years, longer duration of chemotherapy infusion, severe post-treatment NV, extreme anxiety and/or depression, history of susceptibility to motion sickness, and drugs that have associated taste. Of patients receiving chemotherapy 10–44% experience N and/or V before or during chemotherapy infusions.

Methods used to control NV

Nasogastric suction and other non-drug methods

In patients with gastric cancers caused by obstructing tumors, nasogastric suction can help alleviate V. Stomach emptying takes about 6 hours for solid foods and 4 hours for liquid. Agents such as metoclopramide can be used to promote gastric motility and emptying. Gastric aspiration can be used to eliminate regurgitation of stomach contents. Other methods that are useful are listed in Table 27.2.

Table 27.2: Non-drug methods

Method	The problem mitigated
1. Chemotherapy should be given in a quiet and relaxed atmosphere	Anxiety and depression
2. Administer the drug at night, preceded by phenothiazine	Anticipatory NV
3. Behavioral modifications: avoid cooking smells and changes in drug regimens and unpleasant formulations	NV
4. Take short walks before meals, drink separately from meals, eat plain biscuits and dry toast, eat cold foods, reduce very sweet, spicy or fatty food, and drink fizzy drinks	Patients undergoing radiotherapy to the upper GI tract
5. Eat small frequent meals, drink more milk, and eat more milk products (e.g. cheese, cottage cheese) as they are rich in calcium	NV related to chemotherapy or disease state
6. Eat bananas, tomatoes, oranges, apricots, cantaloupe, dates, figs, prunes, and potatoes	Potassium imbalance
7. Hypnosis	NV
8. Sedation	NV

Antiemetic drugs

When selecting antiemetics, the general factors that should be considered include the dose, route of administration, and schedule. Patients who will receive high emetogenic potential chemotherapy may require higher doses of antiemetic therapy. Patients who will return without continued intravenous access, for example, may be better off with sublingual or rectal routes of antiemetic delivery. As the duration of the drug effects varies, the schedule of the antiemetics will directly affect its success. Metoclopramide has a short duration of action (2–3 hours) and therefore should be given frequently. Lorazepam, on the other hand, has a longer duration of action (4–8 hours) and should thus be given less frequently than metoclopramide. When giving combination drugs, each drug must be considered separately. The key to success of antiemetics is to maintain adequate blood levels of a particular drug to prevent NV.

Tables 27.3–27.7 provide summary details. They are based on *Recommendations for Antiemetics in Patients Receiving Chemotherapy 1995–1996*, Stanford University Hospital Pharmacy and Therapeutics Committee.

Table 27.3: Antiemetic drugs

Drugs	Dose	Adverse reactions	Activity
Phenothiazines prochlorperazine	5–10 mg p.o. every 4–6 h 10–15 mg s.r. p.o. every 12 h 25 mg p.r. p.o. every 12 h 5–10 mg i.m./i.v. every 4–6 h Do not exceed 40 mg/day for injections	Sedation Anticholinergic Hypotension Extrapyramidal symptoms	*
promethazine	25–50 mg p.o./p.r. every 4–6 h 25 mg i.m./i.v. every 4–6 h	Sedation Anticholinergic Hypotension Extrapyramidal symptoms	*
thiethylperazine	10 mg i.m./p.o./p.r. every 8 h	Sedation Anticholinergic Hypotension Extrapyramidal symptoms	*
Benzodiazepine lorazepam	0.5–2 mg/m^2 i.v./p.o. every 4 h Reduce dose in elderly patients	Sedation, Amnesia Confusion	**
Butyrophenones haloperidol	1–3 mg i.v. every 2–6 h 1–2 mg p.o. every 3–6 h	Sedation, Confusion Extrapyramidal symptoms	***
droperidol (Inapsine)	0.5–2 mg i.v. every 4 h	Sedation, hypotension	**

(contd)

Table 27.3: (contd)

Drugs	Dose	Adverse reactions	Activity
Benzamide metoclopramide	20 mg i.v./i.m./p.o. every 3–6 h See Table 27.4 for acute emesis and delayed emesis dose	Diarrhea, Sedation Extrapyramidal symptoms	***
Corticosteroid	10–20 mg i.v./p.o. × 1 dose before chemotherapy; optional to follow with 4–8 mg p.o. twice daily	Euphoria	***
dexamethasone	See Table 27.7 for delayed emesis dose	Psychosis	
		Hyperglycemia	
Serotonin antagonists	See Table 27.6 for moderately emetogenic regimens and Table 27.5 for highly emetogenic regimens	Headaches	***
ondansetron		Elevated LFTs	
		Constipation	
		Diarrhea	
granisetron	See Table 27.5 for highly emetogenic regimens		***
Antihistamine diphenhydramine	25–50 mg i.m./i.v./p.o. every 4 h	Sedation	*
dronabinol	5–10 mg p.o. 4–6 times/day	Euphoria Somnolence Paranoid reactions	*/**

Activity for prevention of cisplatin-induced emesis: *, **, ***
LFTs, liver function tests.

Table 27.4: Acute emesis

Metoclopramide
2–3 mg/kg, i.v. push bolus 30 min before chemotherapy, and repeat dose of 2 mg/kg at 1.5 h and 3.5 h after the start of chemotherapy

+

Dexamethasone
10–20 mg, i.v. push bolus, 20 min before chemotherapy × 1 dose.

+

Diphenhydramine
50 mg i.v. before metoclopramide and p.o./i.v./i.m. every 4 h p.r.n. for restlessness or acute dystonic reaction

±

Lorazepam
1–1.5 mg/m^2 (max. 3 mg), i.v. before chemotherapy × 1 dose only, before metoclopramide

Table 27.5: Highly emetogenic regimens

For single doses of chemotherapy:

- Granisetron 10 μg/kg i.v.* × 1 dose + dexamethasone 10–20 mg i.v. for 30 min before chemotherapy. Do not repeat dose for 24 hours for inpatients receiving cisplatin followed with antiemetics for delayed N/V
- Ondansetron 32 mg × 1 dose + dexamethasone 10–20 mg i.v. 30 min before chemotherapy. Do not repeat dose for 24 hours for inpatients receiving cisplatin followed with antiemetics for delayed N/V

For multiple-day chemotherapy regimens: each day a highly emetogenic agent is given

Table 27.6: Moderately emetogenic regimens

Regimen A

- Ondansetron 8–10 i.v. 30 min before chemotherapy × 1 dose

Regimen B

- Ondansetron 8 mg p.o. 30 min before chemotherapy followed by 8 mg ondansetron orally at 4 and 8 h
- Follow with conventional scheduled antiemetic after three doses of p.o. ondansetron are administered for delayed NV
- After 24 h, efficacy of p.o. ondansetron has not been shown to be more effective than alternative regimens. Metoclopramide is more effective for delayed N

Regimen C

Dexamethasone 10–20 mg i.v./p.o. + metoclopramide 1 mg/kg i.v. 30 min before and every 2 h × 3 doses of metoclopramide and every 4 h p.r.n. for restlessness or acute dystonic reaction

Table 27.7: Delayed NV

Regimen A

- Metoclopramide 20–40 mg p.o. scheduled four times daily × 2– 4 days, followed by every 4 h p.r.n.

+

- Dexamethasone 8 mg p.o. twice daily × 2 days, followed by 4 mg p.o. twice daily × 2 days scheduled

+

- Diphenhydramine 50 mg p.o./i.v. every 4 h p.r.n. for restlessness or acute dystonic reaction

or

Regimen B

- Haloperidol 1–2 mg p.o. every 6–8 h scheduled × 2–4 days then p.r.n.

or

(contd)

Table 27.7: (contd)

Regimen C
• Diphenhydramine 50 mg p.o. 1 h before meals, scheduled
and/or
• Lorazepam 0.5 mg p.o. 1 h before meals, scheduled
+
• Prochlorperazine 10 mg p.o. 1 h before meals, scheduled

Case studies

Case study number 1

For radiotherapy-induced emesis, ondansetron has been shown to be very effective. In a single-dose radiation-induced emesis, ondansetron 8 mg orally three times daily provided excellent antiemetic control compared with metoclopramide 10 mg orally three times daily. Ondansetron is also more effective than using prochlorperazine. For hemi-body irradiation, ondansetron 8 mg and dexamethasone 8 mg given orally produced complete control of emesis. A 70-year-old patient with stage II ovarian cancer received abdominal pelvic radiation after optimal surgical debulking. Initial NV were completely controlled by prochlorperazine or by decreasing daily fraction size of radiation. She was then switched to ondansetron with excellent control of NV. The patient was able to complete oral radiotherapy and was alive with evidence of disease for more than 18 months.

Case study number 2

A 26-year-old woman was admitted for her fourth complete cycle of etoposide (VP-16), cisplatin, and bleomycin for her endodermal sinus tumor immature teratoma of the ovary. She had persistent NV during her chemotherapy. She received cisplatin 20 mg/m^2, VP-16 100 mg/m^2, and bleomycin 20 U/m^2. On this admission, the patient was pre-medicated before the bleomycin with dexamethasone 8 mg orally and diphenyldramine 50 mg orally 6 hours and 1 hour before bleomycin. For antiemetics, the patient received granisetron 650 mg i.v. 30 min before cisplatin and was also be on a regimen of metoclopramide 10 mg p.o. four times daily for 4 days, then p.r.n. four times daily. Her NV were controlled with p.r.n. antiemetics with lorazepam, prochlorperazine and diphenyldramine.

NV in cancer patients are either attributable to the malignancy itself or result from cancer treatments such as chemotherapy or radiotherapy. NV still remain acute subjective or observational findings associated with chemotherapy and radiotherapy; however, with new emetics and nonpharmacological methods, health care workers can begin working toward prevention.

CHAPTER 28

Ophthalmology

Ophthalmologists only occasionally encounter patients suffering from nausea and vomiting (NV). These patients' underlying problem usually falls into one of the following four categories:

- Ophthalmic disease
- Neurological disease with ophthalmic manifestations
- Drug effects
- Postoperative complications.

Ophthalmic diseases

Acute elevation in intraocular pressure

Any disorder that results in an acute elevation in the intraocular pressure may cause NV. The most common of these disorders is primary acute angle-closure glaucoma, which is usually seen in the sixth and seventh decades of life in hyperopic individuals. It may be precipitated by topical mydriatics, systemic anticholinergics, or dim illumination (e.g., movie theater). In addition to NV, patients often experience severe eye pain, blurred vision, colored halos around lights, and frontal headache. Signs include closure of the anterior chamber angle, severely elevated intraocular pressure, and corneal edema.

Other disorders that can cause an acute elevation in the intraocular pressure include uveitic glaucoma, traumatic glaucoma, pigmentary glaucoma, and neovascular glaucoma.

Treatment of these disorders is with topical, oral, and parenteral ocular hypotensive medications. A peripheral iridectomy is indicated in cases of primary angle-closure glaucoma. The lowering of intraocular pressure brings prompt relief from NV. Unfortunately, some of the agents used in the treatment of acute glaucoma, particularly the oral hyperosmotics such as glycerin and isosorbide, can themselves exacerbate NV, and must be used with caution (Hoskins and Kass, 1989).

Neurological diseases with ophthalmic manifestations

Migraine headaches

The word migraine is derived from the French term 'hemicraine', meaning one-sided headache. The World Federation of Neurology (1969) has defined migraine headache as 'a disorder characterized by recurrent attacks of headaches of variable frequency, duration, and intensity, which are usually unilateral and usually associated with anorexia, nausea, and vomiting. These attacks may be preceded by neurological or visual symptoms.'

The first attack of migraine usually takes place in the second or third decade of life, but can begin at any age. Most series report a female preponderance of 60–70% (Selby and Lance, 1960). Predisposing factors include stress or emotional upset, hormonal changes (e.g., menstruation or pregnancy), diet-related factors (e.g., foods containing high levels of the amino acid tyramine such as cheeses, yogurt, and liver), and medications (reserpine and nitroglycerin).

Many classification systems have been proposed for migraine headaches. The most useful of these distinguishes between migraine without aura (common migraine) and migraine with aura (classic migraine). The aura usually lasts 5–60 minutes, precedes or occurs concomitantly with the headache, and consists of visual disturbances called scintillating scotomata. N, V, or anorexia occurs in about 90% of cases, although V and anorexia are usually associated with more severe or prolonged attacks.

Treatment of migraine headaches involves a combination of lifestyle modification and medical therapy. The patient should identify specific predisposing factors, including foods and stress, and attempt to reduce or eliminate those factors. Medical treatment of migraine can include three types of drugs: (1) symptomatic, (2) abortive, and (3) prophylactic. Some patients need only one type of drug whereas others require a combination of two or three to control their migraine attacks. Drugs that may be used to reduce or eliminate symptoms during an attack include analgesics, anti-inflammatory agents, antiemetics, and sedatives. Abortive drugs are most useful when the headache is preceded by an aura. The drugs are taken during this aura before the headache begins. The most successful abortive medications are ergotamine tartrate, sumatriptan, nonsteroidal anti-inflammatory drugs (NSAIDs), and calcium channel-blocking agents. Prophylactic drugs are taken daily, whether or not the patient is symptomatic, in order to prevent the onset of migraine attacks. Examples include beta-blocking agents, calcium channel-blocking drugs, tricyclic antidepressants, ergot alkaloids, anticonvulsants, and NSAIDs (Hopp, 1998).

Elevated intracranial pressure

Elevated intracranial pressure resulting from any cause can produce NV, headaches, and cerebrospinal fluid (CSF) rhinorrhea. Visual symptoms can include transient visual obscurations, visual field defects, such as enlargement of the physiological blind spot, diplopia, and loss of central vision. Severe cases can result in loss of consciousness, generalized motor rigidity, and respiratory failure. Swelling of the optic nerve head (papilledema) is often present. The diagnosis is made by demonstrating a high CSF pressure on lumbar puncture. Eye examination and visual field testing are indicated to document and follow visual changes. The differential diagnosis of elevated intracranial pressure is vast and includes intracranial masses, aqueductal stenosis, subdural, epidural, and subarachnoid hemorrhages, brain abscesses, arteriovenous malformations, trauma, meningitis, and pseudotumor cerebri (benign intracranial hypertension) (Miller, 1998). Imaging of the central nervous system is an invaluable tool in determining the etiology.

Other neurological disorders that can present with NV and ophthalmic findings include nystagmus, cerebral vascular aneurysms, paroxysmal vertigo, and paroxysmal torticollis. Detailed discussion of these disorders is beyond the scope of this chapter.

Drug effects

Several drugs commonly used by ophthalmologists can produce NV (Mauger and Craig, 1994).

Carbonic anhydrase inhibitors such as acetazolamide and methazolamide are used in the treatment of glaucoma. Gastrointestinal upset is one of the more frequent causes of intolerance to these drugs, often resulting in discontinuation of treatment.

Symptoms may range from vague abdominal discomfort and a metallic taste to severe N and diarrhea.

Hyperosmotic agents such as glycerol and isosorbide are useful for treating acute elevations in intraocular pressure. They are commonly associated with NV, diarrhea, headaches, pulmonary edema, and cardiac dysrhythmias.

Other drugs used by ophthalmologists that can produce NV include cyclopentolate, fluorescein, demecarium, and echothiophate.

Postoperative NV

NV are infrequently encountered after most types of ophthalmic surgery. However, strabismus surgery has been reported to have higher rates of this postoperative complication, with some authors reporting frequencies as high as 50–60% (Donlon, 1994). Persistent NV are the most frequent reasons for unplanned admission to the hospital after outpatient strabismus surgery. Traction on the extraocular muscles and the depth of anesthesia required for eye muscle surgery have been cited as possible reasons for this association. A systematic review by Tramèr et al. (1995) of randomized controlled trials in squint surgery is summarized in Chapter 6 (page 129). Helveston (1993) reported a rate less than 1% for postoperative persistent V requiring hospitalization. The diminished use of preoperative opioids has probably contributed to the decreased incidence of this problem.

Case study

Migraine

A 24-year-old woman, single mother of two children, was at work as a unit manager in a start-up company when she had the acute onset of photophobia, pressure behind the eyes, and bilateral vision with zig-zag images. Within minutes, she began experiencing a severe, bitemporal, throbbing headache and, shortly thereafter, she complained to colleagues of N. An experienced migraineur, she self-administered, subcutaneously, a 0.5-ml vial of sumatriptan succinate 6 mg. She removed herself to a quiet, darkened room to rest. After an hour, the headache had mostly subsided, and her ocular symptoms abated. A pattern of stress-related onset of migraine was well known to this patient and, although her job requirements were demanding, she had found that the above regimen was usually effective as needed, perhaps every 2–3 months. Only occasionally was the progression of symptoms so rapid that she developed V, and when she did, an additional dose was often effective, 1 hour after the first, in producing sustained relief.

CHAPTER 29

Otolaryngology

Anyone who has gone fishing in a small boat on a rough sea or lake knows of the relationship between certain types of movement and the symptoms of malaise often leading to nausea and vomiting (NV). Seasickness or *mal de mer* has been with us for centuries.

Seasickness and its recent cousins, car, air, and space sickness, are the most common conditions, within the field of ear, nose, and throat (ENT) medicine, that produce NV as a result of unwanted stimulation of the vestibular labyrinth within the inner ear. Other disorders affecting the vestibular labyrinth, its nerve and blood supply, or central nervous system (CNS) connections can also produce NV. However, vertigo is universally a symptom in these conditions with accompanying nystagmus.

There are several causes of NV that occur in the field of ENT medicine that overlap with other fields and are covered in other chapters of this book; they will not, therefore, be discussed here. These include post-anesthetic nausea and the side effects of many prescription drugs. Neurological causes of NV are also seen by otolaryngologists and include migraine, brain tumors (particularly cerebellopontine angle and cerebellar tumors), central vestibular system diseases, and vascular diseases, such as a brain-stem stroke or vertebrobasilar artery insufficiency. These causes are discussed in Chapter 25.

Anatomy

The fluid-filled inner ear or labyrinth, one located on each side of the head, can be divided into two parts, the cochlea or hearing organ and the vestibular labyrinth or balance organ (Anson and

Donaldson, 1973; Baloh and Honrubia, 1990). The vestibular labyrinth can be further subdivided into the three semicircular canals (superior, lateral, and posterior), which are sensitive to rotary motion in the three spatial planes and the otolith organs, the utricle and saccule, which are sensitive to linear motion in these planes.

Sensory receptors composed of specialized hair cells lie within the fluid of each semicircular canal (crista ampularis) and the vestibule (maculae of the utricle and saccule). Movement of the inner ear fluid with movement of the head or body changes the stimuli sent via the vestibular nerve, part of cranial nerve VIII, to the four vestibular nuclei on each side within the brain stem. These nuclei have connections to the cerebellum, oculomotor nuclei, spinal cord, and cerebral cortex. The blood supply comes from end-branches of the vestibular arteries and the cochleovestibular artery. In the head-fixed state, each vestibular labyrinth produces a baseline balanced input to the vestibular nuclei, which changes with changes in head position or movement. Damage or stimulation to one side offsets this balance producing vertigo, usually with NV.

Inner-ear disorders leading to vertigo and NV

The key to the diagnosis of inner-ear-induced NV is the fact that it is regularly accompanied by vertigo, defined as a sensation of space rotating around one or one rotating in space. No other focal neurological signs or symptoms exist; nystagmus is usually present. The symptom of dizziness is differentiated from true vertigo, because it is much less specific (the person feels light-headed, woozy, and faint) and does not have the rotary component. However, patients may have difficulty in explaining the difference to the physician. Spatial disorientation is the feeling that one's balance is not normal, particularly as the person moves his or her head or while walking.

Acute causes

Motion sickness

As mentioned at the start, by far the most common conditions are the easily diagnosed disorders included in the term 'motion sickness.' This can be a serious problem if the individual must perform important tasks, such as flying a plane or piloting a ship. Linear stimulation of the vestibular labyrinth over a period of many minutes or hours is the cause.

Mechanism for NV produced by motion sickness
There is a great deal of individual variation in susceptibility to motion sickness. Furthermore, training and experience can decrease the symptoms (old sailors do better than young sailors); training is used in the space program to decrease the likelihood of space sickness.

Although the combination of movements producing motion sickness in an individual may be complex, and certainly affected by visual input (the driver of a car rarely gets carsick whereas the passengers do), the main cause appears to be repeated linear stimulation of the maculae in the utricle and saccule. This leads to autonomic stimulation, sweating, light-headedness, N, and ultimately V.

Acute labyrinthitis

This condition, thought to be of a viral etiology, is relatively common and follows an upper respiratory infection by 2–3 weeks. The virus apparently reaches the middle ear via the eustachian tube, and then extends into the labyrinth producing inflammation resulting in vertigo and NV. It begins suddenly, is severe, and often requires the patient to remain in bed for several days. It runs a course of 1–2 weeks with gradual improvement over time. Afterwards. the vestibular system usually shows no residual damage. Hearing loss is not present.

Bacterial labyrinthitis is a much more severe disease and is usually a complication of purulent otitis media with the infecting bacteria (commonly pneumococci, staphylococci, and streptococci) extending into the inner ear. Such infections may produce total destruction of the labyrinth and may require longer periods of time before recovery occurs, usually 3-4 weeks. Extension into the CNS may occur, producing meningitis and brain abscess. Hearing loss is regularly present.

Vestibular neuronitis

This condition is poorly understood and appears to be a sudden failure of the peripheral vestibular system on one side. The unbalanced opposite vestibular system produces the symptoms and findings, which mimic the symptoms of viral labyrinthitis. Hearing loss does not occur and the patient recovers in 2–3 weeks (Baloh and Honrubia, 1990).

Ménière's disease

This consists of the triad of fluctuating low-frequency hearing loss, tinnitus, and vertigo. Symptoms are the result of an increase in pressure within the endolymph of the inner car. Again, as in the other inner-ear syndromes producing vertigo, NV may be prominent (Vesterhauge et al., 1995).

Trauma to the inner ear

Destruction of part or all of the inner ear as a result of trauma produces vertigo and hearing loss plus the accompanying NV. This is usually caused by fractures of the temporal bone, which may involve the labyrinth directly or disrupt its nerve or blood supply. The inner ear is well protected from concussion as a result of its location deep in the skull and it takes a severe injury to produce inner-ear disruption.

Benign positional vertigo

This condition is thought to be caused by separation of the otoconia granules from their normal location on the macula of the utricle, so that they float in the endolymph and stimulate the semicircular canal ampulae in certain head positions. It is positional, intense, and short-lived.

Occlusion of the vestibular artery

Small end arteries supply the vestibular labyrinth and occlusion of one or more of these vessels can produce partial or total loss of blood supply, producing vertigo with NV. Depending on the vessel(s) involved, hearing loss may occur as well.

Perilymph fistula

If there is perilymph leakage out of the inner ear with a drop in inner-ear pressure and fluid movement, hearing loss and vertigo with NV may occur. The leak may follow head trauma or rarely after sneezing or straining, which disrupts the round window membrane of the cochlea or the annulus around the footplate in the oval window, producing a leak.

Post-otological surgery

After surgery for otosclerosis (stapedotomy or stapedectomy), which consists of removing the stapes superstructure, making a hole in the oval window, and placing a piston connected to the incus in the hole, there may be a serous labyrinthitis and/or leakage of perilymph. This may produce postoperative vertigo and NV. Labyrinthectomy and vestibular nerve section are used for the treatment of severe inner-ear balance disorders and obviously produce total loss of unilateral vestibular function and postoperative vertigo.

Chronic causes

Presbylibrium

It is well known that the hair cells in the cochlea deteriorate with age, producing a hearing loss (presbycusis). The same thing appears to occur with the hair cells in the vestibular system and leads to a decrease in balance skills with age. When accompanied by decreasing vision, decreased muscle strength, and decreased proprioception, this produces an increase in falls. It can produce a feeling of nausea (Goode, 1981).

Tumors of the acoustic nerve (acoustic neuroma)

These benign tumors are usually slow growing and produce pressure on the vestibular portion of the acoustic nerve, leading to a gradual decrease in hearing and balance on the involved side.

Ototoxic drugs

Streptomycin was one of the original antibiotics that was found to have the side effect of producing toxic effects on the vestibular and cochlear hair cells. Most of the other aminoglycoside antibiotics also have this property as do several of the diuretics, such as ethacrynic acid. The effect is usually dose related but can be idiosyncratic. Vestibular system toxicity occurs before auditory system toxicity. The effect of ototoxic drugs is increased with impaired kidney function and patients on these drugs should have careful monitoring of hearing and balance.

Other non-inner-ear causes

Hyperactive gag reflex

Stimulation of the posterior oral pharynx, as everyone knows, can produce NV. There are some people who cannot go to the dentist without gagging during something as simple as teeth cleaning,

Cervical vertigo

This occurs with whiplash injuries of the neck and produces symptoms of imbalance and occasionally vertigo which may be accompanied by NV. This appears to be secondary to the connections between the proprioceptors in the neck muscles and the vestibular nuclei in the brain stem.

Hyperventilation

Anxious individuals who hyperventilate have light-headedness and dizziness, sometimes with N secondary to lowering of the carbon dioxide blood level.

Treatment

In the case of motion sickness, the best treatment is prevention if at all possible. Don't get on a boat or roller coaster if you don't have to. The less movement, the better. Modern jet aircraft flying at high altitudes do not produce the same inner-ear stimulation as smaller aircraft flying lower in bumpy air. Larger ocean liners have weight and stabilizers to minimize the movement of the ship, and therefore are preferable to small boats. Avoiding sudden head movements or activities that produce vertigo or imbalance should be obvious. Benign positional vertigo can be treated by placing the head into certain positions so the otoconia become trapped and cannot float in the endolymph. Topical anesthetics can decrease the gag reflex. Hyperventilation is treated with education and rebreathing into a paper bag during acute attacks. The underlying anxiety may also need treatment. Removal of the cause is most important, so that if a tumor is producing the symptoms the tumor should be removed.

Medications

Treatment with an antihistamine, such as dimenhydrinate dramamine, meclozine or cyclizine, has been found to be effective in prevention of motion sickness, but must be taken before the stimulus to have a major effect. Anticholinergics such as atropine or scopolamine also help. Scopolamine can now be obtained as a patch which can be worn behind the ear and lasts for 3 days. Again, it needs to be placed before the anticipated motion sickness to have its greatest effect.

Benzodiazpines, such as diazepam, and phenothiazines, such as prochlorperazine, thiethylperazine, and promethazine, are often used; if V is severe, the drugs must be given intravenously, intramuscularly, or rectally. Trimethobenzamide may also be effective in controlling NV. Patients with severe NV must be monitored for dehydration and, if necessary, provided with intravenous replacement of fluids; this may require hospitalization. The antihistamines, phenothiazines, and benzodiazepines unfortunately produce sedation and the patient must be aware of this if they drive or work around moving machinery. Patients with severe vertigo and dizziness should not drive or operate machinery. Methylphenidate can be used to offset the drowsiness. If and when vertigo occurs the patient is advised to stay seated or lie in bed with minimal head movement. Fixation on a target with the eyes is usually better than with the eyes closed. As a result of the accompanying nystagmus, it may be difficult to read or watch television.

Some of the newer drugs developed for the treatment and pretreatment of post-chemotherapy NV have been found to be effective, such as ondansetron. The use of metoclopramide or cisapride can be useful for increasing gastric emptying in the right direction.

Diuretics are used for the treatment of Ménière's disease to decrease inner-ear pressure.

Case report

A 37-year-old female physician woke up and found that she could not get out of bed because the room was spinning clockwise; any movement of her head made the feeling worse. She was nauseous and over the next several hours vomited several times. She remained in bed and had to be helped to the bathroom. There were no other neurological symptoms present. There was no previous history of an upper respiratory tract infection in the past month or an ear infection. There was no weakness of any extremity or headache. She had never had anything like this before and did not notice any ringing in her ears or change in hearing. She was unable to eat, and when she attempted to take liquids or solids she would vomit. Her physical examination revealed her to be clammy with hypotension on sitting up. Nystagmus beating to the left was present. Neurological examination was otherwise negative. She was treated with rectal promethazine and gradually improved over the first 24 hours and was able to take small amounts of liquids. Over the next 4–5 days she continued to get better and was able to walk around. By the end of the week, she was able to drive and returned to work in 8–9 days. However, she was aware that her balance was not perfect.

Approximately 3 weeks afterwards she felt that she had recovered 100% and has had no recurrence in 2 years of follow-up. Based on the history and physical findings, the diagnosis is vestibular neuronitis.

CHAPTER 30

Pediatrics including pediatric oncology

How are nausea and vomiting related to pediatrics?

Nausea and vomiting (NV) are ubiquitous in pediatrics, particularly among infants and young children. There is a vast number of disorders that are associated with NV in pediatrics (Table 30.1). These disorders range from innocuous problems, such as those associated with feeding difficulties, to serious gastrointestinal disorders that require medical or surgical interventions. The wide range of diagnoses and treatments of NV in the field of pediatrics creates a major challenge to the physician caring for a child suffering from NV. The most common approach to diagnosis focuses on a history of the nature of the V and is guided by the age of the patient. Although infants presumably experience nausea, it takes several years before they can identify it and communicate about it. Until then, clinicians, like veterinarians, are forced to rely on vomiting. Physical examinations and laboratory tests are often needed to rule out serious or life-threatening conditions.

Epidemiological studies

These suggest that more than 50% of infants experience spitting, V, or rumination. Approximately 5% of these incidents are associated with significant disease; the remainder are often linked to improper feeding techniques, psychosocial disturbances between parent and infant, or simply physiological immaturity of the gastroesophageal junction. Episodes of V associated with the presence of an abdominal mass, abdominal distention, projectile V, or blood or bile in the vomitus are, however, indications of serious disease that could require hospitalization or surgical emergency.

Table 30.1: Causes of NV in children

Infants	Children	Adolescents
Gastrointestinal	*Gastrointestinal*	*Gastrointestinal*
Regurgitation	Peptic ulcer	Peptic ulcer
Achalasia	Duodenal hematoma	Appendicitis
Gastroesophageal reflux	Gastrointestinal allergy	Pancreatitis
Tracheo-esophageal fistula	Appendicitis	Gastroenteritis
Duodenal stenosis	Achalasia	Hernia
Jejunal stenosis	Adhesive bands	
Ileal atresia	Incarcerated hernia	
Duodenal atresia	Mesenteric vascular obstruction	*CNS*
Intestinal duplication		Intracranial mass,
Gastroenteritis	Paralytic ileus	Esophageal atresia
Duodenitis	Abdominal neoplasm	Head trauma,
Hirschsprung's disease	Crohn's disease	Pancreatitis, Migraine
Midgut volvulus	Gastroenteritis	Cyclic vomiting
Celiac disease	Idiopathic intestinal pseudo-obstruction	Epilepsy
Pyloric stenosis		
Esophageal web	Superior mesenteric artery syndrome	
Diaphragmatic hernia		*Respiratory*
Incarcerated hernia		Common cold
Intussusception		Pneumonia
Meconium ileus	*CNS*	Otitis media
Necrotizing enterocolitis	Intracranial masses	Sinusitis
Congenital bands	Head trauma	Pharyngitis
Acute peritonitis	Intracranial edema	Tonsillitis
Imperforate anus	Migraine	Bronchiolitis
Malrotation of the bowl	Cyclic vomiting	
Hemorrhagic diseases	Epilepsy	
Adynamic ileus	Hydrocephalus	*Genitourinary*
	Pseudotumor cerebri	Pyelonephritis
	Meningitis	Renal colic
CNS	Encephalitis	Urinary tract infections
Hydrocephalus		
Intracranial masses		
Intracranial hemorrhage	*Metabolic*	*Metabolic*
Subdural hematoma	Diabetic ketoacidosis	Uremia
Head trauma	Thyrotoxicosis	
Meningitis		
Diencephalic syndrome		*Other*
	Respiratory	Pregnancy
	Common cold	Drugs
	Pneumonia	Bulimia
	Otitis media	Pelvic inflammatory disease
	Sinusitis	
	Pharyngitis	
	Tonsillitis	
	Bronchiolitis	

Table 30.1: (contd)

Infants	Children	Adolescents
Respiratory	*Genitourinary*	
Pneumonia	Hydronephrosis	
Otitis media	Glomerulonephritis	
Respiratory infection	Pyelonephritis	
	Obstructive anomalies	
Metabolic	Urinary tract infections	
Hypoadrenalism		
Galactosemia		
Adrenogenital syndrome	*Metabolic*	
Fructosemia	Uremia	
Diabetic ketoacidosis	Diabetic ketoacidosis	
Reye's syndrome	Thyrotoxicosis	
Aminoaciduria		
Organic aciduria		
Renal tubular acidosis	*Other*	
	Drugs	
	Poisoning	
Other	Hepatitis	
Improper feeding	Food allergy	
Complications during birth	Diabetes mellitus	
Food allergy	Reye's syndrome	
Sepsis	Mesenteric adenitis	
Poisoning	Hypercalcemia	
Drugs	Munchausen syndrome by proxy	
Nervous vomiting		
Innocent vomiting		
Infant rumination syndrome		
Familial dysautonomia		

Regurgitation or 'spitting up'

This occurs frequently in infants. It is defined as the 'rolling out' of gastric contents through the mouth. Regurgitation is often caused by inadequate feeding; however, it can also be attributed to a lax gastroesophageal sphincter. Regurgitation of this type usually does not interfere with the infant's ability to thrive. In contrast to regurgitation, V is a forceful expulsion of gastric contents that is the result of a complex mechanism controlled by the central nervous system. V is typically preceded by N. N in infants is characterized by failure to suck, restlessness, grimacing, and refusal to refeed after V.

Vomiting in newborns and infants

Nausea is a complex symptom that has a particular meaning to older children and adults, but must be inferred in children and infants. The corollary signs of N, also well known to older children and adults, are lethargy, lack of interest in food despite no recent intake, and repetitive swallowing, usually of excess saliva. Older children may vocalize the negative sensation of 'not feeling good,' or reporting that their 'tummy hurts.' Parents of infants must be reassured that the crying by their infant does not constitute an illness, or necessarily a problem, but an adaptation to a new environment, internally as well as externally. Nevertheless, continuing symptoms consistent with N must be assessed without delay, after a few hours of persistence.

Gastroesophageal reflux

Gastroesophageal reflux (GER) is a common cause of V in many infants, particularly after feeding. GER is typically caused by low esophageal sphincter pressure and increased abdominal pressure. In most infants the condition recedes by 9 months of age without any intervention. Reflux problems of this sort are often aggravated by improper feeding techniques such as overfeeding, failure to burp the infant, and over-stimulating the infant after feeding. GER can be diagnosed by several different methods including fluoroscopy, ultrasonography, upper gastrointestinal scintigraphy, endoscopy, and biopsy of the esophageal mucosa. It is usually not necessary, however, to perform all evaluation techniques on patients with symptoms of GER. In most cases, GER can be adequately managed by using small, frequent feedings, formula thickening, and antireflux positioning. In rare cases of severe GER, which are associated with esophageal structure, aspiration, and failure to thrive, surgical intervention may be necessary.

Parenteral infections and congenital anomalies

These are among the leading causes of NV during the neonatal and infancy period. Respiratory infections (see Table 30.1) are among the major parenteral causes of N throughout early childhood. Gastroenteritis of either viral or bacterial origin is another major cause of NV. The condition is usually characterized by forceful V or bilious V, and often precedes the onset of diarrhea. Management of gastroenteritis typically includes rehydration therapy and systemic antibiotics, once bacterial origin is established.

Pyloric stenosis

This is the most common condition requiring surgical intervention during the newborn period. Epidemiological studies reveal that the condition occurs in one in 700 live births and is five times more likely to occur in male than in female infants. Pyloric stenosis is caused by a hypertrophied pyloric muscle. The condition is characterized by projectile V (beginning between 1 and 6 weeks of age), peristalsis waves from right to left, and palpation of a pyloric tumor or 'olive' in the epigastrium.

Other gastrointestinal anomalies

These include congenital duodenal atresia and duodenal stenosis which are characterized by bilious V and distention of the stomach. These manifestations typically appear 24–48 hours after birth. Similarly, congenital atresia of the ileum, like the two conditions above, is often caused by malrotation of the colon and presents early in life: 24 hours to 4 days of age. Symptoms include V and gaseous distention. In addition, the infant may not experience any bowel movements after passage of the meconium stool. Intestinal tract obstruction is another cause of V which requires surgical intervention. Examples of such conditions include meconium ileus which is characterized by dark-green vomitus caused by intussusception; it occurs most often in male infants aged 3–11 months. Intussusception is usually indicated in an infant who seems to have severe abdominal pain accompanied by V that may become bilious and bloody stools.

Central nervous system

Increased intracranial pressure such as that caused by hydrocephalus and intracranial tumors can produce V that is often projectile in nature and is typically preceded by N. In the infant, the presence of a bulging fontanel and emesis is suggestive of a subdural hematoma or hydrocephalus. Other central nervous systems disorders that present with V include bacterial meningitis and encephalitis.

Functional V disorders

These disorders are V syndromes that mimic organic disease. As many as 20% of infants experience innocent V. They 'spit up' a small amount of stomach contents or expel a large amount in a projectile fashion. This type of V cannot be lessened by changing the position of the patient or changing infant formula. Innocent V does not affect the patient's ability to thrive and usually subsides before the infant is 18 months old. This type of V in infants is often caused by antral dysmotility or pylorospasm. The latter is a condition that results when the pylorus closes more strongly than usual.

Nervous V and infant rumination syndrome

There are two V conditions that are caused by strained parent–infant interactions: nervous V and infant rumination syndrome. Nervous V occurs in infants who are easily aroused by external stimuli. Parents of these infants are often attentive but unable to soothe the infant when she or he becomes excited. The parents usually become distressed when the V continues and the infant begins to lose weight. This type of reaction leads to further breakdown of the parent–infant relationship. Infants with nervous V should be shielded from stimuli that would cause them to become excited, especially during feeding and naps. In contrast, infant rumination syndrome occurs in infants who are not sufficiently stimulated by their parents. Rumination usually begins at 3 months of age and is a form of self-stimulation. It is a rare condition but it can be lethal. Treatment includes ensuring that the baby receives adequate stimulation from the parents or an alternative caregiver.

NV in children

Gastrointestinal disorders

The primary cause of V during childhood is infectious diseases including gastroenteritis and respiratory infections (see Table 30.1) such as pneumonia. Gastrointestinal disorders such as peptic ulcer disease and appendicitis may also present during childhood. V may be a significant manifestation of peptic ulcer disease in the younger patient along with general abdominal pain. In the older child, the most pronounced symptom is abdominal pain. Appendicitis is also associated with V among the pediatric population. Other symptoms may include irritability, loss of appetite, and abdominal distention.

Migraine headache and trauma

In addition to the central nervous system disorders that affect infants, migraine and head trauma commonly cause V in older patients. One study found that V after head trauma was more likely to occur in children over the age of 2. Migraine in children, similar to adults, is often associated with NV and episodes of cyclic V.

Cyclic V syndrome

This syndrome is defined by recurring V episodes that usually begin at night. Other symptoms associated with this syndrome include crampy diarrhea, mild fever, and headache. The onset of the syndrome typically occurs between 2 and 9 years of age. Management through fluid and electrolyte resuscitation is important as the V episodes may last for 12–48 hours.

Ingested poisons

Another important cause of V during childhood is food poisoning caused by various bacterial agents including *Salmonella*, *Shigella*, *Clostridium botulinum* (botulism toxins), and staphylococci. Symptoms often include diarrhea and abdominal pain. Another common toxin ingested is lead obtained from flaking paint in older homes; paint sold during the past 10 years contains no lead. Lead poisoning includes NV, as well as headache, lethargy, and poor appetite. Chronic carbon monoxide poisoning is another cause of NV that occurs during the winter months as a result of faulty ducting of heating sources, and poor venting.

NV in adolescents

Unique causes of NV among patients in this age group, particularly female patients, include pregnancy, pelvic inflammatory disease, and bulimia. Urinary tract infections, suggesting the onset of sexual activity, are also more common in this age group.

Differential diagnosis of NV

Diagnosis of NV in pediatric patients should take into account three major factors: (1) the age of the patient; (2) the sex of the patient; and (3) the description of the V episodes.

Age and sex

The age of the patient can assist the physician greatly in the diagnosis of V disorders. In the newborn period, V after the first feeding is a strong indication of congenital anatomical obstruction such as atresias, esophageal web, and duodenal stenosis. V associated with abdominal distention during this period is also a sign of anatomical obstruction. V in the newborn period may also indicate metabolic disease. In contrast, V that occurs later in infancy may indicate developmental disorders or less severe congenital abnormalities. Pyloric stenosis, meconium ileus, and intussusception are examples of obstructions that emerge during infancy. These conditions are also seen more frequently in males than in females. During the adolescent period, however, physicians should consider pregnancy and eating disorders as a possible cause of V in females.

In infants and young children, feeding techniques, the frequency of the feeding, and the timing of the V with respect to feeding should be considered. Gastrointestinal reflux and functional V disorders such as nervous V can be aggravated by improper feeding techniques.

Acute illness is also a major cause of NV in infants and children. Consequently, associated symptoms should also be considered. For example, V that is associated with diarrhea and abdominal pain usually indicates a parenteral infection such as gastroenteritis. In contrast, V associated with fever and the absence of diarrhea may indicate respiratory infection.

Emesis episodes and vomitus

The nature of the emesis is another important consideration of differential diagnosis of V in pediatrics. A history should include the question of whether or not there was bile, blood, or undigested food in the emesis. Bilious V is associated with postampullary obstructions and should be considered a possible surgical emergency. Blood in the vomitus may indicate gastritis, ulcers, or esophagitis. Undigested food in the vomitus is associated with obstructions proximal to the stomach. Conditions characterized by undigested vomitus include esophageal stenosis and achalasia.

Finally, the force of the V can also be an important indicator of the severity of the V condition. Projectile V is often associated with serious conditions such as intracranial pressure and pyloric stenosis.

When an older child manifests acute vomiting and somnolence, one should always consider Reye's Syndrome (aspirin toxicity), and meningo-encephalitis in the differential diagnosis.

Complications

Persistent V

This can cause a number of complications. The most common health sequelae of V are dehydration and electrolyte imbalance. Other metabolic complications may include alkalosis and sodium and potassium depletion. Aspiration pneumonia may also be a complication of chronic V. Persistent forceful V may result in a tear in the juxtaesophageal gastric mucosa (Mallory–Weiss tear), esophageal rupture, and peptic esophagitis. During infancy, failure to thrive can be a serious complication of chronic V.

Treatment

Treatment of V can include control of sequelae, treatment of the specific condition causing the V, and antiemetic therapy. Dehydration associated with persistent V should be treated with oral rehydration therapy. More serious metabolic disturbances such as hypochloremic alkalosis with secondary hypokalemia requires intravenous fluid therapy.

Management of gastrointestinal reflux during infancy usually includes use of small, frequent feedings, formula thickening, and antireflux positioning. In more severe cases, antireflux surgery may be required. Surgical intervention is necessary in other conditions that cause NV including anatomical obstructions such as pyloric stenosis or appendicitis.

Antiemetics should not be prescribed to infants; however, they may be useful for management of persistent V in children and adolescents. Antiemetics include antihistamines, anticholinergics, β-adrenergic antagonists, dopamine antagonists, and miscellaneous agents (Table 30.2). Antihistamines such as promethazine, dimenhydrinate, and cyclizine are typically used to manage V associated with motion sickness. V associated with vestibular disorders or stimulation can be treated with scopolamine (hyoscine). Metoclopramide, a dopamine antagonist, is useful in treating conditions that arise from poor gastric emptying. The drug acts on the chemoreceptor zone and enhances motor activity of the stomach, duodenum, and small intestine. Other dopamine antagonists such as prochlorperazine and chlorpromazine are prescribed in adults for V that is associated with surgery, drugs, or radiation. These drugs, however, have side effects such as extrapyramidal reactions and blood dyscrasias.

Anticipatory NV, which occurs in 20% of chemotherapy patients, can be controlled by diazepam. V associated with migraine headaches can be managed by propranolol and chlorpromazine.

Conclusion

NV are associated with many pediatric diseases and disorders. They can be caused by genetic disorders, developmental disorders, and

Table 30.2 Commonly used antiemetics

Antihistamines
Promethazine
Dimenhydrinate
Cyclizine
Anticholinergics
Scopolamine (hyoscine)
β-Adrenergic antagonists
Propranolol
Dopamine antagonists
Metoclopramide
Prochlorperazine
Chlorpromazine
Thiethylperazine
Perphenazine
Other
Phosphorylated carbohydrate solution
Lorazepam
Diazepam

infectious diseases, as well as disorders of almost every major organ system. Disorders associated with NV range from innocuous problems that require no intervention to serious disorders that may require surgery. Consequently, early diagnosis of the cause of NV in pediatrics is of vital importance. All diagnoses should take into account the age and sex of the patient, and the nature of the V episodes. In addition, physical examination and laboratory tests may be needed to rule out serious or life-threatening conditions. Treatment and diagnosis of pediatric NV can pose a serious challenge to physicians. This chapter identifies common disorders and characteristics of NV in pediatrics in an effort to assist caregivers in determining the underlying cause of the symptoms.

CHAPTER 31

Psychiatry

Important conditions that present nausea and vomiting (NV) in psychiatric practice include the eating disorders, anorexia nervosa and bulimia, anticipatory NV (as in chemotherapy treatment), and psychogenic V and rumination. Side effects and overdose of medication constitute iatrogenic precipitants for NV and can induce behavioral dysfunctions. The serotonin syndrome must be included when considering NV in emotionally disturbed or otherwise referred patients.

Eating disorders

The eating disorders, including anorexia nervosa and bulimia, are characterized by a preoccupation with body shape and weight, and food intake. A profound disturbance occurs in body image. Being thin is pursued to the point of starvation. The anorectic person is intensely afraid of gaining weight and fails to maintain a minimally normal body weight; the weight criterion is 15% or more below the normal body weight. In women, persistent amenorrhea results, attributable to an altered secretion of the hypothalamus in regulating gonadotropin-releasing hormone (GnRH).

Classification and description

Anorexia nervosa is classified as one of two subtypes: restricting eating and binge eating/purging types. Restrictors accomplish weight loss by dieting or excessive exercise, whereas the binge/purgers engage in weight loss through self-induced V or the misuse of laxatives, diuretics, or enemas, or by excessive exercise. At least 50% of anorectic patients eventually develop bulimic symptoms (Casper et al., 1980).

In bulimia nervosa there are recurrent episodes of eating large quantities of food in a short period of time, accompanied by a feeling of a lack of self-control. To prevent weight gain, these persons regularly engage in recurrent, inappropriate compensatory behaviors. Such episodes, e.g., laxative use, are typically followed by feelings of guilt, depression, and an awareness that one's behavior is abnormal.

Anorectic patients typically are reluctant to seek help and may frequently deny any problems. They tend to be rigid, energetic, and disciplined. People with anorexia who used both restricting and purging techniques display more psychopathology than those who confined their diet activities exclusively to the restriction of energy intake (Garner et al., 1993).

People with bulimia tend to be more popular, more gregarious, and of normal weight, and are often stimulus seekers. Self-esteem tends to depend on family and friends. People with bulimia who employ more than one strategy for purging were found to be more disturbed on a number of psychiatric indices, including state and trait depression (Tobin et al., 1990).

Physical complications

Physical complications of bulimic behaviors include electrolyte, mineral, and fluid imbalances. V can result in hypokalemic/hypochloremic alkalosis. Low levels of potassium can lead to fatigue, generalized muscle weakness, seizures, heart arrhythmias, and kidney damage. Abnormalities in sodium may lead to convulsions, particularly in individuals who consume large quantities of alcohol in their binges. Death from aspirated vomitus can occur and there may be fractures.

V leads to gastric and esophageal irritation and bleeding, and some may develop hiatus hernia with abdominal pain. Repeated V may cause esophageal or gastric dilatation and can result in a fatal rupture (Mallory–Weiss). Large binges may produce pancreatic dysfunction, leading to pancreatitis, and there may be immune system compromise.

Swelling of the parotid glands results in elevated levels of the enzyme amylase in the blood. The level of amylase and the extent of salivary gland enlargement are related to both the frequency and type of V. The usefulness of amylase levels in the assessment of patients with bulimia is under debate. Calluses on the back of the hands and erosion of dental enamel with marked decay may also occur.

Estimates are that 7–10% of outpatients in North America with eating disorders use ipecac to purge (Humphries et al., 1992; Greenfield et al., 1993). Patients who induce V by abusing ipecac may develop a cardiomyopathy because emetine, the active ingredient in ipecac, destroys heart muscle fibers. Ipecac abuse can also lead to gastrointestinal (GI) toxicity and peripheral muscle weakness. Discontinuation of ipecac usually results in recovery from these harmful effects (Vabin, 1992).

The following are complications associated with starvation in anorexia nervosa:

- Cardiac: loss of cardiac muscle, cardiac arrhythmias, and bradycardia
- Hypotension
- Inverted T waves, ST segment depression, and longer QT interval
- Endocrine: amenorrhea; low levels of luteinizing hormone (LH), and low levels of follicle-stimulating hormone (FSH)
- Gastrointestinal: delayed gastric emptying, bloating, constipation, and abdominal pain
- Other: hypothermia, dependent edema, leukopenia, lanugo (the appearance of neonatal-like hair).

Eating disorders plague up to 25% of diabetic adolescent girls and young women. This interferes with glucose control and increases the risk for diabetic complications (Goldman, 1996a). Over 80% of young diabetic women with an eating disorder aged between 12 and 18 had retinopathy, compared with 13% who had threshold disorders and 24% of young diabetic women without an eating disorder (Tucker, 1995).

Treatment

Treatment interventions aim first to correct nutritional deficiencies and second to restore normal eating patterns. Longer-term goals include resolving associated psychological, family, and social conflicts and behaviors in order to prevent relapse. This two-prong approach includes pharmacological and psychotherapeutic interventions. Antidepressants have been shown to reduce the bulimic symptoms of bingeing and vomiting (monoamine oxidase inhibitors, tricyclics, and serotonin-specific reuptake inhibitors), but have a far more limited role in the treatment of anorexia nervosa.

Psychotherapy alone outperforms medications alone. Adding medications to psychotherapy provides only modest, if any, improvement over psychotherapy alone (Mitchell et al., 1993). The most successful psychotherapeutic approaches involve behavioral or cognitive–behavioural approaches whether individual or group.

Attitudes about food, weight, and body image need to be explored. As the therapy progresses, discussion shifts away from food and weight to the more difficult areas involving self-esteem and self-awareness. For those with anorexia, family therapy is recommended as well. In those with bulimia, adjunctive therapies such as light therapy and guided imagery have been successful in relieving some of the symptoms (Tucker, 1996).

Anticipatory NV

Anticipatory NV (ANV) are the NV that occur after there has been initial exposure to chemotherapy, occurring before later episodes of chemotherapy. Although NV after treatment are common responses to the radiotherapy and chemotherapy used in cancer, ANV are less common. The prevalence rates of ANV range between 21% and 67% of patients. NV also varies according to the particular chemotherapy used.

Etiology

ANV seem to be learned; some risk factors are identified other than treatment variables themselves.

Complications: indirect mortality

ANV may add such discomfort that it may prevent the patient from continuing treatment. The discomfort of the ANV may lead to anorexia and malnutrition; these might have adverse effects on the immunity system. The V may lead to esophageal tears and bone fractures.

Treatment

ANV respond to behavioral treatments but do not typically respond to antiemetic medications (Morrow and Morrell, 1982). Particular behavioral techniques that have proved useful include:

- progressive relaxation training with imagery
- hypnosis

- systemic desensitization
- anti-motion medications.

Relaxation training with guided imagery were found not only to reduce anticipatory N, but also to reduce blood pressure, heart rate, and anxiety and depression (Lyles et al., 1982). Some researchers found that cognitive distraction was as effective as relaxation training in reducing pre-treatment N and blood pressure after treatment. The treatment was equally effective for those with high or low anxiety levels (Vasterling et al., 1992).

The best intervention is to seek to control the development of emesis throughout chemo- or radiotherapy. Antiemetics are useful (but by no means always successful) in reducing N after treatment.

Psychogenic V

In cases where no organic cause of V can be found, a psychopathological cause, i.e., psychogenic V, should be considered. The symptoms are neither voluntary nor explained by any physical condition. The symptoms may function to keep an internal conflict hidden from the consciousness. They can also serve as secondary gain to manipulate others in the patient's social environment. V can be a way of communicating: a learned behavior, a means of displacing anger, a somatic equivalent of anxiety, and a means of escape.

All physical disorders have a psychological component or are affected by psychological factors. Hence, in some cases, V may be caused by a mixture of organic and psychological factors. For example, it has been postulated that V is secondary to a disorder in gastrointestinal motility which is a response to psychological stress (*Lancet* editorial, 1992).

As V may be a symptom of serious disease, psychogenic V is diagnosed after organic etiologies have been excluded. Patients with this disorder often have little insight into their condition and are either unaware or have difficulties expressing their emotions. They tend to have a high incidence of hostile and antagonistic relationships with others in their lives (Wruble et al., 1982).

The V is usually chronic although it may remit for periods of time. In contrast to many organic causes of V, psychogenic V typically occurs at meal times, and often occurs just after the meal has begun. It rarely occurs in public places. Many patients can suppress the V but feel nauseous until it is allowed. Thereafter, the patient can return to complete a meal. Most patients do not have N but, in those who do, it does not interfere with their appetite. Weight loss is not significant. Maintaining the appetite in the presence of N is a feature suggesting a nonorganic etiology. Remember, N without V is quite common and also psychogenic, such as that resulting from stress or fatigue. One tends to classify the widespread stress N separately from the rarer 'true psychogenic' N.

For both N and V, women have a higher prevalence. Although psychogenic patients complain of dysphoria and appear to be unhappy, only a minority are clinically depressed.

Treatment

Rapport and support are essential. A constructive clinical strategy is to explain the role of tension and psychological factors (true for any illness). If a patient accepts the idea of a 'nervous stomach,' exploring the cause of the stress that exacerbates it is often productive. Patients should be encouraged to speak openly about life stresses. Antiemetics can be given cautiously. Patients should also be helped to deal with the stress in their lives. Relaxation training, hypnosis, and physical exercise are adjunctive measures.

These patients should receive a thorough clinical evaluation to rule out organic etiologies and to gain the confidence of the patient. As most patients believe that they are seriously ill, negative findings may be met with a combination of relief and resentment. Resen-t-ment and defensiveness are common when a diagnosis implies that a condition might be all 'in your head.'

Rumination

Rumination is a rare, but potentially fatal, disease found in babies and rarely in children and adults. Its incidence is much increased in those with severe learning disorders. There is no associated nausea or GI illness. In this disorder the abdominal muscles contract after ingesting a meal, and the meal is regurgitated back into the mouth. Associated risks include failure to maintain a normal weight, ma-l-nutrition, dehydration, and a failure to thrive.

It typically begins between the ages of 3 and 12 months and may be hard to distinguish from normal V. It may appear to be a voluntary act because the infant will strain to bring the food to his or her mouth. Treatment consists of behavioral techniques such as aversive conditioning. For example, a shock, loud noise, or squirt to the mouth may be administered when the regurgitation occurs.

NV as side effects of medication

Most psychotropic medications including antidepressants, some antipyschotic medications, and mood stabilizers have the side effects of NV. Other medications lead to NV when a toxic level or an overdose is taken. NV can occur when a medication is discontinued abruptly. Psychotropic medications can also have antiemetic properties. Paradoxically, some have both.

Antidepressant medications

Serotonin-specific reuptake inhibitors

Incidence

The serotonin-specific reuptake inhibitors (SSRIs) include fluoxetine, sertraline, paroxetine, and fluvoxamine. They are effective in major depression, obsessive–compulsive disorder, and panic disorder.

NV are common side effects. N rates have been estimated to fall between 9.6% and 38%, and V rates between 2.4% and 14%. N with the SSRIs was found to be dose related. The rate of V increases by two- or threefold when the dose of fluoxetine is increased from 20 mg to 60 mg. N with fluvoxamine becomes more bothersome at doses greater than 150 mg per day; however, tolerance to N develops over time.

Treatment

Patients troubled by irritation of the gastric mucosa, resulting in heartburn, N, and V, can have these alleviated by taking medicine with food, milk, an antacid, or an H_2-antagonist. N may be reduced by dividing the dose into smaller doses or by pre-treatment with one of the $5HT_3$ antagonists, mirtazapine (Goodwin, 1996) or cisapride (Bergeron and Blier, 1994), with the latter probably combating N by several different means.

Nefazodone

Incidence

Nefazodone is active as a serotonin 2 ($5HT_2$)-selective antagonist and a weak norepinephrine/serotonin reuptake blocker. It inhibits the reuptake of both serotonin and norepinephrine. It also has an affinity for α_1-adrenergic receptors. Rates of N and/or V have been estimated to be between 21% and 32%. N appears to be dose related

(Preskorn et al., 1992), with rates of 14% for a low-dose range compared with 13% for placebo and 21% for a high-dose range. N declines rapidly over time. However, the rate of N may still be greater than placebo therapy in the long run.

Treatment

N may be mitigated by taking nefazodone with meals. Food delays absorption, however, and may limit it by as much as 20% (Gelenberg, 1996). N may be minimized by starting at a low dose and increasing the dose gradually.

Venlafaxine

N is a common side effect of venlafaxine: estimates range between 29% and 37% (Montgomery, 1993). It is dose related and patients adapt to this side effect. By the fifth and sixth week the prevalence of N is reduced by 80%, and approximates the incidence of N in placebo groups.

Treatment

N may be mitigated by taking venlafaxine with meals. The incidence of N appears to be related to the magnitude of the initial dose and of the increments during titration, rather than to the total daily maintenance dose.

Other antidepressant medications

N has occasionally been reported with the use of tricyclic antidepressants. The rate of N has been estimated to fall between 2.5% and 22%. Bupropion and monoamine oxidase inhibitors (MAOIs) have also been associated with N.

Antidepressant withdrawal

N can be associated with a rapid discontinuation of the tricyclic antidepressants (as a result of cholinergic rebound) and venlafaxine. The reasons for this are not known.

Antipsychotic medications

Clozapine

Clozapine is an antipsychotic medication that has fewer parkinsonian side effects than some of this group, and it is thought to be more effective in treating the negative symptoms of schizophrenia. About 11% patients experience N and/or V. N may be managed by dose reduction or the use of antacids. Metoclopramide has been suggested, but others recommend avoiding metoclopramide because of the increased risks of extrapyramidal symptoms (Yesavage, 1992).

Newer antipsychotics

Risperidol (risperidone) also presents with an increased incidence of NV. Antipsychotic medications, not yet used in the USA, and that are associated with N include olanzapine, sertindole, and ziprasidone.

Anti-anxiety medications

Buspirone can produce NV in a minority of patients.

Mood stabilizers

Lithium

Lithium is used in bipolar disorder, intermittent explosive disorder, and as an adjunctive medication in depression and schizophrenia. N is a common side effect that is dose related and often occurs early in treatment, or when the dose is raised. It can be averted by raising the lithium dose slowly. Episodic N after each dose, when caused by local gastric irritation, may be relieved by: taking lithium with food, milk, or an antacid; dividing lithium into more frequent but slower doses; or by utilizing a slow-release preparation. The slow-release preparation increases the risks of diarrhea.

GI symptoms (along with a coarse tremor, dysarthria, ataxia, neuromuscular irregularities, and irregularities on electroencephalogram) may herald an impending lithium toxicity. In such a case, lithium levels must be carefully monitored. V for any reason may exacerbate any dehydration which would worsen lithium toxicity.

Carbamazepine

Carbamazepine is an anti-seizure medication used in bipolar disorder and impulse control disorders, particularly intermittent explosive disorder. It has been used as an alternative/adjunct treatment in schizophrenia and depressive disorders. NV are the most common side effects. Nausea is dose related and transient, and ordinarily can be reversed by decreasing the dose.

Valproate

Valproate or valproic acid is an anti-seizure medication used in bipolar disorder, intermittent explosive disorder, and schizoaffective disorder. It has also been used in depression, panic disorder, post-traumatic stress disorder, and alcohol and sedative hypnotic or anxiolytic withdrawal. Twenty-five percent of patients report N and 5% complain of V. NV are most common in the first month of treatment. N subsides over time and is treated by reducing the dose, raising the dose slowly, taking it with meals, or switching to the enteric-coated preparation.

Medication overdoses

Overdoses of lithium, carbamazepine, and valproate can present with NV, as well as change in mental status or changes in psychomotor activity.

With lithium and carbamazepine, there may be dysarthria, lack of coordination, tremors, changed deep tendon reflexes, and seizures. In this case, blood levels should be tested. Do not hesitate to send the patient to the emergency room if necessary.

Overdoses of the SSRIs, trazodone, buspirone, clonidine, nefazodone, and occasionally the tricyclic antidepressants can also present with N as one of the symptoms. Antacids and H_2-antagonists are beneficial.

Psychotropic medications with antiemetic properties

Anti-anxiety medications

- Hydroxyzine hydrochloride used as an anti-anxiety medication
- Lorazepam
- Antipsychotic medications
- Butyrophenone
- Haldoperidol
- Droperidol
- Phenothiazines
  - chlorpromazine

– perphenazine
– prochlorperazine
– trifluoperazine.

Serotonin syndrome

Symptoms include altered mental status, occasional V restlessness, myoclonus, hyperreflexia, diaphoreses, shivering, and tremor. This syndrome usually develops within several hours, but may take several weeks. The treatment stops the medication and offers supportive measures. The syndrome usually resolves within 24 hours after treatment has been started, although confusion may last for days (Sternbach, 1991).

CHAPTER 32

Sports and space medicine

Nausea and vomiting (NV) in sports and space medicine are not often documented in the available research. However, there is reason to mention the concerns because NV can be a serious problem for athletes in sports and for crew members in space. This chapter will indicate the different reasons for NV that have been noted from available research and discussions with physicians.

Although these two areas of medicine are quite different and unrelated, it is important to note that there are some common reasons for NV that will be mentioned here (i.e., pregnancy and drug toxicity), but will not be addressed in detail because they are covered extensively in other chapters.

It is possible that drugs (legal or illegal) are involved if a patient presents symptoms of N and/or V. In sports, many athletes resort to using stimulants such as caffeine to increase their energy levels. Overdosing on stimulants and other drugs can cause both N and V. Diagnosis of drug abuse or overuse can be determined from the patient's history and blood or urine tests. Treatment of drug-induced NV should follow a course of action outlined in Chapter 19.

In addition to the two causes of NV mentioned above, there are a number of causes that are specific to sports medicine and to space medicine as well. These causes will now be separately discussed.

NV in sports

NV in sports can be detrimental to the physical and mental state of an athlete. Psychological stress, poor food intake before athletic competition, heat exhaustion, extreme pain injuries including head traumas, sickness when training or competing at an unfamiliar altitude, and compression sickness when diving under water can all lead to NV. In addition, the growing number of athletes who suffer from anorexia and bulimia make it necessary to include these concerns in this chapter on NV and sports medicine.

Potential causes of NV

Stress and nutrition

Before competition, athletes in all areas of sports occasionally experience NV caused by stress and other psychological reasons. In many cases, the problem is worsened by a full stomach or a meal that is not appropriate before a competition. Athletes need nutritional meals before the competition that will not interfere with their activity. Identifying stress and/or nutrition as the reason for NV requires asking the athletes to remember what they ate before the competition as well as determining whether the problem occurs frequently. If NV are a common occurrence, then it may be a result more of nervousness and stress than of a poorly chosen precompetition meal.

Heat exhaustion

Heat exhaustion can be caused by too much exercise as well as by exercise in a warm climate. Heat exhaustion can be a result of sodium depletion, dehydration, or, usually, both. The second edition of the *Office Sports Medicine* (1996) outlines the symptoms of the two causes of heat exhaustion.

The symptoms of low-sodium heat exhaustion include fatigue, profound weakness, lightheadedness, sweating, and muscle cramps. Temperature elevations are moderate if they are present. The athlete will likely exhibit tachycardia and possibly hypotension. Often 'flu-like symptoms occur including headache, myalgia, NV, and diarrhea. Mental status is usually unaffected or mildly impaired; a loss of consciousness is rare. The symptoms of dehydration include intense thirst, some decrease in the ability to sweat, headache, mild anxiety, agitation, and confusion. Muscle weakness, generalized fatigue, and neuromuscular incoordination may be present. Water-depleted athletes are generally febrile with reduced skin turgor. Tachycardia and hypotension are particularly marked in severe cases.

As most cases of heat exhaustion result from both sodium depletion and water depletion, it is not as important to diagnose the cause as being one or the other as it is to recognize that, when an athlete is overworking the body or working in warm temperatures, NV might result. It is essential to begin treatment immediately to alleviate the NV symptoms of heat exhaustion.

Extreme pain injuries including head traumas

NV often accompany an injury that involves severe pain. They are especially common in traumatic head injuries. Physicians who treat athletes are often present at the competitions and can watch out for when a head trauma or other injury has occurred. If direct observation does not occur, diagnosing the cause of the NV requires asking the athlete or someone who was present at the event whether there was a painful injury or a direct injury to the head.

Altitude sickness (see also Chapter 23, p 408)

Mountain climbers and athletes who train and compete at high altitudes are working in thinner air where there is reduced alveolar oxygen pressure. As a consequence, respiration increases with possible hyperventilation and increased blood flow. These effects can lead to what is called 'mountain sickness' or 'altitude sickness.' In addition, water loss is increased at higher altitudes which can increase the risk of heat exhaustion.

At altitudes of 3000 meters or higher, many people exhibit temporary symptoms of altitude sickness. The symptoms are especially prevalent if climbers ascend too rapidly without gradually acclimatizing themselves to the different altitudes. The symptoms of altitude sickness are headache, dizziness, NV, dimness of vision, insomnia, and generalized weakness. In addition, the appetite may be suppressed during the early stages (McArdle et al., 1991)

Most climbers and athletes are aware of the dangers of working at high altitudes, and train and prepare themselves for thc potential problems. However, it is possible that someone who is inexperienced will suffer from altitude sickness and need treatment. Physicians who work in mountainous areas, and who follow events and competitions that occur at high altitudes, should be aware of the potential problems and treat patients accordingly.

Decompression sickness and other diving concerns

Scuba divers must go through extensive training before they can be licensed to ensure that they are aware of the myriad problems that diving may present. Diving instruction involves reading about proper procedures and experiencing at first hand the effects of breathing oxygen from a tank and the pressure that water exerts on the body at specific depths. The problems that may cause NV during scuba diving include decompression sickness and water pressing externally against the torso, affecting lung excursion and compressing the stomach.

Decompression sickness (the 'bends') occurs when a diver ascends too rapidly. The symptoms of decompression sickness include dizziness, N, itchy skin, and pain in the legs and arms. If an inexperienced diver ascends rapidly, the symptoms of decompression sickness will usually occur within 4–6 hours after the dive. However, if all ascending procedures are ignored (e.g., when a diver runs out of tank air and must ascend immediately), the symptoms usually present straight-away and can progress to paralysis within minutes (McArdle et al., 1991).

Decompression sickness occurs because dissolved nitrogen moves out of solution and forms bubbles in the body tissues and fluids. Bubbles in the lungs can cause choking and asphyxia. Bubbles in the brain or coronary arteries can block blood flow and cause strokes or heart attacks. Therefore, it is essential that divers are adequately prepared for the potential problems that can occur so that decompression sickness is not a factor that needs to be diagnosed.

Another concern that has been reported by experienced divers is that the pressure under water will often feel very painful and can press against the lungs and stomach, causing unaware divers to feel as if they are choking or make them want to vomit. Unfortunately, if a diver vomits under water while using scuba gear, the result is often fatal. If a diver feels dizziness, N, or the effects of water forcing the stomach to empty, returning to the surface as quickly and safely as possible is mandatory.

Anorexia nervosa and bulimia

Athletics requires physical and mental abilities and often strict weight control. Combined with the prevailing social pressures of sustaining an ideal weight this often causes many athletes, male and female, to resort to starving themselves (anorexia) or throwing up (bulimia) to ensure that they will not gain weight. Unfortunately, it is difficult to diagnose anorexia or bulimia because often the individual looks quite healthy.

As a result of the difficulty in determining anorexia and/or bulimia as the cause of NV in athletes, it is frequently essential to talk to coaches, team mates, team psychologists, and parents to establish whether the problems are more than just an isolated experience. The common warning signs of anorexia nervosa are dramatic loss in weight, preoccupation with food, calories, and weight, wearing layered or baggy clothing, mood swings, avoiding food-related activities, and excessive exercise. The common warning signs for bulimia nervosa are noticeable changes in weight, excessive concern about weight, bathroom visits after meals, depressive moods, strict dieting followed by binges, and increasing criticism of one's own body (Mellion, 1996)

Warning those closely associated with the athlete about the signs to watch for may enable them to diagnose anorexia or bulimia as the cause of NV and other associated problems. Once the pattern is established, appropriate measures can be taken to ensure that the athlete gets help. Without help, the effects of anorexia and bulimia can be life threatening.

Patients who suffer from anorexia and/or bulimia may experience many medical problems. Evaluation of adolescents shows that there can be derangement in every organ system. There are frequently cardiovascular abnormalities, including bradycardia, prolonged corrected QT intervals, dysrhythmias, and marked orthostatic pulse. Hypothermia is also common. Bulimic patients experience electrolyte imbalances. Hypokalemia is most common, but there is often hypocalcemia and hypophosphatemia (Mellion, 1996). As a result of the risk of these medical complications, it is imperative that athletes and anyone who is suffering from anorexia or bulimia receive education and surveillance.

Treatment and prevention methods

Stress and nutrition

If NV can be determined to be caused by nutrition and food, it is necessary to ensure that the events will not be repeated. Reducing the amount of fat in precompetition meals will result in the stomach emptying faster, decreasing the problem of a full stomach. A liquid meal will have similar results. In addition, keeping a food diary may enable an athlete to identify the specific foods that cause stomach discomfort before a competition.

If the cause of NV can be attributed to stress and nervousness, then the treatment and prevention are more personal and may require psychological help. Precompetition NV may be reduced if athletes try to calm themselves and keep their minds off the events by doing such things as meditating, deep breathing, or other activities or diversions. However, for some people the effects of stress before an event never stop.

Heat exhaustion

The treatment for heat exhaustion involves rest, rapid cooling, and fluid and electrolyte replacement. Often, moving an athlete into the shade or inside a cool building will help to decrease the problems. Immediate intake of water is essential to cool the body and replenish lost fluids. Adding a small amount of salt to water or ingesting popular sports drinks will help to replace lost electrolytes. If the problems are severe, then hospitalization may be required so that fluid and electrolyte replacement can be monitored carefully.

Extreme pain injuries including head traumas

Treatment of pain injuries that do not involve the head requires taking care of the injury by any means necessary. Assuming that the NV result from the pain stimuli, then treating the injury and stopping the pain should eliminate the associated problems. If the injury involves a head trauma, treatment requires careful observation.

As head injuries can be life threatening, it is essential to rule out possible problems such as swelling or internal bleeding. Motor problems, unequal pupil dilatation, inability to speak, disorientation, and unconsciousness indicate a serious problem. Computed tomography may be necessary to ensure that there are no major complications.

Altitude sickness

If a climber or athlete experiences altitude sickness while training or competing at a high elevation, the treatment involves resting, decreasing exercise, and eating a diet low in salt and high in carbohydrates. As the rate of water loss increases with increasing altitude, drinking balanced fluids may help to alleviate the symptoms. The best method for treating altitude sickness is, however, to prevent it from occurring at all. Slow acclimatization to moderate altitudes below 3000 meters will diminish the chance of the onset of altitude sickness.

Decompression sickness and other diving concerns

Unfortunately, treatment of decompression sickness is difficult without a recompression chamber. As a result of the severity of compression sickness, it is essential that divers know the procedures and are aware of the consequences.

Anorexia and bulimia

The treatment of an anorectic or bulimic person involves medical and psychological help. A physician needs to make sure that the patient is getting the necessary nutrition; however, the problem needs to be addressed completely by everyone involved. Professional psychological help may be necessary.

Case study

A professional football quarterback (QB) sustained a serious blow to the head during a game. The team physicians witnessed the tackle where the defensive player's knee collided with the QB's head. The QB did not get up after the play, and the physicians went out on to the field to determine the extent of the injury. When the QB indicated that he was feeling nauseous and dizzy, the physicians decided that he could not continue playing.

It was determined from examination of the QB's pupils and monitoring of his mental status that he had sustained a concussion. The physicians carefully watched and asked questions for the next few hours to make sure that no other serious problems had resulted from the head trauma. Eventually, after rest and careful observation, the N diminished and the head trauma was not considered to be life threatening.

The concerns of NV in space travel

NV can be a serious concern for astronauts who travel into space. Crew members must follow a strict time schedule which can be radically affected by any debilitation of the crew. In addition, crew members do not have access to physician and hospital care while in space, thus making any illness a serious affair. It is important, therefore, to identify the potential causes of NV in space so that the appropriate preventive and/or treatment measures can be taken to ensure the health and well-being of the crew.

The occurrence of NV in space can be caused by any number of things with the most common and easily organized concerns being improper nutrition, radiation poisoning, and motion sickness. Research, technology, and experience can help to reduce the occurrence of N and/or V as it relates to all three of these concerns; however, because each individual has a unique reaction to foreign environments and stimuli, it is difficult to predict the onset of NV in space. The following discussion illustrates the possible causes and currently known methods for treating and preventing NV in space.

Potential causes of NV

Nutrition

Regardless of whether on earth or above the atmosphere in space, it is essential for every individual to have a diet that can supply essential nutritional and caloric needs. In addition, when a person is required to be active and perform physical and strenuous tasks during each day, increasing the nutritional intake is advisable. A diet low in nutrition can cause temporary and permanent problems to an individual's physical and mental state. Research regarding space travel and activities of crew members states that diets low in nutrition diminish morale, lower performance levels, and can cause N (Brown, 1963).

Proper caloric intake with the necessary vitamins, minerals, and fluids is an important concern in space travel. It would be extremely costly to send astronauts into space to perform certain tasks only to have NV resulting from poor nutrition render them unable to function comfortably. Therefore, before each mission, individual crew members work directly with dietitians to select nutritionally balanced menus. Food designed for space travel needs to combine good taste and nutrition with the importance of minimizing preparation time and waste. In addition, food needs to be lightweight while eliminating the chance of microbial infection from the ambient-temperature storage conditions.

Through research and experience, scientists and nutritionists have determined that minimum energy needs are approximately 1.6 times (for women) and 1.4 times (for men) the crew members' basal energy expenditure (Nicogossian et al., 1994). This amount of food, which is carefully determined to contain the right nutritional supplements, should allow each crew member to perform tasks and to function comfortably. As of now, no allowances are made considering the effects of weightlessness on nutrition and energy needs; however, research is under way to determine whether there is a need to alter food intake.

With all this in mind, if NV occur, it is usually a result of an individual not eating necessary daily rations or some of the other factors presented below.

Radiation exposure

When a spacecraft leaves the atmosphere of the earth it is exposed to a certain amount of radiation. Every craft is equipped with a protective layer to help reduce the amount of radiation that will reach the crew members inside. However, a spacecraft cannot be rendered completely impenetrable to radiation because such protection would make the craft too heavy. Therefore, each craft allows some radiation to penetrate and this therefore reaches the astronauts inside.

The most important concern is protecting the crew members from excessive radiation exposure. The expected amount of exposure depends on the length of the trip and the radiation environment in which they will live. From prior experience with space travel and the known information about radiation exposure, it is possible to establish guidelines and proper procedures to protect crew members from the expected radiation exposure, as well as the potential accidental exposure that may occur.

Initial reactions to radiation exposure can be separated into two groups: gastrointestinal (GI) reactions and neuromuscular reactions. The GI reactions include anorexia, NV, diarrhea, cramps, salivation, dehydration, and weight loss. The neuromuscular reactions include easy fatiguability, apathy or listlessness, sweating, fever, headache, and hypotension followed by hypotensive shock. All of these signs are not usually seen at once unless the dose is in the supralethal range. At around the median lethal dose (about 3 Gy) the principal symptoms are anorexia, NV, and fatiguability. Diarrhea, fever, and hypotension seem to be signs reflecting doses beyond the lethal range (Langham, 1967).

Research and experience have shown that it is possible essentially to eliminate the GI reactions by providing lead chest 'jackets' to protect this area from exposure. If these jackets are used, the only way the GI reactions would be detectable would be if there were an accidentally large or extended dose to the brain.

Space motion sickness

The last area of space medicine that may lead to NV is probably the most common and the most important. This area of concern involves all the sensory problems that cause 'space sickness' or what is more commonly known as 'motion sickness.' The sickness that some people experience on boats or in cars is almost, but not exactly, the same as occurs to individuals who travel in space.

Motion sickness was reported by 48% of cosmonauts in the Russian Space Program. In the history of the US Space Program, 35% of Apollo crew members, 60% of Skylab crew members, and 67% of Space Shuttle crew members flying for the first time reported cases of space motion sickness (Nicogassian et al., 1994). The main symptoms of motion sickness are apathy, headache, stomach awareness, pallor, perspiration, NV, and prostration, usually in that order of occurrence. These symptoms usually present themselves in the first 3–4 days while the astronauts are acclimatizing themselves to the new sensory stimuli.

Motion sickness is the result of incongruous sensory stimulation. The 'sickness' can affect anyone in almost any situation where motion stimuli, visual stimuli, and sometimes sound stimuli do not blend together in a logical way for an individual. This means that motion sickness can occur while a person is flying in space, standing on a boat, or even watching a movie of heaving boats on the ocean.

Motion sickness is, at the most basic level, a vestibular problem. However, motion sickness can result from various stimuli that can include things that are not associated with the vestibular organs. Abnormal stimulation of the semicircular canals (any rotating motion) especially combined with Coriolis stimulation can cause sickness. Stimulation of the utricle and saccule alone (any bouncing or heaving motion) and stimulation of both the semicircular canals and the otolith organs (any bobbing or swinging motion) can cause motion sickness. In addition, motion sickness can occur if there is motion without vision (standing below deck on a ship during a storm), if there is visual stimulation without complementary vestibular stimuli (watching a movie of a heaving ocean), or if the visual and vestibular stimuli do not match (a house in an amusement park which has a slanted floor).

Although motion sickness does not occur just in space, the effect of weightlessness in space adds to the sensory problems that can occur in any type of flight or movement. Sweating is more common in space motion sickness. Flushing is more common than pallor. Although the symptoms of malaise, anorexia or loss of appetite, lack of initiative and irritability are universal, there is usually an increase in stomach awareness; V (usually sudden and infrequent with no dry heaves), headache, impaired concentration, lack of motivation, and drowsiness are more common with motion sickness in space. Recovery is reported to be more rapid in space compared with the resolution of motion sickness on earth (Nicogossian et al., 1994).

Treatment and prevention methods

Nutrition

As was mentioned earlier, NV as related to nutrition are easily prevented if the proper nutritional and energy needs are established and a dietitian helps to create a healthful and palatable menu. If NV occur and the symptoms can be tied to nutrition, it is usually a result of a loss of appetite caused by NV relating either to radiation exposure or (more commonly) to motion sickness. If the problems have not stopped when the crew members return to earth, then the patients should be treated to ensure that they are receiving the proper nutrition.

Radiation exposure

The prevention of radiation exposure includes proper clothing and craft design. However, there have been causes of accidental exposure that can be treated (as in many cancer patients who are exposed to radiation for treatment). Radiation poisoning can be treated with radioprotectants such as immunodulators and vitamins A and C. If there is a case of accidental total body irradiation, therapeutic treatments such as bone marrow transplantations are an option.

Space motion sickness

The prevention of motion sickness is an integral part of space training. As it appears that the occurrence of space sickness decreases with each time a crew member takes part in a mission, the training programs have integrated methods to acquaint potential crew members with the stimuli that they will experience. In addition, there are mechanical and electrical devices such as pressurized insoles that are utilized to trick the body into believing that there is gravity present. In case none of these procedures is effective, there are pharmaceutical methods for treating the occurrence of NV.

From the third edition of *Space Physiology and Medicine* (Nicogossian, 1994), the list of various drugs that have been tested to decrease NV are anticholinergics, antihistamines, sympathomimetics, sympatholytics, and natural treatments such as ginger. The anticholinergic drug scopolamine (hyoscine) appears to work well with a dose of 0.3–1.2 mg being 27–95% effective. Antihistamines have some benefit, but the most effective, promethazine, has a 25-mg dose comparable to a 0.6-mg dose of scopolamine. The sympathomimetic and sympatholytic drugs appear to be only marginally effective. Drug combinations such as scopolamine (0.3–1.2 mg) with *d*-amphetamine (5–10 mg) (aka 'scope-dex') seem to produce a 30–188% increase in tolerance. There are contradicting studies which say that ginger may or may not be effective for preventing motion sickness. However, considering that the other drugs may have side effects such as drowsiness and dizziness, ginger may be the safer alternative.

Case study

To illustrate how serious NV can be to crew members aboard a spacecraft, all one needs to do is research the Apollo IX mission which had all activity delayed for 24 hours while the crew suffered from a debilitating case of space motion sickness (DeHart, 1985).

Part VI

In closing

CHAPTER 33

Essay and assay

In this summary chapter we review some major points and build upon others. We become attentive primarily to thoughts relevant for new perspectives. We begin with some reminders, proposals and offer commentary.

A few reminders

Nausea and vomiting (NV) are important. They are, for most sufferers, quite painful and disabling, and, as a public health, economic matter, they are immensely costly in terms of time lost.

Women are much more vulnerable. Throughout their lives they are at risk of experiencing from three to four times more NV incidents, across the range of 'causative' or precipitating events, than men.

For almost all women (and, we presume, men as well) N is much more common, usually feels worse, is more disabling, and lasts longer than V. Most research on NV control is on V, not N; therefore, claims for drugs that control NV research is at best incomplete and insensitive to the patient's typical situation.

Research has concentrated on iatrogenic V (such as that following cancer treatments, operations, etc.) and has ignored that N which appears the more common, i.e., NV in daily life. For women, fatigue, stress, pregnancy, work situations, as well as precipitating odors, food tastes and odors, etc., are typical precipitants. One knows from good research that, for iatrogenic NV, environmental features play a major part – including who is present in surgery, at what hospital, etc. Situational as well as interacting psychobiological features are present as N risks.

There appears to be a propensity to, a predisposition for, and perhaps a learned vulnerability to NV which varies individually for women. No studies on men have been done. For women, having frequent experiences with one kind of N predicts a greater risk of having NV from some other perturbation. Heretofore, individual risk factors have been listed rather accidentally as clinical observations; only a few major studies attend to them. One must add to risk appraisal the general propensity of personal history and psychobiological process in an environmental interaction. For immediately practical work, one would learn whether general propensity variation from group to group predicts the 'best' kinds of antiemetic (AE) care. For cancer patients, this work on one kind of 'pattern' particularly beckons as having early pain remedial potential.

Pharmacological treatments for NV are frequently overrated with clinical findings that tend to be derived from poor research designs. Measurements have been primarily of V after iatrogenic NV because these are relatively easily (although often unreliably) measured by nurses. Almost nothing has been done with respect to treatment trials which include a variety of efforts, from complementary medicines to food and music. Nurses and mothers usually do these things 'instinctively'; physicians and researchers have held aloof, clinging to the rules of the 'medical model.' Pharmacognosy has contributed much from plant and folk healing observation, so that people do achieve NV reduction from 'herbals' – although to what extent beyond the reduction by placebo is unknown. There is evident reason to test herbals further. This implies the ever-present duty to consumer education and disclosure.

Treatment, i.e. clinical trials, can show that a mixture, a 'cocktail,' of AEs works better than just one prescribed compound. Even here one does not know the statistically identified risk factors that best predict patient V control by one, multiple, or no drugs. Knowledge of actual drug–drug interactions is almost nil. To date, the initial claims of great success for single neurotransmitter antagonists have generally proven disappointing. Exceptions obviously exist, for example, as with antihistamine treatments for motion sickness. But you only need to talk to those who receive no relief to learn the limits of even this 'simple' antagonist drug. There are no comparison studies with complex designs comparing mixes of treatments, including unconventional ones. For example, the success of acupressure, the reports of which seem to be based on good work, are not only inexplicable, but have not encouraged workers to try acupressure in a mixture of treatments.

Our finding of a significant link between risk of hyperemesis gravidarum (HG) and earlier migraine, if replicated, would move research beyond acknowledgment of commonalities in the two conditions, and of the known role of reproductive cyclicity as affecting incidence, to a profound interest in what is for some women perhaps a sequential process. Patterning strongly indicates HG to be a quite different set of events from pregnancy nausea and vomiting (PNV), when carefully discrimin-ated. What substrate variables either predisposing to migraine and its initiation of a later HG risk, or expressive of that pathology as a function of continuing pregnancy itself, would clearly be questions here. And would migraine pharmacotherapeutics be usefully examined for HG? Upon verification of a relationship, as a reality, and not a 'blip,' traditional endocrinological, biochemical research must be furthered.

The greater reminder is what opportunities there are for thought and then important research in the NV field. Some work is at the level at which undergraduates, properly educated and supervised, may well make contributions. We believe that NV opportunities show that science is demonstrably not dying, or dull and, when nourished by interdisciplinary wisdom, creativity is exciting and fun.

Animal research, often brilliantly done, has learned about 'plasticity' and individual differences, even in ablated ferrets or shrews. Neurotransmitters are central to NV, and antagonists for those compounds participating in NV processes strongly affect outcomes. Yet even under heavy doses of emetics, varying responses occur. Neuropeptides and endocrine compounds are of course active, although what their actions are is more conjecture than knowledge. Some of the best workers, using newer methods, such as *c-fos* expression and brain imaging, show an ever-expanding set of neural networks, brain regions, and 'sensoria' involved in NV. What is involved in N by no means needs to be what is involved in V, although one allows, in speculation, that V may function, or try to, as a 'cure' for N. An inclusive view of NV must allow for neural networks which are active even at the unquestionably accurate mid-medullary level of that final common pathway of motor pattern generation, with its efferent V signals to the gut, respiratory muscles, and the autonomic nervous system (ANS). The ANS, in turn, whether or not involved sequentially in precipitating NV as a baseline augmentation, has its own response to patterns generated, and effects ranging from cardiac to consciousness.

Consciousness in humans is essential for N, and for that V not defined as aspirated. The refinements of terminology come to bear here, as in animal studies of 'fictive' V. Consciousness appears important in animals not only for dramatically affecting rates of emesis in response to compounds administered to intact animals, but for that behavior which is inferred to be 'feeling sick' (paws up, appetite loss, face drooping, etc.). As neuropharmacologists, not psychologists or neuroscientists, have been doing the NV research, and as gastroenterologists, not humanists, have been primarily attending to V, consciousness and all of its underlying brain regions and functions have been left out. But not for the sufferer and therefore not for the clinician.

The further contribution of humanists to the development of insights into the experience and meanings of N and V is one bridge to interdisciplinary science. Thus, it becomes psychosomatically and biologically informed, literate humanistic psychology which is scientifically erudite, and poetic in evocation and empathy. We suspect progress will be the domain of broadly talented individuals who are not restricted by disciplines. The remarkable insufficiency of previous attention to the subjectively consequential must itself be examined. We have proposed that the sickness or revulsion that is NV primitively repels interest in it.

If C.P. Snow's bridge between science and the humanities is to be built, those in both schools must be the new piers. Implied as traffic over the bridge is an integrated value, that 'unity of knowledge' which physicist Weyl (see biographical review by medalist J.A. Wheeler, 1986) personified and appreciated in which art, history, literature, mathematics, physics (and for us biology, medicine, and social and environmental sciences) were aspects of the 'community of knowledge.' As Wheeler quotes him: '. . . the realm of Being is not closed but open.' The NV field will be an open enterprise.

Theories have been singularly lacking pertaining to NV process, or for AE control (except for the single neurotransmitter one, which varies by year of popularity, manufacturer, hospital, etc.). Accepted doctrines (e.g., 'toxin expulsion' evolutionarily functionally effective in humans; 'reflex' or 'psychogenic' generally; for pregnancy as 'endocrines') are not just too simple, they are unsupported by observations of any kind in living, conscious humans. In the same way, to consider NV as one category of event, unified, sequential, etiologically and 'reflexively' as only one linear transmission, is to be obtuse.

As much of what occurs in NV is 'inaccurately predictable' (as risk, precipitant, treatment, and locatable 'places' for action), it is our view that NV must be examined anew. We have found it useful to think in multidisciplinary frames of reference. Data and (right now more importantly) *ideas* from all biopsychological levels are required and must be integrated. No one level of inquiry is proven superior to another when each observance is pertinent to the phenomenon (Sapolsky and Balt, 1996). Perhaps, because in NV only reductionist levels, or clinical trials, are in vogue, a probabilistic view is required. For example, dynamic patterns may well be part of the NV process along with linear transmissions and specific but interacting neuropeptide release. For competent scientists, clinicians, students, and sufferers who wish to protect themselves from NV or its incompetent 'professional' treatment, the next era for research on NV will enjoy greater complexity, ambiguity, and novelty of thought.

We now turn to specific reminders or concepts as queries deserving final comment.

N and V, although often joined temporally and etiologically, do not necessarily arise from the same events or involve identical processes. They occur as part of, or are themselves, different patterns, yet they may also be sequential and considered part of a larger whole. Syndromes have yet to be clearly identified, but unfolding patterns can be diverse. We posit that these differentiated outcomes result from differing internal processes; those 'mechanisms' should one day respond to pattern-tailored treatments. As of today, treatments that work for iatrogenic V are less likely to work for iatrogenic N; N treatments other than folk remedies, over-the-counter treatments, are limited. Some women claim their home remedies to be better than prescription AEs. One does not rush to conclusions.

The combination of complexity and uncertainty rules out, for now, the pretense of complete understanding or accurate prediction. It is our view that one is dealing in part with dynamic, 'non-linear' processes which have spontaneity intrinsic to their apparently fluid self-organization. If this is so, much of what occurs in NV will require attention to event spaces, time sequences, and levels of focus. Also invoked are pattern flow transitions, some of these being the 'synergetics' of Haaken (1988), an approach well presented and experimentally demonstrated for brain–behavior processes by Kelso (1995). Gibson's (1950) work on perception is also central, because so much of N or V is a sensory response which, like perception, reflects external and internal interaction with the environment.

Disorganizing perceptions?

Gibson understood perception, which is in essence what the mind makes of and imposes upon sensations in a personal–environmental context. Viewed in this way NV are both a simplified psychosomatic definition of a sensation and the sensation itself. Perception is the sensory–cognitive apparatus at work assessing available environmental structures in relationship to the organism. It is, as research has shown on sensory end-organ filtering, an outreaching, selective, shaping, feedback-sensitive, actively focused as well as dominantly responsive activity. Ecologically, it leads organism-controllable events to restructuring environmental relationships. (Purely cognitive components can lead to the same.) It defines what is response and attention-worthy information, at an aware and subliminal, but by definition potentially conscious and therefore cerebral cortical, level. But NV themselves, as response train, also restructure the environment as a change in the organism itself or a structure in relationship to others. Thus the event train remains interactive.

Our use of 'perturbation' has been like the semantics of 'stress' in the literature: it is the response to that which has created it. As tautology, the perturbation is the perturbing. But a response may well define the event, as in medical practice where one awaits the response to treatment to diagnose the disease. Thus, there can be helpful usage as well as sloppy thinking. For this, one introduces Aristotle's 'universals' as higher-level abstractions across a sequence of particulars, and therefore permeably bounded commonalities within one context, and the question of whether commonalities can be 'real.' A related delineation challenge arose as we considered how it might be that migraine to HG might reflect a singular but changing, underlying pathological process. Or when we propose that NV, in perturbing an environment, semantically mirror the generating disorganizing perturbation, a sequence becomes circular. One sees this well-known positive feedback as cascading oscillation in epilepsy (kindling, cascades or entrainment). Motor pattern-generated V may include, one speculates, respiratory–enteric feedback to the medullary midline.

Viewing NV as a perceptual event, one can see that neither perceptual processes at the nuclei level nor the final NV response itself self-organizes to 'competence,' i.e., there is at best a limited and costly adaptive assessment and response. Diffuse and primitive, in humans NV rarely 'work.' However, in proposing an evolutionary biology in process, we allow another adaptive possibility, that NV, as a response mostly to man-made events, are adaptive in so far as they mobilize social support, action toward problem-solving. And, in a Grand Design they are also a strong warning signal.

Another tautology or reification is obvious, in that NV are a response to a disequilibrating event, but, again, any impinging event is, just as Hans Selye said, 'Life is stress.' It is more discriminating to propose that every instance of NV defines an event, internal or external, where the human, sensitive to sensed adverse alterations in the internal/external environment, is not able to respond 'Cannonically,' i.e., with fight or flight, but regressively, as a kind of defensive, communicative, expressive dysfunction in humans. In this, NV parallel but are not as functional as a 'stress' and pain response with ANS components.

One proposes that NV as a sequence of event–sensation–perceptual, effort-diverse, internal processes cannot involve any adequate sensory definitional integrative apparatus, and so no competent organizing perceptual response and no subsequent coping one. As with the gut wall's serotonin receptor response (Raybould et al., 1995), a toxic event characterized by raised serotonin levels is sensed, but nothing competent by way of coping or protection can be done about it. The NV that occur are not helpful and are thus further maladaptive, except as a distress signal, the premises of the unexamined theories of 'toxin expulsion' thesis being to the contrary. Indeed the coping failure may be to the sensory definitional integrative failing one not the external event. It may be a failure in 'knowing' about that which disallows itself because of human perceptual apparatus deficiencies. The perception of perturbation, at conscious or enteric levels, is intrinsic to the sequence that ends, however repetitively, with the NV response itself.

In this sense NV are a debilitating and maladaptive reaction to sensations that are not sufficiently organized to become competently interactive, or potentially environmentally controlling perceptions, i.e., a motor or mind activity. As an overreaction, it is a total, although failed, mobilization in which the conscious awareness may be only to NV as destabilizing. But it is not a definition of mortal threat that is ordinarily involved (with the exception of post-Hiroshima or Chernobyl radiation, terminal metastatic gut blockage, or terminal baroreceptor-impinging brain tumors). Motion sickness is, after all, only 'felt' to be deadly; it is the sensory apparatus that fails to 'contain' it as destabilizing movement or conflicting cues elicit this failure to cope. Cisplatin, although killing cells, does not, properly administered, kill people. One proposes that the sensory integrative apparatus is itself faulty, overwhelmed, i.e., it cannot integrate and respond in an adaptive manner to the information detected. The perceptual system does not work, nor does an entrained motor or immediate symbolic one.

As to what constitutes a perturbing event for the individual, or for humankind, the range is theoretically almost infinite, although as-yet-to-be constructed probability curves will be able to forecast, for individuals and like groups, prevalence by charting predisposing characteristics. This definition is the basis for one kind of new treatment research. The traditional medical model for that research has been partially successful (e.g., sea sickness control); one does not suggest its abandonment. Parallel work in modern psychology and ecology is, however, also successful. To move to that notional chaos theory close to the dynamics of Kelso, one allows descriptive schemes using nonlinear approaches. For a general view of the now-too-popular chaos theory, see Gleick (1987).

More on meanings

One does not know whether the expressive, communicative, and therefore meaningful aspects of NV are only secondary functions resting on self-awareness of the painful and ugly, or whether something is 'happening' evolutionarily which may have selective features. But as a meaning, NV are not without adaptive value. They define events known or often unknown to the self and others, i.e., 'that's disgusting,' as a signal that alerts oneself, ranging from medical intervention for NV to the sympathetic helpfulness of a PNV woman's partner or other family. It can be, as Erving Goffman would have said, a 'presentation of self.'

One may assume that, with meanings so deeply rooted in personal experience, the interpersonal drama will be normatively cast; there is a high likelihood of agreement on how the other person (in the Parsonian sociological sense) is feeling or what 'statement' she and her body are making. These reactions of others will be sensitive to history and cue. The nurse of the cancer chemotherapy patient will read NV differently from the mother of the chronically 'sick' child who may feel inadequate, or guilt-laden, or possibly hostile toward her child. (The child's pediatrician and the by-now-referred psychologist already know that the kid is playing her like a drum.)

There has been no count of the range and circumstances to which NV are put to interpersonal use. One illustration is the case of a Munchausen-by-proxy syndrome where the child was induced to vomit by the mother giving him ipecac so that the mother then took the child to the doctor for attention. These days of quantification in sociology, psychology as neuroscience, psychiatry as psychopharmacology, and the linear model in medicine do not invite case histories – except perhaps for short journal notes. But Wolf is right (see Chapter 4): case histories are good learning tools. For NV, where there is so much to be learned about previously ignored semeiotics, from pheromones to expressive behavior, one proposes that sensitive case histories are worthy ways to learn. Let us bring back the declining population of practitioner–researchers!

Implicit in a view of NV as interactive communication is a study of their 'environmental impact.' Can a pursuing predator be put off by the smell of Cannon's (thus canonical?) flight vomitus in the prey? For whom is the smell of another's vomitus a pheromonic precipitant of contagious V? Is there a greater risk of that in the child of an alcoholic, V parent?

NV 'being' the meaningful language of perturbation

Perturbation versus stress

We have distinguished between 'perturbation' and 'stress response' in two ways. Clearly 'perturbation' is redundantly defined in our usage as inference from the occurrence of any NV, whereas 'stress' cannot be inferred thereby. Another is that NV are not only a response to perturbation, whether or not that perturbation meets the definition of stress, but, with a few exceptions, have and provide an aware meaning to self and others that the behavior is perturbation as rejection/revulsion. It constitutes a semeiotic chemical and body language or, philosophically placed, a context of in-being as perturbed. Its experience is one of being upset, perturbed, just as one uses the term 'perturbation' to describe the initiating conditions for NV.

NV most surely have meanings to those who experience, observe, or contemplate them. These are powerful, whether as learned (anticipatory NV, the manipulative child), as a symbol and expression of revulsion, or as pheromonically communicative. At the very least the smell of another's vomit, the sight and sound of that expressively cyclical expulsion induces aversion if not sympathetic, contagious mimicry. N or V is a feeling, a communication about a feeling, a communication as to the nature of that initiating perturbation. There may be no more powerful communication, however involuntary, in the primitive vocabulary of expressive sounds, smells, and movement. NV have meanings. Think 'puke.' To speak of these is to integrate a mass of different input contexts, and arrays under one aggregate response, function, and possible set of interpersonal responses. Addressing the interpersonal, nonchemical pheromonic 'semeiotics' of NV is certainly many levels away from G proteins or sectioning the vagus of a ferret to learn which of several ordinarily emetic compounds might trigger fictive V, depending on the network conditions producing 'plasticity.'

This level of interpretation, as an accident become esthetic, become meaningful, become biologically consensual communication, become capable of interpersonal use and manipulation, simultaneously and in parallel as chemical semeiotics, is quite useful at a conceptually integrative level. Thus, we have proposed imaginative research that might begin with identification of brain-imaging events, begun by Miller et al. (1996), peculiar either to N or its prodromal shifting brain pattern states. If such could be a reliable differentiation from other processes, one would have a measure of incipient as well as experienced N, where awareness levels as well as gastrointestinal (GI) tract motility might well vary. Given the luck of such a find, one would examine a range of environmental, symbolic, interpersonal events for their capacity to induce the prodromal imaged states. Whether using positron emission tomography (PET), single photon emission computed tomography (SPECT), functional magnetic resonance (fMR), or magnetic resonance imaging (MRI), one expects cerebral areas and old-brain olfactory–pituitary–hypothalamic ones projecting to thalamic, limbic ones to be predictably involved.

Research foci

To date NV research has been of many kinds. One well-known technique involves pharmacological studies aimed either neuropharmacologically or anatomically at finding rational drug treatments or through clinical trials that test treatments against one another for the major 'causal' situations. The regions most studied anatomically are those that are final motor or enteric pathways in the central nervous system (CNS) or ANS, and, for the latter, NV-generative at GI and medullary levels as well. Particular attention has been paid to the places and sequences apparently generating motor patterns constituting V. This is understandable for any linear model would hope to find AEs that act specifically on such critical final paths. As the work continues, the linear model is intact, although the area postrema

(AP) is now placed conceptually but neuroanatomically as acting through projection to the nearby nucleus tractus solitarius (NTS). For Miller and Leslie (1994), the NTS is a likely beginning of the final pathway 'by which different emetic inputs trigger vomiting.' The NTS as 'the vomiting center' continues to dominate.

Miller and Leslie are careful to state that various inputs initiate action at the motor level. By implication, the chemoreceptor trigger zone (CTZ) and AP are integrative centers as well. Work on GI pharmacology (see Gaginella, 1995) appears attentive to 'input' from sources other than local sensing tissue, i.e., CNS, enteric nervous system (ENS), and motor regions, ANS, neuromessengers, etc. These are conceivably either operating to influence signals via the vagus to the AP or modulating the AP, NTS, and other medullary regions. The capacity of the bowel to govern its own motility through the ENS is probably responsible for the premise that the GI tract is autonomous: a theory not without problems. Roarty and McCallum (1995) and Raybould et al. (1995) provide summary data which allow overview and indicate contradictions. Indeed, inconsistency among studies of serotonin levels, and disappointments regarding clinical trial results with respect to the prevalent $5HT_3$ V single trial theory, now lead to the new pathway heralded, involving natural killer 1 (NK1) receptors (Kris, 1997). We forecast that, as before, this single-mindedly decided pathway will have the same fate as all earlier sole convictions.

The paraventricular and midline medullary reticular regions, the AP, CTZ, NTS (these, with the vagal motor nucleus, are termed the 'dorsal vagal complex'), other midline medullary reticular regions, and the vagus and splanchnic nerves as such dominate research interests. The overlying interest has been efferent innervation to muscles involved in V, through enteric and respiratory pathways. The methods have been surgical with, typically, various emetics and AEs of differing chemistry, and lesions or sectioning in order to define the conditions under which often fictive ('as if') V is observed. The work, at least until the mid-1980s and some continuing, assumes linear sequencing with respect to innervation. Earlier, such work partook of the 'reflex' paradigm, and therefore the 'circuitry' that can be used as the template for animal research considering V initiation and expression. Experimentally, this is to be produced by the direct stimulation of a 'motor pattern generator' as the AP has long been characterized (with only loose accuracy). The CTZ and AP can receive circulating messengers in the cerebrospinal fluid (CSF) and 'toxins,' should they exist even as large molecules, may be detectable in this region which is outside the blood–brain barrier. This notion of stimulation required for V coexists with a direct enteric–plexus–vagus–AP route that initiates V. Miller and his group (1994) have pioneered new and most instructive activation assessment methods in this circumventricular (also paraventricular) region, using deoxyglucose uptake and *c-fos* expression upon stimulation with AEs. And, most recently (1996), methods on brain-imaging activity shown with individual variation in the inferior frontal gyrus. Plasticity remains the rule even within individuals (Miller et al., 1994).

Little work has been done on N which, in any event, can only be inferred from a conscious and intact animal's behavior. N is the more important for humans, with greater diversity of events leading to it and (obvious from the gastroenterological as well as self-report and humanities literature) much greater variation in measurable gastric events accompanying the N. Animal work on V has tended not to speculate on the involvement of higher CNS regions, or on sensory input and mediating processes by which brain regions, messengers, possible nonlinear neural events, and states of awareness are implicated in human NV. Work on animal models, from fish through monkeys but mostly on shrews, cats, and ferrets, is the standard. (Be reminded that they differ as species one from another, among themselves individually, and considerably from humans.)

The NV 'reflex': an old model not in keeping with patterns, plasticity, or cyclicity

In the conventional textbook, and some reviews, not only are NV simply actions ready to be 'triggered' unless replaced by current 'motor pattern generator' terminology, but 'reflex' describes the action route for at least V, if not for NV together. These usages are all comfortingly automated, located, and specific. It is a neat 'model T Ford' world. It does not work.

Considering epilepsy and NV: a quick journey from neurons gone 'awry' to turbulence of mind and philosophy

Epilepsy allows the question, one without foundation except for curiosity, about whether there are any similarities to NV that would be more than an analogy, i.e., they would suggest observational foci in terms of pattern organization. Epilepsy is an uninvited, disabling, dysfunctional, uncanalized, entropic phenomenon without evidence of any earlier adaptive evolutionary role. It is brain and then body in disarray. It can be triggered environmentally. Rhythmic stereotypical oscillations follow. Is the underlying process more than analogy?

The motor to consciousness analogy

With epilepsy as an example, we have asked whether V motor pattern generation is not the expressed regularity of a linear command system doing its job in the homeostasis-maintaining hypothalamus (think of the optimistic parallel of *Candide's* Pangloss, voicing the philosopher Leibnitz's view of the 'best of all possible worlds' but here schemas), but on the contrary motor pattern generation in extremis, at the excruciating limits of morphological and energy boundaries. This of course is the typical subjective, phenomenological experience of the extreme pain of NV (for some, at least). Self-awareness of an uncontrollable extreme reaction should not be dismissed as a possibly accurate cognitive/symbolic characterization of the midline medullary phenomenon that in fact generates it. Here would be an instance of Aristotlean universality of particulars, an aware picture of neural network 'reality' as the Hegelian 'Mind' knowing. It may be as close to a 'bridge' between neurons and perception as humans, including scientists, can get. One is returned to considerations of mind as emergent from neural structures (see Uttal, 1996, or Sperry, 1993).

Mind and emotion are central to any person or patient, or in integrating the theoretical perspective of NV, whether or not the processes are located at the level of neuronal inhibitory/excitatory neurons, or whether they can be shown to involve neuromodulators or levels even within G-cell protein messengers. The mind is an observer, sometimes an instigator, always a respondent, and typically the emergency control seeking and coping, and usually the 'copeless' awareness of NV. In stating this as a thesis, we exclude current cognitive science that is uncomfortable with the mind. By incorporating the obvious, we express our interest in NV psychologically. To place psychology and ecology and expressive meanings within medicine is to be psychosomatic but also 'holistic,' because we understand how painful, disabling, and dehumanizing NV are. It is likely that our environmental responsiveness, if not our motor pattern generation – that epilepsy parallel – has all gone awry. There is a place for the 'mind' and empathy in NV studies and treatment.

One is reminded of the thrust of Vico's observation, about 1700 (discussed by Berlin, 1980), that we know ourselves and others 'from the inside.' Our sameness, expressed in empathy and intuitive understanding (as opposed to that which we understand as the 'other' of natural physical reality), sets our understanding of one another apart from the harder work of understanding objects and their relationships. Thus the mind experiences NV, and likewise 'experiences' the NV of others. As the mind is integral, whether subjective, objective, or in its most central Hegelian self-knowing role, it is the business of philosophy. Or at least with Plato, his student Aristotle, and until early Wittgenstein and later deconstructivism, it had as its business a harmonizing function. This requires perspective, and as such in early overview perhaps becomes a 'theory of theories.' Neither clinician, student, scientist nor sufferer should eschew philosophy in considering ecopsychobiological processes. Such considerations become but one more level, or one more feature of the intellectually appraised environment, to consider as one examines the remarkably extensive processes of NV. One hopes to arrive one day at a tested theory of NV that incorporates its various levels. Its empirical demonstration in behavioral neuroscience is powerful, and it is in that arena that we would place some of a new research direction.

The proposal is that NV studies not only allow the 'mind' to be as 'real' as anything else the mind is aware of, but also encourage the biopsychological mind to work at philosophical levels. It is an elaborated effort to apply meanings and organization to NV phenomena, and to do so in the context of how and where lives are lived and examined. Indeed, science itself, by no means a mansion with only one agreeable room, is only one philosophy of knowing and – as we see with NV – with considerable unsupportable disagreement if one advocates one level of work over another. We propose that these 'knowings' about NV must be expanded – at least as an aspect of human awareness about self in the context of environmental interactions. These are the meanings thereof to the philosopher and as cogitation upon this sector of the universe.

Motor pattern generation as an extreme information-degrading reaction to combined inhibitory and excitatory output

Return now to Kupferman's observations on the role of conflict in the onset of abnormal motor pattern generation. There may well be a parallel between such conflict situations in animal studies and in 'psychogenic' human NV. Kupferman's closely defined usage is rather more exact than the usage found in NV anatomical studies, where pattern generators are defined neither as carefully nor with the oscillating self-organizing features suggested by Kleinfeld and Chiel (1990). In either event, simple characterizations of motor pattern generators as mechanistic buttons is not adequate and, given Kupferman's observations on conflict as 'vacuum' activity generative, one may ask if there is commonality to perturbations leading to V as measurable at the levels of the motor pattern generator region. Note that psychodynamic conflict may induce seizure (Laidlaw).

The separate investigations of Abeles, Fetz, Gerstein and Singer (1998, a discussion) emphasizes that neuron assemblies contain patterns as information expressed in synchronic firing. The neurons in such assemblies are not 'fixed' in networks, neurons may change the assembly of which they are a part. At smaller levels, as within cell G protein instructions as well as among cells, the view of the malleable assembly of information processing also holds (Zuker and Ragnatnan, 1999). Macromolecular assemblies show functional diversity and modular reorganization as signaling complexes. 'Centers' at all levels are constantly, responsively, 'intelligently,' processing as 'plasticity' observed.

A further picture of brain functioning fit for NV as we know it

For those used to thinking in terms of work on less complex animals, there may be an unexamined assumption that regions patterned as triggering V are 'command' neurons, thus invoking hierarchical simple structures. Kupferman indicates that this is not the schema for mammals. As with Kelso, and Kosslyn and Koenig, hierarchical systems are less likely to be assumed to be 'givens' within the nervous system, although there may be particular neuronal–efferent roles. These inputs generate response patterns that are learned (see Stein and Meredith, 1993a) inter- and intraneuronally, and may thus be seen as neuronally generated, not as single command centers but in coordinated or 'conductance' organization. Implicit in this function is malleability over time (in contrast to 'hardwiring'). The work of Ungerleider (1994) and others implies that neurons do not necessarily have fixed functions but may be recruited into new networks as learning occurs.

Brain neurons also die, and this in itself is possibly selective as restructuring. But substitutability of function ('neuron recruitment') continues to be demonstrated, not just for the apparently simple 'pathways' of V, but also for emotional functions, such as learned fear in the amygdala which can be 'relearned' when the amygdala is ablated (Davis, cited in Hickok and Morrow, 1993). This is important for NV not only because the amygdala appears to be involved in their processes, but because much of NV is now shown to be emotionally precipitated as well as to precipitate emotion when they occur. The data encourage exploration of the role of learning, cognition, and emotion in NV cause, process, and potential relief, and of reciprocal even reverberating neural network activity among brain structures.

'Computational' but flexible patterning

Kosslyn and Koenig's work (1992) also assumes fluid but limited patterning allowing malleability that NV appear to reflect. Theirs is a computational network approach to brain function; patterns are recurrently appearing in network expressions. In the case of homeostatic control function or patterns generated by smaller functions that are somewhat autonomous (although hypothalamically 'governed'), one nevertheless expects multiple functions and participation of each in several subsystems. Organized 'crosstalk' at many levels, implied or actual, there will be simultaneous input to regions, nuclei that are involved perhaps only in part in motor patterning. Consider a fluctuating system where incoming information is not exact in determining output. Instead, it may generate altered activity. Variation even in self-organization does characterize network assemblies and conductance therein. The work of Lawes (1990), Zuker (1990), Abeles et al. (1998) demonstrates nicely this interconnected organization which also requires neuronal group self-organization to reach signalling thresholds for action. Said differently, these activities constitute critical instabilities that induce new organizations in and as the medullary V centers.

Uncertainty is implicit in the arena of sensation or perception, and response thereto is 'opportunistic,' to use Kosslyn and Koenig's term. With regard to pattern recognition as the basis of sensory response, grouping, and transmission, there are receptor 'fits' and 'nonfits' and 'moderate fits;' among the nonfits there are those that matter both functionally and adaptively, and those that are discards. Both imply the intrinsic matching of the sensing system – a genetic template into which major learned data are introduced, with demonstrable neuronal and response change. Such matching can be entirely dependent upon experience (i.e., blind persons becoming sighted but not 'seeing' or the development of immune system memory to expand competence). For V, one may assume that, within the networks of motor pattern-generating conductances, a category of signals emerges which, changing over time as risk studies show, come to define the adverse response, and behaviorally as N or V. That 'decision,' N or V or both, is a mystery.

This language, computationally idiomatic when it draws on Kosslyn and Koenig, but molecularly biological with Zuker is consonant with the dynamic conceptions of Haaken–Kelso in which intrinsic self-organization of patterns 'pulled' by attractants occurs, i.e., organizing energy flows, or, as an analog, information exchange occurs involving (via pathways of transmitters, hormones, neuropeptides) field neuromodulation. Viewed conceptually, motor pattern generator regions should be found to be sequential, parallel, interacting, and malleable, self-organizing (in part only!) (see Lawes), and productive of event cascades (the strength or weakness of which will constitute thresholds for the behaviorally observable event of V). Not exactness or precision, not on–off states, not self-contained units, but pattern organizing to cascade via instabilities to other pattern-organizing stages. This is one way to view the otherwise perplexing 'plasticity' and inconsistency that experimenters encounter in NV.

One inevitable circumstance for human V: is touching believing?

We are told that there is one intervention by which neurosurgeons can 'inevitably' produce V. It is surgery touching the region of the floor of the fourth ventricle, i.e., that area where and near to which the array of networks exists whose function is to generate the muscular activity and accompanying sympathetic nervous system (SNS) expressions of V. In no other situation is one likely to find these V-initiating, 'limited' neural networks directly in contact with environmentally originating, sudden and massive physical insult, such as the surgeon's scalpel and the exposed brain. The array of alien events may be likened to, but is greater than, the presence of a tumor, trauma, or intraventricular CSF pressure. The aggregate of intrusive stimuli includes touch, pressure, movement, milieu fluid, air, temperature change, and their reverberating consequences in nearby tissue, biochemicals, CSF, and blood. We would like to find a neurological study that describes outcomes, even in the fourth ventricle, in which there are diverse surgical and pathological situations, risk factors, brain anomalies, and varying kinds and degrees of anesthesia and the like.

In dramatic contrast, we are also advised by surgical colleagues that neurosurgical ablation of the human AP, however great its risk for other homeostatic function, has been done, and 'inevitably' prevents any future V. We have seen that the animal literature is not supportive of anything 'inevitable.' Our search of the literature for such human cases, and particularly for follow-up, has been fruitless. Keeping in mind the sensitivity of modern neuropsychological measures, what one must recommend is much closer cooperation in finding these rare cases, so that the investigator and the neurosurgeon can become consistent cooperators in future NV research, much in the tradition of Goldstein, Vigotsky, Penfield, Myers, and Sperry.

Yet V does not occur during surgery. Clinicians may be heard accounting for this in terms of anesthesia that suppresses nuclei efferent signal activity, causes muscle flaccidity or chemical inhibition, or that which imposes changes in vascular blood supply to vagal and splanchnic nerves, reducing the SNS capacity. But one notes from Chapter 8 that V pathways appear to exist beyond these major nerves and might still operate unless these other messenger systems are also rendered non-functional. This 'common knowledge' of anesthetic impact – which 'should' vary with level of anesthesia – does not exclude the possibility that other and higher CNS centers are also required to function for V to occur.

Arguing again for breadth

Obviously we are arguing for an expanded set of locales, and a much more extensive definition of NV. It is the definition of 'locale' which in one way defines reductionism and pharmacology versus cognitive neuroscience and the categorical aggregate of events research on NV. It is pragmatically the research itself that confirms the utility of defining locales, and of events therein selected for attention. For NV, the presence of dominant neuropharmacological prior research, as we have seen in the analysis of clinical trials, has yielded utility and insight, but these are neither as comprehensive nor as efficacious as scientists, healers, and patients might like. Nor, for theorists at the broader neuroscientific or psychological level, has there been any feast of NV research. If the striking and inventive study of Sapolsky and Balt (1996) is prodromal, work by the reductionist on the pharmacology/neuroanatomy of closed systems, ecologists on open ones, pattern dynamicists on critical instabilities and psychologists on the role of perceptions, mind, and meanings, will all be equally useful. If ever integrated, there could be a satisfying picture of NV in all their complexity.

As psychosomatics

Plasticity at a holistic level means that the CNS–enteric plexus and cells do not respond predictably, that regions and paths can be substituted, and that the molecular structure of one or another emetic or AE alters certain outcomes. Most NV involve a 'plastic' process as opposed to being a linear, stimulus–response (S-R) reflex. But both kinds occur, and lead to the conclusion that there are quite different processes at work. They share at the holistic level only a few common elements: the reported behavioral outcome of NV, the meanings that these have to sufferer and observer, and that consciousness involved in the aware observer. We continue to stake a claim for psychosomatics for what has yet to emerge in the integration of the sciences as a useful approach to NV.

An analogue, the 'sex reflex'?

The multiple level from awareness to cellular processes of NV, considered to be a reflex by most neuropharmacologists, anatomists, and gastroenterologists, may be compared with a rather similar simplification of sex. Axiomatic for many sexologists is the thesis of a universal human sexual response cycle (HSRC) which emphasizes physical–genital and linear behavioral–physiological events. Regan (1996), in a review of Tiefer's book, *Sex is not a Natural Act and Other Essays*, comments that '. . . a cursory examination of even the most recent human sexuality textbooks reveals . . . exact depictions of human sexual anatomy, and more than anyone could possibly want to know about the genital and physiological events associated with arousal, but very little about the meanings that men and women place on these sexual phenomena.' It is, of course, more understandable that a psychologist would protest the exclusion of mind from sex (wherein the presumption of mind, pleasure, is primary as opposed to NV). But today's rendition of the scientific sexology text appears to draw from the same mechanical, reductionist schema, although one where for NV the microlevels are, unlike sex, felt as initial conditions.

Control at the level of mind and comfort is a medical preference. Preferences are a problem of the imposed logical model. What if we must accept uncertainty in multilevel research? Absent control can lower immune system competence in animals and humans. Maybe it can also make patients sick. For whether primate or rat, absent predictability and control can increase 'stress,' morbidity, and reduced immunological competence. At present it is hard on the recruitment of scholars to study NV.

Awareness as emergency and potential problem-solving

Consciousness of NV is preoccupying and painful for most, again with the exception of the unusual projectile or other sudden V. Given the dominant role of consciousness, even if argued as reactive, awareness is nevertheless integral. This is not only phenomenological but potentially adaptive because it arouses the information-gathering capability as an emergency response which NV is felt to compel. What is 'repulsive, sickening' is to be recognized as such and subsequently avoided, altered, or dispatched. The aware brain has evolved to do much of the complex, novel work of completing the nonautomated tasks of living in a complex environment, where the complexity is mostly of our own human doing. This is the job it is stuck with, even if it was not evolved for that (see Ornstein, 1991; Baynes and Caramazza, 1998; Allman, 1999) and even if the brain is a mosaic of by no means always integrated, sometimes competing and contradictory evolutionary discrete domains, when it organizes as a priority to warn via NV there is little beyond that which the brain can do. NV are a novelty that one can always do without, because it is a warning of perturbations about which one can do little.

NV are integrated with consciousness because this is the way the human brain is designed to deal with complex, novel problems that require total capability mobilization. Unfortunately, in NV the capability is to feel miserable and wretched. These, however, may have communicative functions. The study of NV is incomplete without considering the information exchange within the CNS and ANS, and incomplete psychosomatically without examining functions and meanings. Attention to NV requires consideration of possible perturbations occurring in the cerebral cortex, or those sometimes less self-conscious 'emotional' limbic structures, hippocampal memory, and reptilian old-brain olfactory and hormonal influences which are initial conditions for the occurrence of N and V. The perturbations often prove the brain to be incapable of any short-term aware control, although one has rushed to the medicine chest or chamomile tea box, or pressed the nurse's call button. Subjectively, then, NV have certain meanings expressed through experience, language, and, sometimes, intent.

Toward entropy

N and V seem loosely channeled as a chaotic structural flow, tumultuous, disrupting, and exhausting energy. N or V moves toward entropy. All 'body' work is exothermic (for the body is not a closed system), but in healthy metabolism or higher-level thought and behavior one looks toward a life-maintaining, homeostatic balance to move toward greater complexity, and more patterned, organized products. Not NV. No higher organization emerges, and at best there is a return to earlier stability. In the dynamic terms of Schrodinger (see Elitzur, 1995), NV are, metaphorically, philosophically, and energetically, not a move toward self-organizing life but a move toward death. They represent entropic information degrading *in extremis* at morphological and energy limits. Similarly, the Haaken–Kelso scheme requires dissipation of energy in disequilibrium and limits the availability of self-organizing options as a mathematical condition easily met by the psychobiological reality encountered in V.

A flow of critical unstable states?

With N as an extremely unstable state, one argues that, from the initial sensory perception, there begins a succession of acute pattern changes and critical transformations, which go through sensorium–nerves–messenger systems (here only of a semantic and phenomenological equivalence, because the levels of time and space vary remarkably) through the multiple brain regions. Do not assume that there is an exactness in routing or activation. Miller in a personal communication (1997) showed there can even be activation of the inferior frontal gyrus in the temporal–frontal cortex.

V may be described as a flow of unstable phase transitions, energy organizing, propelling toward a given field and morphological conditions, or as being 'pulled' or 'attracted to' more stable states defined by V's termination. Homeostasis, competence, and freedom from distress are system inherent 'curative' attractants implicit in genetic, developmental and volition design.

Non-linear brain, epileptic analog, might defibrillating patterns treat NV?

The foregoing description of critical flows of unstable states, if posed at a morphologically limiting boundary for cascade effects and excitatory energy release, are apt characterizations for epileptic cascades and their motor expression. We have earlier proposed the epileptic phenomena as one alternative and disorderly schema for considering motor pattern generation for V. Mackay (1997) with others in discussing the non-linear brain provide us the conceptual language of electrochemical fields under extreme excitation as a dynamic landscape of energy–space exchange applicable to the epilepsy-prone brain. Two theories are offered; one is that of single network firing where both of two possible neuronal states are stable, predictably altered by electrical change. (Be reminded, change may be intracellular generated over gradients as well as externally so.) Cowan in that discussion allows that waves of excitation spread through bistable neuronal networks leading to non-linear synchronies, where the nature of synchrony depends upon 'switching probabilities' which we infer to be state change propensities, in turn milieu dependent. Think of these as sets of initial conditions with, given morphology and energy impositions, constrained process pathways.

An alternative conception set forth in the discussion – see Mackay – offered by Schiff, So, Gluckman and Sauer invokes a requirement for irregularities in firing patterns in order to maintain ('trap' is their word) the brain in normal thus non-seizure states. They emphasize the role of a variety of unstable periodic orbits as possibly intrinsic (our inference) to brain tissues. We derive these to function as anti-rhythms, interference with extreme synchrony, restraining instabilities of oscillation which, by varying periodicities, disallow intra-cell generated, joined cellular one-phase enhancement to exaggeration, thus, kindling or cascade. Cf. the Apollonian admonishment, 'all things in moderation' as rhythm's homeostat. Put another way, one may think of self-organization at neuron and network level as including periodic disorganizing or constrained random, anti-symmetry activity. So far so good; were it so medullary locally in NTS, AP, CTZ etc., the 'compulsion' to V would occur only in states of shared oscillation, symmetry as, statistically and clinically obvious, abnormal. Just as in epilepsy, V activity could come only when neuron and network do not within their energy structures oppose extremes of network symmetry, one might say the fibrillating raptures of the swaying mob.

This concept, in turn, might provide a notion of a new treatment, test, or, (what do you know?) one explanation for the inexplicable but established success of electrical acupuncture in NV treatments. While in cardiac function it is automated atrial rhythms one needs, and the treatment for dysrhythmia is a defibrillating electrical shock, for NV the foregoing schema suggests that for the treatment of V, (N as well insofar as it is related) the application of a defibrillating minor shock external to the brain (not by any means as strong as electroshock therapy, Cerletti treatments applied as heroic measure to depression) might be helpful. In electrical impulse acupuncture, current applications are far downstream; the Chinese neurological charting is not at all like our Western one. Upstream currents, that is afferent stimulation, is invoked. Is there a better neuroanatomy for interrupting NV electrically? One does suspect so. It is surely worth a much expanded test of single and multiple stimulating current locations, including those nearer the brain itself. As it is, the voltage delivered in electrical acupuncture is so minimal as to be homeopathic. Conservative, we distrust that.

Stereotypy, periodicity, and the structure of degrading orderly disorder

Goldberger (1997) takes a new perspective applicable across diseases. It is of simplified order. When morphologically similar at differing levels of complexity (neuron to network to structure to pathway) these may be viewed as fractals, as in chaos theory. Antithetical to scale-free fractal thus multiple systems are those dominated by but one scale, hence singly periodic. This means that a disease state contains less information and is less capable of an adaptive response.

While calling attention to such regular 'irregularities' as Cheyne-Stokes cyclical breathing – one may be reminded of V or felt waves of N – Goldberger emphasizes the stereotypy arising from the loss of complexity in disease. Thus, there are new periodical structures shared among severely ill persons with a variety of diagnoses. 'Many diseases are better conceptualized as part of a dynamic reordering … often a loss of fractal multi-scale complexity (showing instead) highly (simple) periodic behavior.'

To focus on syndrome similarities as cross-disease 'output repetition' is easy for Parkinsonism or other tremor disorder, sinusoidal heart rate oscillations in fetal distress syndrome, etc. but we extend Goldberger's thoughts to NV. Considering NV thereby becomes not disorder but malfunctioning order characterized by simpler periodicity at, presumably, various processing levels. And NV, most obviously stereotypical pulsing V, are information degraded phenomena common to many diseases and environmental maladaptations. Compared to normal gastric, respiratory, esophageal, brain awareness and communicative functions, NV are obviously simpler 'single scale' behaviors of exaggerated rhythms and periodicity.

We have earlier termed NV events 'primitive', which is equivalent to single (not multiple) scales, less complexity. Often now we have thought of it as at least analogous in V to epilepsy, the events of which impose an expressively radical degrading simplicity on adaptive capabilities. Goldberger's emphasis on the commonalties of disease conceived as fractal structures of reduced information content suggests another means of one day measuring simultaneous processes in, and leading to, NV motor response.

A tolerant 'theory of almost everything' or a helpful nonlinear schema?

Brown's (1911) discovery of an autonomic reflexive spinal motor patterning as a 'mechanism' clearly does not apply to most NV. But is continuing ignorance of what occurs our only reason to entertain dynamic theory or is it really a useful way to conceive of NV event flows and then self-pattern generators? Are we just being fashionable?

If there is a value in the alternative approach to NV, then an overview of principles will be useful. We rely on Kelso whose superb study and exegesis of dynamics is applied to the brain and behavior in *Dynamic Patterns* (1995). Future NV workers who may wish to follow and test the utility of these concepts will surely wish to become more familiar with its mathematics and logic from which, for example, regularities within changing brain-imaging sequences should be identifiable as classes of events forecasting NV and correlating with its awareness. Kelso's 'elementary concepts and conditions for self organization' (pages 16–17) are as follows:

1. Patterns arise spontaneously as the result of large numbers of interacting components . . . the nature of such interactions must be nonlinear.
2. The system must be dissipative and far from thermal equilibrium. Dissipation is equivalent to a kind of attraction that may take several forms.
3. Relevant degrees of freedom . . . (those as) collective variables or order parameters . . . created by the coordination between the parts (characterizes the system's) circular causality.
4. Order parameters are found near nonequilibrium phase transitions, where the loss of stability gives rise to new or different patterns and/or switching.

5. Fluctuations are continually robbing the system, allowing it to feel its stability and providing an opportunity to discover new patterns.
6. Parameters that lead the system through different patterns (unlike order parameters) may be quite unspecific in nature; in no sense do they act as a code or a prescription for the emerging patterns. On the other hand, in biological systems, boundary conditions may be quite specific in an information sense, especially when a particular pattern is required.
7. The order parameter of dynamics, the equation, may have simple (fixed point, limit cycle) or complicated solutions including determinist chaos and stochastic (random) aspects thereby giving rise to enormous behavioral complexity.

The complexity of sequences, constrained and generated by the capabilities of morphological structures and information exchange, gives rise to less complex parameter dynamics. These in turn are capable of generating enormous behavior complexity, so that (quoting Nobelist Gell-Mann):

> . . . the central idea is that understanding of any level of organization starts with the knowledge of basically three things: the parameters acting on the system (which are sometimes equated with the term 'boundary conditions'), the interacting elements themselves, and the emerging patterns or modes to which they give rise . . . especially in biological systems, constraints and borders are constantly being created and dissolved . . . the scheme is level independent and hierarchical, but not . . . unidirectional.

Esthetics again

When considering PNV earlier, we proposed that it is an olfaction-based psychobiological, or sociobiological esthetic. It defines the environment, indeed her momentary ecological niche which is becoming ugly and repulsive. This notion of a biological template is Platonic, Kantian, Chomskian, and 'classical.' It is also, when one relies on Arnheim's work on the psychology of esthetics, gestaltist. It accepts a dominant hedonism in biology, which transforms to Darwinian adaptation as 'rational' and reinforcing, and also rather Hebrew–Christian because 'progress' and higher levels are implicit, right or wrong.

For gestaltists, the brain organizes perception with constraints and in predictable directions. The framework easily allows for self-organization in genetic and cell morphology, and a 'not so hidden' teleology. Implied is the truth of ugliness and, given the data and the proposition, that women are more pheronomically competent judges. Out of this philosophy come research designs. The arguments as to whether men or women are the 'best' art critics (please do review the studies on gender esthetics in the PNV chapters) will be edified but not solved by research.

Cascading instabilities 'attracted' to a final structured, reinforcing pattern of N to V

Consider the possibility that, viewed dynamically, both N and V are phases of instability, each 'pulled' to more unstable patterns that are morphologically constrained, leading then toward a more stable state which V initiates as subsidence. One observes V as transitional and subjectively is glad this is so. One does not readily imagine a well human maintaining life were V to be chronic, as it tends to be in tabetic terminal cancers with GI metastases. Keep in mind that V spasms tax morphological limits which invite rupture, hemorrhage, asphyxiation, collapse, or, given potentiating drugs, convulsion.

The logic of transitional space–time implicit in dynamic theory is 'pulled' by the more dissipative, less constrained instability of V behavior. The logic of V as a naturally selected 'self-cure' for N is equally entertained, because one conceives that an animal beset by N over time is more disabled than one relieved by V. From a functional standpoint one notes a role for N as a warning of incipient V. Given N and knowledge of impending V, one tries prevention via breathing control or diversion. It is so untidy otherwise.

Little NV conditioned taste aversion in humans

The literature and experience seem to prove that conditioned taste aversions (CTAs) do not necessarily occur when humans have N or V. Yet dramatic learning of the single trial sort can be demonstrated in mammals – in Norwegian rats or coyotes, for example. Perhaps one can understand the absence of CTA in humans as a result of the variety in our daily diet, and, when food poisoning does occur, the long S-R delay leading to no proximal S for short-term memory. Conceivably empirical knowledge of possible causes is also operative, because we learn that much more than tainted foods make us ill. Indeed, much food poisoning is unrecognized because, given the S-R delay, no CTA, and a faith in mass food industry sanitation, we are probably more likely to think it is the 'flu. That is a common self-misdiagnosis. In any event, NV are prevalent in humans but CTA seems rare, just as animal experimentation shows little by way of consistent NV–CTA relations. Given the reduction of NV risk with aging, or experience with motion, it is more likely that 'controls' can be learned (we have discussed this and the opposite sensitization; but one avenue underexplored for NV control is biofeedback as part of behavioral medicine).

CTA, olfaction, and the biology of esthetics

Olfaction

An esthetic experience will be learned. This seems to occur in anticipatory NV, or in such CTA that may derive from NV. Of all the immediately 'teaching' senses it is olfaction that involves biochem-ically the least-transformed energy, most immediate to ancient brain mechanisms (traversing no nuclei), most often hedonistic, and most often connected to an adverse judgment. To those who are sensitive, much of a new situation smells bad. The world of the olfactory brain is more often understood as urgent and inundated. It is that path, almost straight to the amygdala, which becomes mindfully unpleasant. This wisdom is fitting to the earlier savage and fecund world in which our ancient 'reptilian' brain performed. It is only refined and elaborated savagery differentiating our modern world from the pre-human one.

It would be a simple theory were most NV to be consistently olfactorily induced. Not so. Beyond NV being caused by repugnant smell, the evidence shows that olfactory precipitation is most common only in pregnancy and, speculatively (Blum, 1988), for radiation synesthesia. One encourages a theory-derived search for neural projections expected to be interacting to and from the various V-involved brain regions. The frontal lobe is already 'in,' thanks to Miller et al. The role of olfaction in NV, in spite of its obvious structural–biochemical relationship to the pituitary, hippocampal, thalamic, and limbic areas, seems (along with the ignored problem of how baroreceptors respond to induced NV) to have been a little regarded modality, even though the fine work of Dodd and Castellucci in Kandel et al. (1991), Engen (1982), Keverene and Rosser in Muller-Schwarze and Silverstein (1986), Moncrieff (1944), Serby and Chobar (1992), Stoddart (1990), Van Toller and Dodd (1988), and, by no means unrelated, Arnheim (1986, 1991) provides enticing hints. One should be mindful of the strong role of the hippocampus in learning, where some CTA 'plans' must be placed.

Futuristic biofeedback?

It appears that humans learn to recognize NV perturbations from immersive contexts such as sea sickness, automobiles on curvy roads, smells, sights, and cancer treatment rather than via CTA or of irritations in the GI tract. What humans learn about cancer and chemotherapy from NV is that it is awful and that returning for treatment may be more awful and can actually yield anticipatory nausea and vomiting (ANV). Olfaction is a different case. Odorant molecules, including those that sicken (such as putricine), can be immediately learned through long-term recognition, labeling, and associations. The history of biofeedback allows a bit of optimism that enteric processes may be brought to lowered threshold levels and thus sensed and controlled.

A parallel case exists wherein radiation is olfactorily sensed and can lead to discrimination and learning in rats and humans (Blum, 1988). This allows for some optimism in biofeedback discrimination and control studies, such as self-control when NV are caused by self-dosing, concentration on images, etc. But it is a less accessible epithelium of the GI tract that contains the sensing cells in a nervous–glandular–motor apparatus which is so self-regulating that the enteric nervous system (ENS) is rightly classified as intrinsically separate from the CNS and ANS (see Gershon, 1995).

The ENS is remarkably self-organizing and exerts control over other structures such as sympathetic ganglia. Serotonin (5HT) acts as a peristalsis-controlling neurotransmitter in the ENS and also has analgesic properties. Whether even the most futuristic of biofeedback projections will allow conscious sensing, or learned and willful control of serotonin activity, others will learn. The application of biofeedback to gut activity is worthy over a range of disorders, stress responses included, but it is difficult to anticipate any immediate NV control benefit. Perhaps a first try would be toward a discrimination for cancer cytogen presence/absence if any autonomic or enteric self-awareness markers can be identified in well subjects. With any success, one would seek in patients a sense of ENS awareness with at least some self-control over what might be conditioned serotonin activation leading to ANV.

Correlated immune mobilization activity?

NV function behaviorally and, were they competent gastointestinally, they would be a biological defense demonstrating alarm functions. Pain is a parallel alarm system which interconnects, however diffusely, to activate NV or be activated by NV. Under these general conditions of alarm, there may be a simultaneous immune system activation. It is a reasonable hypothesis, but we find no studies that examine this possibility. One may expect suppression of immune competence under a chronic NV situation, as in the repeat-cycle cancer or psychogenic patient. But as NV are themselves stressful, the identification of a well-defined independent variable, i.e., 'cause,' will be difficult. Were any adaptive role for NV to be found, as, for example, if patients with *Salmonella* who experienced NV were shown to have a faster recovery time attributable to NV-stimulated immune competencies (microphages, etc.), one would have found (if not the Holy Grail!) an NV function that does have an adaptive or selective advantage.

Our hunch that (some) NV affects immune competence draws on the gender differences in NV's parallel in immune function, i.e., the greater risk of women also to experience auto-immune disease (Whitacre et al., 1999). Immune environments within men and women differ for reasons as unknown as NV real differences. What is known is that the primary immune response is more 'vigorous.' At present, estrogen receptors within immune cells and prostaglandin roles in immune modulation – both also suspect in PNV – are observed. Future research on PNV-immune responsivity, for example some obstetric advantage that PNV may confer, beckons.

Baseline augmentation and interactive system influences

Prior experience leading to learning may be a major formative process in NV. It is not simply the Pavlovian models associated with ANV, but it is neuronal learning of multisensory proximities for the interconnected cells constituting the superior colliculus; these cells are informative interconnections which interact with potential perturbations, altering NV risk. Important, for example, are the ANS, resting states, and reactivity levels along with the levels of compounds [adrenocorticotropic hormone (ACTH), norepinephrine] associated with these circula-ting hormone levels, neuropeptide levels (vasopressin, oxytocin, endogenous peptide Y), personality traits, or environmentally linked conditions (pain, stress, fatigue) – all of which enter into NV process equations. Also as baseline conditions, there are those NV-initiating processes of pregnancy. As pregnancy obviously involves major hormonal changes, the specific alterations accounting for PNV have been sought as a function of various hormone levels. No reliable hormonal 'absolute' or triggering levels have emerged; thus one continues to view the dispositions in pregnancy for NV as an aggregate category.

NV as a nonadaptive but emergency signal to self and others

As interpretive perceptual or internal traumatic (irritable) response, and as subjective experience, NV are evidence that, with Candide, this is not the best of all possible worlds. With NV we experience a psychologically disruptive emergency signal mirroring the perturbations that lead to NV. The meanings of the perturbation and subjective/behavioral events, while occurring in different time–space dimensions, are quite the same – a psychosomatic tautology. With the rare exception of the less than 4% V-induced treatments in poisoning centers, the NV phenomena are a signal and simultaneous response with only the rarest adaptive value. One must reject optimism about any current biopsychological, 'functional utility' with a possible exception for PNV. One rejects the older Darwinian premise of the evolutionary progress and the expanding adaptability of humans as NV might reflect that. We are looking instead at phenomena expanded in humans in terms of inductive stimuli, precipitating conditions (compared with fish or primates and excluding regurgitative feeding in canines). This expansion (as well as any basic function except that cited above as the rare imposed medically, bulimically, or N terminating willed human NV) is nonadaptive; it is not simply an evolutionary flop but, in Darwinian terms, inexplicable. A different view emerges if one allows unselected chancc and subsequent, even if accidentally initiated, self-organization as evolutionary principles. To adhere to the premiss of human NV's conserved and continued adaptive function in humans is to look at it wrongheadedly.

Poison treatments: when 'reflex' works

The V capacity, as an induced reflex, can occasionally be tissue or life saving when induced. Poison treatment is the best example. In 1993 (Litovitz et al., 1994) over 1750 000 poison exposure cases were reported. For only 3.7% of these was treatment with ipecac advised, this figure representing a continuing decline over preferred therapies. Yet 65 000 cases justified induced V as treatment, even if one that is rarely employed at poison centers. In some cases, the patient, usually a young child, has taken some time to be transported there, and ipecac itself, although intended to produce immediate V, may take some time to do so. Upon the advice of poison centers, therefore, ipecac is most often used at ingestion sites, because 90% of cases occur at home.

As medicines used as AEs can sometimes also, depending on sequence, dosage, and timing, be emetics – quite paradoxical (remember, Wolf administered ipecac with suggestion and controlled V) – it is obvious that emetic effects are uncertain, although the treatment data make it appear that AE effects are the more difficult to predict (in so far as emetics limited by definition to chemical compounds appear to have more immediate and, thus, reflexive action). Animal studies may show, on what is a tentative principle for emetic and AE effects, when surgical–chemical interference has occurred with existing anatomical structures. The work of Knox (1993) illustrates this. Specificity of action seems to be dependent on the nerve or brain region ablated, and which one of the many diversely acting AEs is administered. Such work generally shows an extremely high specificity for emetics, i.e., strong constraints on the predictability of emesis. Even that is reduced by tolerance and changes over time in responsivity. And among experimental animals (whether cat, dog, ferret, shrew, etc.) considerable individual differences are found.

Cultural again: the 'ordeal bean'

The uncertainty of induced V is used in African trials and presumes guilt controls fatal reactions to strong emetics. Duke (Callaway pers. comm.) describes, citing anthropologists studying Nigerian tribal witchcraft detection devices, the 'ordeal bean' (*Physostigma venenosum*), wherein a naturally occurring form of physostigmine, an anticholinesterase, crosses the blood–brain barrier, having central as well as peripheral effects (as one suspects of most AEs as well as an unknown number of emetics – Martindale, 1993). An effusion is given to those suspected of witchcraft, who will believe in its discriminating efficacy, very much like modern polygraph lie detection depends on faith in the otherwise quite faulty procedure. Those guilty, knowing this, do not vomit but die of the ordeal instead. The innocent will signal his innocence, lift his hand, and vomit, thereby seeking to rid himself of the toxin. Even here V may not work and, if poisoning is observed to be killing the innocent, extraordinary measures (excrement mixed with water used to wash female genitalia) are employed. These may fail. Callaway (pers. comm.) interprets the report to show that a critical mass of toxin must be retained to produce death, whereas the innocent presumably can allow the irritant to work as an emetic. Note well, both the raised hand and the V are communications and have the meaning of innocence.

We see that as a 'reflex' the 'ordeal bean' is useful when another's healing beliefs, knowledge, or consciousness invokes the capability – V by using an emetic. The ecological, sociobiological schema here obviously cannot ignore that V in immediate poisoning control is the end-product of historical knowledge accumulated and, at least in poison centers, institutionalized interpersonal processes. A 'reflex' that begins with 'folk' knowledge of physostigmine is an ecologically sophisticated reflex indeed

Reminder: individual differences

Individual differences abound in the acuity, sensitivity, pattern recognition, and sensory organ shaping as well as internal processing of that patterned time–space energy which is a sensory message. We have seen that there are consistent sex differences in sensory styles and capabilities, especially that of the olfactory. Nor are sensory channels in any way independent; what is happening in one shapes whether another modality's message will be augmented or ignored. The old masters, Ramon y Cajal, Sherrington, and Lashley, identified these interacting flexible processes to which the current term 'plasticity' in part alludes. Environmental events that are perceptually interpreted often initiate internal processes, some of which will in turn initiate further assessing environmental interactions (sniffing, searching eyes toward information gathering) which can precipitate NV. We are not aware of an active modality that does not inform on events capable of becoming NV; NV in turn generate subjective responses and environmental impacts which alter the sensorium. Olfactory, visual, vestibular, nociceptor, tactile, kinesthetic, pain, sexual, ANS, enteric – all can be at work. Investigated the least are baroreceptors presumed to be responsive to edema, tumor growth, perhaps even to irritability – and worth testing – to circulating metastasized cells. NV occur in many instances of tumor and head injury and in some hypertension, and perhaps from genetic olfaction–immune system chromosomal linkage, if there is a relationship between NV and immune response (either as enhancement or suppression). Against such a hypothesis are clinical data on bone marrow transplants, indicating that autoimmune rejection seems not to exaggerate risks of NV under operative procedures.

'Soft' holism

It is likely that, at humanist, 'holistic' levels, the evocative categories of literature, folk language, esthetics, and possibly philosophy are particularly attractive, at least for those not schooled in medical or biopsychological science. Whether they are negatively charged in the eyes of the 'hard' scientists is not known. It would seem the case that broader categories, subsuming many referents or none, readily lose predictive or explanatory power when heard in the loose conceptions of practitioners of holistic healings, curbside psychoanalysis, or trendy MDs. They are no better able to be extended to levels of observation or analysis from which they are not derived than would microbiological terms prove helpful to a philosopher viewing NV. But don't ignore philosophy, or fail to view NV as a disharmonious response to an unharmonious world. We are the intellectual children of Plato and Aristotle.

Keep in mind that Plato considered philosophy not simply a love of wisdom, but an effort to devise systems that would work toward an ideal human harmony. The philosopher might well employ NV as evidence of a person's momentary relationship to the cosmos, or as a person–environmental perturbation, an esthetic judgment about the extreme unattractiveness of structures (more likely nonstructures) in the environment. It could be a descriptor of the sufferer's disharmonious relationship with those structures, or the subjective experience as a consummate definition of one's being in the moment. Each such statement of disharmony is evidence, at this level, that NV are antithetical to Plato's conception of the good.

In consequence, for the 'research philosopher,' NV may be a good measurement of disharmony as it may, epidemiologically, mark the risky life situations of the impoverished young adult, or the painful vulnerability of women, particularly pregnant women, to levels of perturbation. There would seem to be no less richness in a philosophical theory of NV than in the GI pharmacologist's model of $5HT_3$ action on enterochromaffin serotonin receptors. Sapolsky and Balt might not countenance such an approach as ours, because they understandably restricted themselves to the scientific enterprise. We may, however, rely upon their insightful methods and findings to reiterate that NV deserve study across disciplines and modes of thought.

Again, evolutionary speculation

If one posits an intellectually evolved Darwinism as accurately portraying principles of evolution, including self-organization (see Depew and Weber, 1995), one can find an NV 'purpose,' i.e., adaptive utility in the subsequent intelligent action where the mind, experiencing NV, organizes planned action. This may be individual, as in aversive learning where, in order to avoid NV, one does not drink as much beer, relies on a doctor or pharmacist for a prescription, or on mother for her folk remedy, or one simply ingests soda crackers or rests.

The sixth extinction?

Many (probably almost all) of the perturbations to which NV are the response are to modern conditions as discoveries and inventions and their aftermath. Consider NV precipitants that were not part of earlier hominid life: agricultural production of alcohol and opiates, medicines capable of inducing NV, surgery (which goes back to Egyptian times), and other interventions yielding both health and NV. With urbanization and new technology there was abundant food sufficient for some to overindulge. Thus Roman feasting and bulimia, and good storage and transportation, and mass production (compare *E. coli*). Mark the invention of vehicles to challenge vestibular eye coordination (from chariots, sea-going vessels to space ships) and the development by bureaucratic specialization and refined power hierarchies of governments. Siu, the founder of the Panetic Society which encourages research on the infliction of suffering, shows that governments – the bureaucracy of which is of urban origin – inflict far more suffering than do individuals: power and policy, war and torture, industrial expansion, population and industrial growth encouragements, date government to the rise of urban civilization some 8000+ years ago, and assuring its exponential with the nation state over the last few centuries. Are governmental side effects sickening? They are balanced, of course, by public health and medical advance, all of the amenities, security, and richness of the modern world. But modern NV do appear to be a side effect as well as a warning. Margaret Mead said that the primitive Arapesh had no PNV. Twenty-five percent of the women in our study said that their workplace stress makes them sick. In health surveys poor working young men were at great risk. What does this tell us about modern working and life situations? Not good!

The 'bloomin', buzzin' confusion,' which James characterized as the natural environment that the newborn infant confronts, may well be what all living in any but an isolated preliterate society confront as adults today. One can speculate that the peculiar cruelties and studied inflictions of pain, whether Roman crucifixion, Dutch flailing, Sabine mass rape, witch burnings, Iron Maidens, the Chinese death of 1000 cuts, etc., would seem also to be inventions. The Marquis de Sade signifies them as refinements of the resourceful, the pain of, view, and reflection upon which are more likely to invoke NV as an event. We can also credit to invention our long lifespans, which generate chronic diseases of older age (in ancient Rome the life expectancy was 40, albeit longer for the wealthy) which, in turn, are risk conditions for NV. The most common of these, cardiovascular disease and cancer, are both NV precipitants in their natural state and through iatrogenesis. And both of these major illnesses arise in part from no complaint but we are living longer through environmental mastery, but also as a result of stressful lifestyles and environmental exposures.

The cerebral cortical awareness, which allows thinking, planning, assessment, and overall control, is the maximum informational processing organ, and thus the one most 'optimistically' employed for long-term avoidance and control via consciousness and planning. The functional implication of control is also arguably present because the response itself carries simultaneous external meanings of alarm for the human as a social animal. These are able to invoke community mobilization as, for example, where PNV demonstrably works to get psychological family support for the pregnant woman.

The most readily adaptive state is the unstable one – what Kelso calls intrinsic chaos in the brain as diverse systems are interconnected, and ideally coherent and cooperating. Regional neuronal conductance is a localized illustration, especially in its interaction with the environment. It is fair enough to describe environmental change as a rugged landscape in the sense of unpredictability to which the alert, flexible, and resourceful animal must be ever ready to respond. One may think of interactions in a fluctuating ecological structure and, when the animal and the consequential environment survive or even prosper, it is as a self-organizing one made up of its network of structures. But humans have not only created landscapes intending them to be controlled, safe, and bountiful, but, as a side effect, environmentalists forecast the demise of our species. NV, however primitive, appear to be a most expressive personal measure of its accumulated, acute unharmonious impact.

Stress response, like human NV, may well be increasingly nonadaptive when responsive to aspects of modern environments. Awareness of stress – which must often be mediated by schemes offered by third parties (such as in psychotherapy or after an annual physical) – may take on inescapable and repulsive meanings. The NV behavior and feelings immediately define the situation expressively, in consciousness and as a biological esthetic. The stress comes about over time and must initially be defined, symptomatically, in language, and culturally as aversive, and the symptoms of ANS arousal need have no hedonistic, esthetic tone. Both are psychobiological, both are 'irritable' as essential life signs, and one may 'cause' the other. People in these situations may experience later learned ANV, or shame at having vomited publicly, or fear that N will continue to prevent them going to work.

The arrow and path from stress to NV are strong and wide. [Refer to discussions by Caccioppo and Tassinary (1990) and to chapters therein by Stern and Sison, by Walker and Sanman, by Johnson and Anderson, by Kennedy, Glaser, and Kiecolt-Glaser, and by Reed, Harver and Katkin.] GI symptoms are the most common bodily response to stress, with the GI tract itself exquisitely engaged in control and integration, and with the ENS having more neurons than the spinal cord. The ENS and CNS, not excluding the 'decision-making' immune system (see Kennedy, Glaser, and Kiecolt-Glaser), interact not simply via nerve tracts but with direct or mediated, circulating interactive messengers including neuropeptide endocrines such as cholecystokinin (CCK), somatostatin, vasopressin, vasoactive intestinal peptide (VIP), etc. Furthermore, serotonin receptors so densely distributed in the GI tract are also found in some of the same medullary, paraventricular regions active in NV motor pattern commands (AP, CTZ, NTS), and so serotonin is thought to play an important role in psychiatric disorders. Intrinsic organ and learned predispositions exist so that GI symptoms occur more often as a stress-vulnerable site, leading some people to stereotyped or psychophysiologically response–hierarchical signs.

The fact that more than 1400 physicochemical changes have been shown to be associated with stress responses is a reminder of how difficult it is to expect to move from a laboratory observation to knowing what might be a stress–GI–NV process in a particular patient, or to develop any NV theory limited to stress reactions. As Reed et al. (1990) remind us, research on viscerosensory areas of the cortex has been neglected, but it is known that enteric afferents reach the hypothalamus, cerebral cortex, and thalamus. And one learns (Caccioppo and Tassinary, 1990; Reed et al., 1990) that, in about half of a sample of patients with unexplained NV and in half with anorexia, there was abnormal GI activity, but none in the other halves. What does one do to account for stress-imposed GI disturbance, one that requires some predictive GI transit and motility changes, or, for anorexia, a GI somatic correlate? This is rather typical of the research problem in NV. One may well get back, as Wolf (1985) advises, to clinical studies.

A more than experiential pain relationship?

Pain may also be more than analogy. Pain is a central human experience phenomenon defined not only by subjective clinical or social–philosophical focus (the International Society of Panetics) but by brain space. The cerebral cortical sensory area for pain is much larger than that for visceral experience processing. We have seen in our epidemiological sample that some people describe NV as forms of intense pain. Pain can trigger NV, a not uncommon event in sports or orthopedic injury (Andrews, 1992). In postoperative NV, pain is more likely to be reported leading to an N than to a V outcome. Andrews cites work showing that only 10% of postoperative patients, having pain and having had general anesthesia, had V without N, whereas almost two-thirds had N without V.

The work of Iadarola and Caudle (1997) stimulates speculation that there may be more than parallels and cross-over triggers, feelings between pain and NV, including approaches to treatment. Just as at one time evolutionary V did have a 'good' toxic expelling function, and NV do yet teach animals via CTA wise food aversions, pain has an obvious warning function, compelling attention, problem-solving for source removal. But pain may also have an inappropriate continuing presence as a maladaptive response called 'neuropathic' (Recall, one definition of 'stress' is also a continuing ANS and perhaps felt response to stimuli, situations that are also no longer adaptive where the response now generates dysfunction or pathology.)

Neuropathic pain is typical after physical injury. When pain itself generates pain pathway cell membrane learning, i.e. changes as increased sensitivity, continuing signaling, pain experience is more readily reinvoked by the same or similar stimuli at lower thresholds, or it may persist without stimulation. It is a molecular phenomenon, which alters pathway cell membranes. It involves gene transcription or neuropeptide encoding, one of which is substance P, which is already implicated in some NV processes. There are a number of neuroactive compounds released at synapses in pain pathways, just as it appears multiple information carriers are involved in NV events. For pain, the NK-1 receptor binds substance P. Upon adverse stimulation – the range of events capable of producing pain but most likely surgery for the neuropathic – NK-1 becomes self-generating, 'internalized;' more autonomously active or reverberating (think of the Sorcerer's Apprentice). This receptor perseverance led Ladarola and Caudle to conceive of means to interrupt. They injected a protein inactivator, a toxin ligand compound into the cerebral spinal fluid (CSF), the result of which was a reduction in pain sensitivity of the experimental animal, attributable to chronic or overactive substance P release, that noxious NK-1 downstream pathway spread. Other toxin fusion proteins were found to work in the same way.

Of interest is that an aspect of neuropathic pain is a 'mix-up,' one could say a ganglionic 'misinterpretation' of pain signals. This 'allodynia' means that normally inconsequential, in other humans normally painless, touch produces extreme pain. 'Hyperalgesia' describes such an exaggerated response. In this experimental work with pain a functionally maladaptive neural signal processing inadequacy is present, whether or not 'learned' at the cellular, pathway level. One wonders if this is more than a conceptual analogy to NV, for neuropharmacologists are now looking at NK-1 receptors for further evidence of their involvement as significant NV messengers. Of course, the same or similar transmitters have multiple functions, messages (think of the ubiquity of 5HT receptors) and so NK-1 involvement by no means assures a pain–NV equivalence at the substance P protein binding level. Yet one does ask what are the differences in NK-1 and substance P activities from NV and neuropathic or hyperalgesic pain. Here is research for traditional neuropharmacology.

Here, in the injections of Ladorola and Caudle may also be inferential evidence for the control value of imposing irregularities on expanding network recruitment of neurons to synchrony, as discussed in Mackay by Schiff and others. By injecting a protein inactivator these workers have interrupted autonomous, self-organizing and perpetuating intracellular periodicities at transcription-encoding-membrane-pathway levels and in so doing blocked a process moving toward Goldberger's degraded, simplified, single state periodicity of disorder? Obviously a toxin ligand entering the CSF, diffusing to block NK-1 substance P binding spread yields linear chains of biochemical events. However action site selectivity through diffusion may require probabilistic mapping. But does it help us to think of such biochemical blockades in simultaneous non-linear ways? The ideas and work of readers, and their students, may tell that tale.

Iatrogenesis

Iatrogenic NV comes from surgery, prescriptions, cancer therapies, and psychiatric drugs. Learned NV, including hospital surroundings and interpersonal actions that exacerbate NV distress, are probably less common than the NV of ordinary living, PNV included. It may be that medical interventions – the research has yet to be done – yield higher rates, incidence and duration, and intensities of NV. The best-known risks are bone marrow transplant, strabismus and abdominal surgery, cisplatin and radiation, with neurosurgical insult to the fourth ventricle floor as perhaps the supreme example of humanly engineered, and therefore rational, intrusion on brain tissue in the region where there is tissue involving the motor pattern of V.

Iatrogenesis, including its settings and patient-ascribed meanings, is a major proximate 'cause' for NV. As it is doctor generated in a situation where physician and nurse are responsible, and where the patient is available for at least short-term NV treatments, those treatments occur. We cited the paradoxical outcomes of some 'antiemetics' as emetics, but warn of side effects which can include tardive dyskinesias, fatal malignant neurolytic syndrome, and cardiac arrest.

Examples of procedures, which were widespread until outcome measures were made and iatrogenic causes were identified to be related, were newborn oxygen administration leading to blindness, intestinal resections for obesity which led to water and nutritional deficit, casual but worldwide prescription of chloromycetin leading to blood dyscrasias and fatalities, routine childhood tonsillectomy/adenoidectomy, circumcision, thalidomide prescription, etc. There has as yet been no systematic review of all cases of severe postoperative NV (PONV) in a single hospital to conclude which surgeries might have been avoided, or performed with a lesser anesthetic load, or of cancer treatments recommended and pursued where even that 6 weeks of extended life, which studies suggest can be precious to the terminally ill, was not likely to be obtained. For many, as terminal illness is often NV infested, one asks whether a less NV-disrupted and thus more dignified death might have been possible.

Bogner (1994), examining human error in medicine, estimates that about 100 000 fatalities occur in the USA annually from such errors, 70% preventable, mostly through institutional rather than individual change. We find dramatic differences at all levels of management, quality control, staff selection, morale, and thus organizational competence, between high- and low-malpractice rate hospitals, and quality control outcome between high- and low-rate physicians whom we also carefully evaluated.

With respect to NV themselves, it has not been thought of sufficient consequence to make retrospective measures of medical or nursing procedures. The guidance would not simply be for NV prevention but as quality control for wrongful procedures, prescriptions, and institutional surroundings with happy consequences for cost and pain reduction well beyond NV themselves. Sometimes alternative procedures or the same procedures better performed or prescribed are definitely better options. Yet any such approach to quality control meets resistance of the 'I can do no wrong' syndrome. Requiring drug efficacy evidence via meta-analysis is by no means an accepted rule of practice. Grant that most of what argues for the art of medicine is sensible. 'Whistle blowing' comes hard in close-knit professions, and new rules for caution come hard in institutions run by cherished traditions of professional latitude. Health maintenance organizations (HMOs), in restricting that latitude for reasons of profit, are not, however, sure ways to improve care. Quality reviews, retrospective for a random selection of procedures leading to NV, constitute a preventive approach to NV. Sampling cannot be limited to hospital cases.

Our earlier discussion of meanings, the subjective pain of N, and the ethical imperative of practice, 'do no wrong,' leads to a reminder that philosophy is not irrelevant; it is not simply bioethics but the structure of assumption, however unexamined and implicit, of most of us as observers. We have frameworks for organizing our view of the world. Deconstructivists would say they are all 'relative,' and that science doesn't matter. Eleans, from Democritus through Archimedes, then Aristotle, and Bacon, allow for insight, theory, and experiment. Schools for ontological, theological, existential, cynical, Platonic, and Kantian thought exist. These frameworks provide invested meanings for interpreting events, and, one suspects, particularly striking and unpleasant ones such as NV. This is God's hand? Luck of the draw? Our own fault? Deterministic linear sequencing as electrochemical transactions? Probabilities in an essentially unknowable and approximated world? A strict template for all brains, thus allowing Platonic form? Or just worry about the logic of the observer's text? We are not ourselves free of contexts, nor are NV.

Following thinkers such as Goethe, Hartshorn, Hesse, and

Charles Pierce, one may add the earlier Heidegger and modern Salthe (1993) in the discussion that human NV are existentially the character of some critically salient relationship, constituting at a moment all of the evolved and immediate self *in* the world. It is the being of the 'self world' and of the self in the world. This context is only approximated in psychobiology when the higher organization of process complexity expresses phase transitions leading cognitively to emergency awareness. An evolutionary direction can only be imputed – primitive but from adaptation toward recognition and control. NV as one sees them in humans are a conserved variant of the primitive single-cell avoidance and retreat. But, viewed in terms of meanings, the body and symbolic language of revulsion and rejection, NV could be interpreted as rejection of that which is revolting within the self, that which should become otherness by expulsion, expressing the biological esthetic of unwanted and ugly. It is what has unwantingly intruded upon or become oneself that is sought to be repudiated in its existential symbolism.

Hopelessness is one term for it, self-revulsion another. One turns to philosopher novelists at this point, specifically Jean Paul Sartre and his novel, *Nausea.* It entirely opposes Hegel's optimism as to God, Mind and resolutions as synthesis. For the existentialist self dominates and is meaningless or may invent its own values. This is much more pessimistic, isolating, and deconstructive than the God-fearing Kierkegaard for whom self is in relation to God. Sartre is a nothingness-out-of-suffering sort of man, and 'nausea' is Roquentin's symbolic psychosomatic view of the world.

Roquentin is the hero, and is sensible to the detestability of existence, that 'nauseated consciousness of nothing.' His thoughts, Hayden Carruth reminds us, 'culminate in a pervasive overpowering feeling of N which spreads at the bottom of the vicious puddle, at the bottom of our time – the time of purple suspenders and broken chair seas . . . at the edge, like an oil stain.'

Perhaps this angry cynical and helpless personal and philosophical development, the pointlessness of existence, was anticipated earlier in Kafka's writing on the awesome private terror of man's incomprehension and helplessness. In the nineteenth century Russian literature, there was Goncharov's energyless, purposeless, slothful character Oblomov who could do nothing in, for, or about the nineteenth century world which was already then overwhelming. These circumstances led to a surrender, to passivity, where, but for cynicism, Roquentin musters no action compatible with a view of a happy, adaptive, constructing, organizing life. In the face of the modern world, he comprises only 'sickness.' No framework for belief or faith; the world is disorganized and disorganizing. Roquentin abandons understanding and any hope of that control, any purposefulness as an autonomous practitioner of life. At the very start N is the state *and* statement about life

It is increasingly so. In evolutionary terms humans experience more varied NV than other animals, with PNV as the distinguishing marker. In cultural developmental terms there are more NV-precipitating circumstances now – those modern inventions of ours and the diseases derived from them – than in preurban societies. In so far as we are all somewhat Kafka or Roquentin children overcome by the impact of it all, easily tired and stressed, we experience NV as an ecological psychobiological response. In so far as we may show revulsion to a world increasingly beyond our control, with our brain no match for what our sorcerer's apprentices have accomplished, our N is increasingly a compulsory condition. Most apropos are Stephen Hawking's March 1998, White House remarks on the need to change our DNA so as to cope with our inventions. When we are not experiencing it and are thus competent to do so, we would do well to pay more attention to what, at many levels, it signifies.

Chapter 34
On using the Internet for knowledge acquisition

An information crisis faces medical professionals today. Over 360 000 articles are published annually in medical journals! Diffusion of information is slow; poor access to resources, ignorance of availability, cost, lack of time, and poor organization contribute to the problem. Along with readily-available book resources at one's finger tips, electronic resources are evolving into more useful methods for acquiring information. The Internet is a large collection of information, mostly unorganized, that sits in telephone-linked computers, called servers, anywhere in the world. This information is available to any equipped computer, called a client, at any time, if the remote server is turned on. A host of browsers such as Netscape Navigator and Microsoft Explorer, and search engines, such as Yahoo!, Infoseek, Excite, have been developed to find the information that a seeker may wish; Yahoo! has a medical section. None are as developed for medical information retrieval as the following sources, but one is pleasantly surprised occasionally!

Excellent sources of information

Ready access to organized, medical information is offered by The National Library of Medicine, at the National Institutes of Health in Bethesda, Maryland, USA. The NLM has made its extensive MEDLINE service free of charge, a 9-million-record bibliographic database, as well as full-text articles, compiled from 30 years of publications. The Oregon Health Sciences University maintains a site called CliniWeb that is directed toward assisting medical practitioners to find answers about clinical problems. A commercial source, Medical Matrix, is another source of information catalogued by clinical topic, available from Slack, Inc. Medscape is another excellent commercial source particularly emphazing women's health.

The URLs (Uniform Resource Locators) for these sites are:

http://nlm.nih.gov/ for Medline, PubMed
http://www.ohsu.edu/clinweb/ for Clinweb
http: //www. slackinc. com. matrix/ for Medical Matrix
http://www.medscape.com/ for Medscape.

As an example, searching Medscape's keywords database for the word 'nausea' turned up 205 referenced articles that include this word.

Other interesting sites:
http://gen.emory.edu/MEDWEB/medweb.html
http://www.nih.gov/health/ (for HSTAT, clinical practice guidelines, National Cancer Institute)
http://www.nih.gov/cgi-bin/cnetsrchp/?keywords= Nausea+and+Vomiting) (for the CancerNet resources)
http://altmed.od.nih.gov/ (for alternative medications)
http://wellweb.com (for general wellness)
http://www.healthworld.com (for broad health issues)
http://nhic-nt.health.org/ (for the National Health Information Center)

One of the authors (WLH) currently maintains the following web site:

http://www .stanford.edu/group/whpu/

which individuals may contact for information about clinical problems and health promotion information.

Appendix
Apothegms: expert views

We have collected some apothegms as pithy sayings, adages, that are pertinent to the nausea and vomiting (NV) field. You will see that some authorities' comments directly contradict those of others. The flavor of the current endeavor is thus conveyed.

To keep in mind

. . . there are deep unifying principles underlying human behavior and the brain (Kelso, 1995)

. . . the neurology of vomiting has been fairly well elucidated (Hickok and Morrow, 1993)

[processes] by which all these diverse stimuli culminate in a final common act is unknown (Andrews and Hawthorne, 1988)

Most of an organism most of the time is developing from one pattern to another not from homogeneity into a pattern (A.J. Turing)

Pattern is at the heart of great science and art (Kelso)

. . . all we are left with is dynamics, self sustaining and persisting on several space time scales, at all levels from the single cell up (Kelso, 1995)

It is a myth that the great majority of [cancer chemotherapy] patients can enjoy complete control of NV (paraphrasing Martin, 1992)

With respect to the treatment of NV, most oncologists are unread (paraphrasing Van Hoff et al., 1991)

Most [primary care providers] believe that NV is sufficiently covered in their primary care or general medicine texts (Winters, Senior Editor, Lippincott Raven, personal communication, 1995)

5HT antagonists . . . do not confer any significant benefit [in treatment of acute chemotherapy NV] compared with traditional agents, and they have not shown any benefit in the prevention of delayed symptoms (Roarty and McCallum, 1995)

As a single agent $5HT_3$ receptor antagonists are the most effective anti-emetics . . . for controlling radiotherapy and chemotherapy induced emesis. The superior activity [of OND] has been demonstrated (Hawthorne, 1995)

. . . no unique well identified group of labeled neurons that might function as a vomiting center could be identified (Miller and Ruggiero, 1994)

. . . no consensus yet exists concerning the detailed mechanism of the initiation and control of most clinically relevant forms of vomiting (Davis et al., 1986)

The brain is fundamentally a pattern-forming, self organized, dynamical system poised on the brink of instability (Kelso, 1995)

The importance of enteric serotoninergic systems as a target for drugs to treat gastrointestinal disorders is illustrated by the success of ondansetron . . . as we learn more about variations in the protein structure of the receptors, new opportunities will arise (Gaginella and Galligan, 1995)

Reductionism alone is bankrupt, and systems models . . . are so full of holes the Emperor might as well be naked (Kelso, 1995)

The tendency to retch from a fetid odor is immediately strengthened in a curious manner by some degree of habit (Darwin, 1872)

Roquentin . . . a man living at an extraordinary metaphysical pitch . . . discovers that all essences are volatile . . . reality itself reduced to pure existence [is] disgusting and fearsome, [thus] the detestability of existence (from Carruth's Introduction to Sartre's *Nausea* – [Editor's expansion: the essence of philosophical existentialism is set forth in Sarte's best novel, *Nausea*, where Roquentin's 'thoughts culminate in a pervasive, over-powering feeling of nausea' . . .])

In sum, and to the point

There is no phenomenon, no matter how complex, that after careful examination does not turn out to be more complex (D. Kretch, cited in Caccioppo and Tassinary, 1990)

From Horgan, *The Death of Science* (1996) we offer the following quotations:

> Harold Bloom eminent in the humanities, said 'because no poet can hope to approach, let alone surpass the perfection of [his forebears such as Milton, Shakespeare, Dante] "modern poets are all essentially tragic figures, latecomers, and their burden is much heavier than poets".'

Citing Gunther Stent on Henry Adams' law of acceleration:

> . . . certain fields of science . . . are limited . . . by the boundedness of their subject matter

arguing that, with a few other questions to solve, once one understands

> . . . how the nervous system processes information ... the basic task of pure biology will be completed.

However, he quotes Stent:

> . . . physiological therory can never really explain consciousness.

And on Arthur Langton of the Santa Fe Institute:

> . . . he [is] frustrated with the linearity of scientific language . . . . Poetry is a very non-linear use of language . . . [with respect to science], . . . there's stuff to explain out there that is more than the sum of its parts . . . [the linear summing of parts] . . . is not going to be adequate for capturing the essence of many systems . . . there's going to be something like poetry in the future of science.

Glossary: acronyms and abbreviations

ACTH	adrenocorticotropic hormone
ANS	autonomic nervous system
ANV	anticipatory nausea and vomiting
AP	area postrema
ATP	adenosine triphosphate
AVP	arginine vasopressin
CCK	cholecystokinin
CSF	cerebrospinal fluid
CMV	cytomegalovirus
CNS	central nervous system
CTA	conditioned taste aversion
CTZ	chemoreceptor trigger zone
CVS	cardiovascular system
DMV	dorsal motor nucleus of the vagus
DVC	dorsal vagal complex
ENS	enteric nervous system
FDA	Federal Drug Administration
fMRI	functional magnetic resonance imaging
GABA	gamma-aminobutyric acid
GnRH	gonadotropin-releasing hormone
hCG	human chorionic gonadotropin
HG	hyperemesis gravidarum
HMO	health maintenance organization
IOP	intraocular pressure
LOS	length of stay
MeAP	medial preoptic nucleus
MOB	main olfactory bulb
N	nausea
NA	nucleus ambiguus
NCI	National Cancer Institute

NIH	National Institutes of Health
NTS	nucleus tractus solitarius
NV	nausea and vomiting
OED	*Oxford English Dictionary*
OTC	over the counter
PDR	*Physician's Desk Reference*
PET	positron emission tomography
PNS	parasympathetic nervous system
PNV	pregnancy nausea and vomiting
PONV	postoperative nausea and vomiting
QALY	quality adjusted life year
QoL	quality of life
SNS	sympathetic nervous system
SPECT	single photon emission computed tomography
SQUID	superconducting quantum interference device
S-R	stimulus–response
SUMC	Stanford University Medical Center
UHC	University Hospital Consortium
V	vomiting
VIP	vasoactive intestinal polypeptide
VP/AVP	vasopressin

References

Aapro, M. (1993) Methodological issues in antiemetic studies. *Investigational New Drugs* **11**: 243–53.

Abeles, M. et al. (1998) Listening in on the brain. Research News: *Science* **280**: 376–7.

Abney, S.E. (1985) Nausea and vomiting during pregnancy. Unpublished manuscript.

Adachi, A. et al. (1991) Chemosensitive neurons in the area postrema of the rat and their possible functions. *Brain Research Bulletin* **26**: 137–40.

Ader, R. and Cohen, N. (1981) *Psychoneuroimmunology*. New York: Academic Press.

Ader, R. et al. (1991) *Psychoneuroimmunology*, 2nd edn, San Diego: Academic Press.

Aghababian, R. and Fleisher, G. (eds) (1992) *Emergency Medicine,* 2nd edn, Vols 1 and 2. Boston: Little, Brown.

Aikins Murphy, P. and Cruikshank, S.H. (1995) *Drug Treatment in Gynaecology*, 2nd edn. Oxford: Isis Medical Media.

Alba, E. et al. (1989) Anticipatory nausea and vomiting: prevalence and predictors in chemotherapy patients. *Oncology* **46**: 26–30.

Allman, J.M. (1999) *Evolving Brains*, New York: Scientific American Library.

American Nurses Association (1980) *Nursing: A Social Policy Statement.* Kansas City, MO: American Nurses Association.

American Psychiatric Association (1994) *Diagnostic and Statistical Manual of Mental Disorders,* 4th edn. Washington DC: American Psychiatric Association.

Ames, B.N. et al. (1987) Ranking possible carcinogenic hazards. *Science* **236**: 271–80.

Ames, B.N. et al. (1990) *Dietary Pesticides (99.9% All Natural).* Washington DC: National Academy of Science.

Amos, S.P. (1978) Personality differences between established and less established male and female creative artists. *Journal of Personality Assessment* **42**: 274–377.

Andrews, P.L. (1992) Physiology of nausea and vomiting. *British Journal of Anaesthesia* **69**: 2S–19S.

Andrews, P.L. and Hawthorne, P.L. (1988) The neurophysiology of vomiting. *Baillière's Clinical Gastroenterology* **2**: 141–68.

Andrews, P.L. and Sanger, G.J. (1993) *Emesis in Anti-Cancer Therapy: Mechanisms and Treatment.* London: Chapman and Hall.

Andrews, P.L. et al. (1990) The abdominal visceral innervation and the emetic reflex: pathways pharmacology and plasticity. *Canadian Journal of Physiology and Pharmacology* **68**: 325–45.

Andrykowski, M. (1990) The role of anxiety in the development of anticipatory nausea and cancer chemotherapy: a review and synthesis. *Psychosomatic Medicine* **52**: 458–75.

Andrykowski, M.A. and Redd, W.H. (1987) Longitudinal analysis of the development of anticipatory nausea. *Journal of Consulting and Clinical Psychology* **55**:36–41.

Andrykowski, M.A. et al. (1992) The role of psychological variability in post-chemotherapy nausea: anxiety and expectation. *Psychosomatic Medicine* **54**: 48–58.

Anholt, R.H. (1992) Molecular aspects of olfaction. In: *Science of Olfaction* (Serby, M. and Chobar, K.L., eds). New York: Springer-Verlag.

Anson, B. and Donaldson, J. (eds) (1973) *Surgical Anatomy of the Temporal Bone and Ear*, 2nd edn. Philadelphia: W.B. Saunders Co.

Antonovsky, A. (1980) *Health, Stress and Coping*. San Francisco: Jossey-Bass.

Arnheim, R. (1986) *Toward a Psychology of Art*. Berkeley, CA: University of California Press.

Arnheim, R. (1991) *Entropy and Art*. Berkeley, CA: University of California Press.

Arnheim, R. (1995) *New Essays on the Psychology of Art*. Berkeley, CA: University of California Press.

Baloh, R. and Honrubia, V. (eds) (1990) *Clinical Neurophysiology of the Vestibular System*, 2nd edn. Philadelphia: F.A. Davis Co.

Barber, N. and Raffield, T. (1994) The battle of the sexes and the evolution of social manipulativeness. Unpublished manuscript, cited in Sloan-Wilson et al. (1996).

Barbour, A. (1995). *Curing for Patients: A Critique of the Medical Model*. Stanford, CA: Stanford University Press.

Barnes, J.H. (1984) The physiology and pharmacology of emesis. *Molecular Aspects of Medicine* **7**: 309–18.

Barnes, N.M. et al. (1991) The actions of fentanyl to inhibit drug-induced emesis. *Neuropharmacology* **10**: 1073–83.

Barnes, D.M. and Kimura, S. (1988) Sex hormones linked to task performance. *Science* **242**: 1509.

Barnes, J.M. (1988) Reserpine, para-chlorophenylalanine and fenfluramine antagonist cisplatin-induced emesis in the ferret. *Neuropharmacology*: 783-90.

Barron, S.L. and Thomson, A.M. (1983). *Obstetrical Epidemiology*. London: Academic Press.

Barsky, A.J. (1979) Patients who amplify bodily sensations. *Annals of Internal Medicine* **91**: 63–9.

Baynes, K. and Caramazza, A. (1998) Writing, speech separated in split brain. *Science* **280**, 827.

Beck, T.M. et al. (1993) Efficacy of oral ondansetron in preventing emesis in outpatients receiving cyclophosphamide based chemotherapy. *Annals of Internal Medicine* **118**: 407–13.

Becker, K. (1990) *Principles and Practice of Endocrinology and Metabolism*. Philadelphia: Lippincott.

Beecher, H.K. (1955) The powerful placebo. *JAMA* **159**: 1602–6.
Behrman, C.A. (1990) Nausea and vomiting in teenage pregnancy; effects on birth weight. *Journal of Adolescent Health Care* **11**: 418–22.
Belluomini, J. (1994) Acupressure for nausea and vomiting of pregnancy; a randomized blind study. *Obstetrics and Gynecology* **84**: 245–8.
Benson, R.C. (1984) *Current Obstetrics and Gynecological Diagnosis and Treatment*. Los Altos, CA: Lange.
Bergeron, R. and Blier, P. (1994) Cisapride for the treatment of nausea produced by selective serotonin reuptake inhibitors. *American Journal of Psychiatry* **151**: 1084–6.
Berlin, I. (1980) *Against the Current: Essays in the History of Ideas*. New York: Viking.
Bertling, M.H. (1948) Some psychic aspects of dysmenorrhea and nausea and vomiting in pregnancy. *American Journal of Obstetrics and Gynecology* **56**: 723–37.
Bes, A. et al. (1981) Effects of a dopaminergic agonist (Piribedil) on CBF in migraine patients. *Journal of Cerebral Blood Flow Metabology* **1**: S549–50.
Biederman, G.B. and Davey, V.A. (1993) Antisickness conditioning using a nausea producing nondrug cue. *Behavioral Neuroscience* **107**: 315–17.
Bilgrami, S. and Fallon, B.G. (1993) Chemotherapy induced nausea and vomiting: easing patients' fear and discomfort with effective antiemetic regiments. *Postgraduate Medicine* **94**: 55–8, 62–4.
Blau, J.N. and Solomon, F. (1985) Smell and other sensory disturbances in migraine. *Journal of Neurology* **231**: 275–6.
Bleiberg, H. (1992) Antiemetic agents. *Current Opinions in Oncology* **4**: 597–604.
Bleiberg, H. (1994) Cost effectiveness analysis of antiemetic treatment. *Support Care Cancer* **2**: 145–9.
Bloom, H. (1998) *Shakespeare: The Invention of the Human*. New York, Penguin Putnam, Inc.
Blum, R.H. (1958) The prevention of patient dissatisfaction. Paper presented before ENT section of the American Medical Association, June 27.
Blum, R.H. (1960) *Management of the Doctor–Patient Relationship*. New York: McGraw-Hill.
Blum, R.H. (1988) A new basis for sensory-behavioral pretreatments to ameliorate radiation-therapy-induced nausea and vomiting?' *Cancer Treatment Reviews* **15**: 211–27.
Blum, R.H. and Blum, E. (1965) *Health and Healing in Rural Greece*. Palo Alto, CA: Stanford University Press.
Blum, R.H. and Blum, E. (1970) *The Dangerous Hour: A Socio-Psychological Study of the Lore of Crisis and Mystery in Rural Greece*. London: Chatto and Windus.
Blum, R.H. and Heinrichs, W.L. (1988) *Helping Women Keep Well*. New York: Irvington.
Blum, R.H. et al. (1972) *Horatio Alger's Children: Role of the Family in the Origin and Prevention of Drug Risk*. San Francisco: Jossey-Bass.
Blum, R.H. et al. (1981) *Pharmaceuticals and Health Policy: An International Perspective on Provision and Control of Medicines*. London: Croom Helm.
Boakes, R.A. et al. (1993) Prevalence of anticipatory nausea and other side-effects in cancer patients receiving chemotherapy. *European Journal of Cancer* **29A**: 866–70.
Bodis, S. et al. (1994) The prevention of radiosurgery induced nausea and vomiting by ondansetron. *Surgical Neurology* **42**: 249–51.

Bogardus, S.T. et al. (1995) Alimentary agony: allergy and the gut. *Perspectives in Biology and Medicine* **39**: 394–404.

Bogner, M.J. (ed.) (1994) *Human Error in Medicine*. Hillsdale, NJ: Erlbaum.

Bongard, F and Sue, D. (1994) *Current Critical Care, Diagnosis, and Treatment*. Norwalk, CT: Appleton Lange.

Bonneterre, J. et al. (1991) Tetracosactrin vs methylprednisolone in the prevention of emesis in patients receiving FEC regimen for breast cancer. *European Journal of Cancer* **27**: 849–52.

Boodman, S.G. (1995) Emergency contraception; 'morning after' pill has long been available. Health Section. *Washington Post*.

Borison, H.L. and Wang, S.C. (1953) Physiology and pharmacology of vomiting. *Pharmacological Reviews* **5**: 193–233.

Bovbjerg, D.H. et al. (1990) Anticipatory immune suppression and nausea in women receiving cyclic chemotherapy for ovarian cancer. *Journal of Consulting and Clinical Psychology* **58**: 153–7.

Boyse, E.A. et al. (1987) The genetics of body scent. *Trends in Genetics* **3**(4): 97–102.

Bradette, M., Pare, P., Douville, P. and Morin, A. (1991) Visceral perception in health and functional dyspepsia. Crossover study of gastric distention with placebo and domperidone. *Dip Dis Sci* **36**: 52–8.

Brandes, J.H. (1967) First trimester nausea and vomiting as related to outcome of pregnancy. *Obstetrics and Gynecology* **38**: 427–31.

Bruppacher, R. et al. (1988) Abdominal pain, indigestion, anorexia, nausea and vomiting. *Baillière's Clinical Gastroenterology* **2**: 275–92.

Brennan, P. et al. (1990) Olfactory recognition: a simple memory system. *Science* **250**: 1223–6.

Broberg, D.J. (1990) Nausea in bulimic women in response to a palatable food. *Journal of Abnormal Psychology* **99**: 183–8.

Brown, T.G. (1911) The intrinsic factors in the act of progression in the mammal *Proceedings of the Royal Society, London (Biology)* **84**: 308–19.

Brown, J.H.U. (ed.) (1963) *Physiology of Man in Space*. New York: Academic Press.

Bruce, H.M. (1960) A block to fertility in the mouse caused by proximity of strange males. *Journal of Reproductive Fertility* **1**: 96 107.

Bufton, K.E. (1993) Distribution and characterization of the ^{3}H granisetron-labelled 5HT$_3$ receptor in the human brain. *Neuropharmacology* **32**: 1325–30.

Burks, S.L. (1995) *Managing Your Migraine*. Totawan, NJ: Human Press.

Caccioppo, J.T. and Tassinary, L.G. (1990) *Principles of Psychophysiology: Physical, Social, and Inferential Elements*. Cambridge: Cambridge University Press.

Cairns, J. et al. (1988) The origins of mutants. *Nature* **335**: 142–5.

Calamandrei, M. (1994) Effects of ondansetron and metoclopramide on postoperative nausea and vomiting after epidural anesthesia in children. *Canadian Journal of Anesthesiology* **42**: 19–23.

Cameron, J.D. (1995) Hyperemesis. *Interactive Education* **1** (3), 1 November.

Camu, F. et al. (1992) Incidence and aetiology of postoperative nausea and vomiting. *European Journal of Anesthesiology* **9** (Suppl. 6): 25–31.

Carpenito, L.J. (1995) *Nursing Diagnosis Applications to Clinical Practice*, 6th edn Philadelphia: J.B. Lippincott, pp. 218–225, 1041.

Casper, R. et al. (1980) Bulimia; its incidence and clinical importance in patients with anorexia. *Archives of General Psychiatry* **37**: 1030–5.

Casper, R.C. et al. (1998) Placebo and 'nocebo' responses in depressed outpatients: gender differences? Am. College Neuropsychopharm. Croabus, P.R., Dec 1998.

Casti, J. L. and Karlquist, A. (1986) *Complexity, Language, and Life; Mathematical Approaches.* New York: Springer-Verlag.

Cenci, M.A. (1992) Dopaminergic transplants normalize amphetamine and apomorphine induced *fos* expression in the 6-hydroxydopamine lesioned striatum. *Neuroscience* **46**: 432–57.

Chalmers, I. and Richards, M.P. (1977) Intervention and causal inference in obstetrical practice. In: *Benefits and Hazards of the New Obstetrics* (Chard, T. and Richards, M., eds). London: Heinemann.

Chalmers, I. et al. (1989) Effective care in pregnancy and childbirth: taste sensitivity may be used to predict pharmacological effects. *Life Sciences* **7**: 533–7.

Chaput de Saintonge, D.M. and Herxheimer, A. (1994) Harnessing placebo effects in health care. *Lancet* **344**: 995–8.

Chase, S.L. (1993) GI remedies. *RN* 56(October): 30–3.

Christensen, S. et al. (1988) Postanesthetic vomiting in children undergoing strabismus surgery: a comparison of droperidol and lidocaine. *Anesthesia and Analgesia* **67**: S30.

Citron, M.L. (1993) Placebos and principles: a trial of ondansetron. *Annals of Internal Medicine* **118**: 470–1.

Clark, M.M. (1952) *Health in the Mexican American Culture.* Berkeley, CA: University of California Press.

Clark, R.A. and Gralla, R.J. (1993) Delayed emesis: a dilemma in antiemetic control. *Support Care Cancer* **4**: 182–5.

Clarke, D.J. et al. (1988) Psychogenic vomiting among female Asian immigrants to the United Kingdom. *International Journal of Social Psychiatry* **31**: 221–9.

Claybon, L. (1994) Single dose intravenous ondansetron for the 24-hour treatment of postoperative nausea and vomiting. *Anaesthesia* **219**. (Suppl.): 24–9.

Cobb, S.R. and McCrossan, M (1978) A study of foveal tripanopia. *Perceptual and Motor Skills* **46**: 1319–27.

Cochrane Library (database on CDROM and disk) 1997, issue 3. Oxford: Update Software. Updated quarterly. The Cochrane Library includes the Cochrane Database of Systematic Reviews (CDSR), a database of other assessed reviews assembled by the York Centre for Reviews and Dissemination, and the Cochrane Controlled Trials Register (CCTR).

Cohen, J. (1995) News and reports. *Science* **270**: 72.

Cohen, M.M. (1994) The postoperative interview: assessing risk factors for nausea and vomiting. *Anesthesia and Analgesia* **78**: 7–16.

Cohen, M.B. et al. (1994) Severe vomiting and diarrhea: initial measures. *Patient Care* **28**(15 Aug): 92–110.

Coleman, B. (1992) *Diseases of the Nose, Throat, and Ear, and Head and Neck.* New York: Churchill.

Cookson, R.F. (1986) Mechanisms and treatment of postoperative nausea and vomiting. In: *Nausea and Vomiting, Mechanisms and Treatment* (Davis, C.J et al., eds). New York: Springer-Verlag, pp. 120–58.

Cotanch, P.H. (1988) Management of nausea: current basis for practice. In: *Key Aspects of Comfort Management of Pain, Fatigue, and Nausea* (Kunk, S. et al. eds). New York: Springer-Verlag, pp. 243–8.

Creasy R.K. and Resnick, R. (1994) *Maternal Fetal Medicine.* Philadelphia: W.B. Saunders.

Cubeddu, L.X. (1992) Changes in serotonin metabolism in cancer patients: its relationship to nausea and vomiting induced by chemotherapeutic drugs. *British Journal of Cancer* **66**: 198–203.

Culbertson, F.M. (1997) Depression and gender, *American Psychologist* **52**: 25–31.

Cunningham, E.T., Jr et al. (1994) The relationship of efferent projections from the area postrema to vagal motor and brain stem catecholamine-containing cell groups: an axonal transport and immunohistochemical study in the rat. *Neuroscience* **58**: 635–48.

Cunningham, G.F. (1993) *Williams' Obstetrics*. Norwalk, CT: Appleton & Lange.

Dalton, T.C. (1996) The revival of consciousness: a review of Penrose's shadows of the mind. *Contemporary Psychology* 546–7.

Davidoff, R.A. (1995) *Migraine: Manifestations, Pathogenesis and Management*. Philadelphia: Davis.

Davidson, H.I. et al. (1993) Stimulation of gastrointestinal motility by cisplatin in the ferret: activation of an intrinsic cholinergic mechanism dissociated from emesis. *Naunyn Schmiedebergs Archiv für Pharmacologie*. 1993 May; **347**: 506–13.

Davis, C.J. et al. (1986) *Nausea and Vomiting: Mechanisms and Treatment*. Berlin: Springer-Verlag.

Davis, J.H. et al. (1991) *Essentials of Clinical Surgery*. St Louis, MO: Mosby Year Book.

Davis, R.C. (1957) Response patterns. *Transactions of the New York Academy of Science* **19**: 731–9.

Dawkins, R. (1989) *The Selfish Gene*. Oxford: Oxford University Press.

Dawkins, R.K. et al. (1982) *Animal Signals: Information or Manipulation*. Oxford: Oxford University Press.

Decherney, A.H. et al. (1994) *Current Obstetrics and Gynecologic Diagnosis and Treatment*. Norwalk, CT: Appleton and Lange.

Decherney, A.H. et al. (1971) Abortions and unrecognized trophoblastic disease. *New England Journal of Medicine* **285**: 407–8.

De Groot, L. et al. (1985) *Endocrinology*. Philadelphia: W.B. Saunders.

DeHart, R.L, ed. (1985) *Fundamentals of Aerospace Medicine*. Philadelphia: Lea and Febiger.

Del Favero, A. (1992) Nausea and vomiting due to cytarabine containing chemotherapy regiments: an epidemiological study. *Third International Symposium on Supportive Care in Cancer*.

Del Favero, A. (1993) Reducing chemotherapy induced nausea and vomiting: current perspectives and future possibilities. *Drug Safety* **9**: 410–28.

Del Favero, A. et al. (1992) Issues in the measurement of nausea. *British Journal of Cancer* **19** (Suppl.): S69–71.

Depew, D.J. and Weber, B.H. (1995) *Darwinism Evolving: Systems Dynamics and the Genealogy of Natural Selection*. Cambridge, MA: MIT Press.

Depue, R.H. et al. (1987) Hyperemesis gravidarum in relation to estradiol levels, pregnancy outcome, and other maternal factors: a seroepidemiologic study. *American Journal of Obstetrics and Gynecology* **156**: 1137–41.

Devine, E.C. (1992) Effects of psychoeducational care for adult surgical patients: a meta-analysis of 191 studies. *Patient Education and Counselling* **19**: 127–42.

Devine, E.C. and Westlake, S.K. (1995) The effects of psychoeducational care provided to adults with cancer: meta-analysis of 116 studies. *Oncology Nursing Forum* **22**: 1369–81.

Dexter, F. et al. (1995) Analysis of strategies to decrease postanesthesia care unit costs. *Anesthesiology* **82**: 94–101.

DiLorio, C. (1985) First trimester nausea in pregnant teenagers. incidence, characteristics, intervention. *Nursing Research* **34**: 427–31.

DiLorio, C. and van den Lier, D (1989) Nausea and vomiting in pregnancy. In: *Key Aspects of Comfort, Management of Pain, Fatigue, and Nausea.* (Funk, S.G., ed.). New York: Springer-Verlag, p. 259.

DiLorio, C. et al. (1994) Recommendations by clinicians for NV of pregnancy. *Clinical Nursing Research* **3**: 209–27.

Donlon, J.V. (1994) Anesthesia for ophthalmic surgery. In: *Principles and Practice of Ophthalmology*, Chapter 231. Philadelphia: W.B. Saunders, p. 2864.

Dorries, K.M. (1992) Sex differences in olfaction in mammals. In: *Science of Olfaction* (Serby, M. and Chobar, K.L., eds). New York: Springer-Verlag.

Dossey, B. et al. (1988) *Holistic Nursing: A Handbook for Practice.* MA: Aspen, pp. 42–3, 142–83.

Doty, R.L. and Muller-Schwarze, D. (1992) *Chemical Signals in Vertebrates.* New York: Plenum Press.

Doty, R.L. et al. (1981) Endocrine, cardiovascular, and psychological correlates of olfactory sensitivity changes during the human menstrual cycle. *Journal of Comparative and Physiological Psychology* **95**: 45–60.

Douglas, R.J. et al. (1995) Recurrent excitation in neocortical circuits. *Science* **269**: 981.

Dowling, J.E. (1987) *The Retina: An Approachable Part of the Brain.* Cambridge, MA: Belknap Press.

Downs, S. and Blum, R.H. (1993) *Southeast Asian Refugees: Cultural Issues and a New Syndrome.* San Francisco: American Psychiatric Association.

Drewnowski, A. et al. (1994) Eating pathology and DSM-III-R bulimia nervosa: a continuum of behavior. *American Journal of Psychiatry* **151**: 1217–19.

Dundee, J.W. (1990a) Belfast experience with P6 acupuncture emesis. *Ulster Medical Journal* **59**: 63–70.

Dundee, J.W. (1990b) Prolongation of the antiemetic action of P6 acupuncture by acupressure in patients having cancer chemotherapy. *Journal of the Royal Society of Medicine* **83**: 360–2.

Dundee, J.W. (1991a) Local anesthesia blocks the antiemetic action of P6 acupuncture. *Clinical Pharmacological Therapy* **50**: 78–80.

Dundee, J.W. (1991b) Non invasive stimulation of the P6 Neiguan antiemetic acupuncture point in cancer chemotherapy. *Journal of Social Medicine* **84**: 210–12.

Edwards, E.M. et al. (1989) Arginine vasopressin – a mediator of chemotherapy-induced emesis. *British Journal of Cancer* **59**: 467–70.

Egid, K. et al. (1989) The major histocompatibility: complex and female mating preferences in mice. *Animal Behavior* **38**: 548–50.

Elitzur, A.C. (1995) Life and mind, past and future: Schrodinger's vision fifty years later. *Perspectives in Biology and Medicine* **3**: 433–66.

Engel, G.L. (1977) The need for a new medical model: A challenge for biomedicine. *Science* **196**: 129–36.

Engen, T. (1982) *The Perception of Odours.* New York: Academic Press.

Engen, T. (1983) The human uses of olfaction. *American Journal of Otolaryngology* **4**: 250–1.

Erlichman, H. and Bastone, L. (1992) Olfaction and emotion. In: *Science of Olfaction* (Serby, M. and Chobar, K.L., eds). New York: Springer-Verlag, pp. 410–33.

Evans, A.T. et al. (1993) Suppression of pregnancy-induced nausea and vomiting with sensory afferent stimulation. *Journal of Reproductive Medicine* **38**: 603–6.

Eysenck, H. (1992) Introversion and sensitivity. In: *Fragrance: the Psychology and Biology of Perfume* (Van Toller, S. and Dodd, G.H., eds). New York: Elsevier.

Facione, N.C. et al. (1994) Critical thinking in disposition as a measure of competent clinical judgment: the development of the California Critical Thinking Disposition Inventory. *Journal of Nursing Education* **33**: 345–50.

Fainsinger, R. et al. (1991) Symptom control during the last week of life on a palliative care unit. *Journal of Palliative Care* **7**: 5–11.

Fairweather, D.V.I. (1968) Nausea and vomiting in pregnancy. *American Journal of Obstetrics and Gynecology* **102**: 102–25.

Fanciullacci, M. et al. (1980) Hyperresponsiveness of migraine patients to the hypotensive action of bromocriptine. *Headache* **20**: 99–102.

Feldman, M. and Schiller, L.R. (1983) Disorders of gastrointestinal motility associated with diabetes mellitus. *Annals of Internal Medicine* **98**: 378–84.

Feldman, M et al. (1988) Apomorphine-induced nausea in humans: release of vasopressin and pancreatic polypeptide. *Gastroenterology* **95**: 721–6.

Felig, B. et al. (1995) *Endocrinology and Metabolism*. New York: McGraw-Hill.

Ferstl, R. et al. (1992) MHC-related odors in humans. *Chemical Signals in Vertebrates*, Vol 4 (Muller-Schwarze D.A., ed.). New York: Plenum Press, pp. 205–11.

Findlay, M. (1993) Randomised cross over trial of antiemetic therapy for platinum based chemotherapy. *European Journal of Cancer* **29A**: 309–15.

Finlay, B. L. and Darlington, R. B.(1995) Linked regularities in the development and evolution of mammalian brains. *Science* **268**: 1578–84.

Fischer-Rasmussen, W. (1991) Ginger treatment of hyperemesis gravidarum. *European Journal of Obstetrics and Gynecology and Reproductive Biology* **4**: 19–24.

Fitzgerald, C.M. (1984) Nausea and vomiting in pregnancy. *British Journal of Medical Psychology* **57**: 159–65.

Fitzgerald, J.P. (1956) Epidemiology of hyperemesis gravidarum. *Lancet;* 660–2.

Flood, J.F. et al. (1987) Modulation of memory processing by cholecystokinin: dependence on the vagus nerve. *Science* **236**: 832–4.

Foster, D.W. (1992) Eating disorders: obesity and anorexia nervosa. In: *William's Textbook of Endocrinology*, 9th edn (Wilson, J. and Foster, D., eds). London: W.B. Saunders.

Franklin, H.R. (1994) Toxicity grading systems: a comparison between the WHO scoring system and the Common Toxicity Criteria when used for nausea and vomiting. *Annals of Oncology* **5**: 113–17.

Fredrikson, M. et al. (1996) Gender and age differences in the prevalence of specific fears and phobias. *Behavior Research and Therapy* **34**: 33–9.

Freedman, D.A. (1992) The search body, mind, and human purpose. *American Journal of Psychiatry* **149**: 858–66.

Fuchs, V.C. (1993) *The Future of Health Policy*. Cambridge, MA: Harvard University Press.

Fukai, J. et al. (1993) Involvement of 5-HTR$_3$ receptors and vagal afferents in copper sulphate and cisplatin induced emesis in monkeys. *European Journal of Pharmacology* **250**: 193.

Funk, S.G. (1989) *Key Aspects of Comfort: Management of Pain, Fatigue, and Nausea*. New York: Springer-Verlag.

Gaginella, T.S. (1995) *Regulatory Mechanisms in Gastrointestinal Function*. Boca Raton, FL: CRC Press.

Gaginella, T.S. and Galligan, J.J. (1995) *Serotonin and Gastrointestinal Function*. Boca Raton, FL: CRC Press.

Garcia, V. et al. (1974) Behavioural negation of the milieu interne in man. Food preferences set by delayed visceral effects facilitate memory research and predatory control. *Science* **85**: 824–31.

Garner, D. et al. (1993) Anorexia nervosa 'restrictors' who purge: implications for sub-typing anorexia nervosa. *International Journal of Eating Disorders* **13**: 171–85.

Geldof, H. et al. (1986) Electrogastrographic study of gastric myoelectrical activity in patients with unexplained nausea and vomiting. *Gut* **27**: 799–808.

Gelenberg, A. (1996) Biological therapies. *Psychiatric Newsletter* **19** (May).

Gerhart, D.J. (1991) Emesis, learned aversion and chemical defense in octocorals. *American Journal of Physiology* **260**: 839–943.

Gershon, M.D. (1995) Localization and neurochemical aspects of serotonin in the gut. Cited in Gaginella and Galligan (1995), pp. 11–32.

Ghaly, R.G. et al. (1987) Antiemetic studies with traditional Chinese acupuncture. A comparison of manual needling with electrical stimulation and commonly used antiemetics. *Anaesthesia* **42**: 1108–10.

Gibson, T.R. et al. (1986) Autoradiographic localisation and characterisation of atrial natriuretic peptide binding sites in the rat central nervous system and adrenal gland. *Journal of Neuroscience* **6**: 2004–11.

Gibson, J. (1950) *The Ecological Approach to Visual Perception*. Boston: Houghton-Mifflin.

Gilbert, A.N. et al. (1986) Olfactory discrimination of mouse strains (*Mus musculus*) and major histocompatibility types by humans (*Homo sapiens*). *Journal of Comparative Psychology* **100**: 262–5.

Gilman, A.G. et al. (eds) (1993) *Pharmacological Basis of Therapeutics*. New York: McGraw Hill.

Giorgi, D. et al. (1998) Distribution of olfactory receptor genes in the human genome. *Nature Genetics* **18**: 243–50.

Gleicher, N. (1992) *Principles and Practice of Medical Therapy in Pregnancy*. Norwalk, CT: Appleton and Lange.

Gleick, J. (1987) *Chaos: Making a New Science*. New York: Pantheon.

Godsey, R.K. and Newman, R.B. (1991) Hyperemesis gravidarum: A comparison of single and multiple admissions. *Journal of Reproductive Medicine* **36**: 287–90.

Gold, G. (1996) Research news. *Science* **274**: 500–1.

Goldberger, A.L. (1997) Fractal variability versus pathologic periodicity; complexity loss and stereotype in disease, *Perspectives in Biology and Medicine* **40**: 543–61.

Goldman, E. (1996a) Eating disorders plague many teens with IDDM. *Pediatric News* **3**: 30.

Goldman, E. (1996b) Eating disorders on the rise in preteens, adolescents. *Clinical Psychiatry News* (Feb.): 10.

Goode, R.L. (1981) The effect of aging on the ear. In: *Management of Common Problems in Geriatric Medicine* (Ebaugh, E.B. Jr, ed.). London: Addison Wesley Publications.

Goodwin, B. (1994) *How the Leopard Changed its Spots: The Evolution of Complexity*. New York: Scribner.

Goodwin, G. (1996) How do antidepressants affect serotonin receptors? The role of serotonin receptors in the therapeutic and side effect profile of the SSRIs. *Journal of Clinical Psychiatry* **57** (Suppl. 4): 9–13.

Goodwin, T.M. (1991) The role of chorionic gonadotropin in transient hyperthyroidism of hyperemesis gravidarum. *Transactions of the Society of American Physicians* **104**: 233–7.

Goodwin, T.M. et al. (1994) Increased concentration of the free beta-subunit of human chorionic gonatropin in hyperemesis gravidarum. *Acta Obstetrica et Gynecologica, Scandinavica* **73**: 770–2.

Goodwin, T.M. et al. (1997) Hyperthyroidism due to inappropriate production of human chorionic gonadotropin. Clinics in Obstetrics and Gynecology **40**: 32–44.

Gould, S.J. (1989) *Wonderful Life*. New York: W.W. Norton.

Gould, S.J. and Lewontin, R.C. (1979) *The Spandrels of San Marco and the Panglossian Paradigm*. New York: W.W. Norton.

Gran, L.B. et al. (1990) Nausea in cancer patients – an analysis of its frequency and an evaluation of its treatment in a Norwegian population. *Tidsskrift for den Norske Laegeforening (Oslo)* **110**: 63–5.

Graves, T. (1992) Emesis as a complication of cancer chemotherapy: pathophysiology, importance, and treatment. *Pharmacotherapy* **11**: 337–45.

Gray, R.H. and Doyle, P.E. (1983) The epidemiology of conception and fertility. In: *Obstetrical Epidemiology* (Barron, S.L. and Thomson, A.M., eds). London: Academic Press, pp. 25–54.

Greenfield, D. et al. (1993) Ipecac abuse in a sample of eating disordered outpatients. *International Journal of Eating Disorders* **13**: 411–14.

Greenspan, F.S. and Baxter, J.D. (1994) *Basic and Clinical Endocrinology*, 4th edn. Norwalk, CT: Appleton & Lange.

Greenspan, F.S. and Forsham, P.H. (1986) *Basic and Clinical Endocrinology*, 2nd edn. Los Altos: Lange.

Haaken, J. (1988) Field dependence research: a historical analysis of a psychological construct. *Signs* **13**: 311–30.

Hameroff, S. (1989) *Ultimate Computing: Biomolecular Consciousness and Nanotechnology*. Amsterdam: Elsevier.

Hammerstein, P. (1996) Darwinian adaption, population genetics and the streetcar theory of evolution. *J Math Biol* **34**: 511–32.

Hammerstein, P. (1996) Theoretical biology (on game theory and multiple gene trait control). *Science* **271**: 1365–6.

Hare, J.W. (1986) *Signs and Symptoms in Endocrine and Metabolic Disorders*. Philadelphia: Lippincott.

Harlan, R.T. et al. (1983) Midbrain microinfusion of prolactin increases the estrogen dependent behaviour. *Science* **218**: 1451–3.

Harris, A.I. and Cantwell, B.M.S. (1986) Mechanisms and treatment of cytotoxic-induced nausea and vomiting. In: *Nausea and Vomiting, Mechanisms and Treatment* (Davis, C.J. et al. eds). New York: Springer-Verlag, pp. 78–109.

Hartl, D.L. (1988) *A Primer of Population Genetics*, 2nd edn. Sunderland, MA: Sinauer Associates, Inc.

Hawkins, D.F. and Stern, L. (1991) *Drug Treatment in Obstetrics*, 2nd edn. New York: Chapman & Hall.

Hawthorne, J. (1995) *Understanding and Management of Nausea and Vomiting*. Oxford: Blackwell Science.

Helveston, E.M. (1993) *Surgical Management of Strabismus*. St Louis, MO: Mosby Yearbook.

Hen, R. (1993) *Science* (November).

Henderson, K.H. (1917) *The Order of Nature*. Cambridge, MA: Harvard University Press.

Henkin, R.I. (1974) Sensory changes during menstrual cycle. In: *Biorhythms and Human Reproduction* (Ferin, M. et al., eds). New York: Wiley.

Herrstedt, J. (1994) Treatment of drug induced nausea and vomiting. *Ugeskr Laeger* **24**(156): 453–60.

Hershman, J.M. (1980) *Management of Endocrine Disorders*. Philadelphia: Lea & Febiger.

Herxheimer, A. et al. (1994) Harnessing placebo effects in health care. *Lancet* **344**: 995–8.

Hickish, G. (1985) *Ear, Nose and Throat Disorders*. New York: Churchill.

Hickok, J.T. and Morrow, G.R. (1993) A biobehavioral model of patient reported nausea: implications for clinical practice. *Advanced Medical Psychotherapy* **6**: 227–30.

Hikasa, Y. (1992) Alpha adrenoceptor subtypes involved in the emetic action in dogs. *Journal of Pharmacological and Experimental Therapy* **261**: 746–54.

Hilgetag, C.C. et al. (1996) Indeterminate organization of the visual system. *Science* **271**: 776–7.

Hinkle, L.E. and Wolff, H.G. (1957a) Health and the social environment: experimental investigations. In: *Explorations in Social Psychiatry*, New York: Basic Books, pp. 104–37.

Hinkle, L.E. and Wolff, H.G. (1957b) The nature of man's adaptation to the total environment and the relation of this to illness. *Archives of Internal Medicine* **99**: 442–60.

Hirsch, J. (1994) Impact of postoperative nausea and vomiting in the surgical setting. *Anaesthesia* **49** (Suppl.): 30–33.

Ho, R.T. (1990) Electro acupuncture and postoperative emesis. *Anaesthesia* **45**: 327–9.

Hokavaara, P. (1991) Nausea and vomiting after gynecological laparoscopy depends upon the phase of the menstrual cycle. *Canadian Journal of Anesthesiology* **38**: 876–9.

Hollingsworth, C. (1996) Physical and proximate irritation of the vagus nerve from different anesthetics in the thoracic cavity as a possible source of postoperative nausea and vomiting. Schema presented to faculty of OB/GYN research course 399, Stanford University, April 1996.

Hollis, K.L. (1997) Contemporary research on Pavlovian conditioning: a 'new' functional analysis *American Psychologist* **52**: 956–65.

Hopp, S.L . (1998) *Walsh and Hoyt's Clinical Neuroophthalmology*, Vol. 3, Chapter 56. Baltimore, MD: Williams & Wilkins,.

Hoskins, H.D. and Kass, M. (1989) *Becker-Shaffer's Diagnosis and Therapy of the Glaucomas*. St Louis, MO: Mosby Yearbook.

Hoyenaga, K.B. and Wallace, B (1979) Sex differences in the perception of autokinetic movement of an afterimage. *Journal of General Psychology* **100**: 93–101.

Humphries, L.L. et al. (1992) Ipecac misuse in clinical and non-clinical samples. *International Journal of Eating Disorders* **11**: 361–7.

Hursti, T.J. et al. (1993) Endogenous cortisol exerts antiemetic effect similar to that of exogenous corticosteroids. *British Journal of Cancer* **68**: 112–14.

Iadarola, J.M. and Caudle, R.M. (1997) Good pain, bad pain. *Science* **278**: 239–40.

Italian Group for Antiemetic Research (1994) On the relationship between nausea and vomiting in patients undergoing chemotherapy. *Support Care Cancer* **2**: 161–6.

Jarnfelt-Samsioe, A. (1985a) Gallbladder disease and related use of oral contraceptives and nausea in pregnancy. *Southern Medicine* **78**: 1040–3.

Jarnfelt-Samsioe, A. (1985b) Some new aspects on emesis gravidarum. *Gynecology and Obstetrics Investigation* **19**: 174–86.

Jarnfelt-Samsioe, A. (1986) Steroid hormones in emetic and non-emetic pregnancy. *European Journal of Obstetrics, Gynecology and Reproductive Biology* **21**: 87–99.

Jarnfelt-Samsioe, A. (1987) Nausea and vomiting in pregnancy: a review. *Obstetrical and Gynecological Surgery* **41**: 422–7.

Jenkins, M.L. and Shelton, B.J. (1989) The effectiveness of self care actions in reducing 'morning sickness'. In: *Key Aspects of Comfort Management of Pain Fatigue and Nausea* (Funk, S. et al. eds). New York: Springer-Verlag, pp. 267–75.

Jewell, D. and Young, G. (1996) Treatments for nausea and vomiting in early pregnancy. In: *Pregnancy and Childbirth* (Neilson J.P. et al. eds). Module of the Cochrane Database of Systematic Reviews [updated 5 December 1996]. Available in The Cochrane Library.

John, E.R. (1980) Multipotentiality: a statistical theory of brain function – evidence and implications. In: *The Psychobiology of Consciousness* (Davidson, B.H and Davidson, R.J., eds). New York: Plenum Press, pp. 129–96.

Johnson, A.K. and Anderson E.K. (1990) Stress and arousal. In: *Principles of Psychophysiology: Physical, Social, and Inferential Elements* (Caccioppo, J.T. and Tassinary, L.G., eds). Cambridge: Cambridge University Press, pp. 216–62.

Jordan, V. et al. (1998) Hyperemesis gravidarum in European and Samoan women is associated with increase in acidic hCG isoforms. Abstracts of the Endocrine Society, June, P1-137, p. 190.

Joss, R. et al. (1981) Nausea und Erbrechen bei der Chemotherapie maligner Tumoren. *Schweizerische Medizinische Wochenschrift* **III**: 1614–22.

Jovanovic, M. (1989) Area postrema and emesis. *Metabolism and Brain Disease* **4**: 55 60.

Joyce, C.R.B. and Weldon, R.M.C. (1965) The objective efficacy of prayer; a double-blind clinical trial. *Journal of Chronic Diseases* **18**: 367–77.

Joyce, C.R.B. et al. (1968) Taste sensitivity may be used to predict pharmacological effects. *Life Sciences* **7**:533–7.

Joyce, C.R.B. et al. (1970) Relationships between taste threshold for drugs and clinical progress in a varied group of psychiatric patients. *British Journal of Psychiatry* **117**: 653–9.

Kaba, H. et al. (1988) Hormonal enhancement of neurogenesis and its relationship to the duration of olfactory memory. *Neuroscience* **24**: 93–8.

Kaiser, L. (1992) A survey of the costs of chemotherapy induced nausea and vomiting at 5 Canadian cancer centers. *Proceedings of the Annual Meeting of the American Society for Clinical Oncology* **11**: A1381.

K'all, E.B. (1987) Hyperemesis during pregnancy and delivery outcome: a registry study. *European Journal of Obstetrics and Gynaecology* **26**: 291–302.

Kandel, E.R. et al. (1991) *Principles of Neural Science*. East Norwalk, CT: Appleton & Lange.

Kanigel, R. (1983) Magic medicine, the placebo. *Johns Hopkins Magazine* **13**: 18–32.

Kaplan, R. (1994) The Ziggy Theorem: toward an outcome focused health psychology. *Health Psychology* **13**: 451–60.

Kapur, S. and Remington, G. (1996) Serotonin–dopamine interaction and its relevance to schizophrenia. *American Journal of Psychiatry* April: 153–4.

Kaufmann, M.A. (1994) Prophylactic antiemetic therapy with patient controlled analgesia. *Anesthesiology and Analgesia* **78**: 988–94.

Kauffman, S.A. (1992) *Origins of Order: Self-Organization and Selection in Evolution.* Oxford: Oxford University Press.

Kauffman, S.A. (1995) *At Home in the Universe: The Search for the Laws of Self Organization and Complexity*. Oxford: Oxford University Press.

Kelly, D.D. (1991) Sexual differentiation of the nervous system. *Principles of Neural Science*: 960–73.

Kelso, J.A. (1995) *Dynamic Patterns: The Self Organization of Brain and Behavior.* Cambridge, MA: MIT Press.

Keverne, E.B. and Rosser, A.E. (1986) The evolutionary significance of the olfactory to pregnancy. In: *Chemical Signals in Vertebrates*, Vol 4. (D. Muller-Schwarze, D. and Silverstein D.M., eds) New York: Plenum Press, pp. 433–9.

Khojasteh, A. (1993) Transdermal scopolamine patch (TSP) for prevention of chemotherapy induced delayed emesis. *Proceedings of the Annual Meeting of the American Society for Clinical Oncology* **12**: A1576.

King, J.R. (1988) Scientific status of aromatherapy. *Perspectives in Biology and Medicine* **37**: 409–15.

King, J.R. (1988) Influence of neostigmine on postoperative vomiting. *British Journal of Anaesthesiology* **61**: 403–6.

Kish, L. (1994) Letters. *Science* July 25 (**265**).

Klebanoff, M.A. et al. (1985) Epidemiology of vomiting in early pregnancy. *Obstetrics and Gynecology* **66**: 612–16.

Kleinfeld, D. and Chiel, V. (1990) Cited in Research news on individual motor pattern activity as network self organization. *Science* **250**: 206–7.

Klopfer, F.J. (1978) *More Than Meets the Eye: Spatial Visualization and Sex Differences.* RIE.

Knox, A.P. (1993) Behavioral studies of emetic sensitivity in the ferret. *Brain Research Bulletin* **31**: 477–84.

Koch, K.L. (1990) Gastric dysrhythmias and nausea of pregnancy. *Digestive Disease and Science* **35**: 961–8.

Koga, T. and Fukuda, H. (1990) Characteristic behavior of the respiratory muscles, esophagus, and external anal and urethral sphincters during straining, retching, and vomiting in the decerebrate dog. *Japan Journal of Physiology* **40**: 789–807.

Kosslyn, S.M. and Koenig, O. (1992) *Wet Mind. The New Cognitive Neuroscience.* New York: Free Press.

Krasnow, S.H. (1989) Problems in antiemetic trial design and interpretation. *Oncology* **3**: 5–10.

Kris, M.G. (1997) Use of an NK1 receptor antagonist to prevent delayed emesis after cisplatin. *Journal of the National Cancer Institute* **89**: 817–8.

Kucharczyk, J. et al. (1991) *Nausea and Vomiting: Recent Research and Clinical Advances.* Boca Raton, FL: CRC Press.

Kunz-Kostokomanolakis, M et al. (1987) Hypokalemia as the principal symptom of recurrent vomiting. *Deutsche Medizinische Wochenschrift.*

Kupferman, I. (1991a) Genetic determinants of behavior. In: *Principles of Neuroscience*, 3rd edn. (Kandel, E.R. et al., eds). East Norwalk, CT: Appleton & Lange, pp. 996–7.

Kupferman, I. (1991b) Hypothalamus and limbic system. Peptidergic neurons, homeostasis, and behaviour. In: Kandel, E.R., et al., *Principles of Neuroscience*, 3rd edn. East Norwalk, CT: Appleton & Lange, pp. 735–60.

Kvale, G. and Hugdahl, K. (1994) Cardiovascular conditioning and anticipatory nausea and vomiting in cancer patients. *Behavioural Medicine* **20**: 78–83.

Kvale, G. et al. (1991) Anticipatory nausea and vomiting in cancer patients. *Journal of Consulting and Clinical Psychology* **59**: 894–8.

Lambas-Schas, L. et al. (1985) Distribution of dopamine, noradrenaline and adrenaline in coronal sections of the rat lower brainstem. *Brain Research* **347**: 306–12.

Lancet Editorial (1992) **339**: 279.

Langham, W.H. (ed.) (1967) *Radiobiological Factors in Space Flight*. Washington, DC: National Academy of Science.

Laupacis, A. et al. (1992) How attractive does a new technology have to be to warrant adoption and utilization? Tentative guidelines for using clinical and economic evaluations. *Canadian Medical Association Journal* **146**: 473–81.

Lawes, I.N. (1990) The origin of the vomiting response: a neuroanatomical hypothesis. *Canadian Journal of Physiology Pharmacology* **68**: 254–9.

Le Magnen, J. (1986) *Hunger*. Cambridge: Cambridge University Press.

Leahey, T.H. (1994) Is this a dagger I see before me? Four theorists in search of consciousness. *Contemporary Psychology* **39**: 575–81.

Leakey, R. and Lewin, R. (1995) *The Sixth Extinction: Heroes of Human Life and the Future of Mankind*. New York: Doubleday.

Leathem, A.M. (1986) Safety and efficacy of antiemetics used to treat nausea and vomiting in pregnancy. *Clinical Pharmacology* **5**: 660–768.

Ledward, R.S. et al. (1995) *Drug Treatment in Gynaecology*. Oxford: Isis Medical Media.

Ledward, R.S. et al. (1991) *Drug Treatment in Obstetrics*. New York: Chapman & Hall.

Lee et al. (1989) *Textbook of Otolaryngology and Head and Neck Surgery*. New York: Elsevier.

Lee, B. et al. (1993) *Wintrobe's Clinical Hematology*. Philadelphia: Lea & Febiger.

Lehner, J.P. (1993) Gender differences in long term odor recognition memory: verbal vs sensory influence and the consistency of label use. *Chemical Senses* **18**: 17–26.

Lenski, R. (1994) Genetic mistakes. *Research News* **265**: 3183–90.

Lerman, C. (1990) Effects of coping style and relaxation on cancer chemotherapy: side effects and emotional responses. *Cancer Nursing* **13**: 308–15.

Leslie, R.A. et al. (1990) Evidence for presynaptic 5-hydroxytryptamine$_3$ recognition sites on vagal afferent terminals in the brainstem of the ferret. *Neuroscience* **38**: 667.

Letters (1992) Ondansetron and chest pain. *Lancet* **340**: 1107, 1410.

Liebenberg, B. (1969) Expectant fathers. *Child and Family* **8**: 269–70.

Lindblad, T. (1989) Increased incidence of postoperative nausea and vomiting in menstruating women. *Canadian Journal of Anesthesia* **36**: 78–9.

Lindley, C.M. (1992) Quality of life: consequences of chemotherapy induced emesis. *Quality of Life Research* **1**: 331–40.

Lindley, M. (1989) Incidence and duration of chemotherapy induced nausea and vomiting in the outpatient oncology population. *Journal of Clinical Oncology* **7**: 1142–9.

Link, B. and Phelan, J.C. (1996) Understanding sociodemographic differences in health. *American Journal of Public Health* **86**: 471–2.

Litovitz, T. et al. (1994) Toxic exposure surveillance system. *Annual Report of the American Journal of Emergency Medicine* **12**: 494–555.

Llimas, R.R. (1988) The intrinsic electrophysiological properties of mammalian neurones: insights into central nervous system function. *Science* **242**: 1654–69.

Logothetis, J. et al. (1959) The role of estrogens in catamenial exacerbation of epilepsy. *Neurology* **9**: 351.

Lomas, J. (1993) Diffusion, dissemination and implementation: who should do what? In: *Doing More Good than Harm: The Evaluation of Health Care Interventions* (Warren, K.S. and Mosteller, F., eds), pp. 226–337. New York: New York Academy of Sciences.

Lord, T. K. and Kasprzak, M (1989) Identification of self through olfaction. *Perceptual and Motor Skills* **69**: 219-4.

Lundberg, U. and Frankhauser, M. (1980) Pituitary-adrenal and sympathetic adrenal correlates of distress and efforts. *Journal of Psychosomatic Research* **21**: 125–30.

Lydiard, B. et al. (1994) Panic disorder and gastrointestinal symptoms: findings from the NIMH Epidemiological Catchment Area Project. *American Journal of Psychiatry* **151**: 64–70.

Lyles, J.N. et al. (1982) Efficacy of relaxation training and guided imagery in reducing the aversiveness of cancer chemotherapy. *Journal of Consulting and Clinical Psychology* **50**: 509–24.

McArdle, W.D. et al. (eds) (1991) *Exercise Physiology*. Philadelphia: Lea & Febiger.

McGrath, J.E. (ed.) (1970) Setting measures and themes. An integrative review of some research on social–psychological factors in stress. In: *Social and Psychological Factors in Stress*. New York: Rinehart & Winston.

McKeique, P.M. et al. (1994) Bendectin and birth defects. *Teratology* **50**: 27–37.

MacLean, P.D. (1949) Psychosomatic disease and the 'visceral' brain. Recent development bearing on the Papez theory of emotion. *Psychosomatic Medicine* **11**: 338–53.

McLean, J.H. and Shipley, M.T. (1992) Neuroanatomical substrates of olfaction. In: *The Science of Olfaction* (Serby, M.J. and Chobar, K., eds). New York: Springer-Verlag, pp. 126–71.

Magee, L.A. and Redman, C.W. (1996) An N-of-1 trial for treatment of hyperemesis gravidarum. *British Journal of Obstetrics and Gynaecolology* **103**: 478–80.

Maiworm, R.E. and Langthaler, W.U. (1992) Influence of androstenol and androsterone on the evaluation of men of varying attractiveness levels. In: *Chemical Signals in Vertebrates*. New York: Plenum Press, pp. 575–9.

Makale, M.T. and King, G.L. (1992) Surgical and pharmacological dissociation of cardiovascular and emetic responses to intragastric $CuSO_4$. *American Journal of Physiology* **263**: 284–91.

Martin, M. (1992) Myths and realities of anti emetic treatment. *British Journal of Cancer* **660** (Suppl. 19): 46–51.

Martin, R.J. (1991) The regulation of body weight. *American Scientist* **79**: 528–41.

Martindale (1993) *The Extra Pharmacopoeia* 30th edn (Reynolds J.E.F., ed). London: Pharmaceutical Press.

Marty, M. et al. (1993) Antiemetic effect of ondansetron in recurrent chemotherapy with cisplatin. *Bulletin of Cancer* **80**: 618–23.

Marx, J.L. (1987) Polyphosphoinositide research updated. *Science* **235**: 974–6.

Masoni, S. et al. (1994) The couvade syndrome. *Journal of Psychosomatic Obstetrics and Gynecology* **15**: 125–31.

Matsuki, N., et al., (1993) Emetic responses of Sorex unguiculatus. *Jikken Dobutsu* **42**: 225–8.
Matthews, R. (1997) Drug trial results thrown into doubt. *The Sunday Telegraph*, 28 September, p. 19.
Mauger, T.F. and Craig, E.L. (1994) *Havener's Ocular Pharmacology*. St Louis, MO: Mosby Yearbook.
Mead, M. (1935) *Sex and Temperament in Three Primitive Societies*. New York: William Morrow.
Meehl, P.E. (1960) *Clinical US Statistical Prediction*. Minneapolis: University of Minnesota Press.
Mellaart, J. (1967) *Catal Hüyük: a Neolithic Town in Anatolia*. London: Thames and Hudson.
Menashian, L. et al. (1992) Improved food intake and reduced nausea and vomiting in patients given a restricted diet while receiving cisplatin chemotherapy. *Journal of the American Dietetic Association* **92**: 58–61.
Mellion, M. (ed.) (1996) *Office Sports Medicine*. St Louis, MO: Mosby Yearbook.
Melzack, R. and Wall, P.D. (eds) (1994) *Textbook of Pain*, 3rd edn. New York: Churchill Livingstone.
Michaloudis, D. et al., (1993) Postoperative nausea and vomiting: a comparison of anti-emetic drugs used alone or in combination. *Journal of the Royal Society of Medicine* **86**: 137–8.
Milano, S. (1991) In vitro release and tissue levels of ileal serotonin after cisplatin induced emesis in the cat. *Clinical Autonomic Research* **1**: 275–80.
Milheiro, A. et al. (1995) Acute pancreatitis: an analysis of 91 consecutive cases (1988–1991). *Acta Medica Portuguesa* **8**: 269–77.
Miller, A.D. (1994) Plasticity of emesis to a $5HT_3$ agonist: effect of order of visceral nerve cuts. *NeuroReports* **14**: 986–8.
Miller, A.D. and Nonaka, S. (1992) Mechanisms of vomiting induced by serotonin 3 receptor agonists in the cat: effect of vagotomy, splanchnicectomy, or area postrema lesion. *Journal of Pharmacology and Experimental Therapeutics* **260**: 509–17.
Miller, A.D. and Leslie, R.A. (1994) The area postrema and vomiting front. *Neuroendocrinology* **15**: 301–2.
Miller, A.D. and Ruggiero, D.A. (1994) Emetic reflex arc revealed by expression of the immediate-early gene c-*fos* in the cat. *Journal of Neuroscience* **14**: 871–8.
Miller, A.D. et al. (1990) Human cortical activity during vestibular and drug induced nausea detected using MSI. *New Directions in Vestibular Research* **781**: 670–2.
Miller, A.D. et al. (1994) Brain areas essential or non essential for emesis. *Brain Research* **647**: 255–64.
Miller, A.D. et al. (1996) Modulation of vomiting by the medullary midline. *Brain Research* **737**: 51–8.
Miller, N.E. (1995) Clinical experimental interactions in the development of neuroscience. *American Journal of Psychology* **50**: 901–11.
Miller, N.R. (1998) *Walsh and Hoyt's Clinical Neuroophthalmology*, Vol. 1, Chapter 10. Baltimore, MD: Williams & Wilkins.
Minabe, Y. (1991) The $5HT_3$ receptor antagonists LY 277359 and granisetron potentiate the suppressant action of apomorphinogen on the basal firing rate of ventral tegmental dopamine cells. *European Journal of Pharmacology* **209**: 143–50.

Miner, W.D. and Sayer, G.J. (1986) Inhibition of cisplatin-induced vomiting by selective 5-hydroxytryptamine M-receptor antagonism. *British Journal of Pharmacology* **88**: 374.

Minturn, L. et al. (1984) The influence of diet on morning sickness: a cross cultural study. *Medical Anthropology* **8**: 71–5.

Mitchell, J.E. et al. (1993) A review of the controlled trials of pharmacotherapy and psychotherapy in the treatment of bulimia nervosa. *International Journal of Eating Disorders* **14**: 229–47.

Mitchelson, F. (1992) Pharmacological agents affecting emesis: a review (Part I). *Drugs* **43**: 295–315.

Moncrieff, R.W. (1944) *The Chemical Senses*. New York: Wiley.

Money, K.F. (1970) Motion sickness. *Physiology Reviews* **50**:1–39.

Montgomery, S.A. (1993) Venlafaxine: a new dimension in antidepressant pharmacotherapy. *Journal of Clinical Psychiatry* **54**: 119–26.

Morrow, G.R. and Morrell, C. (1982) Behavioural treatment for the anticipatory nausea and vomiting induced by cancer chemotherapy. *New England Journal of Medicine* **307**: 1476–80.

Morse, C.A. and Van Hall, E.U. (1987) Psychosocial aspects of infertility: a review of current concepts. *Journal of Psychosomatics* **6**:156–64.

Mulrow, C.D. (1987) The medical review article: state of the science. *Annals of Internal Medicine* **106**: 485–8.

Murakawa, M. (1994) Activation of the cortical and medullary dopaminergic systems by nitrous oxide in rats: a possible neurochemical basis for psychotropic effects and postanesthetic nausea and vomiting. *Anesthesia and Analgesia* **78**: 376–81.

Nasser, M. (1993) A prescription of vomiting: historical footnotes. *International Journal of Eating Disorders* **13**: 129–31.

Naylor, C.D. (1996a) Users' guide to the medical literature. XI. How to use an article about a clinical utilization review. *JAMA* **275**: 1435–9.

Naylor, C.D. (1996b) Users' guide to the medical literature. X. How to use an article reporting variations in the outcomes of health services. *JAMA* **275**: 554–8.

Nerenz, D. R. et al. (1986) Anxiety and drug taste as predictors of anticipatory nausea in cancer chemotherapy. *Journal of Clinical Oncology* **42**: 224–33.

Nicogossian, A.E. et al. (eds) (1994) *Space Physiology and Medicine*. Philadelphia: Lea & Febiger.

Nussey, L.L. et al. (1988) The responses of plasma oxytocin and arginine vasopressin to nausea induced by apomorphine and ipecacuanha. *Clinical Endocrinology (Oxford)* **28**: 297–304.

O'Brien, B. et al. (1993) Impact of chemotherapy-associated nausea and vomiting on patients' functional status and costs: survey of five Canadian centres. *Canadian Medical Association Journal* **149**: 296–302.

O'Kelly, C. (1980) Sex-role imagery in modern art: an empirical examination. *Sex Roles* **6**.

Oliver, I.N. (1992) Antiemetic study design: desirable objectives, stratification and analyses. *British Journal of Cancer* **195** (Suppl.): 30–33.

Oliver, I.N. et al. (1994) The roles of patient and observer assessments in anti-emetic trials. *European Journal of Cancer* **30A**: 1223–7.

Orem, D.E. (1985) *Nursing Concepts of Practice*, 3rd edn. New York: McGraw-Hill.

Ornstein, R. (1993) *The Evolution of Consciousness.* New York: Simon & Schuster.

Oster, M.W. (1991) *American Journal of Diseases of Children* **145**: 773–8.

Pater, J. (1994) Inconsistency of prognostic factors for post chemotherapy nausea and vomiting. *Support Care Cancer* **2**:161–6.

Pennebaker, J.W. (1982) *The Psychology of Physical Symptoms.* New York: Springer-Verlag.

Pennebaker, J.W. (1984) Accuracy of symptom perception. In *Social Psychological Aspects of Health. Handbook of Health Psychology*, Vol. IV (Taylor, S.E. and Singer, J.E., eds). Hillsdale, NJ: Erlbaum, pp. 189–217.

Penrose, R. (1994) *Shadows of the Mind: A Search for the Missing Science of Consciousness.* Oxford: Oxford University Press.

Perez, E.A. (1995) Review of the preclinical pharmacology and comparative efficacy of 5-hydroxytryptamine receptor antagonists for chemotherapy-induced emesis. *Journal of Clinical Oncology* **13**: 1036–43.

Peroutka, S.J. (1995) *(Esfa) Spectra Allelic Profile Analysis.* Menlo Park , CA.

Porter, R.H. and Moore, J.D. (1981) Human kin recognition by olfactory cues. *Physiology and Behavior* **27**: 493–5.

Potts, W.K. et al. (1993) Evolution of MHC genetic diversity: a tale of incest, pestilence and sexual preference. *Trends in Genetics* **9**: 408–12.

Powledge, T.M. and Rose, M. (1996) The great DNA hunt. *Archaeology* Sept/Oct: 36–44.

Preskorn, S.H. et al. (1992) Advances in the pharmacotherapy of depressive disorders. *Principles and Practice of Psychopharmacotherapy* (1) (Spring).

Price, A et al. (1996) Asian women are at risk of gestational thyrotoxicosis. *Journal of Clinical and Endocrinological Metabolism* **81**: 1160–3.

Profet, M. (1991) The function of allergy: Immunological defense against toxins. *Quarterly Review of Biology* **66**(1): 23–62.

Profet, M. (1992) Pregnancy sickness as adaptation: a deterrent to maternal ingestion of teratogens. In *The Adapted Mind* (Barkow C.T., ed.) Oxford: Oxford University Press, pp. 327–57.

Profet, M. (1995) Your news. *Science* **270**: 1299–300.

Rain, B. and Hunt, W. (1992) Relationship between vomiting and taste aversion learning in the ferret; studies with ionizing radiation, lithium chloride and amphetamine. *Behavioral and Neural Biology* **58**: 83–93.

Rao, N. (1992) Sex differences in the disposition of substituted benzamides; pharmacokinetics of a gastroprokinetic agent. *Biopharm Drug Dispos* **13**: 68–91.

Raybould, H.E., Grundy, D. and Andrews P.L. (1995) Serotonin and the afferent innervation of the gastrointestinal tract. In *Serotonin and Gastrointestinal Function.* Boca Raton, FL: CRC Press.

Redd, W.H. et al. (1982) Hypnotic control of anticipatory emesis in patients receiving cancer chemotherapy. *Journal of Consulting and Clinical Psychology* **50**: 14–19.

Redd, H. et al. (1989) Behavioural side effects of adjuvant chemotherapy. *Recent Results in Cancer Research* **115**: 272–8.

Redd, W.H. et al. (1993) Nausea induced by mental images of chemotherapy. *Cancer* **72**: 629–36.

Reed, S.D. et al. (1990) Interoception. In: *Principles of Psychophysiology: Physical, Social, and Inferential Elements* (Caccioppo, J.T. and Tassinary, L.G., eds). Cambridge: Cambridge University Press, pp. 253–94.

Regan, P.C. (1996). Book review of *Sex is not a Natural Act*, by Treter, L. *Contemporary Psychology* **41**: 9.
Regan, E.C. and Price, K.R. (1994) The frequency of occurrence and severity of side effects of immersion virtual reality. *Aviation Space and Environmental Medicine* **65**: 527–30.
Renaud, L.P. et al. (1984) Characterization of noradrenergic afferents to hypothalamic magnocellular neurons. In: *Endocrinology* (Labrie, T. and Proulx, L., eds). New York: Excerpta Medica.
Rhodes, V. (1990a) Predictors of antineoplastic chemotherapy nausea and vomiting. *Oncology Nurses Forum* **17**: 177.
Rhodes, V. (1990b) Nausea, vomiting and retching. *Nursing Clinics of North America* **24**: 885–90.
Rice, W.R. (1966) Flies unmask evolutionary warfare between the sexes. *Science* **272**: 953–4.
Roarty, T.P. and McCallum, R.W. (1995) The clinical application of 5-HT agonists and antagonists in gastrointestinal disease. In *Serotonin and Gastrointestinal Function.* Boca Raton, FL: CRC Press.
Roberts, A.H. (1995) The powerful placebo revisited. *Mind/Body Medicine* **1**: 26–43.
Roberts, K.A. et al. (1995) Autoradiographic identification of brain angiotensin IV binding sites and differential *c-fos* expression following intracerebroventricular injection of angiotensin II and IV in rats. *Brain Research* **682**: 13–21.
Robertson, G.L. (1989) Regulation of vasopressin secretion. *Baillière's Clinical Endocrinology* **3**: 513–30.
Robins, L.N. and Regies, (eds) (1991) *Psychiatric Disorders in America.* New York: Free Press.
Roila, F. et al. and the Italian Group for Antiemetic Research (1995) Dexamethasone, granisetron, or both for the prevention of nausea and vomiting during chemotherapy for cancer. *New England Journal of Medicine* **332**: 1–5.
Rosenwaks, Z. et al. (1987) *Gynecology: Principles and Practice.* New York: Macmillan.
Roser, B. et al. (1991) Excretion of transplantation antigens as signals of genetic individuality. In *Chemical Senses: Genetics of Perception and Communication* (Kare W., ed.) New York: Dekker **86**: 41–5.
Rubenstein, E.E. (1994) Pharmacoeconomic analyses: whose perspective counts and costs the most? *American Journal of Hospital Pharmacology* **51**: 1564–9.
Rudd, J.A. and Nayiro, R.J. (1992) Pharmacology of ondansetron. *European Journal of Anesthesiology* **6**: 3–10.
Russell, D. (1996) Green light for steroid hormones. *Science* **272**: 370–1.
Sackett, D.L. et al. (1991) *Clinical Epidemiology.* Boston: Little, Brown.
Salthe, S.N. (1993) *Development and Evolution: Complexity and Change in Biology.* Cambridge, MA: MIT Press.
Sancilio, L.F., Pinkus, L.M., Jackson, C.B. and Munson, H.R. Jr (1991) Studies on the emetic and antiemetic properties of zacopride and its enantiomers. *European Journal of Pharmacology* **192**: 365–9.
Sandler, M. (1990) *Migraine: A Spectrum of Ideas.* Oxford: Oxford University Press.
Sapolsky, R. and Balt, S. (1996) Reductionism and variability in data, a meta-analysis. *Perspectives in Biology and Medicine* **39**: 193–203.
Sartre, J.P. (1964) *Nausea.* New York: New Directions.
Sawin, C.T. (1969) *The Hormones: Endocrine Physiology* Boston: Little, Brown & Co.
Scarantino, C.W. (1992) Radiation induced emesis; effects of ondansetron. *Seminars in Oncology* **19**: S38–43.

Schaoxiang, L. et al. (1991) Magnetic disk applied on Neiguan point for prevention of cisplatin-induced nausea and vomiting. *Journal of Traditional Chinese Medicine* **4**: 181–3.

Schiller, L.R. and Feldman, M. (1990) Gastrointestinal complications of diabetes. In: *Principles and Practice of Endocrinology and Metabolism* (Becker, K., ed.). Philadelphia: Lippincott, p. 1146.

Schleidt, V. (1992) *The Semiotic Relevance of Human Olfaction: A Biological Approach.*

Schorr-Lesnick, B. et al. (1991) Liver diseases unique to pregnancy. *American Journal of Gastroenterology* **86**: 659–70.

Schrier, R.W. and Goldberg, T.P. (1980) The physiology of vasopressin release and the pathogenesis of impaired water excretion in adrenal, thyroid and edematous disorders. *Yale Journal of Biological Medicine* **53**: 525–41.

Schulz, K.F. et al. (1994) Assessing the quality of randomization from reports of controlled trials published in obstetrics and gynecological journals. *JAMA* **272**: 125–8.

Schwartz, C. et al. (1992) *Principles and Practice of Emergency Medicine.* Philadelphia: W.B. Saunders.

Science (1998) How the genome readies itself for evolution. *Science* **281**: 1131–4.

Scott, J. et al. (1994) *Danforth's Obstetrics and Gynecology.* Philadelphia: Lippincott.

Seely, T.D. (1989) The honey bee colony as superorganism. *American Scientist* **77**: 546–54.

Segal, N.L. et al. (1995) Twin analysis of odor identification and perception. *Physiology and Behavior* **57**: 605–9.

Selby, G. and Lance, J.W. (1960) Observations on 500 cases of migraine and allied vascular headaches. *Journal of Neurology, Neurosurgery and Psychiatry* **23**: 23–32.

Serby, M.J. and Chobar, K. (1992) *The Science of Olfaction.* New York: Springer-Verlag.

Ship, J.A. et al. (1993) Age, gender, medical treatment, and medication effects on smell identification. *Journal of Gerontology* **48**: M26–32.

Shivers, B.D. et al. (1989) A subset of neurons containing immunoreactive prolactin is a target for estrogen regulation of gene expression in rat hypothalamus. *Neuroendocrinology* **49**: 23–7.

Silberstein, S.D. (1995) Migraine symptoms: results of a survey of self-reported migraineurs. *Headache* **35**: 387–96.

Silver, N.C. and Ferrante, R. (1995) Sex differences in colour preferences among an elderly sample. *Perceptual and Motor Skills* **80**: 920–2.

Silverman, W.A. (1995) Effectiveness, efficiency, and subjective choice. *Perspectives in Biology and Medicine* **38**: 480.

Sivilotti, L. and Colquhoun, D. (1995) Acetylcholine receptors: too many channels, too few functions. *Science* **269**: 1681–2.

Sloan-Wilson, D. et al. (1996) Machiavellianism: A synthesis of the evolutionary and psychological literatures. *Psychology Bulletin* **109**: 285–99.

Soules, M.R. (1980) NV of pregnancy: a role of human chorionic gonadotropin and 17-hydroxyprogesterone. *Obstetrics and Gynecology* **55**: 696.

Soussignan, R. (1996) Children's facial responsiveness to odors: influences of hedonic valence of odor, gender, age and social presence. *Developmental Psychology* **32**: 367–79.

Speroff, L. (1975) An autoregulatory role for prostaglandins in placental hemodynamics: their possible influence on blood pressure in pregnancy. *Journal of Reproductive Medicine* **15**: 81.

Sperry, R.W. (1993) The impact and promise of the cognitive revolution. *American Psychology* **48**: 878–85.

Spierings, E.L. (1995) *Migraine: Questions and Answers.* Coral Springs, FL: Merit Publishing.

Stannard, D. (1989) Pressure prevents nausea. *Nursing Times* **85**: 33–4.

Starr, P. (1982) *The Social Transformation of American Medicine.* New York: Basic Books.

Steadman, C.J. (1992) Selective 5 hydroxytryptamine type 3 receptor antagonism with ondansetron as treatment for diarrhea predominant irritable bowel syndrome. *Mayo Clinical Procedures* **67**: 732–8.

Steadman, C.J., Talley, N.J., Phillips, S.F. and Zinsmeister, A.R. (1992) Selective 5-hydroxytryptamine type 3 receptor antagonism with ondansetron as treatment for diarrhea-predominant irritable bowel syndrome: a pilot study. *Mayo Clinical Procedures* **67**: 732–8.

Stefanek, M.C. et al. (1988) Anticipatory nausea and vomiting: does it remain a significant clinical problem? *Cancer* **62**: 1654.

Stehling, M.K. (1991) Echo-planar imaging : MRI in a fraction of a second. *Science* **254**: 43–50.

Stein, B.E. and Meredith, M.A. (1993a) *The Merging of the Senses.* Cambridge: MIT Press.

Stein, B.E. and Meredith, M.A. (1993b) Converging influences from visual, auditory and somatosensory cortices onto output neuron of the superior colliculus. *Journal of Neurophysiology* **69**: 1797–809.

Sternbach H. (1991) The serotonin syndrome. *American Journal of Psychiatry* **148**: 705–13.

Stevens, R.F. (1991) The role of ondansetron in paediatric patients: a review of three studies. *European Journal of Cancer*, **27** (Suppl. 1): S20–2.

Stewart, W.F. et al. (1992) Prevalence of migraine headache in the U.S.: relation to age, income, race and other sociodemographic factors. *JAMA* **276**: 64–9.

Stoddart, D.M. (1990) *The Scented Ape.* Cambridge: Cambridge University Press.

Stott, J.R.R. (1986) Mechanism and treatment of motor illness. In: *Nausea and Vomiting Mechanisms and Treatment* (Davis, E.J. et al., eds). New York: Springer-Verlag, pp. 110–29.

Strauss, E. (1998) Writing, speech separated in split brain. *Science Research News* **280**: 827.

Strohman, R. C. (1993) Ancient genomes, wise bodies, unhealthy people: limits of a genetic paradigm in biology and medicine. *Perspectives in Biology and Medicine* **37**: 112–45.

Strominger, N.L. et al. (1994) The connectivity of the area postrema in the ferret. *Brain Research Bulletin* **33**: 33–47.

Sundeen, S. J. et al. (1994) *Nurse–Client Interaction*, 5th edn. St Louis, MO: Mosby Yearbook, pp. 2–7.

Tareen, A.K. et al. (1995) Thyroid hormone in hypermesis gravidarum. Journal of Obstetrics and Gynaecology **21**: 497–501.

Tarkkila, P. and Isola, J. (1992) A regression model for identifying patients at high risk of hypotension, bradycardia and nausea during spinal anesthesia. *Acta Anaesthesiologica Scandinavica* **36**: 554–8.

Tedeschi, D.N. and Tedeschi, R.E. (1968) *Importance of Fundamental Principles in Drug Education.* New York: Raven Press.

Thom, R. (1988) Organs and tools: a common theory of morphogenesis. In

Complexity, Language and Life: Mathematical Approaches (Casti, D.K., ed.). New York: Springer-Verlag.

Thomas, J.H. (1994) The mind of a worm. *Science* **264**: 1698–9.

Tierson, F.D. et al. (1986) Nausea and vomiting of pregnancy and association with pregnancy outcome. *American Journal of Obstetrics and Gynecology* **155**: 1017–22.

Tigerstedt, I. (1988) Double blind comparisons of transdermal scopolamine, droperidol, and placebo against postoperative nausea and vomiting. *Acta Anaesthesiologica Scandinavica* **32**: 454–7.

Tobin, D.L. et al. (1990) Divergent forms of purging behavior in bulimia nervosa patients. *International Journal of Eating Disorders* **11**: 17–24.

Todes, D.P. (1997) From the machine to the ghost within: Pavlov's transition from digestive physiology to conditional reflexes. *American Psychologist* **52**: 947–55.

Tonato, M. (1994) Antiemetics in cancer chemotherapy: historical perspective and current state of the art. *Support Care Cancer* **2**:150–60.

Tramèr, M. et al. (1995) Prevention of vomiting after paediatric strabismus surgery: a systematic review using the numbers-needed-to-treat method. *British Journal of Anaesthesia* **75**: 556–61.

Tramèr, M. et al. (1996) Omitting nitrous oxide in general anaesthesia: meta-analysis of intraoperative awareness and postoperative emesis in randomized controlled trials. *British Journal of Anaesthesia* **76**: 186–93.

Tramèr, M. et al. (1997a) Propofol anaesthesia and postoperative nausea and vomiting: quantitative systematic review of randomized controlled studies. *British Journal of Anaesthesia* **78**: 247–55.

Tramèr, M. et al. (1997b) Meta-analytic comparison of prophylactic antiemetic efficacy for postoperative nausea and vomiting: propofol anaesthesia vs omitting nitrous oxide vs total i.v. anaesthesia with propofol. *British Journal of Anaesthesia* **78**: 256–9.

Tramèr, M. et al. (1997c) Impact of duplicate publication on meta-analysis: a case study. *British Journal of Medicine* **315**: 635–40.

Trethowan, W.H. and Colon, M.F. (1965) The couvade syndrome. *British Journal of Psychiatry* **3**: 937–50.

Triesman, M. (1977) Relationship between taste threshold for drugs and clinical progress in a mixed group of psychiatric patients. *British Journal of Psychiatry* **117**: 653–9.

Triggs, W.J. et al. (1992) Neuropsychiatric manifestations of defect in mitochondrial beta oxidation response to riboflavin. *Journal of Neurology, Neurosurgery, and Psychiatry* **55**: 209–11.

Troesch, L.M. (1993) The influence of guided imagery on chemotherapy related nausea and vomiting. *Oncology Nursing Forum* **20**: 1179–85.

Tucker, M.E. (1996) Psychotherapy for bulimia gets boost. *Psychiatric News* (July).

Tucker, M.E. (1995) Eating disorders put young diabetics at risk of medical complications. *Clinical Psychiatry News* (April): 13.

Turner, J.A. et al. (1994) The importance of placebo effects in pain treatment and research. *JAMA* **271**: 1609–14.

Tyers, M.B. (1992) Pharmacology and preclinical antiemetic properties of ondansetron F. *Seminars in Oncology* **10**(suppl): 1–8.

Ummenhofer, W. et al. (1994) Effects of ondansetron in the prevention of postoperative nausea and vomiting in children. *Anesthesiology* **81**: 804–10.

Ungerleider, L.G. (1994) Functional brain imaging studies of cortical mechanisms for memory. *Science* **270**: 769–74.

Uttal, W.R. (1996) Do theoretical bridges exist between perceptual experience and neurophysiology? *Perspectives in Biology and Medicine* **40**: 280–301.

Vabin, J.R. (1992) Ipecac abuse – danger. *Journal of American College Health* **40**: 237–8.

van Hoff, J. et al. (1991) A survey of antiemetic use in children with cancer. *American Journal of Diseases of Children* **145**: 773–8.

van Lier, D. (1993) Nausea and fatigue during early pregnancy. *Birth* **20**: 193–7.

Van Toller, S. and Dodd, G.H. (1988) *Perfumery: the Psychology and Biology of Fragrance.* London: Chapman & Hall.

Van Toller, S. and Dodd, G.H. (1992) *Fragrance: the Psychology and Biology of Perfume.* New York: Elsevier.

Vasterling, J. et al. (1992) Cognitive distraction and relaxation training for the control of side effects due to cancer chemotherapy. *Journal of Behavioural Medicine* **16**(1): 65–80.

Vellacott, I.D. (1988) Nausea and vomiting in early pregnancy. *International Journal of Gynaecology and Obstetrics* **1**: 57–62.

Velle-Weiert, W. (1987) Sex differences in sensory functions. *Perspectives in Biology and Medicine* **30**: 490–522.

Verbalis, V.G. et al. (1974) Vasopressin release in response to nausea-producing agents and cholecystokinin in monkeys. *American Journal of Physiology* **252**: 749–53.

Verbalis, J.G., Richardson, D.W. and Stricker, E.M. (1987) Vassopressin release in response to nausea-producing agents and cholecystokinin in monkeys. *American Journal of Physiology* **252**: R749–53.

Vermeulen, L.C. et al. (1994) Evaluation of ondansetron prescribing in U.S. academic medical centers. *Archives of Internal Medicine* **154**: 1733–40.

Vesterhauge, S. et al. (eds) (1995) *Ménière's Disease.* 16th Danavox Symposium. Scanaticon Kolding, DK.

Vickers, A.J. (1996) Can acupuncture have specific effects on health? A systematic review of acupuncture antiemesis trials. *Journal of the Royal Society of Medicine* **89**: 303–11.

Voda, A.M. and Randall, M.P. (1982) Nausea and vomiting of pregnancy: 'morning sickness'. In: *Concept Clarification in Nursing* (Norris, C.M., ed.). Rockville, MD: Aspen Systems Corporation.

Vutyavanich, T. et al. (1995) Pyridoxine for NV of pregnancy: a randomized, double-blind, placebo-controlled trial. *American Journal of Obstetrics and Gynecology* **173**: 881–4.

Walder, A.D. et al. (1994) Antiemetic efficacy of metoclopramide when included in a patient-controlled analgesia infusion. *Anaesthesia* **49**: 804–6.

Walker, A.R.P et al. (1985) Nausea and vomiting and dietary cravings and aversions during pregnancy in South African women. *British Journal of Obstetrics and Gynaecology* **92**: 484–9.

Warner, L.O. et al. (1988) Intravenous lidocaine reduces the incidence of vomiting in children after surgery to correct strabismus. *Anesthesiology* **68**: 618–22.

Warren, K.S. and Mosteller, F. (eds) (1993) *Doing More Good than Harm: The Evaluation of Health Care Interventions.* New York: New York Academy of Sciences.

Wasserstein, A.G. (1996) Death and the internal milieu: Claude Bernard and the origins of experimental medicine. *Perspectives in Biology and Medicine* **39**: 313–26.

Watson, W.J. and Seeds, J.W. (1990) Acute fatty liver of pregnancy. *Obstetrics and Gynecology* **45**: 585–91.

Weatherall, D.J. et al. (1996) *Oxford Textbook of Medicine.* New York: Oxford University Press.

Wedekind, C. et al. (1995) MHC-dependent mate preferences in humans. *Proceedings of the Royal Society*. London B Biol Sci **260**: 245–9.

Weigel, M.M. and Weigel, R.M. (1988) The association of report history, demographic factors and alcohol and tobacco consumption with the risk of developing nausea and vomiting in early pregnancy. *American Journal of Epidemiology* **127**: 562–70.

Wilkinson, A. R. (1989) Preoperative transdermal hyoscine for the prevention of postoperative nausea and vomiting. *Anesthesiology Intensive Care* **17**: 285-289.

Wheeler, B.L. (1985) Relationship of personal characteristics to mood and enjoyment after hearing live and recorded music and to musical taste. *Psychology of Music* **13**(2): 81–92.

Wheeler, J.A. (1986) Herman Weyl and the unity of knowledge. *American Scientist* **7**: 366–75.

Whitacre, C.C. et al. (1999) A gender gap in autoimmunity *Science* **283**: 1277–8.

Whitehead, S.A. et al. (1992) Characterization of NV in early pregnancy: a survey of 1000 women. *Journal of Obstetrics and Gynecology* **12**: 364–9.

Williams, N. (1997) Biologists cut reductionist approach down to size. *Science* **277**: 476–7.

Wilson, D.S. et al. (1996) Machiavellianism: a synthesis of the evolutionary and psychological literatures. *Psychology Bulletin* **119**: 285–99.

Witlin, A.G. and Sibai, B.M. (1998) Magnesium sulphate therapy in preeclampsia and eclampsia. *Obstetrics and Gynecology* **92**: 883–9.

Wolf, S. (1959) Placebos. Association for Research in Nervous and Mental Disease 1959; U37: 147–61.

Wolf, S. (1985) The stomach's link to the brain. *Federation Proceedings* **44**: 2889–93.

Wood, W.W. (1994) Dose and dose intensity of adjuvant chemotherapy for stage II, node positive breast carcinoma. *New England Journal of Medicine* **330**: 1253–9.

World Federation of Neurology (1969) Research Group on Migraine and Headache. *Hemicrania* **1**: 3–4.

Wruble, L.D. et al. (1982) Psychogenic vomiting: a review. *American Journal of Gastroenterology* **77**: 318–21.

Yamazaki, K. et al. (1983) Recognition of H-2 types in relation to the blocking of pregnancy in mice. *Science* **221**: 186 8.

Yamazaki, K. et al. (1988) Familial imprinting determines H-2 selective mating preferences. *Science* **240**: 1331–2.

Yamazaki, K. et al. (1990) Odor types determined by the major histocompatibility antigens and susceptibility to disease. *Annual Review of Microbiology* **33**: 201–13.

Yerushalmy, J. and Milkovich, L. (1992) Pregnancy sickness as adaptation. In: *The Adapted Mind* (Barko, J. et al., eds). Oxford: Oxford University Press.

Yesavage, J. (1992) *Clozapine: A Compendium of Selected Readings.* Sandoz Pharmaceutical Corporation, USA.

Yoshimura, M. et al. (1995) Thyrotropic action of human chorionic gonadotropin. *Thyroid* **5**: 425–34.

Yousfi-Malki, P. (1994) Induction of Fos-like protein in neurons of the medulla oblongata after stimulation of the vagus nerve in anesthetized rabbit. *Brain Research* **635**: 317–22.

Zavazava, N. et al. (1990) Characterization of soluble HLA molecules in sweat and quantitative HLA differences in serum of healthy individuals. *Journal of Immunogenetics* **17**: 387–94.

Zbrowski, M. (1952) Cultural components on response to pain. *Journal of Social Issues* **8**: 16–30.

Zbrozek, A.S. et al. (1994) Pharmoeconomic analysis of ondansetron vs. metoclopramide for cisplatin-induced nausea and vomiting. *American Journal of Hospital Pharmacy* **51**: 1555–63.

Zibell-Frisk, D. (1990) Use of parental nutrition to maintain adequate nutritional status in hyperemesis gravidarum. *Journal of Perinatology* **10**: 390–5.

Zola, I. (1973) Pathways to the doctor from person to patient. *Social Science and Medicine* **7**: 677–89.

Zuker, C. and Ranganathan, R. (1999) The path to specificity *Science* **283**: 650–1.

Further reading

Abel T.L. (1987) Gastric electromechanical and neurohormonal function in anorexia nervosa. *Gastroenterology* **93**: 958–65.

Abel, T.L. (1992) Nausea and vomiting of pregnancy and the electrogastrogram: old disease, new technology. *American Journal of Gastroenterology* **87**: 689–91.

Adams, R. and Victor, M. (1993) *Principles of Neurology*. New York: McGraw-Hill.

Adams, S.L. (1990) Alcoholic ketoacidosis. *Emergency Medical Clinics of North America* **8**: 749–58.

Agnati, L.F. et al. (1992) Volume transmission in the brain. *American Scientist* **80**: 362–73.

Aguglia, E. et al. (1993) Double-blind Study of the Efficacy and Safety of Sertraline versus Fluoxetine in Major Depression. *International Clinical Psychopharmacology* **8**: 197–202.

Ahles, T.K. and Hegel, M.T. (1992) Behavioral analysis and treatment of reflexive vomiting associated with visceral sensations. *Journal of Behavioral Therapy* **23**: 237–42.

Ahn, M.J. (1994) A randomized double-blind trial of ondansetron alone versus in combination with dexamethasone versus in combination with dexamethasone an lorzepain in the prevention of emesis one to cisplatin-based chemotherapy. American Journal of Clinical Oncology **17**: 150–6.

Alexander, I.E. and Rushton, L.P. (1993) *Contemporary Psychology* (38): 968–72.

Altmaier, E.M. et al. (1982) A Pilot Investigation of the Psychologic Functioning of Patients with Anticipatory Vomiting. *Cancer* **49**: 201–4.

Alvarez, M.M. et al. (1988) Gender Differences in Visual Attention to Television Form and Content. *Journal of Applied Developmental Psychology* **9**: 459–75.

Alvarez-Gonzales, P. (1962) *Yerbas Medicinales*. Mexico DF: El Libro Español.

Amico, J.A. (1993) Oxytocin and vasopressin secretion in monkeys administered apomorphine and a D2 receptor agonist. *Life Science* **52**: 1301–09.

Anand, A. (1994) Nausea induced by mental images of chemotherapy. *Cancer* **73**: 755–6.

Andrykowski, M. A. et al. (1985) Development of Anticipatory Nausea: A Prospective Analysis. *Journal of Consulting Clinical Psychology* **53**: 447–454.

Annanth, C.V. and Rao, P.S.S. (1993) Epidemiology of nausea and vomiting of pregnancy and its relation to fetal outcome in a rural area. *Journal of Tropical Pediatrics* **39**: 313.

Arrington, D.B. (1987) A Jungian-based Study of Selected Visual Constructs Preferred by Women. *Dissertation Abstracts International* **48**(5B): 1541

Avery, M.E. and First, L.R. (eds.) (1989) Pediatric Medicine. Baltimore, MD: Williams and Wilkins, pp. 408–703.

Babyak, M.N. (1992) Anger and Fear as Human Experience. *Contemporary Psychology* **37**: 407.

Bachevalier, J. et al. (1989) Gender Differences in Visual Habit Formation in 3-month-old Rhesus Monkeys. *Developmental Psychobiology* **22**: 585–99.

Backon, J. (1991) Ginger as an antiemetic; possible side effects due to its thromboxane synthetase activity. *Anaesthesia* **46**: 705–06.

Bailey P.L. (1990) Transdermal scopolamine reduces nausea and vomiting after outpatient laproscopy. *Anesthesiology* **72**: 977–80.

Bailey, J.E. et al. (1995) The 5–HT_3 Antagonist Ondansetron Reduces Gastrointestinal Side Effects Induced by a Specific Serotonin Reuptake Inhibitor in Man. *Journal of Psychopharmacology* **19**: 137–41.

Bains, J.S. et al. (1992) Angiotensin II actions in paraventricular nucleus: functional evidence for neurotransmitter role in efferents originating in subfornical organ. *Brain Research* **599** (2)(Dec. 25): 223–9.

Bakowski, M.T. (1984) Advances in Anti-emetic Therapy. *Cancer Treatment Reviews* **11**: 237–56.

Bakwin, H. (1971) Carsickness in twins. *Developmental Medicine and Child Neurology* **13**: 310.

Baldwin, D.S. et al. (1996) A multicenter double-blind comparison of nefazodone and paroxetine in the treatment of outpatients with moderate-to-severe depression. *Journal of Clinical Psychiatry* **75** (Suppl. 2): 46–52.

Ballard, H.S. (1992) Ondansetron and Chest Pain. *Lancet* **340**: 1107.

Ballatori, E. (1994) Cost efficacy analysis of two antiemetic treatments: the Italian experience from hospital perspective. *Proceedings of the Annual Meeting of the American Society for Clinical Oncology* **13**: A615.

Baltzer, L. (1993) High dose ondansetron plus dexamethasone for the prevention of nausea and vomiting with multiple day cisplatin chemotherapy. *Proceedings of the Annual Meeting of the American Society for Clinical Oncology* **12**: A1607.

Baltzer, L. (1994) The addition of ondansetron to the combination of metoclopramide, dexamethazone and lorazepram did not improve vomiting prevention in patients receiving high dose cisplatin. *Cancer* **73**: 720–23.

Bannister, R. (1992) Brain and Bannister's Clinical Neurology. New York: Oxford University Press.

Barbero, G.D. et al (1993) Pyloric stenosis. In: *Current Pediatric Therapy*, Vol 8 (Kagan, G., ed.): Philadelphia: W.B. Sanders, pp. 203–04.

Barinaga, M. (1990) The Mind Revealed? *Science* **249**: 856–58.

Barinaga, M. (1990) Technical Advances Power Neuroscience. *Science*: 908–09.

Barinaga, M. (1990) Research News. *Science* **248**: 1603–605.

Barinaga, M. (1991) Research News. *Science*, 1296–297.

Barinaga, M. (1992) How Scary Things Get That Way. *Science* **258**: 887–88.

Barinaga, M. (1994) Watching the Brain Remake Itself. *Science* **266**: 1475–476.

Barinaga M. (1997) New imagery methods provide better view into the brain. *Science* **276**: 1974–976.

Barkin and Rosen. (1992) Emergency Medicine: Concepts and Clinical Practice, Vols 1, 2 and 3, 3rd edn. St. Louis, MO: Mosby Yearbook.

Barnes, D.M and Kimura, S (1988) Sex Hormones Linked to Task Performance. *Science* **242**: 1509.

Barnes, J.M. (1988) Reserpine, para-chlorophenylalanine and fenfluramine antagonist cisplatin-induced emesis in the ferret. *Neuropharmacology* **27**: 783–90.

Barnes, K.L. et al. (1984) Participation of the Area Postrema in Cardiovascular Control in the Dog. Federation Proceedings **43**: 2959.

Bartholomew, U. and Klapp, B.F. (1992) Inpatient psychotherapy of hyperemesis gravidarum: a case report. *Z Geburtshilfe Perinatol* (May–June) 196: 134–9.

Baylis, J.M. et al. (1983) Persistent Nausea and Food Aversions in Pregnancy. Oxford: Blackwell Scientific Publications.

Beattle, W.S. (1991) The incidence of postoperative nausea and vomiting in women undergoing laproscopy is influenced by day of menstrual cycle. *Canadian Journal of Anesthesiology* **38**: 298–302.

Beauchamp. G. et al. (1985) The Chemosensory Recognition of Genetic Individuality. *Scientific American* **253**: 86–92.

Beaumont, J.S. et al. (1992). Anesthesia and Perioperative Complications. St Louis, MO: Mosby Yearbook.

Beccaro, M.A. (1991) Severe gastric distension in 7 patients with cerebral palsy. *Developmental Medicine Child Neurology* **33**: 912–16.

Beckman, C. B. et al. (1995). Obstetrics and Gynecology for Medical Students. Baltimore, MD: Williams & Wilkins.

Beer, A.E. et al. (1985) Pregnancy Outcome in Human Couples With Recurrent Spontaneous Abortions. *Experimental Clinical Immunogenetics* **2**: 137–53.

Begley, S. (1995) Gray matters. *Newsweek* (March 27): 48–54.

Beleslin, D.B. (1989) Area postrema: cholinergic and noradrenergic regulation of emesis. *Arch. Int. Physiology Biochimie* **9**: 107–15.

Beleslin, D.B. (1991) Selective effect of ethanol on norepinephrine and nicotine induced emesis in cats. *Alcohol* **8**: 499–501.

Beleslin, D.B. (1992) Differential inhibition of ethanol of norepinephrine and clonidine induced emesis in cats. *Alcohol* **9**: 389–93.

Bergin, P.S. and Harvey P. (1992) Wenicke's encephalopathy and central pontine myelinosis associated with hyperemesis gravidarum. *British Medical Journal* **305**: 517–518.

Bernstein, L. (1986) Higher pregnancy levels of estradiol and sex hormone binding globulin in hyperemetic women: a case control study. *American Journal of Epidemiology* **124**: 409.

Bhandari, P. (1992) The neuropharmacology of loperamide induced emesis in the ferret; the role of the area postrema, vagus, opiate and $5HT_3$ receptors. *Neuropharmacology* **31**: 735–42.

Bhandari, P. and Andrews, P.L. (1993) Resinferatoxin, an ultrapotent capsaicin analogue, has antiemetic properties in the ferret. *Neuropharmacology* **32**: 799–886.

Bittetti, J. and Weintraub, H. (1992) Nausea and vomiting. In: Anesthesia and Perioperative Complications (Beaumont, J. and Saichman, L., eds). New York: Mosby Yearbook, pp. 396–412.

Boericke and Tafel (1988) The Family Guide to Self Medication: Homeopathic, Alexandria, V.A., *National Center for Homeopathy*.

Bohen, S.P. (1995) Hold em and fold em: chaperones and signal transduction. *Science* **268**: 1303–04.

Bondarenko, M.Y. et al. (1994) Sexual Dimorphism in Formation and Extinction of Aversion Developed to Familiar and Unfamiliar Taste. *Fiziologicheskii Zhurnal SSSR* **80**(5): 75–83.

Bone, M.E. (1990) Ginger root - a new antiemetic: the effect of ginger root on post-operative nausea and vomiting after major gynecological surgery. *Anaesthesia* **45**: 669–71.

Borod, J.C. et al. (1988) The Effects of Emotion and Ocular Dominance on Lateral Eye Movement. *Neuropsychologia* **26**: 213–20.

Bossert, S. et al. (1991) Visual Palatability of Food in Patients with Eating Disorders and Dieting Women. *Behaviour Research and Therapy* **29**: 337–41.

Bountra, C. (1993) Anti emetic profile of a non peptide neurokinin NKI receptor antagonist CP 999 994 in ferrets. *European Journal of Pharmacology* **249**: 74–6.

Bourne, G.H., (Ed.) (1963) Medical and Biological Problems of Space Flight. New York: Academic Press.

Boyce, R.A. (1992) Enteral nutrition in hyperemesis gravidarum: a new development. *Journal of the American Diet Association* **92**: 733-6.

Bradette, M. (1991) Visceral perception in health and function dyspepsia. Crossover study of gastric distension with placebo and domperidone. *Digestive Diseases Science* **36**: 52–8.

Bradley, D.W. et al. (1990) Assessing Two domains for Communicating Romance: Behavior Context and Mode of Interaction. *Communication Research Reports* **7**: 9499.

Bradley, W. (1991) Neurology in Clinical Practice. Boston: Butterworth-Heinemann.

Braude et al. (1986) Infectious Diseases and Medical Microbiology. New York: W.B. Saunders Co.

Braunwald, E. et al. (1992) Harrison's Principles of Internal Medicine. New York: McGraw-Hill.

Bravemann, D.Z. and Morali, G.A (1990) Abnormal liver enzymes and ketonuria in hyperemesis gravidarum: a retrospective review of 80 patients. *Journal of Clinical Gastroenterology* **12**: 303–5.

Braybiel, J.R. et al. (1994) Use of promethazine to hasten adaptation to provocative motion. *Journal of Clinical Pharmacology* **34**: 644–51.

Breefeld, D. (1993) Ipecac abuse in a sample of eating disordered outpatients. *International Journal of Eating Disorders* **13**: 411–4.

Brennes, L. (1994) Herbs. London: Dorling Kindersley.

Brizzee, K.R. (1990) Mechanics of Vomiting: a review. *Canadian Journal of Physiology and Pharmacology* **68**: 221–9.

Brody, D. (1991) Olfactory identification deficits in HIV infection. *American Journal of Psychiatry* **148**: 248–9.

Brosvic, G.M. et al. (1995) Conditioned taste aversions and latent inhibition in Egyptian spiny mice and Long-Evans rats. *Perceptual and Motor Skills* **80**: 995–8.

Brown, N.J. (1993) Granisetron and ondansetron; effects on the ileal brake mechanism in the rat. *Journal of Pharmacy and Pharmacology* **45**: 521–4.

Brown, R.E. (1991) Effects of rearing condition, gender, and sexual experience on odor preferences and urine marking in Long-Evans rats. *Animal Learning and Behavior* **19**: 18–28.

Browner, et al. (1992) Skeletal Trauma. Philadelphia: W.B. Saunders Co.

Bunce, K. and Tyers, M.B. (1992) The role of 5HT in postoperative nausea and

vomiting. *British Journal of Anaesthesiology* (Suppl.) **1**: 6–2.
Burish, T.G. and Lyles, J.N (1981) Effectiveness of relaxation training in reducing adverse reactions to cancer chemotherapy. *Journal of Behavioral Medicine* **4**: 65–78.
Burish, T.G. et al. (1987) Conditioned Side Effects Induced by Cancer Chemotherapy: Prevention Through Behavioural Treatment. *Journal of Consulting and Clinical Psychology* **55**: 42–8.
Burks, S.L. (1995) Managing Your Migraine. Totawan, NJ: Humana Press.
Burton, L.A. and Levy, L. (1989) Sex Differences in the Lateralized Processing of Facial Emotion. *Brain and Cognition* **11**: 210–28.
Bush, F.M. et al. (1993) Analysis of Gender Effects on Pain Perception and Symptom Presentation in Temporomandibular Pain. *Pain* **53**: 73–80.
Bushong, M.E. and Mann, M. (1994) Gender and Intrauterine Position Influence Saccharin Preference in Mice. *Hormones and Behavior* **28**: 207–18.
Cahill, L. and McGaugh, J.L. (1991) Amygdaloid complex lesions differentially affect retention of tasks using appetitive and aversive reinforcement. Behavioral *Neuroscience* **104**: 532–43.
Calignano, A. et al. (1993) Endogenous nitric oxide modulates morphine-induced changes in locomotion and food intake in mice. *European Journal of Pharmacology* **231**: 415–9.
Campora, E. (1991) The incidence of narcotic induced emesis. *Journal of Pain Symptom Management* **6**: 428–30.
Camposano, S.L. (1992) Effects of Stimulation Intensity, Gender and Handedness Upon Auditory Evoked Potentials. *Arquivos de Neuro-Psiquiatria* **50**: 43–9.
Cantu, R.C. (1985) Neurology in Primary Care. New York: MacMillan.
Capan et al. (1991) Trauma, Anesthesia, and Intensive Care. Philadelphia: Lippincott.
Carnrike, C.L. and Carey, M.R (1990) Assessing nausea and vomiting in adult chemotherapy patients: review and recommendations. *Annals of Behavioral Medicine* **12**: 79–85.
Carpenter, D.O. (1990) Neural mechanisms in emesis. *Canadian Journal of Physiology and Pharmacology* **68**: 230–6.
Carrieri-Kohlman et al. (1993) Pathophysiological Phenomena in Nursing: Human Responses to Illness. Philadelphia: W.B. Saunders.
Carty, J.L. (1990) Relaxation with imagery: an adjunctive treatment for anticipatory nausea and vomiting. *Dissertation Abstracts International* **51**(5B).
Cavaliere, S. (1994) Gender may be a prognostic factor for emesis only in high dose cisplatin chemotherapy. *Proceedings of the Annual Meeting of the American Society for Clinical Oncology* **13**: A438.
Cella, D.F. et al. (1986) Persistent Anticipatory Nausea, Vomiting, and Anxiety in Cured Hodgkin's Disease Patients After Completion of Chemotherapy. *American Journal of Psychiatry* **143**: 641–3.
Chadwick, D. (1989) Medical Neurology. New York: Churchill Livingstone.
Chadwick, P.R. and McCann, R. (1994) Transmission of a small round structured virus by vomiting during a hospital outbreak of gastroenteritis. *Journal of Hospital Infection* **26**: 25–9.
Challis, G. and Stam, H. (1992) A longitudinal study of the development of anticipatory nausea and vomiting in cancer chemotherapy patients: the role of absorption and autonomic perception. *Health Psychology* **11**: 181–9.

Chalmers, I. et al. (1968) Effective Care in Pregnancy and Childbirth: Taste Sensitivity May be Used to Predict Pharmacological Effects. *Life Sciences* **7**: 533–7.

Chin, R.K. (1989) Antenatal complications and perinatal outcome in patients with nausea and vomiting. *European Journal of Obstetrics Gynecology and Reproductive Biology* **33**: 215–9.

Chiodera, P. (1993) Reduction in the arginine vasopressin response to metoclopramide and insulin induced hypoglycemia in normal weight bulimic women. *Neuroendocrinology* **57**: 907–11.

Chiodero, P. et al. (1991) Abnormal arginine vasopressin response to cigarette smoking and metoclopromide (but not to insulin-induced hypoglycemia) in elderly subjects. *Journal of Gerontology* **46**: 6–10.

Chouinard, G. (1985) A Double-blind Controlled Clinical Trial of Fluoxetine and Amitriptyline in the Treatment of Outpatients with Major Depressive Disorder. *Journal of Clinical Psychiatry* **46**: 32–7.

Christenson, J. (1944) Defining the irritable bowel syndrome. *Perspectives in Biology and Medicine* **8**: 21–35.

Cioffi, D. (1991) Beyond attentional strategies: a cognitive perceptual model of somatic interpretation. *Psychology Bulletin* **109**: 25–41.

Claussen, D.W. (1994) Zofran injection. *Gastroenterology Nursing* **16**: 184–6.

Clifford, W.M. (1991) Is there a role for amines other than histamines in the etiology of scombrotoxicosis. *Food Additives Contamination* **8**: 641–51.

Cohen, H. and Furget, K (1995) Auditory Cerebral Lateralization Following Cross-gender Hormone Therapy. *Cortex* **31**: 565–73.

Cohen, M.I. (1992) Weakness of short term synchronization among respiratory nerve activities during fictive vomiting. *American Journal of Physiology* **263**: 339–47.

Cohn, C.K. et al. (1990) Double-blind, Multicenter Comparison of Sertraline and Amitriptyline in Elderly Depressed Patients. *Journal of Clinical Psychiatry* **51**(Suppl. B): 28–33.

Cohn, J.B. (1985) A Comparison of Fluoxetine, Imipramine, and Placebo in Patients with Major Depressive Disorder. *Journal of Clinical Psychiatry* **46**: 26–31.

Coles, W. (1989) Opthalmology: A Diagnostic Text. Baltimore, MD. Williams and Wilkins.

Collman, P.I. et al. (1993) The central fagal efferent supply to the esophagus and lower esophageal sphincter of the cat. *Gastroenterology* **104**: 1430–8

Committee for Pharmacy and Therapeutics (1993–94) Recommendations for Anti-Emetics in Patients Receiving Chemotherapy. Stamford, CA: Stanford University Hospital.

Condes-Lara, M. et al. (1994) Correlation between oxytocin neuronal sensitivity and oxytocin-binding sites in the amygdala of the rat: electrophysiological and histoautoradiographic study. *Brain Research* **637**: 277–86.

Conroy, T. (1994) Acute antiemetic efficacy and safety of dolasetron mesylate, a $5HT_3$ antagonist, in cancer patients treated with cisplatin. *American Journal of Clinical Oncology* **17**: 97–102.

Cooper, S.J. and Barber, D. (1993) Effects of d fenfluramine, MK 212 and ondansetron on saline drinking in two choice tests in the rehydrating rat. *Pharmacology Biochemistry and Behavior*: 593–610.

Coons, H.L. et al. (1987) Anticipatory Nausea and Emotional Distress in Patients Receiving Cisplatin-based Chemotherapy. *Oncology Nursing Forum* **14**: 31–5.

Costall, B. and Naylor, R.J. (1992) Neuropharmacology of emesis in relation to clinical response. *British Journal of Cancer* (Suppl.) (Dec 19): 2–7.

Cotanch, P.H. (1991) Use of Nonpharmacological Techniques to Prevent Chemotherapy-related Nausea and Vomiting. *Recent Results in Cancer Research* **121**: 101–7.

Craig and Mauger (1994) Havenger's Ocular Pharmacology. St Louis, MD: Mosby Yearbook.

Crampton, G.H. and Lucot, J.B. (1991) Animal models: cats for motion sickness. Dayton, OH: Wright State University Department of Pharmacology.

Crosson. B. (1993) Subcortical Functions in Language and Memory. New York: Guilford.

Cubeddu, L.X. (1993) Participation of serotonin on early and delayed emesis induced by initial and subsequent cycles of ciplatinum based chemotherapy. *Journal of Clinical Pharmacology* **33**: 691–7.

Cupchik, G.C. et al. (1992) Judgments of Similarity and Difference Between Paintings. *Visual Arts Research* **18**: 37–50.

Dancer, J. et al. (1994) A Cross-sectional Investigation of Speechreading in Adults: Effects of Age. Gender, Practice, and Education. *Volta Review* **96**: 31–40.

Davey, G.B. (1993) Evolution and "anti-sickness": the role of taste in emesis 99. *Behavioral Neuroscience* **107**: 215–7.

Davis, D. et al. (1994) Comparison of Related Perceptual Tests. *Perceptual and Motor Skills* **79**: 399–402.

Davis, Z.A., (ed.) (1992) Atlas of Pediatric Physical Diagnosis. New York: Gower Medical Publishing.

Dawe, S. and Corballis, M. (1986) The Influence of Gender, Handedness and Head-turn on Auditory Asymmetries. *Neuropsychologia* **24**: 857–62.

Day, H.E. et al. (1994) Evidence that cholecystokinin induces immediate early gene expression in the brainstem, hypothalamus and amygdala of the rat by a CCKA receptor mechanism. *Neuropharmacology* **6**: 719–27.

De Wet, M. (1993) Factors predisposing to incomplete control of emesis in patients receiving repeat cycles of cytostatic therapy: a logistic regression analysis of 416 cycles of granisetron. *Proceedings of the Annual Meeting of the American Society for Clinical Oncology* **12**: 1542.

Defilippi, C. (1989) Relationship between small intestinal fasting motility and vomiting in dogs. *Clinical Diagnostic Ultrasound* **24**: 707.

Del Favero, D. (1990). "Assessment of nausea." European Journal of Clinical Pharmacology(38): 115-120.

Demitrack, M.A. (1990) CSF oxytocin in anorexia nervosa and bulimia nervosa: clinical and pathophysiologic considerations. *American Journal of Psychiatry* **147**: 882–6.

Derlaga, V.J. et al. (1989) Gender Differences in the Initiation and Attribution of Tactile Intimacy. *Journal of Nonverbal Behavior* **13**: 83–96.

Desai, K.M. (1994) $5HT_3$ receptors do not mediate vagally induced relaxation or contraction of the isolated stomach of the guinea pig. *British Journal of Pharmacology* **111**: 346–50.

Devita, L.V. et al. (1993) Cancer Principles and Practice of Oncology, 4th edn: Philadelphia: Lippincott.

Devitt, N.F. (1991) Hyperemesis gravidarum: a case report suggesting new concepts and research needs. *Family Practical Medical Journal* **11**: 279–82.

Dienstbier, R.A. (1989) Arousal and physiological toughness: implications for mental and physical health. *Psychological Review* **96**: 84–100.

Dilly, S.G. (1994) Contribution of dexamethasone to antiemetic control with granisetron is greatest in patients at high risk of emesis. *Proceedings of the Annual Meeting of the American Society for Clinical Oncology* **13**: A1500.

Dion, K.L. and Dion, K.K. (1976) The Honi Phenomenon Revisited: Factors Underlying the Resistance to Perceptual Distortion of One's Partner. *Personal Social Psychology* **33**: 170–7.

Dolgin, M.J. et al. (1985) Anticipatory Nausea and Vomiting in Pediatric Patients. *Pediatrics* **75**: 547–52.

Doty, R.L. (1976) Reproductive Endocrine Influences Upon Human Nasal Chemoreception: A Review. Mammalian Olfaction, Reproductive Processes, and Behavior. R.L. Doty. New York: Academic Press: 295–321.

Doty, R.L. et al. (1994) Tests of Human Olfactory Function: Principal Components Analysis Suggests that Most Measure a Common Source of Variance. Perception and Psychophysics 56: 701–7.

Duhaney, A. and McKelvie, S.J. (1993) Gender Differences in Accuracy of Identification and Rated Intensity of Facial Expressions. *Perceptual and Motor Skills* **76**: 716–8.

Duke, J.A. Handbook of Medicinal Herbs. Boca Raton, FL: CRC Press.

Dun, N.J. et al. (1994) Nitric oxide synthase immunoreactivity in rat pontine medullary neurons. *Neuroscience* **59**: 429–45.

Dunlop, D.J. (1990) Hypothalamic pituitary responses in induced emesis: relationship to chemically induced emesis. *British Journal of Cancer* **62**: 524.

Dunn, W. (1994) Performance of Typical Children on the Sensory Profile: An Item Analysis. *American Journal of Occupational Therapy* **48**: 967–74.

Dunner, D.L. et al. (1992) Two Combined Multicenter Double-blind Studies of Paroxetine and Doxepin in Geriatric Patients with Major Depression. *Journal of Clinical Psychiatry* **53** (Suppl.): 57–60.

Dwivedi, C.B. and Singh, I.L. (1978) Effects of Shock Inputs on Perceptual Vigilance. *Perception Motor Skills* **47**: 1207–12.

Dykstra, L. (1992) Psychopharmacology: Gastric Mechanisms and Applied Interventions. Washington D.C.: American Psychology Association.

Edelman, G. (1989) The Remembered Present: A Biological Theory of Consciousness. New York: Basic Books.

Edelman, G.M. (1992) Bright Air, Brilliant Fire: On the Matter of Mind. New York: Basic Books.

Edwards, R. (1995) Pleasant aromas chase away those bitter moods. *APA Monitor* (March 18–19).

Eichenbaum, H. (1993) Thinking about brain cell assemblies. *Science* **261**: 993–4.

Elkins, R. et al. (1992) Continued development and unconditioned stimulus characterization of selectively bred lines of taste aversion prone and resistant rats. *Alcoholism, Clinical and Experimental Research* **16**: 928–34.

Elkins, R.L. (1991) An appraisal of chemical aversion approaches to alcoholism treatment. *Behavioral Research and Therapy* **29**: 387–413.

Ellermeier, W and Wolfgang, W. (1995) Gender Differences in Pain Ratings and Pupil Reactions to Painful Pressure Stimuli. *Pain* **61**: 435–9.

Endo, T. (1990) Emesis related biochemical and histopathological changes induced by cisplatin in the ferret. *Journal of Toxicological Science* **15**: 235–44.

Evans, A.T. (1994) Suppression of pregnancy induced nausea and vomiting with sensory afferent information. *Obstetrics and Gynecology Survey* **49**: 155–6.

Evans, W.J. et al. (1995) Olfactory Event-related Potentials in Normal Human Subjects: Effects of Age and Gender. *Electroencephalography and Clinical Neurophysiology* **95**: 293–301.

Fabre. L.F. (1992) A 6-week, Double-blind Trial of Paroxetine, Imipramine, and Placebo in Depressed Outpatients. *Journal of Clinical Psychiatry* **53** (Suppl. 2) 40–3.

Fairbanks, L.A. (1993) What is a good mother? Adaptive variation in maternal behavior of primates. *Current Directions in Psychological Science* **2**: 180–4.

Feiger, A. et al. (1996) Nefazodone vs. Sertraline in Outpatients with Major Depression: Focus on Efficacy, Tolerability and Effects on Sexual Function and Satisfaction. *Journal of Clinical Psychiatry* **57** (Suppl. 2): 53–62.

Feighner, J.P. et al. (1985) Double-blind Comparative Trials of Fluoxetine and Doxepin in Geriatric Patients with Major Depressive Disorder. *Journal of Clinical Psychiatry* **46**: 20–5.

Fein, G.B. and Fein, F. (1987) Gender Differences in Pattern Reversal Evoked Potentials in Normal Elderly. *Psychophysiology* **24**: 683–90.

Feine, J.S. et al. (1991) Sex Differences in the Perception of Noxious Heat Stimuli. *Pain* **44**: 255–62.

Feldman, P.D. et al. (1995) Cardiovascular effects of serotonin in the nucleus of the solitary tract. *American Journal of Physiology* **269**: R48–56.

Feldman, R.G. (1984) Neurology, the Physician's Guide. New York:

Felts, J.A. (1990) Nitrous oxide, nausea and vomiting after outpatient gynecologic surgery. *Journal of Clinical Anesthesiology* **2**: 168–71.

Fernandez-Fewell, G.D. et al. (1994) c-fos Expression in Vomeronals Pathways of Mated or Pheromone Stimulated Male Golden Hamsters: Contribution from Vomeronasal Sensory Input and Expression Related to Mating Performance. *Journal of Neuroscience* **14**: 3643–54.

Fernandez, E. and Turk, D.C. (1992) Sensory and affective components of pain: separation and synthesis. *Psychological Bulletin* **112**: 205–17.

Ferrando, S. and Eisendrath, S. (1991) Adverse neuropsychiatric effects of dopamine agonist medications. Misdiagnosis in the medical setting. *Psyhosomatics* **32**: 426–32.

Fetting, J.H. (1992) Noradrenergic activity in anticipatory nausea. *Psychosomatic Medicine* **54**: 641–7.

Fetting, J.H. et al. (1983) Anticipatory Nausea and Vomiting in an Ambulatory Medical Oncology Population. *Cancer Treatment Reports* **67**: 1093–8.

Feudtner, C. (1996) A disease in motion: diabetes history and the new paradigm of transmuted disease. *Perspectives in Biology and Medicine* **39**: 158–70. Chicago: University of Chicago Press.

Fink-Jensen, A. (1992) Inhibition of cisplatin induced emesis in ferrets by the non-NMDA receptor antagonists NBQX and CNQX. Neuroscience Letters 30: 173–7.

First, L.R. (1993) Nausea and vomiting. *Current Pediatric Therapy*, Vol 8 (Kagan, G., ed.) . Philadelphia: W.B. Saunders, pp. 196–8.

Fleisher, D.R. (1986) Nausea and vomiting. *Current Pediatric Therapy*, Vol 8 (Kagan, G., ed.) . Philadelphia: W.B. Saunders, pp. 183–7.

Fleisher, D.R. and Matar, M.J. (1993) The cyclic vomiting syndrome: a report of 71 cases and literature review. *Journal of Pediatric Gastroenterology and Nutrition* **17**: 361–9.

Forgie, M.L. et al. (1988) Contributions of Taste Factors and Gender to Opioid Preference in C57BL and DBA Mice. *Psychopharmacology* **95**: 237–44.

Forsyth, P.A. et al. (1993) Headaches in Patients with Brain Tumors. *Neurology* **43**: 1678–83.

Francis, G. et al. (1991) Munchausen Syndrome by Proxy 1990: A Portent for Problems. *Clinical Pediatrics* **30**: 112–6.

Fredrikson, M. (1993) Conditioned nausea after cancer chemotherapy and autonomic nervous system conditionability. *Scandinavian Journal of Psychology* **34**: 318–27.

Fredrikson, M. et al. (1992) Nausea in cancer chemotherapy is inversely related to urinary cortisol excretion. *British Journal of Cancer* **65**: 779–80.

Freeman, A.J. (1992) Selectivity of $5HT_3$ receptor antagonists and anti emetic mechanisms of action. *Anticancer Drugs* **3**: 79–85.

Freeman, A.J. and Tyers, M.B. (1992) Mechanism of the anti emetic activity of $5HT_3$ receptor antagonists. Oncology 49: 263–8.

Freeman, A.J. et al. (1993) The vomiting reflex and the role of $5HT_3$ receptors. *Anticancer Drugs* **4** (Suppl. 2): 9–15.

Freeman, F.G. et al. (1995) Lateralized Processing of Centrally Presented Verbal and Spatial Tasks: Effects of Attention, Gender, and Hand Used. *Neuropsychiatry, Neuropsychology, and Behavioral Neurology* **8**: 88–98.

Friedman, C. (1994) Incidence of delayed emesis after complete prevention of acute symptoms by granisetron. *Proceedings of the Annual Meeting of the American Society for Clinical Oncology* **13**: 410.

Fromm, D. (1985) Gastrointestinal Surgely. New York: Churchill Livingstone.

Frye, C.A. et al. (1994) Menstrual Cycle and Dietary Restraint Influence Taste Preferences in Young Women. *Physiology and Behavior* **55**: 561–7.

Frye, R.E. et al. (1992) Bilateral and Unilateral Olfactory Sensitivity Relationship to Handedness and Gender. *Chemical Signals in Vertebrates*. New York: Plenum Press: 559–64.

Fuchs, K. (1989) Treatment of hyperemesis by hypnosis. *Australian Journal of Clinical Hypnotherapy and Hypnosis* **10**: 31–42.

Fukuda, H. and Koga, T. (1991) The Botzinger complex as the pattern generator for retching and vomiting in the dog. *Meirpsco Research* 12: 471–85.

Fukui, H. (1992) Vagal afferent fibers and peripheral $5HT_3$ receptors mediate cisplatin induced emesis in dogs. *Japanese Journal of Pharmacology* **59**: 221–6.

Fukui, H. (1993) Emetic effects of anticancer drugs and involvement of visceral afferent fibers and $5HT_3$ receptors in dogs. *European Journal of Pharmacology* **250**: 281–7.

Fullerton, D. (1988) Differences in the plasma beta endorphin levels of bulimics. *International Journal of Eating Disorders* **7**: 191–200.

Fullerton, D. (1991) Prolonged nausea and vomiting associated with buprenorphine. *Pharmacotherapy* **11**: 90–3.

Fullerton, D. (1992) Persistent functional vomiting. *International Journal of Eating Disorders* **12**: 229–33.

Furst, C.J. (1992) Control of cisplatin induced emesis; a multidisciplinary intervention strategy. *Medical Oncology and Tumor Pharmacotherapy* **9**: 81–6.

Gabuzda, T. and Erslev, A. (1987) Pathophysiology of Blood. Philadelphia: W.B. Saunders.

Gai, W.P. et al. (1995) Nitric oxide-synthesizing neurons in the central subnucleus of the nucleus tractus solitarius provide a major innervation of the rostral nucleus ambiguus in the rabbit. *Journal of Comparative Neurology* **357**: 348–61.

Ganguly, D.K. et al. (1994) Involvement of gamma aminobutyric acid in the stimulatory effect of methocloapramide on gastrointestinal motility. *Life Sciences* **54**: 253–9.

Gao, J.-H. et al. (1996) Cerebellum Implicated in Sensory Acquisition and Discrimination Rather Than Motor Control. *Science* **272**: 545–6.

Gapro, M. (1993) Granisetron compared with granisetron plus desamethasone; a placebo controlled double blind randomized cross over study. *Proceedings of the Annual Meeting of the American Society for Clinical Oncology* **12**: 540.

Gazzaniga, M.S. (1989) Organization of the human brain. *Science* **245**: 947–52.

George, M.S. et al. (1991) Brain activity during transient sadness and happiness in healthy women. *American Journal of Psychiatry* **152**: 341–51.

Geraud, G. et al. (1983) Clinical Value of a Dopaminergic Agonist Administration in Migraine Patients. *Headache* **123**: 191–2.

Ghelardini, C. (1992) Involvement of central cholinergic neurotransmission in metoclopramide analgesia. *Pharmacology Research* (Suppl. 1): 25–6.

Gilroy, J. (1979). Medical Neurology. New York, MacMillan.

Glanville, E. et al. (1965) Taste Perception and the Menstrual Cycle. *Nature* 205: 930–1.

Glasbreen, B. (1991) *Gastroenterology* **29**: 163–6.

Glass, L. and Young, R.E. (1979) Structure and dynamics of neural network oscillators. *Brain Research* **179**: 207–18.

Golazewski, T.M. et al. (1994) Treatment of hyperemesis gravidarum, by electrical stimulation of the vestibular system. *American Journal of Obstetrics and Gynecology* **171**: 588.

Golden, R.N. et al. (1988) Amoxapine treatment of psychogenic vomiting and depression. *Psychosomatics* **29**: 352–4.

Gonzalez-Heydrich, J. (1991) Testing the psychogenic vomiting diagnosis: four pediatric patients. *American Journal of Diseases of Children* **145**: 913–6.

Goodrich, G.A. et al. (1993) Gender Differences in Piagetian Visual-spatial Representation of Verticality and Horizontality. *Journal of Genetic Psychology* **154**: 449–58

Goodwin, T.M. (1992) Transient hyperthyroidism and hyperemesis gravidarum clinical aspects. *American Journal of Obstetrics and Gynecology* **167**: 648–52.

Gottfraeothsdottir, M.S. (1993) Effects of retrobulbar bujpivacaine on postoperative pain and nausea in retinal detachment surgery. *Acta Opthalmology* **71**: 544–7.

Gotz-Karl, O. et al. (1979) A New Visual Aesthetic Sensitivity Test: 1 Construction and Psychometric Properties. *Perceptual and Motor Skills* **49**: 795–802.

Grahame-Smith, D.G. (1990) The Multiple Causes of Vomiting: Is there a Common Mechanism? *Canadian Journal of Physiology and Pharmacology* **68**: 1–8.

Gralla, R.J. (1991) Does serotonin mediate chemotherapy induced emesis. *Proceedings of the Annual Meeting of the American Society for Clinical Oncology* **10**: Al 142.

Gralla, R.J. (1992) Antiemetic drugs for chemotherapeutic support. *Cancer* (Suppl. 4): 1003.

Green, K.P. et al. (1991) Integrating Speech Information Across Talkers, Gender, and Sensory Modality: Females Faces and Male Voices in the McGurk Effect. *Perception and Psychophysics* **50**: 524–36.

Grelot, L.M. et al. (1994) Vomiting - Its ins and outs. *NIPS* **9**: 142 –7.

Grimsely, S.R. et al. (1992) Paroxetine, Sertraline, and Fluoximine: New Selective Serotonin Reuptake Inhibitors. *Clinical Pharmacy* **1**: 930–55.

Gross, S. (1989) Maternal weight loss associated with hyperemesis gravidarum: a predictor of fetal outcome. *American Journal of Obstetrics and Gynecology* **160**: 906–9.

Grunber, S.M. (1989) Advances in the management of nausea and vomiting induced by non-cisplatin containing chemotherapeutic regimens. *Blood Reviews* **3**: 216–21.

Grunberg, N.E. and Straub, R.O. (1992) The Role of Gender and Taste Class in the Effects of Stress on Eating. *Health Psychology* **11**: 97–100.

Gu, Y. (1993) Expression of *c-fos* in brain subcortical structures in response to nausea, lithium chloride and osmotic pressure in rats. *Neuroscience Letters* **1**: 49–52.

Guerrini, R. (1994) Occipitotemporal seizures with ictus emeticus induced by intermittant photic stimulation. *Neurology*: 253–9.

Guikontes, E. (1992) Ondansetron and hyperemesis gravidarum. *Lancet* **339**: 1228.

Gullikson, G.W. (1991) Relationship of serotonin 3 receptor antagonist activity to gastric emptying and motor stimulating actions of prokinetic drugs in dogs. *Journal of Pharmacology and Experimental Therapy* **258**: 103–10.

Gupta, Y.K. (1989) Role of endogenous opioids and histamine in morphine induced emesis. *Indian Journal of Experimental Biology* **27**: 52–5.

Gur, R.Z. et al. (1995) Sex differences in regional cerebral glucose metabolism during a resting state. *Science* **267**: 528–31.

Hachinski, V. (1992) Challenges in Neurology. Philadelphia: F.A. Davis Co.

Hagine, Y. et al. (1994) Effects of systemically administered ceruletide on the in vivo release and metabolism of dopamine in the medial prefrontal cortex of awake, freely moving rats: an in vivo microdialysis study. *Brain Research* **644**: 40–6.

Haighy, C.G. (1993) Nausea and vomiting after gynecological surgery: a meta analysis of factors affecting their incidence. *British Journal of Anaesthesiology* **71**: 517–22.

Haisenleder, D. (1991) The effect of transient dopamine antagonism on thyrotropin-releasing hormone-induced prolactin release in female rats during the estrous cycle. *Life Sciences* **48**: 1911–18.

Hall, E.G. and Davies, S. (1991) Gender Differences in Perceived Intensity and Affect of Pain Between Athletes and Nonathletes. *Perceptual and Motor Skills* **73**: 779–86.

Halmi, F.S. (1981) Binge-eating and Vomiting: A Survey of a College Population. *Psychological Medicine* **11**: 697–706.

Hamilton, S. et al. (1991) Emergency medicine: An Approach to Clinical Problem Solving. Philadelphia: W.B. Saunders.

Hampton, K.K. et al. (1991) Elevation of plasma vasopressin in spontaneous migraine. *Cephalalgia* **11**: 249–509.

Hanson, J.S. et al. (1985) The diagnosis and management of nausea and vomiting: a review. *American Journal of Gastroenterology* **80**: 210.

Harding, R.K. (1988) Prodromal effects of radiation: pathways, models, and protection by anti emetics. *Pharmaceutics Review* **335**: 335–45.

Harris, J.G. (1978) Nausea, Vomiting, and Cancer Treatment. *CA A Cancer Journal for Clinicians* **28**: 194–201.

Harris, T.O. (1993) Lack of complete correlation between emetic and T cell stimulatory activities of staphylococcal enterotins. *Infection and Immunology* **61**: 3175–83.

Harrison, M. et al. (1984) Contemporary Neurology. Boston: Butterworths.

Hartley, L.R. (1991) Chlorpromazine increases speed of right hemispheric processing of negative emotional stimuli. *Physiology and Behavior* **50**: 881–5.

Hasegawa, S. (1992) Vestibular, central, and gastral triggering of emesis, a study on individual susceptibility in cats. *Acta Otolaryngologia* **112**: 927–3 1.

Havsteen, H. and Kjaer, M. (1991) Double blind randomized cross over trial comparing methylprednisone with placebo in chemotherapy induced nausea and vomiting: a study with special reference to efficacy parameters. Anticancer *Drugs* **2**: 571–9.

Hawthorn, J. and Andrews, P.L. (1988) The neurophysiology of vomiting. *Clinical Gastroenterology* **2**: 141–68.

Heaton, J.P. et al. (1995) Recovery of Erectile Function by the Oral Administration of Apomorphine. *Urology* **45**: 200–6.

Hedrick, P.W. (1994) Evolutionary Genetics of the Major Histocompatibility Complex. *The American Naturalist* **143**: 945–64.

Heilmeyer, L. and Begemann, H. (1989) Atlas of Clinical Hematology, Berlin: Springer-Verlag.

Helson, L. (1992) Total control of chemotherapy induced emesis. *Anticancer Research* **12**: 2243–4.

Herbst, J.J. (1993) Gastroesophageal Reflux. *Current Pediatric Therapy*. G. Kagan, 14: Baltimore, MD: Mosby Yearbook, 194–6.

Herkenham, M. (1990) Cannabinoid receptor localization in the brain. *Proceedings of the National Academy of Science* **87**: 1932–6.

Herman, A. et al. (1993) Transsexualism and Sex-related Differences in Hemispheric Asymmetry. *Acta Neurobiologiae Experimentalis* **53**: 269–74.

Herman, Z.S. and Hvzarska, M. (1993) Chronic treatment with atypical neurolopetics with sulpiride and metoclopromide increase striatal enkaphalins in rat brain. *Polish Journal of Pharmacology* **45**: 493–502.

Herrstedt, J. et al. (1993) Interaction of the antiemetic metopimazine and anticancer agents with brain dopamine. *Cancer Chemotherapy Pharmacology* **33**: 53–6.

Herxheimer, A. et al. (1993) Wanted: a Formulary for Self-Care. *The Pharmaceutical Journal* (August 7): 179.

Herzog, D.B. et al. (1993) A Follow-up Study of 33 Subdiagnostic Eating Disordered Women. *International Journal of Eating Disorders* **14**: 261–7.

Hesketh, P.J. (1993) A randomized double blind comparison of intravenous ondansetron alone and in combination with IV dexamethasone in the prevention of nausea and vomiting associated with high dose cisplatin. *Proceedings of the Annual Meeting of American Society for Clinical Oncology* **12**: A1491.

Heverly, L.L. et al. (1986) Neurodevelopmental and Racial Differences in Tactile-Visual (Cross-Modal) Discrimination in Normal Black and White Children. *Archives of Clinical Neuropsychology* 1: 139–45.

Hikasa, Y. (1989) Evidence for the involvement of alpha 2 adrenoreceptors in the emetic action of zyalizine in cats. *American Journal of Veterinary Research* **50**: 1348–51.

Hikasa, Y. (1992) Central alpha adrenoceptor subtypes involved in the emetic pathway in cats. *European Journal of Pharmacology* **15**: 241–51.

Hinks, G. et al. (1995) Changes in hypothalamic cholecystokininA and cholescystokininB receptor subtypes and associated neuropeptide expression in response to salt-stress in the rat and mouse. *Neuroscience* **3**: 765–81.

Hirsch, J.D. and Lindley, C.M. (1992) Nausea and vomiting and cancer patients' quality of life. *British Journal of Cancer* (Suppl. 19): 26–9.

Hoeprich, L, and Ronald (1994) Infectious Diseases: A Treatise of Infectious Processes. Philadelphia: J.B. Lippincott.

Hoffman et al. (1995) Hematology: Basic Principles and Practice. New York: Churchill Livingstone

Holtmann, S. (1989) The anti motion sickness mechanism of ginger: a comparative study with placebo and dimenhydrinate. *Acta Otolaryngologia* **108**: 168–74.

Honig, W.K. and Fetterman, J.R (1992) Cognitive Aspects of Stimulus Control. Hillsdale, NJ: Erlbaum.

Hooper, S.L. and Moulins, M. (1989) Switching of a neuron from one network to another by sensory induced changes in membrane properties. *Science* **244**: 1587–9.

Houston, H.G. and McClelland, R.J. (1985) Age and Gender Contributions to Intersubject Variability of the Auditory Brainstem Potentials. *Biological Psychiatry* **20**: 419–30.

Hovorka, J. (1990) The experience of the person ventilating the lungs does influence postoperative nausea and vomiting. *Acta Anesthesiologica Scandinavica* **34**: 203–5.

Howell, R. (1990) Mechanisms for the emetic side effect of xanthine bronchiodilators. *Life Sciences* **46**: 563–8.

Hsu, D. and Witter, F.R. (1993) Fetal sex and severe hyperemesis gravidarim. *International Journal of Gynecology and Obstetrics* **40**: 63–4.

Hudzik, T.J. (1992) Signaling and induced emesis in the pigeon. *Pharmacology Biochemistry and Behavior* **41**: 215–7.

Hudzik, T.J. (1993) Sigma receptor mediated emetic response in pigeons: agonists, antagonists, and modifiers. *European Journal of Pharmacology* **236**: 279–87.

Humphrey, N. (1992) A History of Mind. New York: Simon and Schuster

Hutton, L.V. (1992) Using statistics to assess the performance of neural network classifiers. *APL Technical Digest* **113**: 291–9.

Iadarola, M.J. and Caudle, R.M. (1997) Good pain, bad pain. *Science* **278**: 239–40.

Iatrakis, G. (1988) Vomiting and Nausea in first 12 weeks of pregnancy. *Psychotherapy and Psychosomatics* **49**: 22–4.

Imamura, Y. (1991) Opposite effects of metoclopramide and propantheline on intestinal absorption of imipramine in rats. *Journal of Pharmacobiodynamics* **14**: 66–71.

Inall, F.C. and Naylor, R.J. (1994) The physiology and pharmacology of postoperative nausea and vomiting. *Anaesthesia* (Suppl.): 2–5.

Ingise, L.H. and Kase, N.G. et al. The Premenstrual Syndromes. New York: Churchill Livingstone.

Ingle, R.J. et al. (1984) Conditionability of Cancer Chemotherapy Patients. *Oncology Nursing Forum* **11**: 97–102.

Insnetsov, V.V. (1992) The central neurophysiological and neurochemical mechanisms of vomiting: a review of the literature. *Aviakosm Ekolog Medizin* **26**: 10–18.

Ivanova, S.F. and Bures, L. (1990) Conditioned taste aversion is disrupted by prolonged retrograde effects of intracerebral injection of tetrodotoxin in rats. *Behavioral Neuroscience* **104**: 948–54.

Iyoya, M. (1992) Management of chemotherapy induced nausea and vomiting. *Focus on Cancer.*

Jeffrey, H.F. (1991) An unusual case of tear of spleen. *Canadian Journal of Surgery* **34**: 315.

Jenkins, I.H. (1992) Impaired activation of the supplementary motor area in Parkinson's disease is reversed when akinesia is treated with apomorphine. *Annals of Neurology* **32**: 749–57.

Jia, Y.S. et al. (1994) Nitric oxide synthase expression in vagal complex following vagotomy in the rat. *Neuroreport* **5**: 793–6.

Jibson, M.D. et al. (1996) A Summary of Research Findings on the New Antipsychotic Drugs. *The Psychiatry Forum* **16** (May).

Jin, K. et al. (1995) Reproductive Failure and the Major Histocompatibility Complexes. *American Journal of Human Genetics* **56**: 1456–67.

Johns, T. (1986) Detoxification Function of Geophagy and Domestication of the Potato. *Journal of Chemical Ecology* **12**: 635–46.

Johnson T.M. (1993) Vomiting as a manifestation of borderline personality disorder in primary care. *Journal of the American Board of Family Practitioners* **6**: 385–94.

Johnson, W.H. (1993) Motion sickness, vascular changes accompanying pseudo-coriolis-induced nausea. *Aviation, Space, and Environmental Medicine* **64**: 367–9.

Jones, A.L. (1992) The budgetary impact of $5HT_3$ receptor antagonists in the management of chemotherapy induced emesis. *British Journal of Cancer* (Suppl. 29A): 51–6.

Jones, D.T. and Reed, R.R. (1989) Golf: an olfactory neuron specific G protein involved in odorant signal transduction. *Science* **244**: 790–5.

Jonsson, L. and Green, G. (1993) Nausea: the most important factor determining length of stay after ambulatory anesthesia; a comparative study of isoflurane and/or propofol techniques. *Acta Anaesthesiologica Scandinavica* **37**: 742–6.

Jordan, L.N. (1989) Effects of fluid manipulation on the incidence of vomiting during outpatient cisplatin infusion. *Oncology Nurses' Forum* **16**: 213–8.

Julius, D. (1989) Ectopic expression of the serotonin lc receptor and the triggering of malignant transformation. *Science* **244**: 1057–62.

Juneja, M.M. (1991) Epidural morphine pruritus reduction with hydroxyzine in parturients. *Journal of the Kentucky Medical Association* **89**: 319–21.

Kaitz, M. (1992) Recognition of Familiar Individuals by Touch. *Physiology and Behavior* **52**: 565–7.

Kalaska, J.F. and Crammond, D.J. (1992) Cerebral cortical mechanisms of reaching movements. *Science* **255**: 1517–23.

Karnato, T. (1993) Mechanisms of cisplatin and *m*-chlorophenylbiguanide induced emesis in ferrets. *European Journal of Pharmacology* **20**: 369–76.

Kase, N. et al. (1990) Principles and Practice of Clinical Gynecology. New York: Churchill Livingstone.

Katz, P. et al. (1990) Gender Processing and Person Perception. *Social Cognition* **8**: 186–202.

Kauffman, S.A. (1991) Antichaos and adaptation. *Scientific American* **265**: 78–95.

Kaye, W. (1989) The effect of binging and vomiting on hormonal secretion. *Biological Psychiatry* **25**: 768–80.

Kennedy, R.I. (1992) Thyrotoxicosis and hyperemesis gravidarum associated with a serum activity which stimulates human thyroid cells in vitro. *Clinical Endocrinology* **36**: 83–9.

Kenny, G. et al. (1994) Risk Factors for Postoperative Nausea and Vomiting. *Anaesthesia* **49** (Suppl.): 6–10.

Kerlin, P. (1989) Postprandial antral hypomotility in patients with idiopathic nausea and vomiting. *Gut* **30**: 54–9.

Khoo, D. (1994) Palliation of malignant intestinal obstruction using octreotide. *European Journal of Cancer* **30A**: 28–30.

Kiev, A. (1992) A Double-blind, Placebo-controlled Study of Paroxetine in Depressed Outpatients. *Journal of Clinical Psychiatry* **53** (Suppl. 2): 27–9.

King, A.J. (1993) Review of 'Merging of the Senses'. *Science* **261**: 928–9.

King, C. and Hall, W.G. (1991) Developmental change in unilateral olfactory habituation is mediated by anterior commissure maturation. *Behavioral Neuroscience* **105**: 796–807.

King, G.L. and Landauer, M.R. (1990) Effects of zacopride and BMY25 80 (batanopride) on radiation induced emesis and locomotor behavior in the ferret. *Journal of Pharmacology Experimental Therapy* **253**:1026–33.

King, G.L. and Makale, M.T. (1993) Plasticity of autonomic control of emesis in irradiated ferrets. *American Journal of Physiology* **265**: 1092–9.

Kipala, L. (1989) Sex differences in olfactory function in schizophrenia. *American Journal of Psychiatry* **146**: 1320–2.

Kirouac, G.J. and Ganguly, P.K. (1995) Topographical organization in the nucleus accumbens of afferents from the basolateral amygdala and efferents to the later hypothalamus. *Neuroscience* **67**: 625–30.

Klauser, A.G. et al., (1991). A 28-year-old patient with chronic vomiting and diarrhea. *Z Gastroenterology Verh* **26**: 307–8.

Klaustermeyer, W.B. (ed.) (1983) Practical Allergy and Immunology. New York: John Wiley & Sons.

Klein, K. et al. (ed.) (1990) The Doctor's Book of Home Remedies. Emmaus, PA: Rodale Press.

Knudsen, A. et al. (1995) Upper gastrointestinal symptoms in third trimester of the normal pregnancy. *European Journal of Obstetrics and Gynecology and Reproductive Biology* **60**: 29–33.

Kobler, J.B. et al. (1994) Innervation of the larynx, pharynx, and upper esophageal sphincter of the rat. *Journal of Comparative Neurology* **349**: 129–47.

Kobrinsky, N.L. (1988) Regulation of nausea and vomiting in cancer chemotherapy: a review with emphasis on opiate mediators. *American Journal of Pediatrics, Hematology, and Oncology* **10**: 209–13.

Koella, W.P. and Czicman, L. (1966) Mechanism of the EEG synchronizing action of serotonin. *American Journal of Physiology* **211**: 926–34.

Koga, T. (1992) Neurons in the nucleus of the solitary tract mediating inputs from emetic vagal afferents and the area postrema to the pattern generator for the emetic act in dogs. *Neuroscience Research* **14**: 166–79.

Koga, T. and Fukuda, H. (1992) Non respiratory neurons in the Botzinger complex exhibiting appropriate firing patterns to generate the emetic act in dogs. *Neuroscience Research* 14: 180–94.

Koga, T. and Fukuda, H. (1993) Hypercapnia, and hypoxia which develop during retching participate in the transition from retching to expulsion in dogs. *Neuroscience Research* **17**: 205–15.

Kohl, R.L. (1991) Control of nausea and autonomic dysfunction with terfenadine, a peripherally acting antihistamine. *Aviation, Space, and Environmental Medicine* **62**: 392–6.

Kolarikova, O. (1985) Differentiation of Interest Preferences in Dependence on Extraversion-Introversion and Sex. *Ceskoslsovenska Psychologie* **29**: 201–14.

Kornberg, A. and Dolgin, L. (1991) Pediatric ingestions. *Annals of Emergency Medicine* **6**: 648–51.

Koski, E.M. (1990) Double blind comparison of transdermal hyoscine and placebo for the prevention of postoperative nausea. *British Journal of Anaesthesiology* **64**: 16–20.

Koslow, R.E. (1987) Sex-related Differences and Visual-spatial Mental Imagery as Factors Affecting Symbolic Motor Skill Acquisition. *Sex Roles* **17**: 521–7.

Kovats, S. et al. (1990) A Class I Antigen, HLA-G, Expressed in Human Trophoblasts. *Science* **248**: 220–3.

Krebs, J.R. et al. (1976) Behavioral Ecology: An Evolutionary Approach. Oxford: Blackwell.

Kucharezyk, J. and Harding R.K. (1990) Regulatory peptides and the onset of nausea and vomiting. *Canadian Journal of Physiology and Pharmacology* **68**: 289–93.

Kulynych, J.J. et al. (1994) Gender Differences in the Normal Lateralization of the Supratemporal Cortex: MR1 Surface-rendering Morphometry of Heschl's Gyru and the Planum Temporale. *Cerebral Cortex* **4**: 107–18.

Kunz, J. (1993). Ice Cream Preference: Gender Differences in Taste and Quality. *Perceptual and Motor Skills* **77**: 1097–8.

Kuschinsky, K. (1991) Electroencephalographic Correlates of the Sedative Effects of Dopamine Agonists Presumably Acting on Autoreceptors. *Neuropharmacology* **30**: 953–60.

La Rocca. G. (1992) Neurally mediated effects of metoclopramide on pigeon esophageal muscle. *Italian Journal of Gastroenterology* **4**: 198–202.

La Wall, C. (1927) The Curious Lore of Drugs and Medicines: Four Thousand Years of Pharmacy. Garden City, NY: Lippincott.

Lader, M.H. (1996) Tolerability and Safety: Essentials in Antidepressant Pharmacotherapy. *Journal of Clinical Psychiatry* **57** (Suppl. 2): 39–44.

Ladurelle, N. (1991) Stimulation of D1 and D2 dopamine receptors produces additive anorectic effects. *Fundamental Clinical Pharmacology* **5**: 481–90.

Laeng, B. et al. (1993) Pleasantness of a Sweet Taste During Hunger and Satiety: Effects of Gender and 'Sweet Tooth'. *Appetite* **21**: 247–54.

Laidlaw, R. and Chadwick, D.W. (1993) A Textbook of Epilepsy. New York: Churchill Livingstone.

Lang, I.M. (1993) Pharyngeal, esophageal, and proximal gastric responses associated with vomiting. *American Journal of Physiology* **265**: 963–72.

Lao. T.T. and Chin, R.K. (1988) Low birth weight and hyperemesis gravidarum. *European Journal of Obstetrics and Gynecology* **28**: 179–83.

Larkjani, G.E. (1994) Postoperative nystagmus and nausea. *Annals of Pharmacotherapy* **8**: 179–81.

Laszlo, L, (ed.) (1983) Antiemetics and Cancer Chemotherapy. Baltimore, MD: Williams and Wilkins.

Lawless, J. (1992) The Encyclopedia of Essential Oils. Trowbridge: Barnes and Noble.

Le Moine, C. and Bloch, B (1995) Dl and D2 dopamine receptor gene expression in the rat striatum: sensitive cRNA probes demonstrate prominent segregation of D1 and D2 mRNAs in distinct neuronal populations of the dorsal and ventral striatum. *Journal of Comparative Neurology* **355**: 418–26.

Lee, B.H. et al. (1992) Calcitonin gene-related peptide in nucleus ambiguus motoneurons in rat: viscerotopic organization. *Journal of Comparative Neurology* **320**: 531–43.

Legros, J. et al. (1992) Apomorphine stimulation of vasopressin- and oxytocin-neurophysins: Evidence for increased oxytocinergic and decreased vasopressinergic function in schizophrenics. *Psychoneuroendocrinology* **17**: 611–7.

Leijsma, M.K. (1994) Effects of ondansetron on symptoms and gastric emptying in carcinoid patients. *Proceedings of the Annual Meeting of the American Society for Clinical Oncology* **13**: A548.

Len, J. (1991) The regulating effect of electroacupuncture on gastroenteric electric activity in guinea pigs peripheral vomiting. *Chem Tzu Yen Chiu* **16**: 69–72.

Lentz, J.M. and Collins, W.E. (1977) Genetical and developmental aspects of susceptibility to motion sickness and frost bite. *Human Heredity* **20**: 507.

Leopold, J.S. (1992) Pharmacologic/pharmacokinetic evaluation of emesis induced by analogs of RSU 1069 and its control by antiemetic agents. *International Journal of Radiation, Oncology, Biology and Physics* **22**: 549–51.

Lewis, R.K. et al (1987) Sex Differences in Spatial Task Performance of Patients With and Without Unilateral Cerebral Lesions. *Brain and Cognition* **6**: 142–52.

Lewkowicz, D.J. (1996) Infants' Response to the Audible and Visible Properties of the Human Face: Role of Lexical-syntactic Content, Temporal Synchrony, Gender, and Manner of Speech. *Developmental Psychology* **32**: 347–66.

Li, Z. and Ferguson, A.V. (1993) Subfornical organ efferents to paraventricular nucleus utilize angiotensin as a neurotransmitter. *American Journal of Physiology* **265**: 302–9.

Lichter, I. (1993) Results of antiemetic management in terminal illness. *Journal of Palliative Care* **9**: 19–21.

Lifsey, D.S. (1993) Electrocardiographic changes with serotonin antagonist eanitietis rate of occurrence and clinical relevance. *Proceedings of the Annual Meeting of the American Society for Clinical Oncology* **12**: 1611.

Locher, P.J. (1995) A Measure of the Information Content of Visual Art Stimuli for Studies in Experimental Aesthetics. *Empirical Studies of the Arts* **13**: 183–91.

Lockard, I. (1992) Desk Reference for Neuroscience. New York: Springer-Verlag.

Lucas, R. (1966) Nature's Medicines. New York: Parker Publishing.

Lucto, J.B. and Takeda, N. (1992) Alpha fluoromethylhistidine but not diphemhydramine prevents motion induced emesis in the cat. *American Journal of Otolaryngology* **13**: 176–80.

Luh, K.E. et al. (1994) Left-and-Right-Handers See People Differently: Free-Vision Perceptual Asymmetries for Chimeric Stimuli. *Brain and Cognition* **25**: 141–60.

Lumb, A.B. (1993) Mechanism of antiemetic effect of ginger. *Anaesthesia* **48**: 118.

Lydiard, R.B. (1993) CSF cholecystokinin octapeptide in patients with bulimia nervosa and in normal comparison subjects. *American Journal of Psychiatry* **150**: 1099–102.

Lynch, M.R. and Woo, L. (1991) Enhanced haloperidol-induced prolactin stimulation with chronic neuroleptic treatment in the rat. *Life Sciences* **49**: 1721–9.

Mailleus, P. et al. (1994) Delta 9 tetrahydrocanabinol regulates substance P and enkephalin mRNAs levels in the caudate-putamin. *European Journal of Pharmacology* **15**: 267.

Malcolm, K. (1992) Supersensitivity psychosis with concurrent episodic vomiting. *British Journal of Psychiatry* **161**: 407–9.
Mallakh, R.H. (1990) Hyperemesis gravidarum as conversion disorder. *Journal of Nervous and Mental Disorders* **178**: 655–9.
Malm, K. et al. (1993) Regurgitation as a weaning strategy: a selective review on an old subject in a new light. *Applied Animal Behavior Science* **36**: 47–64.
Mandell et al. (1990) Principles and Practice of Infectious Diseases. New York: Churchill Livingstone.
Mangi, H.K. (1992) G proteins: implications for psychiatry. *American Journal of Psychiatry* **149**: 746–60.
Marin, J. (1990) Clinical guidance to anti emetics. *General Pharmacology* **21**: 1–10.
Marsden, D.C. (1989) Clinical Neurology. New York: Raven Press.
Martin, M. (1990) The natural course of emesis after carboplatin treatment. *Acta Oncologica* **29**: 593–5.
Martin, M. and Diaz, R. (1990) Emesis during past pregnancy: a new prognostic factor in chemotherapy. *Annual Oncology* **1**: 152–3.
Marvig, J. and Lang, I.M. (1989) Functional localization of specific receptor mediating gastrointestinal motor correlates of vomiting. *American Journal of Physiology* **256**: 92–99.
Masters, P. and Coyle, S. (1993) Wernicke's encephalopathy and hyperemesis gravidarum. *British Medical Journal* **305**: 1095.
Mataruski, M.R. (1990) Effects of steroids on postoperative nausea and vomiting. *Nurses' Anesthesiology* **1**: 183–8.
Matsuki, N. (1993) Effects of iron and deferoxamine on cisplatin induced emesis: further evidence for the role of free radicals. *European Journal of Pharmacology* **248**: 329–31.
Matsuki, N. (1993) Emetic responses of *Sorex unguiculatus*. *Jikken Dobutsu* **42**: 225–8.
Matta, S.G. et al. (1993) Nicotine stimulates the expression of *c-fos* protein in the parvocellular paraventricular nucleus and brainstem catecholaminergic regions. *Endocrinology* **132**: 2149–56.
Maturana, H.V. (1987) The Tree of Knowledge: The Biological Roots of Human Understanding. Boston: New Science Library.
McBride, M.R. (1989) Self-reports on Suprathreshold Taste Stimuli of Mature and Older Adults. *Annals of the New York Academy of Sciences* **561**: 322.
McCaskill-Stevens, M. (1994) Phase III study of ondansetron, chlorpromazine plus dexamethasone on day 1 and 2 vs 4 and 5 in chemo naive germ cell tumor patients with multiple day cisplatin based chemotherapy. *Proceedings of the Annual Meeting of the American Society for Clinical Oncology* **13**: A1556.
McCondalt (1993). *British Medical Journal* **307**: 1167–71.
McDermott, J.L. et al. (1994) Effects of Estrogen Treatment on Sensorimotor Task Performance and Brain Dopamine Concentrations in Gonadectomized Male and Female CD-1 Mice. *Hormones and Behavior* **28**: 16–28.
McGuiness, D. (1976) Away from a Unisex Psychology: Individual Differences in Visual, Sensory, and Perceptual Processes. *Perception* **5**: 279–94.
McHugh, P.R. and Smith, G.P. (1967) Gastric secretory response to amygdaloid or hypothalamic stimulation in monkeys. *American Journal of Physiology* **211**: 604–44.
McIntyre, A. (1997) The Apothecary's Garden. London: Piatkus.
McKenzie, S. (1994) Hypnotherapy for vomiting phobia in a 40 year old woman. *Contemporary Hypnosis* **11**: 37–40.

McLaughlin, J.P. et al. (1994) Preference for Profile Orientation in Portraits. *Empirical Studies of the Arts* **12**: 1–7.

McQuay, H.J. and Moore, R.A. (1998) Postoperative analgesia and vomiting, with special reference to day-case surgery: a systematic review. *Health Technology Assessment* **2**: 1–236.

McRoberts, G.W. and Saunders, B. (1992) Sex Differences in Performance and Hemispheric Organization for a Nonverbal Auditory Task. *Perception and Psychophysics* **51**: 118–22.

McWilliams, E. (1991) Post-op NV treatment with hypnosis. *Dissertation Abstracts.*

Meek, L.R. (1994) Effect of Vomeronasal organ Removal on Behavioral Estrus and Mating Latency in Female Meadow Voles. *Biology of Reproduction* **51**: 400–4.

Mehler, W.R. (1983) Observation of the connectivity of the parvicellular reticular formation with respect to a vomiting center. *Brain Behavior Evolution* **23**: 63.

Melmon, K. et al. (1992) Melmon & Merrelli's Clinical Pharmacology: Basic Principles in Therapeutics. New York: McGraw-Hill.

Melzack, R. (1989) Measurement of Nausea. *Journal of Pain and Symptom Management* **4**: 157–60.

Mestel, R. (1997) Feeling a Little Strange? *New Scientist*: 25–8.

Miale (1982) Laboratory Medicine Hematology. St Louis, MO: Mosby Yearbook.

Michaloudis, D. (1990) Postoperative nausea and vomiting. *Journal of the Royal Society of Medicine* **86**: 137–8.

Middleton, E. et al. (ed.) (1993) Allergy: Principles and Practice. St Louis, MO: Mosby Yearbook.

Milano, S. (1990) Vagal induced vomiting in decerebrate cat is not suppressed by specific $5HT_3$ receptor antagonists. *Journal of the Autonomic Nervous System* **31**: 109–18.

Mileson, R.E. (1991) Dopamine receptor 'supersensitivity' occurring without receptor up-regulation. *Brain Research* **561**: 1–10.

Miller, G. (1997) Neural Control of Respiratory Muscle Activities During Vomiting. Neural Control of the Respiratory Muscles. Boca Raton, FL: CRC Press.

Miro Barrachina, M. et al. (1984) Development and Transformation of Personal Significance: An Experimental Study. *Boletín de Psicologia* (Spain) **3**: 47–75

Miyawaki, A. (1994) A Possible Pheromone Carrier Function of Two Lipcalin Proteins in the Vomeronasal Organ. *Embo Journal* **13**: 5835–52.

Mizuimoto, Y. (1994) Studies on hypogeusia in hyperemesis gravidarum. *Nippon Sanka Fujinka Gakkai Zasshi* **46**: 35–41.

Moatles (1991) Progress in Neuropsychopharmacology. *BioPsychiatry* **15**: 105–17.

Mogadam, M. (1992) Perspective as to pathogenesis and management of hyperemesis in pregnancy. *American Journal of Gastroenterology* **87**: 806–7.

Money, K. F. et al. The Vestibular System. Nunton, R. (ed.). New York: Academic Press.

Monkovic, I. (1988) Substituted benzamides: potential non dopaminergic antagonist of chemotherapy induced nausea and emesis. *Journal Medicinal Chemistry* **31**: 1548–58.

Montgomery, E. (1986) Principles of Neurologic Diagnosis. Boston: Little Brown.

Monti-Bloch, I. et al. (1994) The Human Vomeronasal System. *Psychoneuroendocrinology* **19**: 673–86.

Moore, et al. (1991) Trauma., 2nd ed. San Mateo, CA: Appleton & Lange.

Moossa, A.R. et al. (1991) Comprehensive Textbook of Oncology: Philadelphia: Lippincott 1604–07 and 1710–12.

Morant, R. et al. (1994) Sandostatin can blunt chemotherapy induced secretion of 5OH indoleacetic acid. *Proceedings of the Annual Meeting of the American Society for Clinical Oncology* **13**: A1599.

Morariu, M. (1979) Major Neurological Syndromes. Springfield, IL: Thomas.

Morraco, G. et al. (1982) Anticipatory Nausea and Vomiting in Chemotherapy Patients. *New England Journal of Medicine* **306**: 431–2.

Morrow, G.R. (1982) Prevalence and Correlates of Anticipatory Nausea and Vomiting in Chemotherapy Patients. *Journal of the National Cancer Institute* **68**: 585–8.

Morrow, G.R. (1984) Susceptibility to Motion Sickness and the Development of Anticipatory Nausea and Vomiting in Cancer Patients Undergoing Chemotherapy. *Cancer Treatment Report* **68**: 1177–8.

Morrow, G.R. (1990) Autonomic changes resulting from chemotherapy induced nausea and vomiting in cancer patients. *Proceedings of the Annual Meeting of the American Society for Clinical Oncology* **9A**: 1238.

Morrow, G.R. (1991) Advances in data assessment: application to the etiology of nausea reported during chemotherapy. *Cancer* **967**: 780–7.

Morrow, G.R. (1992) Autonomic changes during cancer chemotherapy induce nausea and vomiting. *British Journal of Cancer* (Suppl. 19): 42–5.

Morrow, G.R. (1992) Cortisol changes with cisplatin and carboplatin induced nausea. *Proceedings of the Annual Meeting of the American Society for Clinical Oncology* **11**: 405.

Morrow, G.R. (1993) Predicting chemotherapy induced nausea in cancer patients by their resting autonomic activity. *Proceedings of the Annual Meeting of the American Society for Clinical Oncology* **12**: 51–81.

Morrow, G.R. (1994) Abnormal clinical tests of autonomic function and nausea related to chemotherapy. *Proceedings of the Annual Meeting of the American Society for Clinical Oncology* **13**: 153–8.

Morrow, G.R. et al. (1992) Comparing the Effectiveness of Behavioral Treatment for Chemotherapy-Induced Nausea and Vomiting When Administered by Oncologists, Oncology Nurses, and Clinical Psychologists. *Health Psychology* 11: 250–6.

Motles, E. et al. (1991) Effects of p-chloro-phenylalanine on the behaviors induced by apomorphine and amphetamine in adult cats. *Progress in Neuro-Psychopharmacology and Biology Psychiatry* **15**: 105–17.

Muhrback, E. (1994) Postoperative nausea and vomiting: a comparison between intravenous and inhalation anesthesia in breast surgery. *Acta Anaesthesiologica* **38**: 52–6.

Mullenix, J.W. et al. (1995) The Perceptual Representation of Voice Gender. *Journal of the Acoustical Society of America* **98**: 3080–95.

Munro, H.M. (1994) Comparison of the analgesic and emetic properties of ketorolac and morphine for pediatric outpatient strabismus surgery. *British Journal of Anaesthesiology* **72**: 624–8.

Munro, P.G. (1993) Dynamic Gender-related Differences in Dichotic Listening Performance. *Neuropsychologia* **31**: 347–53.

Munson, M. (1994) Antinausea Trick. *Prevention* **46**: 34.

Muraoka, M. (1990) Psychogenic vomiting: the relation between patterns of vomiting and psychiatric diagnoses. *Gut* **31**: 526–8.

Myers, P. (1995) Mind/Body Medicine and the Popular Press. *Mind/Body Medicine* **1**: 5–6.

Myosin (1992) Principles of Trauma Surgery. Philadelphia: Lippincott.

Nabers, S. and O'Brien, B. (1992) Nausea and vomiting during pregnancy: effects on the quality of women's lives. *Birth* **19**: 138–43.

Najarian, J.S. and Delany, J. (1989) Progress in Gastrointestinal Surgery. Chicago, Yearbook: Medical Publishers.

Natale, M. (1983) Hemispheric asymmetries in processing emotional expressions. *Neuropsychology* **21**: 555.

Navara (1992) A dual effect of some $5HT_3$ receptor antagonists on cisplatin induced emesis in the pigeon. *Toxicological Letters* (December): 745–9.

Naylor, R.J. and Costall, B. (1992) Neuropharmacology of emesis in relation to clinical response. *British Journal of Cancer* (Suppl. 19): 2–7.

Nelson, L. et al. (1991) Pediatric Ophthalmology. Philadelphia: W.B. Saunders

Nelson, T.J. (1990) Isolation of a G protein that is modified by learning and reduces potassium currents. *Science* **247**: 1479–83.

Nesse, R.M. et al. (1980) Pretreatment Nausea in Cancer Chemotherapy: A Conditioned Response? *Psychosomatic Medicine* **42**: 43–6.

Newman, R.B. and Godsey, R.K. (1991) Hyperemesis gravidarum: a comparison of single and multiple admissions. *Journal of Reproductive Medicine* **36**: 287–90.

Nielsen, L.H. (1990) Gastric emptying and subjective symptoms of nausea; lack of effects of a $5HT_3$ antagonist ondansetron on gastric emptying in patients with gastric stasis syndrome. *Digestion* **46**: 89–96.

Ninane, J. et al. (1995) Variation in the use of ondansetron as an antiemetic drug in children treated with hemotherapy. *Medical and Pediatric Oncology* **25**: 33–7.

Ninomiya, N. (1994) Reproductive and developmental toxicity studies of lactitol: teratogenicity study in rats by oral administration. *Journal of Toxicological Science* **19**: 441S–6S.

Nonaka, S. and Miller A.D. (1991) Behavior of upper cervical inspiratory propriospinal neurons during fictive vomiting. *Journal of Neurophysiology* **65**: 1492–500.

Norfleet, W.S. (1992) Treatment of Motion Sickness in parabolic flight with buccal scopolamine. *Aviation, Space, and Environmental Medicine* **63**: 46–51.

Nyhus, L.M. et al. (1977) Surgery of the Stomach and Duodenum. Boston: Little, Brown.

O'Connor, B.H. (1984) Color Atlas and Instruction Manual of Peripheral Blood Cell Morphology. Baltimore, MD: Williams & Wilkins

O'Neill, et al. (1964) What are we, where did we come from, where are we going? *Science* **263**: 181–3.

O'Reilly, S.A. (1993) Low risk mothers: oral intake and emesis in labor. *Journal of Nursing and Midwifery* **38**: 228–35.

O'Rourke, D.E. et al. (1967) Geophagia during pregnancy. *Obstetrics and Gynecology* **29**: 581–4.

Ogle, C.W. (1992) 5-Hydroxytryptamine 3 receptor blockade protects against gastric mucosal damage in rats. *Acta Physiologica* **80**: 181–8.

Ohkoshi, N. (1994) Wernicke's encephalopathy induced by hyperemesis gravidarum associated with bilateral caudate lesions on computed tomography and magnetic resonance imaging. *European Neurology* **34**: 177–80.

Okada, F. (1994) Antiemetic effects of serotonergic 5HTI receptor agonists in *Suncus murinus*. *Japanese Journal of Pharmacology* **664**: 109–14.

Olhauser, M. (1993) Right hemisphere dominance for the production of facial expression in monkeys. *Science* **261**: 475–8.

Oowaki, K. (1994) Relationship between oral food intake and nausea caused by intravenous injection of iodinated contrast material. *Nippon Igaku Hoshasen Gakkai Aasshi* **25**: 476–9.

Orchinik, M. et al. (1991) A corticosteroid receptor in neuronal membranes. *Science* **252**: 1848–50.

Orihata, M. and Sarna, S.K. (1994) Contractile mechanism of action of gastroprokinetic agents: cisapride, metoclopramide and domperidone. *American Journal of Physiology* **266**: 665–76

Osterkamp, D.S. (1990) Gender and Genre: Similarities and Differences in Pictorial Themes and Images by Adult Women and Men. *Dissertation Abstracts International* **50**: 5869.

Otto, T. (1991) Hippocampus and olfactory discrimination learning: effects of entorhinal cortex lesions on olfactory learning and memory. *Behavioral Neuroscience* **105**: 111–19.

Paarlberg, K.M. et al. (1996) Psychosocial Factors as Predictors of Maternal Well Being and Pregnancy Related Complaints. *Journal of Psychosomatic Obstetrics and Gynecology* **17**: 93–102.

Page, S.R. (1990) The responses of arginine vasopressin and adrenocorticotropin to nausea induced by ipecacuanha. *Clinical Endocrinology* **33**: 761–70.

Palazzo, M. and Evans, R. (1993) Logistic regression analysis of fixed patient factors for postoperative sickness: a model for risk assessment. *British Journal of Anaesthesiology* **70**: 135–40.

Palca, J. (1990) More on brain convergence for representation, theoretical basis for plasticity use. *Science* **248**: 812–4.

Palmer, J.B. (1992) Side effects: more on ondansetron and chest pain. *Lancet* **5**: 340.

Panayiotopoulos, C.P. (1989) Benign nocturnal childhood occipital epilepsy: a new syndrome with nocturnal seizures, tonic deviation of the eyes, and vomiting. *Journal of Children's Neurology* **2**: 141–68.

Park, D.M. and McClellan, L. (1973) Failure to vomit in hereditary ataxia. *Neurology* **23**: 725–8.

Parker, L.A. (1991) Trimethobenzamine an antiemetic in rats. Chin rub in rats may measure sickness as near nausea model in rats. .

Parker, L.A. and MacLeod, K.B. (1991) Chin rub CRs may reflect conditioned sickness elicited by a lithium-paired sucrose solution. Published erratum appears in Pharmacology Biochemistry Behavior 1994 (June, 48(2): 569). *Pharmacology Biochemistry Behavior* 40: 983–6.

Parker, C. (1980) Clinical Immunology. Philadelphia: Saunders.

Parks, C.W. et al. (1988) Dimensions of Thought as a Function of Age, Gender and Task Difficulty. *Imagination, Cognition and Personality* **8**: 49–62.

Parlee, M.B. (1983) Menstrual Rhythms in Sensory Processes: A review of fluctuations in vision, olfaction, audition, taste and touch. *Psychological Bulletin* **93**: 539–48.

Passalacque, R. (1993) Double blind randomized trial for the control of delayed emesis; comparisons of placebo vs. two different doses of adrenocorticotropic hormone (ACTH). *Proceedings of the Annual Meeting of the American Society for Clinical Oncology* **12**: A1513.

Patterson, M.D. (1992). Vomiting. Pediatric Emergency Medicine: Concepts and Clinical Practice. R.M. Barkin. Baltimore, MD: Mosby Yearbook: 755–8.

Peckham, M. (1995). Oxford Textbook of Oncology. Oxford: Oxford University Press.

Pellier, P. (1994) Crossover analysis of efficacy and side effects of granisetron and ondansetron. *Proceedings of the Annual Meeting of the American Society for Clinical Oncology* **13**: A1521.

Perkins, K.A. et al. (1994) Acute Effects of Tobacco Smoking on Hunger and Eating in Male and Female Smokers. *Appetite* **2**: 149–58.

Peroutka, S.J. (1989) Differential interactions of traditional and novel antiemetics with dopamine D2 and 5-hydroxytryptamine 3 receptors. *Cancer Chemotherapy* 24: 307–10.

Peroutka, S.J. and Snyder, S.H. (1982) Antiemetics: neurotransmitter receptor binding predicts therapeutic action. *Lancet* **1**: 658–9.

Petrov, T. et al. (1994) Electrical stimulation of the central nucleus of the amygdala induces *fos*-like immunoreactivity in the hypothalamus of the rat: a quantitative study. *Brain Research Molecular Brain Research* **22**: 333–40.

Pfeiffer, C.A. and Johnston, R.E. (1994) Hormonal and Behavioral Responses of Male Hamsters to Females and Female Odors: Roles of Olfaction, the Vomeronasal System, and Sexual Experience. *Physiology and Behavior* **55**: 129–38.

Pies, R. (1995) New Directions in the Diagnosis and Treatment of Eating Disorders. *Psychiatric Times*(Oct): (Suppl.).

Pisters, K.M.W. et al. (1992) Dose ranging trial of zacopride: the emetic antiemetic? *Journal of the National Cancer Institution* **84**: 717–8.

Poeck, K. (1985) Diagnostic Decisions in Neurology. New York: Springer-Verlag.

Pogun, S. et al. (1994) Nitric oxide inhibits [3H]dopamine uptake. *Brain Research* **641**: 83–91.

Pohjanvirta, R. et al. (1994) TCDD-induced Hypophagia is Not Explained by Nausea. *Pharmacology, Biochemistry and Behavior* **47**: 273–82.

Polk, H.C. et al. (1993) Basic Surgery. St Louis, MO: Quality Medical Publishing.

Posner, L.B. et al. (1957) Pregnancy Craving and Pica. *Obstetrics and Gynecology* **9**:.

Posner, M. I. (1993) Seeing the mind. *Science* **262**: 673–4.

Powsell, C.B. (1990) Dexamethasone as anti emetic inhibits natural cytotoxin cell activity. *Cancer* **65**: 466–72.

Praterelli, M. et al. (1995) Effects of Gender on Perception of Spatial Illusions. *Perception and Motor Skills* **80**: 625–6.

Quinn, A.C. (1994) Studies in postoperative nausea and vomiting—still a problem. *Anaesthesia* **49**: 62–5.

Rabin, B.M. and Hunt, W.S. (1992) Relationship between vomiting and taste aversion learning in the ferret: studies with ionizing radiation, lithium chloride, and amphetamine. *Behavioral Neural Biology* **58**: 83–93.

Raichle, M.E. (1993) Visualizing the Mind. *Scientific American* (April): 58–64.

Rankin-Box, D. (1995) The Nurses' Handbook of Complementary Therapies. New York: Churchill Livingstone.

Rappaport, M. (1990) P300 response under active and passive attentional states and uni and bimodality stimulus presentation conditions. *Journal of Neuropsychiatry* **2**: 399–407.

Reimherr, F.W. et al. (1990) Antidepressant Efficacy of Sertraline: A Double-blind, Placebo-and-Amitriptyline-Controlled, Multicenter Comparison Study in Outpatients with Major Depression. *Journal of Clinical Psychiatry* 51: 18–27.

Reimer, E.J. (1993) Propofol anesthesia reduces early postoperative emesis after pediatric strabismus surgery. *Canadian Journal of Anaesthesiology* **40**: 927–33.

Relling, M.V. (1993) Chlorpromazine with and without lorazepram as antiemetic therapy in children receiving uniform chemotherapy. *Journal of Pediatrics* **123**: 811–6.

Ren, G. et al. (1995) Clinical Efficacy of Sensory Integrative Therapy (SIT). *Chinese Mental Health Journal* **9**: 74–6.

Restrepo, D. (1990) Odor stimuli trigger influx of calcium into olfactory neurons in the channel catfish. *Science* **249**: 1166–8.

Reynolds, D.J. et al. (1991) Cisplatin evoked induction of *c-fos* protein in the brainstem of the ferret: the effect of cervical vagotomy and the anti emetic $5HT_3$ receptor antagonist granisetron. *Brain Research* **29**: 231–6.

Reynolds, D.J. et al. (1994) Evidence for cholinergic vagal afferents and vagal presynaptic M1 receptors in the ferret. Neurochemistry 25: 455–64.

Rhodes, V.A. et al. (1987) Patterns of nausea, vomiting, and distress in patients receiving antineoplastic drug protocols. *Oncology Nursing Forum* **14**: 35–44.

Rich, (ed.) (1996) Clinical Immunology: Principles and Practice. St Louis, MO: Mosby Yearbook.

Richardson, J.T. and Zucco, G.M. (1989) Cognition and olfaction: a review. *Psychology Bulletin* **105**: 352–60.

Richardson, J.T. (1995) Gender Differences in the Vividness of Visual Imagery Questionnaire: A Meta-analysis. *Journal of Mental Imagery* **19**: 177–87.

Rickard, K.M. (1990) The Effect of Feminist Identity Level on Gender Prejudice Toward Artists' Illustrations. *Journal of Research in Personality* **24**: 145–62.

Rickels, K. and Schweizer, E. (1990) Clinical Overview of Serotonin Reuptake Inhibitors. *Journal of Clinical Psychiatry* **51**: 9–12.

Rickels, K. et al. (1992) The Efficacy and Safety of Paroxetine Compared With Placebo in Outpatients with Major Depression. *Journal of Clinical Psychiatry* **53** (Suppl. 2): 30–32.

Riding, M. and Litz, D. Nausea and Vomiting in the Clinical Practices of Radiology and Anesthesia.

Ridings, P. (1994) Reduction in postoperative vomiting after surgical correction of prominent ears. *British Journal of Anaesthesiology* **72**: 592–3.

Riezo, G. (1992) Gastric myoelectrical activity in the first trimester of pregnancy: a cutaneous electrogastrographic study. *American Journal of Gastroenterology* **87**: 702–7.

Rigas, B. et al. (1995) Clinical Gastroenterology: Companion Handbook. New York: McGraw-Hill.

Rinaman, L. et al. (1995) Cholecystokinin activates catecholaminergic neurons in the caudal medulla that innervate the paraventricular nucleus of the hypothalamus in rats. *Journal of Comparative Neurology* **360**: 246–56.

Rittenberg, C.N. (1994) Combinatio antiemetic trials for delayed emesis. *Proceedings of the Annual Meeting of the American Society for Clinical Oncology* **13**: A1565.

Rivest, S. and Laflamme, N. (1995) Neuronal activity and neuropeptide gene transcription in the brains of immune-challenged rats. *Journal of Neuroendocrinology* **7**: 501–25.

Riviere, A. (1994) Dose finding study of granisetron in patients receiving high-dose cisplatin chemotherapy. *British Journal of Cancer* **69**: 965–71.

Roberts, J.T. et al. (1993) A Review of Ondansetron in the Management of Radiotherapy-induced Emesis. *Oncology* **50**: 173–9.

Robinson, D.S. et al. (1996) The Safety Profile of Nefazodone. *Journal of Clinical Psychiatry* 57 (Suppl. 2): 6–9 and 31–8.
Robinson, R.G. (1995) Mapping brain activity associated with emotion. *American Journal of Psychiatry* **152**: 327–9.
Rocklin, R.E. et al. (1976) Maternal-fetal Relation: Absence of an Immunologic Blocking Factor from the Serum of Women with Chronic Abortions. *New England Journal of Medicine* **295**: 1209–13.
Rodgers, C. (1992) Extrapyramidal side effects of antiemetics presenting as psychiatric illness. *General Hospital Psychiatry* **14**: 192–5.
Rogers (1992) Radiology of Skeletal Trauma. New York: Churchill
Roila, F.R. (1993) Persistence of efficacy of ondansetron plus dexamethasone vs. metoclopramide plus EEX and diphenhydramine in acute emesis during three consecutive cycles of cisplatin chemotherapy. *Proceedings of the Annual Meeting of the American Society for Clinical Oncology* **12**: A1490.
Roozendaal, B. et al. (1992) Vasopressinergic modulation of stress responses in the central amygdala of the Roman high-avoidance and low-avoidance rat. *Brain Research* **596**: 35–40.
Roper-Hall (1989) Stallard's Eye Surgery. Woburn, MA: Butterworth-Heinemann.
Rosenau, L. (1994) Serum alkaline phosphate levels in pregnancy. *Journal Gynecology Obstetrics Biological Reproduction* **23**: 175–9.
Rosenberg, R. (1980) Neurology . New York: Grune and Stratton.
Rothenberg, D.M. (1991) Ephedrine as postoperative nausea and vomiting anti emetic. *Anesthesia and Analgesia* **72**: 58–61.
Rowbotham, D.J. (1992) Current management of postoperative nausea and vomiting. *British Journal of Anaesthesia* **69** (Suppl. 1): 46S–59S.
Rupniak, N.M. (1990) Drug induced purposeless chewing: animal model of dyskinesia or nausea? *Psychopharmacology* **102**: 325–8.
Rusinova, Z. (1985) Psychosemantic Analysis of Artistic Perception of Painting. *Psikhologiia* (Bulgaria) **5**: 41–9.
Russell, P.A. et al. (1994) Ranking or Rating? Some Data and Their Implications for the Measurement of Evaluative Response. *British Journal of Psychology* **85**: 79–92.
Russell, S. (1994) Nobel Laureate's Warning on Research. *San Francisco Chronicle* (May 28): A3–A4.
Saetta, J.P. (1991) Gastric emptying procedures in the self poisoned patient. *Journal of Royal Society of Medicine* **84**: 274–6.
Sagan, L.A. (1989) On radiation, paradigms, and hormesis. *Science* **245**: 574–5.
Sahakian, V. (1991) Vitamin B_6 is effective therapy for nausea and vomiting of pregnancy: a randomized double blind placebo controlled study. *Obstetrics and Gynecology* **78**: 33–6.
Salim, A.S. (1993) A new approach to the treatment of nonsteroidal anti inflammatory drugs induced gastric bleeding by free radical scavengers. *Surgery Gynecology and Obstetrics* **176**: 484–9.
Salkind, L.W. (1993) The Relationship of Gender, Age, and Cognitive Style to Preference for Works of Art. *Dissertation Abstracts International* **53**: 2653.
Sallaz, M. and Jourdan, F. (1992) Apromorphine disrupts odor induced patterns of glomerular activation in the olfactory bulb. NeuroReport **3**: 833–6.
Salzman, C.D. and Newsome, W.T. (1994) Neural mechanisms for forming a perceptual decision. *Science* **264**: 231–7.
Sarna, S.K. and Lang, I.M. (1992) The role of adrenergic receptors in the initiation

of vomiting and its gastrointestinal motor correlates. *Journal of Pharmacology and Experimental Therapies* **263**: 395–9, 403.
Scarantino, W. et al. (1994) On the Mechanism of Radiation-induced Emesis: The Role of Serotonin. *International Journal of Oncology, Biology and Physics* **30**: 825–30.
Schatzberg, A. (1995) Initial Treatment. *American Society of Clinical Psychopharmacology* **6**: 4.
Schatzberg, A. (1996) Course of Depression in Adults: Treatment Options. *Psychiatric Annals* **26**: 336–41.
Schatzberg, A. and Nemeroff, C. (1996) Textbook of Psychopharmacology. Washington, DC: American Psychiatric Press.
Schnou, J. (1992) Unclear post operative anesthesia NV reduced by use of muscle relaxants, thiopentone. *Anaesthesiology Reanim* **17**: 70–6.
Schoen, R. and Brandt, L.J. (1993) *Gastroenterology* **104**: 302–9.
Schuman, E.M. and Madison (1994) Locally distributed synaptic potentiation in hippocampus. *Science* **263**: 532–6.
Schwartz, S.I. et al. (1985) Maingot's Abdominal Operations. Norwalk: Appleton Century Crofts.
Schwarz, K.J. and Tessell, T.M. (1991) Principles of Neural Science. New York: Appleton and Lange.
Schweizer, E. et al. (1990) What Constitutes an Adequate Antidepressant Trial for Fluoxetine. *Journal of Clinical Psychiatry* **51**: 8–11.
Selman, W. and Warren, D. (1992). Neuroendocrinology. Baltimore: Williams and Wilkins.
Service, R.F. (1995) Prompting Complex Patterns to Form Themselves. *Science* **270**: 1299–300.
Shakian, V. et al. (1991) Vitamin B_6 is effective therapy for NV of pregnancy: a randomized, Double-blind placebo-controlled study. *Obstetrics and Gynecology* **78**: 33–6.
Sicuteri, F. (1977) Dopamine, the Second Putative Protagonist in Headache. *Headache* **17**: 129–31.
Sicuteri, F. et al. (1982) A New Nonvascular Interpretation of Syncopal Migraine. *Advanced Neurology* **33**: 199-208.
Silva, J.A. and Leogn, G.B. et al. (1991) Misidentification syndrome and male pseudocytes. *Psychosomatics* **32**: 228–31.
Simon, H. A. (1992) What is an explanation of behavior? *American Psychological Society* **3**: 150–61.
Singer, W. (1990) Research News. *Science* **249**: 856–8.
Skerrit, P.J. (1990) Substance P Causes Pain - But Also Heals. *Science* **249**: 625.
Sleissenger, M. et al. (1989) Gastrointestinal Disease: Pathophysiology, Diagnosis, Management. Philadelphia: W.B. Saunders.
Sloley, B. (1991) Selective depletion of dopamine in the goldfish pituitary caused by domperidone. *Canadian Journal of Physiology and Pharmacology* **69**: 776–81.
Smiley, B.A. and Paradise, N.F. (1991) Does the duration of N20 administration affect postoperative nausea and vomiting. *Nurses' Anaesthesiology* **2**: 13–18.
Smith, B.D. et al. (1993) Effects of Caffeine and Gender on Physiology and Performance: Further Tests of a Biobehavioral Model. *Physiology and Behavior* **54**: 415–22.
Smith, T.K. and Macdonald, E.L. (1991) Effect of fusaric acid on brain regional neurochemistry and vomiting behavior in swine. *Journal of Animal Science* **69**: 2044–9.

Sossai, R. Postoperative vomiting in children: a persisting unsolved problem. *European Journal of Pediatric Surgery*.

Speer, F. (1982) Handbook of Clinical Allergy: A Practical Guide to Patient Management. London: John Wright.

Spivak, J.L. and Eichner, E. (1993) Fundamentals of Clinical Hematology. Philadephia: Harper & Row.

Staddon, J.E. and Bueno, J.L. (1991) On models, behaviorism and the neural basis of learning. *Psychological Science* **2**: 3–10.

Stam, C. (1992) A Longitudinal Study of the Development of Anticipatory Nausea and Vomiting in Cancer Chemotherapy Patients: The Role of Absorption and Autonomic Perception. *Health Psychology* **11**: 181–9.

Stark, P.H. et al. (1985) A Review of Multicenter Controlled Studies of Fluoxetine vs. Imipramine and Placebo in Outpatients with Major Depressive Disorder. *Journal of Clinical Psychiatry* **46**: 53–8.

Steriade, M. et al. (1993) Thalamocortical Oscillations in the Sleeping and Aroused Brain. *Science* **262**: 679–85.

Steward, D.J. (1990) Cancer therapy, vomiting, and antiemetics. *Canadian Journal of Physiology and Pharmacology* **68**: 304–13.

Stimson, W.H. et al. (1979) Studies on the maternal immune response to placental antigens: absence of a blocking factor from the blood of abortion-prone women. *British Journal of Obstetrics and Gynaecology* **86**: 41–5.

Stockhorst, U. (1993) Anticipatory nausea in cancer patients receiving chemotherapy: classical conditioning etiology and therapeutical implications. *Integrative Physiology and Behavioral Science* **28**: 177–81.

Stout, C.J. (1990) An analysis of students' questions in college art history classes. *Visual Arts Research* **16**: 58–76.

Strutzenberg, C.A. (1990) Nausea and vomiting during the bone marrow transplantation process; a retrospective chart review. *Oncology Nursing Forum* **17**: 212.

Stux, G.P. and Bruce (1987). Acupuncture: Textbook and Atlas. Berlin: Springer-Verlag.

Sukhani, R. et al. (1994) Proposal for ambulatory gynecologic laproscopy: does omission of nitrous oxide alter postoperative emetic sequelae and recovery. *Anaesthesiology Analgesia* **78**: 831–5.

Suyners, H. (1993) Signs and symptoms of patients with brain tumors presented to the emergency department. *Journal of Emergency Medicine* **11**: 253–8.

Swaminathan, R. (1994) Thyroid function tests are rarely abnormal in patients with severe hyperemesis gravidarum. *Clinical Endocrinology* **40**: 283.

Swischuk, L.E. (1993) Nausea, vomiting and diarrhea in an older child. *Pediatric Emergency Care* **9**: 307–9.

Synnott, A. (1991) A Sociology of Smell. *Canadian Review of Sociology and Anthropology* **284**: 437–59.

Szpir, M. (1994) The smiling brain. *American Science* **82**: 119–20.

Takahashi, T. (1991) Mechanism for the gastrokinetic action of doperidone. *Gastroenterology* **101**: 703–10.

Takeda, J.N. (1993) Neuropharmacology of motion sickness and emesis. *Acta Otolaryngologica* (Suppl.) **501**: 10–15.

Takeda, N. (1993) Pica in rats is analogous to emesis: an animal model in emesis research. *Pharmacology Biochemical Behavior* **45**: 817–21.

Talbot, J.E. (1991) Multiple representations of pain in human cerebral cortex. *Science* **251**: 1355–8.

Tan, E.H. (1994) Control of emesis by intravenous granisetron in breast cancer patients treated with 5FU espirubicin and cyclophosphamide. *Support Care Cancer* **2**: 197–200.

Tan, L. (1976) Acupuncture Therapy: Current Chinese Practice. Philadelphia: Temple University Press.

Tancredi, L.R. and Volkow, N. (1991) Biological correlates of mental activity studied with PET. *American Journal of Psychiatry* **148**: 439–44.

Taubes, G. (1993) Play of light opens a new window into the body. *Science* **276**: 1991–3.

Taubes, G. (1996) Looking for the Evidence in Medicine. *Science* **272**: 22–4.

Taylor, T.V. (1985) Surgical Gastroenterology. Oxford: Blackwell Scientific Publications.

Tepperman, J. et al. (1987) Metabolic and Endocrine Physiology. Chicago: Yearbook Medical Publishers.

Thompson, D. (1942) On Growth and Form. Cambridge: Cambridge University Press.

Thornton, J.F. (1992) Increased vomiting among patients treated with neuroleptics: Letter. *Schizophrenia Research* **7**: 197.

Tiden, E. (1971) Hyperemesis and psychological vomiting. *Journal of Psychosomatic Research* **12**: 85–93.

Todes, D.P. (1997) The machine to the ghost within; Pavlov's transition from the digestive physiology to conditional reflexes. *American Psychology* **52**: 947–55.

Tolstoi, L.G. (1990) Ipecac induced toxicity in eating disorders. *International Journal of Eating Disorders* **9**: 371–5.

Tompkins, S. (1991) Affect, Imagery, Consciousness. New York: Springer-Verlag.

Torem, M.S. (1994) Hypnotherapeutic techniques in the treatment of hyperemesis gravidarum. *American Journal of Clinical Hypnosis* **37**: 1–11.

Torii, Y. (1991) 5-Hydroxytryptamine is emetogenic in the house musk shrew. *Naunyn Schmiedeberg's Archiv für Pharmacologie* **344**: 564–7.

Torii, Y. (1991) Selective blockade of cytotoxic drug induced emesis by $5HT_3$ receptor antagonist in *Suncus murinus*. *Japanese Journal of Pharmacology* **55**: 107–13.

Torii, Y. (1993) Involvement of free radicals in cisplatin-induced emesis in *Suncus murinus*. *European Journal of Pharmacology* **248**: 131–5.

Torii, Y. (1994) Induction of emesis in *Suncus murinus* by pryogallol, a generator of free radicals. *British Journal of Pharmacology* **111**: 431–4.

Torre, E. (1992) Psychosomatic assessment in patients with hyperemesis gravidarum. *Minerva Psychiatry* **33**: 169–75.

Travis, J. (1994) Glia: the brain's other cells. *Science* **266**: 970–2.

Tresquerres, J.A. and Devesa, L. (1991) The role of central dopaminergic pathways in the neural control of growth hormone secretion in normal men: studies with metoclopramide. *Neuroendocrinology* **53**: 143–9.

Trotier, D. et al. (1996) The vomeronasal organ — a rediscovered sensory organ. *Tiddskrift for Den Norske Laegeforening* **116**: 47–51.

Tsukagoish, S. (1993) An outline of $5HT_3$ receptor antagonists in pharmacological actions. *Gan To Kagaku Rycho* **20**: 2108–14.

Tuorila, H. et al. (1994) Role of Sensory and Cognitive Information in the Enhancement of Certainty and Liking for Novel and Familiar Foods. *Appetite* **23**: 231–46.

Uecker, A.O. and Brzut, L.E. (1993) Hemisphere and gender differences in mental rotation. *Brain and Cognition* **22**: 42–50.

Ukai M. et al. (1991) Pentazocine-like discriminate stimulus effects of morphine are blocked by the dopamine DL antagonist SCH23390 but not by the dopamine D2 antagonist sulpiride. *Brain Research* **54**: 146–8.

Ulshen, M.H. (1992) Vomiting. Primary Pediatric Care. R.A. Hoekelman. Baltimore, MD: Mosby Yearbook.

Upchurch, T. (1989) Otolaryngology Problems and Primary Care. Montcalm, NJ: Medical Economics.

Uyenoyama, M.K. (1988) On the Evolution of Genetic Incompatibility Systems: Incompatibility as a Mechanism for the Regulation of Outcrossing Distance. *The Evolution of Sex*. Sunderland, MA: Sinaur Associates: 212–32.

Van Buren, J. (1994) The Engendering of Female Subjectivity. *American Journal of Psychoanalysis* **54**: 109–25.

Van Wyk, M. (1993) Effects of enhancement and antagonism of 5-hydroxytryptamine activity on the influence of metoclopromide on gastric emptying. *Digestion* **54**: 40–3.

Vandenpol, A.N. (1990) Glutamate, the dorminant excitatory transmitter in neuroendocrine regulation. *Science* **250**: 1276–7.

Varanos, D.D. et al. (1968) Taste sensitivity may be used to predict pharmacological effects. *Life Sciences* **7**: 533–7.

Vasar, E. (1991) Caerulein stimulates CCK in mouse brain as antiamphetamine effect. *Psychopharmacology* 105: 393–9.

Victor, M. and Adams, R. (1993). Principles of Neurology. New York: McGraw Hill.

Vlasco, T. (1994) Anticipatory nausea and vomiting are psychological factors adequately investigated. *British Journal of Clinical Psychology* **33**: 85–100

Vogt, T. (1994) Mental health status as a predictor of morbidity and mortality: a 15 year follow up of members of a health maintenance organization. *American Journal of Public Health* **84**: 227–32.

Volkow, N.D. and Tancredi, L.R. (1991) Biological Correlates of Mental Activity Studied With PET. *American Journal of Psychiatry* **148**: 439–43.

Vonderohe, M.R. (1994) $5HT_3$ antagonist corrects the postprandial colonic hypertonic response in carcinoid diarrhea. *Gastroenterology* **106**: 1184–90.

Voyer, D. et al. (1990) Gender, level of spatial ability, and lateralization of mental rotation. *Brain and Cognition* **13**: 18–29.

Vutyavanich, T. et al. (1995) Pyridoxine for NV of pregnancy: a randomized, double-blind, placebo-controlled trial. *American Journal of Obstetrics and Gynecology* **173**: 881–4.

Walden, T.L. (1994) Effect of ondansetron on serotonin levels in patients receive total body irradiation. *Proceedings of the Annual Meeting of the American Society for Clinical Oncology* **13**: A440.

Walker, E.A. (1990) Irritable bowel syndrome and psychiatric illness. *American Journal of Psychiatry* **147**: 565–72.

Walker, E.A. and Fonseca (1991) Oral and Maxillofacial Trauma. Philadelphia: W.B. Saunders.

Wall, B.M. et al. (1994) Characteristics of vasopressin release during controlled reduction in arterial pressure. *Journal of Laboratory and Clinical Medicine* **124**: 501–25.

Wall, H.P. (1977) Acute Vomiting in Infancy and Childhood, Part 1. *Hospital Medicine*: 24–43.

Wall, H.P. (1977) Acute Vomiting in Infancy and Childhood, Part 2. *Hospital Medicine*: 44–67.

Wall, K.M. and Gross, P.M. (1992) Efferent microvascular responses to electrical stimulation of the area postrema in rats. *Brain Research* **579**: 50–8.

Wallis, C. (1995) The estrogen dilemma. *Time* (June 26): 46–53.

Walton, J.N. (1982) Essentials of Neurology. Marshfield: Pitman.

Wang, H.W. (1993) Induction of olfactory receptor sensitivity in mice. *Science* **260**: 998–1010.

Ware, L.M. and Jernigan, S.A. (1991) Reversible quantitative EEG changes in a case of cyclic vomiting; evidence for migraine equivalent. *Developmental Medical Child Neurology* **33**: 80–5.

Watcha, M.F. (1991) Effect of properol on the incidence of postoperative vomiting after strabismus surgery in pediatric outpatients. *Anaesthesiology* **75**: 204–9.

Watcha, M.F. and Whie, P.F. (1992) Postoperative nausea and vomiting: its etiology treatment and prevention. *Anaesthesiology* **77**: 162–84.

Watson, M. et al. (1992) Anticipatory nausea and emesis, and psychological morbidity: assessment of prevalence among out-patients on mild to moderate chemotherapy regimens. *British Journal of Cancer* **66**: 862–6.

Watson, M. et al. (1992) Anticipatory nausea and vomiting among cancer patients: a review. *Psychology and Health* **6**: 97–106.

Weigel, M.M. and Weigel, R.M. (1989) Nausea and vomiting of early pregnancy and pregnancy outcome. *British Journal of Obstetrics and Gynecology* **96**: 1304–11.

Weiner, W.J (1989) Neurology for the Non-Neurologist . Philadelphia: Lippincott.

Weinstein, M.S. (1994) A single dose of morphine sulfate increases the incidence of vomiting after inguinal surgery in children. *Anaesthesiology* **81**: 572–5.

Wekese, K. et al. (1994) Removal of the Vomeronasal Organ Rescues Reproductive Performance and Aggression in Male Prairie Voles. *Chemical Senses* **19**: 35–45.

Weller, A. (1990) Endogenous cholecystokinin reduces feeding in young rats. *Science* **247**: 1589–91.

Weller, A. and Blass, E.M. (1990) Cholecystokinin conditioning in rats: ontogenetic determinants. *Behavioral Neuroscience* 104: 199–206.

Westbrook, C. et al. (1987) Vomiting associated with whole body irradiation. *Clinical Radiology* **38**: 263–6.

Wiedner, E.B. et al. (1995) Localization of nitric oxide synthase in the brain stem neural circuit controlling esophageal peristalsis in rats. *Gastroenterology* **108**: 367–76.

Wilcox, P.M. et al. (1982) Anticipatory Vomiting in Women Receiving Cyclophosphamide, Methotrexate, and 5-FU (CMF) Adjuvant Chemotherapy for Breast Carcinoma. *Cancer Treatment Reports* **66**: 1601–4.

Wild, R.A. et al. (1994) Matriarchal model for cardiovascular prevention. *Obstetrics and Gynecology Survey* **49**: 147–52.

Wilkinson, A.R. (1989) Preoperative transdermal hyoscine for the prevention of postoperative nausea and vomiting. *Anaesthesiology Intensive Care* **17**: 285–9.

Williams, A.R. (1994) The incidence and severity of postoperative nausea and vomiting in patients exposed to positive intra-operative suggestions. *Anaesthesia* **49**: 340–2.

Williams, R. (1985) Textbook of Endocrinology. Philadelphia: W. B. Saunders

Wilson, F.A. et al. (1993) Dissociation of object and spatial processing domains in primate prefrontal cortex. *Science* **260**: 1955–7.

Wilson, G.T. (1991) Chemical aversion condition in the treatment of alcoholism. *Behavioral Research and Therapy* **29**: 415–9.

Wilson, R. (1988) Thyroid function tests are rarely abnormal in patients with severe hyperemesis gravidarum. *Clinical Endocrinology* **37**: 331–4.

Winiarski, M.G. (1989) Effects of distraction on post chemotherapy nausea in cancer patients. *PhD Dissertation*. Florida State University.

Winner, P. and Shiftless, F. (1994) Concomitant administration of antiemetics is not necessary with intramuscular dihydroergotamine. *American Journal of Emergency Medicine* **12**: 138–41.

Wood, C.D. and Graybiel, A. (1972) Theory of antimotion sickness drug mechanisms. *Aerospace Medicine* **43**: 249–52.

Xu, L.H. (1993) Hypothalamic and gastric myoelectrical responses during vection induced nausea in healthy Chinese subjects. *American Journal of Physiology* **265**: 578–84.

Xu, Z. et al. (1994) Regional suppression by water intake of *c-fos* expression induced by intraventricular infusions of angiotensin II. *Brain Research* **659**: 157–68.

Yamada, T. et al. (1991) Textbook of Gastroenterology. Philadelphia: J.B. Lippincott.

Yamamoto, M. (1990) Birth order, gender differences, and language development in modem Japanese pre-school children. *Psychologia: An International Journal of Psychology in the Orient* **33**: 185–90.

Yamazaki, K. et al. (1991) Chemosensory Identity and Immune Function in Mice. In: Chemical Senses: Genetics of Perception and Communication. W.A. Kare. New York: Dekker: 187–209.

Yangihashi, R. (1991) The effects of apomorphine on the hippocampal field potential in freely moving rats: pharmacological evidence of the involvement of D2 receptors. *Neuropharmacology* **30**: 177–82.

Yanovski, A. et al. (1995) Analysis by gender and visual imagery reactivity of conventional and imagery rorschach. *Perceptual and Motor Skills* **80**: 1319–40.

Yen, C.T. and Blum, P.S. (1984) Response properties and functional organization of neurons in midline region of medullary reticular formation of cats. *Journal of Neurophysiology* **52**: 951–79.

Young, W.F. and Vibins, H.G. (1993) Evaluation of gastric emptying using radionuclides. *Annals of Emergency Medicine* **22**: 142.

Zaidel, D. et al. (1994) Sex of the face in Western art: left and right in portraits. Empirical Studies : *Festival of the Arts* **12**: 9–18.

Zhang, J. and Cai, W.W. (1991) Severe vomiting during pregnancy: antenatal correlations and fetal outcomes. *Epidemiology* **2**: 454–7.

Zhang, X. et al. (1992) Vasopressin receptors in the area postrema differentially modulate baroreceptor responses in rats. *European Journal of Pharmacology* **222**: 81–91.

Zitelli, B. and Davis, H. (eds.) (1992) Atlas of Pediatric Physical Diagnosis, 2nd ed. *Gower Medical Publishing*, New York: 17.7–17.13.

Zuckerman, M. et al. (1993) Sensation Seeking and Reactions to Nature Paintings. *Personality and Individual Differences* **15**: 563–76.

Zuñiga, J.R. et al. (1993) Taste Performance on the Anterior Human Tongue Varies with Fungiform Taste Bud Density. *Chemical Senses* **18**: 449–60.

Zunini, G.S. (1990) The inhibitory effect of halothane on the emetic response in the ferret. *Canadian Journal of Physiology and Pharmacology* **68**: 374–8.

Index

DO NOT REMOVE

This is an item
ID tag for lending